KNOW YOUR
OPTIONS

KNOW YOUR OPTIONS

The Definitive Guide to Choosing

The Best Medical Treatments

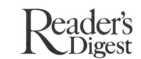

Reader's Digest Association, Inc.
Pleasantville, New York / Montreal

Reader's Digest Health Books

Senior Health Editor
Marianne Wait

Managing Editor
Suzanne G. Beason

Editor in Chief and Publishing Director
Neil Wertheimer

Vice President & General Manager
Keira Krausz

President, North America
Global Editor-in-Chief
Eric W. Schrier

Senior Designers
Judith Carmel
Susan Welt

Production Technology Manager
Douglas A. Croll

Manufacturing Manager
John L. Cassidy

Marketing Director
Dawn Nelson

Address any comments about
Know Your Options to:
Reader's Digest
Editor in Chief, Health Books
Reader's Digest Road
Pleasantville, NY 10570

To order more copies, call
1-800-846-2100.
Visit our website at www.rd.com

Created by Rebus, Inc.

Publisher
Rodney M. Friedman

Project Editor
Sandra Wilmot

Executive Editor
Marya Dalrymple

Senior Editor
Andrea Peirce

Contributing Editor
Carol Weeg

Editorial Assistants
Melissa Coplak, Elizabeth Hooker

Administrative Assisant
James W. Brown, Jr.

Copy Editors
Sarah Rutledge, Patricia Brennan

Indexer
Catherine Dorsey

Chief of Information Services
Tom R. Damrauer

Art Director
Tim Jeffs

Art Production
Mervyn E. Clay

Production Database Designer
Carney W. Mimms III

Production Database Programmer
John Vasiliadis

Illustrators
Rob Duckwall, Judy Speicher

Medical Board of Advisors
Chief Consultant
David Edelberg, M.D.
Internal Medicine

Consultants
Sukhjit S. Gill, M.D.
Cardiology

Robert O. Graham, M.D.
Ophthalmology

Krystyna Kiel, M.D.
Oncology

William Markey, M.D.
Gastroenterology

Michael R. Mintz, D.D.S.
Dentistry

David L. Mutchnik, M.D.
Urology

David M. Shenker, M.D.
Neurology

Richard A. Wilmot, M.D.
Rheumatology

Ronald D. Wise, M.D.
Dermatology

NOVA Graphic Services, Inc.
2370 York Road, Suite A9A
Jamison, PA 18929
(215) 542-3900
President David Davenport
Composition Manager
Steve Magnin
Editorial Director
Sandra Kear
Associate Editor
Kimberly L. Gana
Indexer Kathleen Rocheleau

The Library of Congress has catalogued an earlier version as follows:

Know your options : the definitive guide to choosing the best medical treatments.
    p. cm.
  Includes index.
  ISBN 0-7621-0708-1 (hardcover)

   1. Medicine, Popular. 2. Alternative treatment. I. Reader's Digest Association.

RC82 .K665 2002
610--dc21

2002036881

3 5 7 9 10 8 6 4

Contents

Contents continues on next page

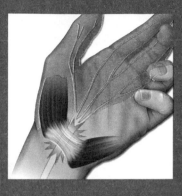

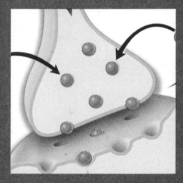

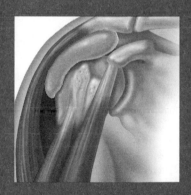

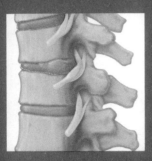

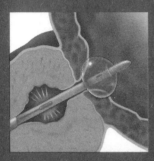

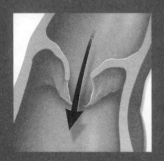

Contents

Part I: Ailments A to Z

Part II: Everyday Complaints

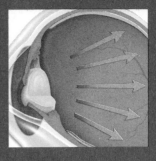

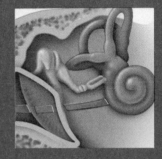

Part III: Preventive Tests

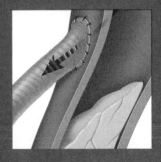

Empowering the Patient

You can probably picture yourself in this scene, which I've been part of countless times during my 25 years as a primary care doctor. Here's the setup: You've come in with some symptoms. I've asked you some questions, done an examination, and ordered some tests. Now you're back for a recap.

I've just told you there's "something." Maybe it's diabetes, high blood pressure, or you may need to be scheduled for a biopsy or major surgery. While I'm talking about what you can expect or how a medication will work, I can see that you're not really hearing what I'm saying.

This is actually quite a normal reaction to the stress of getting upsetting news, especially when you learn you've got a condition that won't go away on its own. My patients tell me they can often remember that moment in minute detail, down to the color of the tie I was wearing. They usually *can't* recall, however, anything else I said. They can't remember what I told them about how the condition came about or what treatment options are now available.

That's why this book has been created. Each entry starts at that pivotal point immediately after diagnosis. Then, in clear conversational style, it lays out exactly what's happening in your body, what your best options are for treating it successfully, and what you can expect from therapy—both the good and the bad. You can read its advice at your leisure, once the shock of learning your diagnosis has worn off.

The information provided here is meant to guide your discussions with your doctors and other members of your healthcare team and to clarify the choices you may have to make. It's not meant to be a blueprint for your own personal care.

To put the book together, we gathered a knowledgeable group of primary care physicians and specialists, doctors who see patients like you every day. We consulted gold-standard sources of information, reviewed the latest clinical research, and then condensed the most relevant information about every sort of treatment option—from simple lifestyle changes and natural approaches to cutting-edge drugs and surgery.

In short, we've given you the ammunition to become an educated, empowered patient, able to control your condition rather than be controlled by it. Personally, I love proactive people who arrive at my office armed with a book, some information they found on the Internet, and a list of challenging questions. They keep me on my toes. More importantly, they make themselves a real part of their medical team.

Ironically, these are probably the best of times *and* the worst of times to be a patient. Best, because diagnostic tests identify diseases at more curable stages. "Wonder" drugs allow people with chronic illness to enjoy many symptom-free years. Microsurgical techniques are the stuff of science fiction. Worst, because under managed care, patients never get to spend enough time with a doctor. Too many people have questions that remain unanswered and sense their doctor doesn't know them very well.

For all these reasons, *Know Your Options* and the wealth of information it contains is sure to be one of the most important and useful books in your library. We hope it will set you on a clear path to managing your health care successfully.

David Edelberg, M.D.

DAVID EDELBERG, M.D., CHIEF MEDICAL CONSULTANT FOR THIS BOOK, IS A PRACTICING PHYSICIAN, A BOARD-CERTIFIED SPECIALIST IN INTERNAL MEDICINE, AND ASSISTANT PROFESSOR OF MEDICINE AT RUSH MEDICAL COLLEGE IN CHICAGO.

Making the Right Health Choices

Modern American medicine offers powerful ways to ease pain and treat disease. Newfound openness to natural methods and effective self-care strategies further widen the vista. The challenge comes in choosing what's best for you.

Have you shopped for apples lately? As grocery stores become bigger and bigger, the variety of apples they stock gets bigger, too. Bramleys. Galas. Empires. McIntoshes. Fujis. Winesaps. Granny Smiths. Once upon a time, an apple was an apple. Today, picking an apple has become an art and a science.

Or how about exercise shoes? Once, you went out and bought plain white sneakers. Now, you have running shoes, walking shoes, hiking shoes, cross-trainers, tennis shoes, basketball shoes, high-tops, low-tops, slip-ons, Velcro® closures, snaps, safety devices, replaceable inserts, color variations—and that's just for one brand. Be prepared to spend hours shopping.

This range of choices applies to most anything you buy today. From spaghetti sauce to televisions, from the socks you wear to the water you drink— the options are often complex and overwhelming. One writer coined a nice phrase for this dilemma: *The tyranny of choice*. We want to feel informed. We want to make the right decisions. But in the face of so many options, staying informed and choosing wisely has become nearly impossible. We can't all be experts on everything. So, we look for what's on sale. We ponder the brand. We prod and poke to get a sense of value. We make sure we like the way it looks. Then we shrug our shoulders and head to the cash register.

The healthcare dilemma

Over the past 20 years or so, this "tyranny of choice" has swept through the world of health. It has done so with the little things—like the seemingly 2,000 variations of vitamin C to be found at the local drugstore—as well as the big things—like the number of treatment options you face when struck with a chronic disease.

We all know that choice is a good thing, particularly where our health is concerned. That's because there are many paths to healing, and we rarely know which is best for any given person. Just as important, our personal preferences must be respected.

The only problem with having lots of choices is that ultimately, we have to choose. Or have someone choose for us. And therein lies the rub.

Health is perhaps our most precious asset. Given all the changes that have occurred in the worlds of medicine and health insurance in recent years, how much control of our decisions do we want to relinquish to others? Even doctors will say that you are in charge of your own health, not them.

So we set out to educate ourselves. We scan newspapers, read magazines, and buy books. We talk with our families and friends. Then we go online and search for information and like-minded communities. As a whole, the American public is stunningly savvy about health. So much so that in many ways, we are leading the world of healthcare, rather than being led by it. It wasn't the demand of hospitals and doctors that got Wal-Mart or Kmart to stock more herbs and nutritional supplements; it was public demand.

As a whole, we have become highly astute healthcare consumers. We ask doctors tougher questions. We know a fair amount about new healing ways and traditional alternative therapies that have recently gained wider approval. But the odd thing about choice is that it seems to beget even more choice. New supplements, new diets, new medical breakthroughs are announced every day. Who can keep up with it all?

We based *Know Your Options* on the premise that each of us at some point encounters health situations in which we need to find out fast what is going on with our bodies and what choices there are to make things right. In his preface to this book, David Edelberg, M.D. notes that when a patient is first told of a health problem by a doctor, a typical response is to freeze up and stop listening. That's easy to understand: Emotions run high when one is told of a disease or injury. But what about a few hours later, when the emotions have settled, the reality has set in, and the hunger for understanding and advice has taken hold?

It is precisely at that moment that this book is most valuable.

To create it, we assembled a team of top-notch health journalists to consult hundreds of health-care experts and research the full gamut of health remedies. We then distilled the information into simple, clear entries that offer the full range of viable healing methods. More important, we put these methods in context. What would a doctor be most likely to recommend? Is that a sensible recommendation? What would other experts tell you? What can you do on your own that the doctor might not have mentioned? What is controversial, what is tried and true?

The end result, we believe, is one of the simplest and most effective health books available. We think you'll agree.

Doctors in perspective

There's irony in all this discussion about health choices: While the number of healing options for any particular problem is on the rise, our freedom to shop around for healthcare is increasingly restricted. With the rise of managed care, more and more of us are finding ourselves in rigid healthcare organizations. For many, no medical treatment is allowed unless first approved by our "primary care provider" and then by our insurer. In most cases, neither of these doors is that hard to pass through. But sometimes, they stick, get locked, or like any door, make a horrible squeaking sound as you push by.

Everyone who worked on this book believes that doctors do an outstanding job. We strongly recommend that your primary care provider be your main partner in healing and health. You will find that the treatment options presented throughout this book are the time-tested therapies your doctor is most likely to recommend.

But don't shirk your own responsibility. Just as your insurance (or lack of it) might constrict your healing choices, your doctor might be restricted in what can be prescribed or approved. It is reasonable and appropriate to question your doctor, to make independent decisions, to research solutions that go beyond what he or she might recommend.

There is little you can do on your own about the complexities of health insurance in America today. Whatever you can control, you should, and control it strongly. That means working in close partnership with your doctor and deciding for yourself if care and recommendations are satisfactory. If spending a little money outside your insurance program gets you the care you truly want, it is money well spent.

Choose Your Doctor Wisely

Whenever you enter a new health plan or move to a new location, you have to choose a new primary care provider for yourself and your family. This is one of the most crucial healthcare decisions you can make.

The doctor you choose will be a major player in every health issue that arises from then on, whether it involves cancer or the common cold. Choosing wisely will make all your future decisions easier to make.

This is the one important health decision that doesn't usually involve time pressure, inherent emotional fallout, or strong-willed outside influences. Just think about it: Most encounters with a doctor occur when someone is injured or ill. In these situations, there's no time to shop, ponder, or explore. You will be emotional, and the insurance rule book must guide your decisions. This is exactly the wrong time to decide that you really don't like your doctor's approach.

So pick your doctor with care. We recommend you apply the same shopping savvy you would for any big-ticket purchase:

- **Determine where you can shop.** Most healthcare plans provide a list of acceptable doctors, medical practices, or local hospitals from which you must choose your primary care provider. Start by screening for location. Most of us don't want to travel beyond a certain distance for routine doctor trips. Then, try to make some sense of the list. Are many of the doctors clustered in the same group practice? Which ones appear to be independent? Which ones work out of hospitals? Determine if any of that matters to you. This preliminary level of screening can winnow your options to a manageable number.

■ **Get good advice.** Ask your co-workers, friends, family members, or acquaintances in the healthcare field about the practices and hospitals on your list. Ask whether they know any of the individual doctors. Hunt through "Best Doctor Listings" from local magazines or newspapers, but be aware that many of these doctors are swamped and may not take new patients.

■ **Be savvy about "brand."** A doctor's background and credentials matter a lot. Find out where the doctor you're considering went to medical school and completed residency. (Just remember that while attendance at a top school or residency program is a clue to the doctor's knowledge and training, it's only one factor to consider.) You can find a lot of this information under the Doctor Finder feature on the American Medical Association's website, www.ama-assn.org. Note which hospitals the doctor is affiliated with. Large teaching hospitals tend to attract high-quality physicians. They also do a lot of the background legwork for you, screening credentials carefully before allowing a new doctor to join the staff. Be sure to look for people who are board-certified: After completing their formal training, they earned extra qualifications by taking a two-day exam that tested their breadth of knowledge. Experience matters too. The longer doctors have been in practice, the more they'll know and the more set in their ways they'll probably be. Some older doctors, for instance, may not readily subscribe to the doctor-patient teamwork approach.

■ **Be sure of the fit.** You try on new clothes. You test-drive new cars. You sample a grape before buying the whole bunch. Likewise, you should stop by the doctor's office and chat with the nurses. Try to interview the doctor before you decide. Choose someone with whom you feel relaxed and communicates well. Do you feel reassured? Are you treated as a healthcare partner who shares in selecting a treatment plan or medicine? Are the doctor's religious and ethical perspectives on end-of-life decisions compatible with yours?

■ **Check out the service.** There's the product. In this case, that's the doctor—and then there's the service. What's the policy for weekends and holidays? Who covers for the doctor during vacations or emergencies? Will the doctor come to see you if you are in the hospital? Is the office

Essential Step: Getting a Second Opinion

Placing all your trust in one doctor—especially when you're weighing different treatment options—can be unnerving, not to mention unwise. Surveys show, for instance, that a treatment popular in one region might be mysteriously unpopular in another.

● **The first rule of thumb:** If life-changing care (such as surgery, chemotherapy, or radiation) is involved, always get a second opinion before going ahead. Many insurance plans actually require this. Know your company's requirements before you decide on a course of treatment, because you can't turn back the clock once you've started. Your doctor will expect to give you referrals; you may also have names of other experts you want to consult. If a second doctor gives you a notably different opinion on how to proceed, especially if your illness is a serious one, consider getting a third perspective from an expert at a nationally recognized center.

● **The second rule of thumb:** If your diagnosis is based on biopsy results (often the case with cancer), always get a second opinion on the biopsy. Every year, 30,000 errors are made in reading and interpreting pathology specimens. These mistakes can lead to wrong treatments and grave complications. To get a biopsy read by a second pathologist, ask your specialist for a referral, or look on the nonprofit website, www.findcancerexperts.com.

location convenient? Do they handle paperwork and billing efficiently?

- **Check out the legal issues.** If you have any reason to question a doctor's ability or you want to be extra careful, you can find out whether the state medical licensing board has ever taken a disciplinary action against him or her. About one in every 200 doctors has been disciplined, according to the Federation of State Medical Boards (contact them at 817-868-4000 or www.docinfo.org to get the number for your area). You can also check in a book called *Questionable Doctors,* published by The Public Citizens' Health Research Group in Washington, D.C. Look for it in your local library or call 202-588-1000 to order the supplement for your state.

Medicine in perspective

Modern healthcare is based on the belief that the scientific method—that is, objective, measurable research—holds the answers to curing disease. When students go to college to become doctors, they learn about the chemistry of the body and how certain medicines can alter that chemistry for the better. They learn about the physiology of the body and how surgical procedures can fix flaws and repair damage. They learn that certain measurements—blood pressure, cholesterol counts, heart rate, blood sugar levels—are strong indicators of health and disease. It is a rational, thoughtful, rigorous mind-set. In most cases, it is quite accurate and effective.

The warriors of modern healthcare are the researchers. Newspapers and magazines constantly report new findings from clinical studies conducted to test new healing hypotheses and methods. Some of the researchers who conduct these investigations are affiliated with universities. Others work for businesses, such as pharmaceutical companies. Watching over it all is the federal government, which works hard to verify that all testing done is valid and comprehensive. On the surface, this world of health research is noble, logical, and successful. Few would debate that the United States leads the world in medical research.

But there are cracks. Those who read the newspapers closely know that the quality of research can vary, and results sometimes conflict. Further, clinical studies rarely provide a complete solution. They advance our knowledge incrementally, and we are left trying to infer the broader application. This is the nature of science. In rare situations, however, the results can be troubling. One need only look at the ever-changing debate over hormone replacement therapy (HRT) for postmenopausal women to see that research does not always deliver the correct or complete answer the first time around.

We must also acknowledge the huge money machine that is the healthcare industry and the influence this flow of dollars can have on those within the field. Was anyone surprised when front-page headlines announced that the federal government would start cracking down on pharmaceutical companies if they continued to give lucrative gifts to doctors and pharmacists who then prescribe their medicines for patients who had been responding to other therapy? The message was clear: Stop putting profits and personal gain before your patients' health.

We don't bring this up to cast doubt on the efficacy of modern health methodologies. We all know the extraordinary wonders being performed every day at hospitals everywhere, using new drugs, lasers, and procedures. The point—and it's an important one—is that the health world is enormously dynamic. Drugs and procedures come and go. Assumptions also come and go.

Using Medications Wisely

Perhaps the most dynamic area of health is pharmaceuticals. The pursuit of new medicine is exciting, exasperating, and expensive. For every breakthrough, there are dozens of near misses. Companies can be made or broken by betting on a single new medicine.

Know Your Options discusses pharmaceuticals in detail. Truth is, medicine is often the first line of attack for doctors. It usually works—fast, safely, and without hassle. We strongly support intelligent use of over-the-counter and prescription drugs. But you need to be part of this decision-making process, too. Ask questions about the medicines you are being told to take. Here are several tips to help you along:

Controlling Your Drug Costs

The soaring cost of pharmaceuticals remains one of the hottest social issues in America. It is a familiar story: seniors forced to pick between medicine or food, pharmaceutical companies complaining about extreme government regulation, consumer advocates grumbling about too-high drug company profits, and politicians vowing to pass new legislation to remedy the situation.

For those lucky enough to have good-quality health insurance, the argument is not very relevant; a relatively small co-payment gets you any prescription drug, no questions asked. But for the millions without prescription drug coverage, the horror of full retail price is real. As the debate stretches on and on in Washington, here are some things you can do on your own:

● **Ask your doctor if generic equivalents are right for you.** Many brand-name drugs (both over-the-counter and prescription) have cheaper, generic alternatives that are just as safe and effective. Despite the implications in drug company advertisements, generics are required by law to be bioequivalent to—behave the same way as—brand-name versions.

● **Shop around.** Every store sets its own price on medicine, as it does for any other product it sells. While it seems odd to price-shop among pharmacies, the savings can be more than worth the effort. Or you can do the "footwork" online: Try Verified Internet Pharmacy Practice (www.nabp.net/vipps/consumer/search.asp). If you take a drug regularly and insurance doesn't pay, you may also be able to save from 15% to 50% by ordering online or by mail.

● **Buy in bulk.** Here again, medicine is like any other retail product—cheaper in bulk. If you are paying out-of-pocket for the medicine and have the cash, consider getting several months'

worth at one time. A caveat: Insurance companies often only cover a certain quantity per month, so if you have a co-pay, ask first. Be wary of expiration dates. If you buy too far ahead, your medicine may lose its oomph by the time you're ready to use it.

● **Split your tablets.** Drug costs are based more on the number of pills you get than on the dosage they contain. So if you take 100 mg, consider buying 200 mg pills and splitting them to save money. This only works on noncoated pills, so check with the pharmacist first.

● **Ask about special programs.** If you don't have insurance (or are underinsured), talk with your doctor about applying for aid from the drug company itself or helpingpatients.org. Contact the Pharmaceutical Research and Manufacturer's Association of America, (202-835-3400), then have your doctor complete the application.

■ **Get the facts.** When your doctor hands you a prescription, ask about its history. When did it hit the market, and have there been any surprises? Is it controversial? How widely is it used? Why this drug and not another? Then ask about what it does, if it has notable side effects, and what to do if you develop a reaction. Find out what to do if you miss a dose.

■ **Speak up.** The FDA reports that up to 21% of people never even fill their prescriptions. Why? It could be cost, fear, laziness, or doubts about the drug's appropriateness or efficacy. Don't let it come to that. If you doubt what the doctor is prescribing, you need to say so. If you fear the drug itself, you need to say so. If you can't afford it, you need to say so.

■ **Report back.** Your doctor will want to know if the medicine is working. Report any side effects. If you're unhappy for some reason, there may well be an alternative.

■ **Work with one pharmacist.** These professionals can be a fantastic source of information on new or alternate drugs. They can also keep track of all the medicines you use and alert you to harmful combinations.

■ **Watch for interactions.** Medications (and supplements) don't always mix well and may even counteract each other. Drugs can also cause symptoms that mimic diseases other than the condition for which they're prescribed. Always let your doctor know about everything you're taking, including prescription medications, OTC drugs, and supplements.

About Clinical Trials

Formal research studies, known as clinical trials, test new medications, treatments, and medical devices. The gold-standard trial is called the "double-blind" test. In it, subjects are split into two groups. One section gets the new medicine or treatment, while the other gets a placebo. Placebos are rarely used in clinical trials involving cancer or other life-threatening illnesses. Participants in these trials are treated with the best currently approved therapy or with an experimental treatment researchers believe will be more effective. Placebos are used only if no standard treatment exists. Neither patient nor doctor is told who got which. So no one can be biased as the test progresses.

From the patient's standpoint, clinical trials are a mixed bag. On the negative side, you might be in the placebo group and go weeks or months without receiving optimal treatment. The new treatment you're testing might have side effects or other problems. But the positives can be compelling: You have access to promising drugs or procedures that otherwise might not be available. Your overall health gets intensively monitored, and you get excellent—and most likely free—medical care.

If you are considering a clinical trial, check the credentials and experience of the key researchers involved. Your doctor may have thoughts about this. Look into the quality of the facility you'll be visiting. Remember, you have the right to withdraw from a clinical trial at any time, for any reason—that's the law.

Ask the Researchers . . .
- What's the purpose of the trial?
- What are the potential benefits—or risks—to me?
- Who is sponsoring the trial?
- What is the primary investigator's track record?
- Do I have to pay? What about for travel to a distant facility? Or for housing?
- What if severe side effects develop or I'm hurt by something that happens in the trial?
- Is there a 24-hour contact person?
- Can I continue the treatment after the trial?

Ask Yourself . . .
- Are my expectations realistic?
- Am I comfortable dealing with the many researchers and other professionals running the study, and with having to (most likely) switch doctors?
- Will I be comfortable with the intense monitoring and attention?
- Do I understand what I'm being asked to do?

■ **Take your medicine.** Many people use how they feel as a barometer for whether or not to take a pill. But doing that disregards the non-symptomatic things going on in your body. Prescription drugs have been tested thoroughly for optimal duration and effect, so when a doctor says take your medications for 10 days, take them for 10 days. If the dosage schedule is complex, try sorting your pills into a monthly, weekly, or daily pillbox. Even an alarm clock can help you keep track.

It's about life

Dean Ornish. Andrew Weil. Deepak Chopra. Christiane Northrup. Nicholas Perricone. Have you heard of these people? They are the new voices of health, the popular doctor-authors who are selling millions of books by showing people how to live good health every day. While each has a unique message and voice, certain themes run through all their books:

■ **Good health is not merely the absence of bad health.** It is a positive attitude about life, a feeling of energy and happiness, an active engagement of mind, body, and yes, spirit.

■ **At the heart of good health is a healthy lifestyle.** Eating well. Losing weight. Being active. Knowing how to relax. Having fun. Having a purpose.

■ **Only you can create good health for yourself.** You control all the things that matter most to your health.

These are powerful notions. They are all true. Numerous clinical trials confirm them.

Five Key Lifestyle Choices

Know Your Options, you will find, embraces the belief that lifestyle adjustments can play a big role not only in being healthy, but in improving most aspects of your health. In particular, you should:

■ **Quit smoking.** This is still just about the best thing you can do for your health. For a few decades now, the government, the health industry, educators, and even social policymakers have been saying this loudly, with a wealth of research to support them. Slowly, the message is sinking in. Yet millions continue to smoke.

- **Choose healthful foods** (and eliminate the junk). Doing so can be a powerful weapon against disease. One example is the DASH diet, which can dramatically lower your blood pressure by limiting sodium and increasing potassium, calcium, and magnesium. This eating plan can be so effective that you may eventually be able to stop taking blood pressure drugs.

- **Lose weight.** This is a key treatment recommendation throughout this book. You'll find it in such diverse entries as back pain, diabetes, arthritis, and heart disease. Excess pounds can profoundly tax your body. Each pound lost lightens your body's workload.

- **Exercise regularly.** You can't go wrong here. Research shows that exercise reduces your cholesterol, keeps you flexible, gives you energy, and improves your mental state. (The latest findings report it may even help raise your tolerance to pain.) All it takes for most adults to get well and stay well is 30 minutes of moderate physical activity every day. Try working exercise into your daily choices: Park farther from the store and walk the extra distance, get out and dig in the garden, or take the stairs. Exercise is good for your pocketbook, too: Experts calculate the annual medical costs for an inactive American are $330 higher than for someone who is active.

- **Sleep well.** Sleep is the best medicine for many ailments. You'll be more alert, of course, but there's more to it than that. Sleep literally heals. When you slip deep into slumber, the demanding job of replenishing your cells, hormones, and entire immune system begins. Myriad physical and mental tensions are ironed out.

Little Changes Make a Difference

It is sad but true that the American way of life is not very healthy. Compared with statistically healthier cultures around the world, we watch more television, work longer hours, eat far more food, and commute longer distances. We also sleep less, relax less, get less exercise, and even seem to have less fun.

Know how to change? You just do it. There's nothing about a more healthful lifestyle that requires approvals, investments, or substantial change. You just turn off the television, go for a walk, and have fruit for dessert instead of cake. You say *no* to the late-night movie. Healthful living, in the end, is about little changes. Make enough of them, and you'll suddenly realize that you've changed in big ways.

Dealing with Stress

Uncontrolled stress is epidemic in American life today, so it's no wonder that most of the entries in this book tell you to do everything you can to reduce your stress levels. Chronic stress wreaks havoc on nearly every system of your body. It precipitates and exacerbates heart disease, muscle pain, fatigue, immune system problems, insomnia, and dozens of other ills.

Don't dismiss stress relief as New Age hooey. Nearly every major cancer clinic in the United States now includes stress-relief training as part of its prescribed healing regimen. The physiological response to stress has been carefully measured and analyzed. The healing power of relaxation has been quantified and confirmed.

There are lots of ways to halt stress and limit the insidious damage it causes. Many popular techniques have been used for centuries—yoga, meditation, and deep breathing, for example. If you recoil at the idea of a "relaxation technique," then just relax the old-fashioned way, with the newspaper on the porch, or with a glass of wine and a symphony on the stereo. Spend an hour baking or playing catch with your kids or grandkids. Take a walk in a park. Beating stress doesn't have to be complicated. What matters is that you let go of your tensions, have a little fun, and feel a little calmer. Do so every day, not just when you find free time on your hands.

The Next Step: Alternative Healing

Flash back about 10 years. Managed care was growing in prominence, Washington was deep into the debate about healthcare reform, and many Americans were increasingly disgusted with the state of medicine in general. Suddenly, alternative healing methods were all the rage. Acupuncture, healing herbs, essential oils, massage, Chinese medicine, and many other "healing modalities" became the stuff of talk shows, newspaper articles, and countless books. People responded with their checkbooks, and a billion-dollar industry was created.

Fast forward to today, and the revolution has quietly achieved victory. Herbs, homeopathic medicines, and all sorts of dietary supplements can be found in most every grocery and drugstore in America. Visits to alternative health practitioners continue to grow, and more and more people now believe that the herb echinacea helps to fight colds or that foods can be used to heal.

Of course, not everyone has embraced this new world of ancient medicine. The gentle, slow healing many of these methods claim can rarely be replicated or confirmed in clinical settings, which continues to make the modern health care establishment skeptical. Most doctors aren't thrilled at the notion that their patients are off trying unproven remedies based on self-diagnoses.

As with any popular movement, the good will stick around and the silly or outrageous will fade away. Indeed, there are many good aspects to these alternative healing methods. The main message—that for minor problems, simple, natural, time-tested solutions should be the first line of attack—is sound wisdom. The anecdotal evidence that vitamins, herbs, and other natural medicines and practices help fight and treat disease seems impressive. Most of all, these alternative methods are extremely respectful of the patient. Naturopaths, homeopaths, and other "alternative" practitioners are renowned—and even in some cases revered—for the time they give to their patients, listening, talking, comforting, and caring.

In *Know Your Options*, we take a measured view of this new/old world of alternative medicine. When credible evidence exists that these methods work, we don't hesitate to recommend them. On the pages that follow, you'll find many such remedies from the apothecaries of yesteryear: licorice wafers for ulcers, valerian for insomnia, and capsaicin cream for muscle strains or arthritis pain. Even though these natural remedies take a while to work, many remain popular because they're often gentler and less likely to cause adverse reactions than powerful modern drugs. When a natural alternative like glucosamine for arthritis or feverfew for migraine

has been shown to be effective and safe, this book mentions it.

The curative effects of many dietary supplements are unproven, however, when it comes to serious medical problems. That is where we draw the line. If the health problem is serious and quick response is appropriate, then it is hard to beat the medicines and procedures of modern health care.

When healing gets serious

Many of the entries in *Know Your Options* deal with everyday problems like colds and flu, but there are entries on more serious and chronic diseases as well. For these, we often suggest treatments that require a hospital stay.

Going to the hospital is hard business. None of us want to be there. No matter how much the personnel work at making it a warm and friendly environment (and some try harder than others), it is still a place with too many negative connotations and implications. In our mind's eye, none of us see ourselves as being hospital-bound. Yet, when serious disease or injury hits, we must go to the hospital.

You cannot allow yourself to surrender to the situation. Do not hand yourself over to the doctors and nurses and say, "Do what you must." Now, more than ever, you need to be assertive—to feel that you are a partner in the decisions and the main force behind your own healing. It's not easy—being in a hospital bed can sap you of energy and spirit. But it shouldn't hinder your thoughts or determination. Be as strong as you can. You will emerge from your hospital stay faster, healthier, and with a sense of control.

Finding the Best Hospital

In choosing a facility, the most common error is to settle for the closest one. Seeking out a first-rate medical center, even if it means travel, extra expense, or switching doctors, could be one of the most important decisions you make.

So-called "general hospitals" treat a wide variety of problems, from hernias to broken arms. A specialized facility may be better for innovative cancer therapy or heart surgery. Here are some issues to explore:

- **Accreditation.** Is the facility evaluated by the Joint Commission on Accreditation of Healthcare Organizations (www.jcaho.org)? This independent group sets standards and tracks treatment success rates; reviews are done every three years.
- **Experience.** Has the hospital been successful in treating conditions like yours? How often does it provide the type of care you need? High volume is linked to quicker recovery, to lower complication and mortality rates, and often, lower costs.
- **Quality.** What's the background of the surgical team? The nurse-to-patient ratio? Are there social workers and patient advocates? Is the facility clean? For reports on hospitals (and nursing homes) nationwide, go to www.healthgrades.com.
- **Ranking.** Do you need specialized care? One good place to begin is the *U.S. News & World Report* (www.usnews.com). Once a year, it ranks 205 top medical centers in 17 different specialties. The highest-rated facilities tend to perform the most difficult procedures and offer the seriously ill the best options.
- **Affiliation.** Is your doctor on the hospital staff? If not, can you have a say in who's assigned to your case?
- **Timing.** Can you choose when to schedule your stay? If so, try to avoid holidays when hospitals tend to be short-staffed, and steer clear of teaching hospitals in early July, when residents begin their formal training.

Pay Attention to Details

What you do before and during your time in the hospital can make a big difference in the length and cost of your stay. To begin, see if a procedure can be done on an outpatient basis or on the same day you're admitted. Schedule it for early in the week to avoid a costly weekend stay. Try to have pre-op tests before admittance, saving hospital charges as you await results. Have copies of previous medical test results so you don't have to pay to have them repeated.

Look closely at your insurance policy. You may be required to provide notification and obtain approval for hospital procedures. You may be responsible for some type of co-payment of the total bill. Be warned: Insurance may cover only what it considers "usual and customary" charges. The insurance company (not your doctor) determines what these charges are.

While you're in the hospital, you or a family member should keep a log of all doctor visits,

Worth the Effort: Selecting a Top Surgeon

Studies show that the more skilled the surgeon, the more likely it is that you'll come through alive and well. To find a top-notch surgeon, look into:

- **More than one name.** No matter how much you trust your doctor, never let your choice of a surgeon rest solely on his shoulders. Friendships, social connections, and economic considerations can subtly influence even the most noble intentions.
- **Qualifications.** Check on board certification (*see page 11*)

and the doctor's acceptance as a fellow of the American College of Surgeons. Affiliation with a first-rate medical center is another good sign.
- **Track record.** Ask how many times the surgeon has performed the particular procedure you're considering; volume matters. How do his or her results (outcomes, such as cure and infection-free recovery) compare with other surgeons? Has his or her license ever been suspended. Has he or she ever been the subject of a professional peer review (and if so, why)? Ask for the names of

some patients you can call to ask about their experiences.
- **Safeguards.** It's very tempting to suppress the thought, but surgeons do make mistakes. Protect against the "oops" factor by discussing exactly what will be done while you're on the table. You and your surgeon should mark the surgical site with a permanent pen. Write "wrong" on the opposing limb (left vs. right knee, for example). Don't be intimidated or reluctant to appear silly in doing this. There are more mix-ups during surgery than you'd like to imagine.

drugs, tests, and services you received you'll want to check against later. Don't pay on exit: Request a bill itemized in plain English to take home. Ask that miscellaneous charges be spelled out and daily expenses be listed.

Billing mistakes do happen. If you think one has occurred, start by immediately alerting the hospital's patient accounts supervisor and your insurance company. If the dispute is not resolved, write to your state's Attorney General's Office of Consumer Affairs. (Be sure to make copies of the bill and your letters.) A private claims assistance professional can help you sort through the paperwork or pursue payment from your insurance carrier, if necessary. Contact the Alliance of Claims Assistance Professionals at www.claims.org.

Using this book

As we've mentioned, *Know Your Options* is meant to be the first resource you turn to when you (or someone close to you) discover that you have an acute illness or chronic condition. We've organized it in three parts:

Part I: Ailments A to Z (*pages 20–340*) includes doctor-reviewed information on more than 100 ailments and conditions, from acne to wrinkles. Each entry gives you a quick overview on how the condition affects your body, then explains the latest treatment options available.

Treatments are divided into four categories: medications (OTC and prescription); procedures (surgical and nonsurgical); lifestyle changes or self-care measures you can undertake; and, when appropriate, natural methods (such as herbs or nutritional supplements) that have been shown to be beneficial for that condition.

These treatment options are presented in the order your doctor would probably recommend them to you as part of an overall recovery plan. For example, if you have borderline high blood pressure (*page 170*), you would most likely be told

to start with some key lifestyle changes, then move on to medications if those steps didn't work. If you have Parkinson's disease (*page 246*), medications would be a first-line treatment.

Part II: Everyday Complaints (*pages 341–348*) covers the more minor health problems—from athlete's foot to yeast infections—that many of us suffer from on occasion but don't always know how best to treat.

Part III: Preventive Tests (*pages 349–367*) features key screening tests (beginning with a routine physical) that adults need to spot problems early and maintain optimal health.

Knowing your options

In the end, *Know Your Options* is devoted to helping you become aware of all the treatment choices you have—along with their benefits and risks. The final decision on what to choose, however, is a very personal one that depends on many factors: your particular problem, what your doctors recommend, and what your gut feelings tell you.

Just like picking the "right" apple at the market or the "right" shoes at a sporting goods store, there is no absolute "right" choice in picking a healing method. You can look at the process two ways. If you're a pessimist, you'll probably despair that whatever you chose, there would have been a better alternative, if only you had known a little more. If you're an optimist, you'll say that the lack of a single solution is liberating. It means you can decide on your own path. If that path is chosen sensibly and with conviction—and with the consultation of a smart, caring health partner like a good doctor—it will be the one most likely to take you where you want to go.

We, of course, advocate the optimistic view, as do most doctors. Trust yourself, listen carefully to your doctor, be thoughtful and clear-headed, and the healing path you choose will most certainly be the right one for you.

Part I
Ailments A to Z

Acne

Even if you sail through your teens with clear skin, you may develop acne when you're an adult. Don't despair. An ever-widening variety of treatment options are available, from powerful medications to surgical techniques to reduce scarring.

LIKELY **First Steps**

- **Daily cleansing routine** to control oil and bacteria.
- For milder acne, **over-the-counter antibacterial products** (lotions, gels, pads).
- For more serious acne, **prescription medications** (topical and oral).

QUESTIONS TO **Ask**

- What is the risk that my mild acne will turn into severe, cystic acne?
- Does it make sense to treat my scars now, as they occur, or should I wait?
- Could a hormonal imbalance be the cause of my premenopausal acne?
- Is it possible that at some point the antibiotic I'm taking won't work anymore? What will I do then?

What is happening

Acne occurs when the oil (or sebaceous) glands under hair follicles—often on your face, neck, chest, or back—get plugged up, inflamed, or infected. Frequently the glands simply secrete too much of a thick waxy lubricant called **sebum** that keeps your skin healthy. Sebum can block the pores and create a perfect breeding ground for bacteria (especially *Propionibacterium acnes*). **Follicles** then get red and inflamed.

Hormonal imbalances can also play a role: Sebum increases with the overproduction of testosterone and other androgens in teenage boys, for instance, or with women's hormonal fluctuations, such as those associated with the menstrual cycle, pregnancy, and menopause. In mild cases of acne (referred to as **acne vulgaris**), whiteheads and blackheads as well as some raised red blemishes appear. In more severe cases (**cystic acne**), pus-filled cysts and deep nodules form around the inflamed follicles, causing unsightly bumps and tenderness, which are often painful.

Treatments

Acne doesn't really last forever (it just seems like it does). It can, however, take time to clear up. Anywhere from several days for a crop of pimples to months or years for some types of cystic acne. For occasional blemishes, applying over-the-counter anti-acne preparations and keeping your skin clean can make a real difference. For an extended outbreak, you'll need to see a dermatologist for prescription medications. Certain office procedures—cyst removal, skin peels, steroid injections—can also be very effective in treating severe cases.

Acne isn't life-threatening, but its ravages can be long term. The best way to prevent disfiguring scars is to treat any lesions promptly. And take heart: If you already have facial scars, cosmetic laser treatments have shown great success in reducing pitting.

Medications

If you have mild to moderate acne, home treatment should begin with **OTC antibacterial drugs**—gels, creams, lotions, and pads. Look for remedies with benzoyl peroxide (Oxy10, Neutrogena, Clearasil products), which fights the *P. acnes* bacteria. Other products (pads by Clearasil, Noxzema 2, Stri-Dex) feature salicylic acid, a derivative of aspirin. Salicylic acid products are a good choice for whiteheads or blackheads (medically known as **comedones**), because they gently dry up and peel away the skin's top layer, unclogging pores.

Treatment options

Medications

OTC antibacterials	Benzoyl peroxide or salicylic acid products.
Oral contraceptives	Maximum benefit seen in 4–6 months.
Antibiotics	Topical: Best if paired with OTC antibacterial. Oral: Effective but promote drug resistance.
Vitamin A derivatives	Tretinoin (topical): Benefits in 3–4 weeks. Isotretinoin (oral): Needs doctor supervision.

Procedures

Comedone removal	Must be done regularly; lasting benefits arguable.
Skin peel	Transitory effect but enhances drug absorption.
Steroid injections	Effective for severe lesions.
Scar lessening	Collagen, dermabrasion, laser treatments.

Lifestyle changes

Cleansing regimens	Keystone of homecare program.

Natural methods

Herbal options	Tea tree oil and chamomile tea cleansers.

If you think your acne flare-ups are related to your period, ask your doctor about **oral contraceptives.** Birth control pills can help because they systematically regulate the release of monthly hormones, preventing the natural imbalances that contribute to acne.

If your acne doesn't improve, you may need to move on to prescription **antibiotics** (topical or oral), which reduce skin bacteria and have an anti-inflammatory effect. You may actually get the best results by combining topical OTC antibacterials with topical antibiotics, such as clindamycin or erythromycin. Oral antibiotics (tetracycline, minocycline, doxycycline) can be very effective at controlling acne when used long term. However, this practice is problematic because bacteria are becoming resistant to the drugs.

For this reason, consider trying a synthetic form of vitamin A known as **tretinoin** (Retin-A, Retinoic Acid). This topical prescription drug unclogs pores by regulating the growth of skin cells; it's often used in combination with benzoyl peroxide. A word of warning: If you use tretinoin, your acne may actually look worse before it gets better. Because your skin will be extra sensitive, you'll also need to stay out of the sun, and be sure to keep the gel or liquid away from your eyes.

Even more effective is the oral vitamin A derivative **isotretinoin** (Accutane), which shrinks the sebum-producing glands attached to hair follicles. Often dubbed a "miracle cure" for severe cystic acne, Accutane requires careful medical supervision because it can have serious side effects (*see box, page 22*).

TAKING Control

■ **Go to a dermatologist,** not a general practitioner, especially if you need to have a procedure done. Skin doctors are specially trained to perform such treatments.

■ **Choose acne products with care.** Expensive medicated cleansers often work no better than mild soap and are not worth the extra cost.

■ **Try a blackhead extractor.** This drugstore device may save you costly trips to the dermatologist. Before using this tool, soften the area with hot, wet compresses for about 10 minutes.

■ **Use water-based makeup.** Look for products labeled "noncomedogenic" or "nonacnegenic." Also, don't overdo on moisturizing. Skip cosmetics completely if your acne is severe.

Promising
DEVELOPMENTS

■ Lasers are the new-wave treatment for acne scars. However, the jury's still out on which procedure is best. One device, the **pulsed carbon dioxide (CO_2) laser,** is particularly effective for revising indented scars. Its heat vaporizes thin layers of depressed skin and tightens collagen fibers. Another so-called "cool" laser treatment, **the Erbium:YAG laser,** uses short bursts of energy that are absorbed by the water in the skin. This permits the precise sculpting of irregular scars.

What about Accutane?

The greatest acne development in 20 years, this potent drug is now used by 500,000 people a year. And 85% of them show great improvement after 4–5 months. Unfortunately, Accutane's negative effects can be equally powerful.

The drug has long been known to cause birth defects. Reports of serious psychiatric problems have also appeared. Depression and thoughts of suicide haunt some people, even weeks after they stop taking the drug.

In response, the FDA has designed a safety net of sorts. Women who use Accutane must agree to use two forms of birth control and have a pregnancy test every month or the prescription cannot be renewed. Every patient is required to sign a consent sheet before a doctor writes a prescription.

The bottom line: This medicine can be amazingly effective, but you'll need to use it with great care.

FINDING Support

■ If you're looking for a skin doctor, the American Academy of Dermatology in Schaumburg, IL can provide referrals to dermatologists in your area (1-888-462-3376 or www.aad.org).

■ For information about acne-related clinical trials and specifics on skin diseases, check with the experts at the NIH's National Institute of Arthritis and Musculoskeletal and Skin Diseases, NIAMS, in Bethesda, MD (877-226-4267 or www.niams.nih.gov).

Procedures

Dermatologists have an arsenal of techniques to help control problem lesions and prevent scarring, however, many of these office procedures must be performed frequently. For **comedone removal**, doctors use a comedo (or loop) extractor to pull bacterial matter out of whiteheads and blackheads, reducing the risk they will develop into troublesome blemishes. (Some patients can learn to do this themselves.) For severe acne, doctors may **inject steroids** (corticosteroid drugs) into cysts and nodules to lessen inflammation and shrink the lesions. Superficial chemical **skin peels** often fail to minimize acne scars, which reflect damage to deeper layers of skin.

If you're among the 1% of acne sufferers who scars—and this depends on various factors, from your skin type to how extensive your inflammation is—new surgical procedures can have dramatic results. For one or two scars, consider **collagen injections,** which insert this natural protein under the skin to "fill out" depressions. For a more extensive problem, **dermabrasion** is an effective surgical treatment that minimizes even deep scars. Under local anesthesia, a high-speed brush removes surface skin and alters the contour of scars. **Laser treatments** are an encouraging new development. They employ various wavelengths and intensities of light to recontour scar tissue, and are now being explored for the treatment of acne. Although your skin may be red for months, your scars will be changed for good.

Lifestyle Changes

In addition to medical treatments, good home care is essential for dealing with acne successfully. Try the following:

■ **Wash your face gently** (no more than twice a day) with a mild soap to remove oil, dead skin cells, and bacteria.

■ **Pay attention to your hair.** Style it away from your face so scalp oils don't irritate your complexion, and avoid greasy styling products. Always pull your hair back when you sleep.

■ **Wear clean, loose-fitting exercise gear.** Working up a sweat in tight, nonabsorbent clothes or a constricting sweatband alters oil production, contributing to acne formation.

■ **Don't squeeze lesions.** Picking at pimples will make the inflammation worse and increase the risk of scars and pitting.

■ **Avoid prolonged exposure to the sun and ultraviolet lamps.** These light sources dry up acne, but they also result in long-term skin damage and can even cause cancer.

Natural Methods*

Some herbal products are useful for drying up acne. Topically applied, **tea tree oil** is a natural alternative to benzoyl peroxide. Wipe on a 10% to 15% strength solution twice a day. The herb **chamomile** has long been used for calming skin inflammations. Make a strong chamomile tea, and wipe the cooled liquid over your face each morning. This effective daily rinse tones and cleanses.

Natural methods are not subject to the same testing and regulation as prescription medications. Please seek your doctor's advice and use caution.

Allergies

For millions of people, sneezing and wheezing, runny noses and itchy eyes, are the natural consequences of opening a window, working in the yard, or petting the cat. Take heart: Relief is at hand, whether you need it when pollen flies or all year round.

What is happening

If you're among the 20% of Americans who suffer from hay fever (medically known as **allergic rhinitis**), you know all about congestion, sneezing, and watery eyes. Such symptoms can be traced to a variety of pollens (from ragweed and grasses to trees and flowers). And sniffling and hacking aren't just springtime problems. They can make you miserable any time of year, depending on what you are allergic to. Trees pollinate from late winter through May. In summer, grasses start, followed by weeds in the fall. And plants aren't the only problem.

Many molds and mildews shed spores that cause allergies year-round, January to December. Dust mites, pet dander, mice, and in cities, cockroaches can cause persistent problems. If you're allergic to substances like nickel (used in watchbands and jewelry) you may develop a rash wherever metal touches your skin. Severe reactions to foods (*see box, page 27*) or to stings from bees or other insects can cover you with hives, or in the worst-case scenario, may even be fatal. Allergies can even trigger asthma, a chronic respiratory disease that kills thousands of people annually (*see Asthma, page 40*).

LIKELY First Steps

- An **antihistamine** to relieve sneezing, itching, watery eyes, and other symptoms.
- A **decongestant** to ease nasal congestion.
- A **nasal spray** (steroid or cromolyn) to reduce inflammation and prevent allergy attacks.
- A **nasal wash** to remove mucus from the nose.
- **Allergy tests** to determine which pollens or molds are causing your allergies (several may be to blame).
- If symptoms persist or are severe or if you have asthma: **allergy shots** to desensitize you to allergy triggers.

QUESTIONS TO Ask

- Should I pull up all the carpeting in my house?
- What can I do about the cat?
- Should I get tested for hidden food allergies?
- Could my allergies ever become something more serious, like asthma?
- Can my allergies just go away?
- Could my allergy symptoms be caused by something else, maybe a drug I'm taking?
- When should I see an allergist? What about an ear, nose, and throat (ENT) specialist?

STAGES OF AN ALLERGIC REACTION

3. Histamine makes the cells in the nasal passages contract, which allows fluid to escape.

4. Nasal passages swell.

5. As a defensive ploy, excess mucus is produced.

2. Immune system mast cells are triggered to release the chemical histamine.

1. An airborne allergen is inhaled through the nose.

6. And the result: An allergy attack, with sneezing, itching, irritation, and general misery.

In susceptible people, hay fever or an allergy begins when tiny allergens such as pollen or dust, set off a cascade of events (*see stages 1–6 above*). This is basically an overreaction by your own immune system.

A

TAKING Control

- **Identify what's causing your allergies.** Keep an allergy diary, recording the times of day and year when symptoms occur and any foods, plants, pets, or other factors that trigger reactions.

- **Close the windows** at night to keep pollen and molds out. Use a central air conditioner equipped with a filter to clean and dry the air. You might even run it off-season with the cooling gauge turned off. Use your car's AC too.

- **Use a dehumidifier** to keep mold counts down.

- **Take a vacation by the sea**. Pollen counts are often lower at the beach.

▶ Should I consider moving somewhere else?

Treatment for allergies is preferable—and a lot more practical—than escape, though depending on what you are allergic to, relocating might provide some relief. Sufferers of ragweed-triggered hay fever do especially poorly in southern cities such as Tampa, Louisville, and Orlando, which top the list of the worst American cities for seasonal allergies. Dust mites, which can cause year-round trouble, thrive in humid conditions and are fairly rare in places, such as the desert Southwest, where relative humidity is under 50%. But once you move, you could develop allergies to other plants, or ragweed could have a banner year in your new location. The only locale where you may be entirely allergy-free is Antarctica!

Treatment options

Medications

Antihistamines	Quick relief: OTC or prescription nasal spray.
Decongestants	Oral drugs and sprays to relieve stuffiness.
Steroid nasal sprays	Reduce inflammation; stop allergic process.
Eye drops	Good for itchy, watery eyes.
Leukotriene antagonists	Asthma drugs used in certain circumstances.

Procedures

Nasal wash	Saline solution to wash mucus from the nose.
Allergy shots	Immunotherapy to reduce allergic reactions.

Lifestyle changes

Stay indoors	Reduce exposure to potential allergens.
Get rid of allergens	Use a HEPA vacuum; change bedding often.

Natural methods

Supplements	Quercetin and stinging nettle.

Allergy symptoms arise because your immune system over-responds to microscopic pollens, molds, and other allergy triggers known as **allergens** (*see illustration, page 23*). If you breathe in or touch a particular allergen to which you are sensitive, it will combine with a component of your immune system called an immunoglobulin E (IgE) antibody. IgE is normally a helpful substance that protects your body against parasites, germs, and other foreign invaders. If you have allergies, however, harmless substances like pollen cause IgE to activate specialized mast cells in your nose, eyes, or other areas that have come in contact with the irritant. As a defense, mast cells then release inflammatory substances, such as histamine, which cause the congestion, itching, sneezing, hives, and other complaints so familiar to allergy sufferers.

Treatments

Identifying your allergy triggers, then doing your best to avoid them is your best bet for preventing an allergy attack. Many drugs are effective at relieving symptoms, allowing you to get on with your daily affairs. Until recently, OTC antihistamines and decongestants were the mainstays of allergy treatment. Antihistamines block the irritating effects of histamine on the nasal passages, eyes, skin, or other tissues and can be very effective at easing symptoms. They are often combined with a decongestant, which shrinks the swollen membranes in the nasal passages.

In recent years, newer nonsedating prescription antihistamines and steroid nasal sprays have proven safe and more effective for the majority of allergy sufferers. Most people with seasonal allergies know

Can Being Too Clean Cause Allergies?

The incidence of allergies is rising, but nobody knows why. Some experts cite the "hygiene hypothesis" as a possible reason. According to this theory, the squeaky-clean kitchen counters, germ-free bathrooms, and well-sealed living spaces in modern homes, combined with antibiotics and vaccinations, may be to blame. More and more children are exposed to fewer and fewer germs at an early age, when their immune systems can properly process them. This ultrahygienic lifestyle, some believe, may throw underutilized immune systems into overdrive, triggering allergic reactions to harmless molds or pollens. That may be one reason why allergies are much more common in developed countries than in rural areas of Africa or Asia. It may also explain why infants who grow up with a dog or cat, younger children in large families, or kids who've had a lot of illnesses are less likely to suffer from allergies when they get older. Other possible causes of the allergy boom include pollutants, an increase in smoking, a decline in breast-feeding, and dietary changes. Any or all of these factors might interact with genetic susceptibilities to bring on allergies.

when their first symptoms appear. That's when to begin their medication programs, which continue for the duration. For more serious cases, specialized medications or procedures like allergy shots can be very effective. If you have allergies all year, you'll have to turn detective to discover what's causing your symptoms. And you may also be more willing to make the prolonged commitment allergy shots require. A number of sensible changes you can make in your daily life can also help keep your allergies in check.

Medications

Most allergy drugs act quickly to relieve symptoms. You'll get considerable relief, for instance, within an hour of taking an **antihistamine,** which helps dry out the sinuses, relieve itching and hives, and prevent sneezing. Such drugs are most effective if taken prior to an allergy attack, say before you plan to go outside. Most older **OTC antihistamines,** such as Chlor-Trimeton or Benadryl, can cause drowsiness or slowed reactions. This can be dangerous if you're driving or handling heavy machinery, but helpful if you want to go to sleep. Newer **prescription antihistamines,** such as desloratadine (Clarinex), cetirizine (Zyrtec), and fexofenadine (Allegra), cause less drowsiness but are more expensive. They too may soon be widely available OTC. An **antihistamine nasal spray** called azelastine (Astelin) is good for nasal congestion and other symptoms.

If allergies have you all stuffed up, **decongestants** can be very useful, and they also help prevent sinusitis (*see page 281*). **Nasal decongestants** come in a multitude of sprays, gels, drops, mists, or vapors. Some, such as oxymetazoline (Vicks Sinex, Afrin, Dristan 12-hour), last up to 12 hours. Others, such as phenylephrine (4-Way, Neo-Synephrine, Dristan Mist-Spray) or naphazoline (Naphcon Forte, Privine), last about four hours. These sprays should not be taken for more than three days in a row. They can lose effectiveness or cause dependence if used for too long. There are also many **oral decongestants** (such as Sudafed or Drixoral), which typically contain pseudoephedrine.

Antihistamines and decongestants may be more effective combined with a **steroid nasal spray**, which works more slowly (some doctors

Promising
DEVELOPMENTS

■ Allergy sufferers in Europe have an exciting new option: Drops, rather than shots, for desensitizing their allergy triggers. Also known as **oral or sublingual ("under-the-tongue") immunotherapy,** the new treatment uses liquid drops with tiny amounts of allergens. The regimen gradually desensitizes you, just as shots do. But you can use drops at home, rather than trekking to the doctor's office. More than a dozen small studies show that drops safely reduce symptoms by 30%, and that people might cut their allergy medications in half. The drops are still undergoing testing in the United States, but some American allergists are beginning to prescribe them as well.

■ A promising new prospect for allergy sufferers is **anti-IgE drugs.** These medications intercept the allergic reaction at an early stage, stopping symptoms before they start. Early tests show that these medications appear to be effective, although they must be taken indefinitely in order to remain beneficial.

Clarinex: Just Claritin in a New Bottle?

Is your new allergy medication simply the same old drug—reformulated, renamed, and re-released—in a snappy new package? That's the concern raised by a 2002 report from the National Institute for Health Care Management. This foundation found that two-thirds of the new medicines released between 1989 and 2000 were simply modified versions of existing drugs, or even the same drug with a new name, rather than truly innovative medications.

Among the drugs cited was Clarinex (desloratadine), a new generation of Claritin (loratadine), the blockbuster allergy medicine now available as a cheaper—and less lucrative for its maker—over-the-counter medication.

The Pharmaceutical Research and Manufacturers of America, the trade association that represents drugmakers, argued that the study was flawed and that many people who do not respond to older drugs may benefit from these new formulations. In addition, it pointed out that the Food and Drug Administration (FDA) extensively reviews and approves new drugs based on their safety and effectiveness, so they must offer some advantages to gain approval.

The bottom line: It remains to be seen whether some of the newer, heavily advertised, so-called "me too" drugs offer advantages that justify their often steep price tags.

recommend using the steroid spray daily). These sprays, which gradually reduce inflammation and block the allergic response, are effective for hay fever. Use daily one week before allergy season starts. Familiar brands include fluticasone (Flonase), beclomethasone (Beconase, Vancenase), flunisolide (Nasalide), triamcinolone (Nasacort), budesonide (Rhinocort), and mometasone furoate (Nasonex). Nasal steroids are safer than oral steroids and have few severe side effects. **Cromolyn nasal sprays,** such as Nasalcrom, quiet inflammation by preventing mast cells from releasing histamine. They're not as effective as steroids, but may relieve symptoms of milder allergies. Children often respond well to these sprays, which have virtually no side effects if given before a reaction begins.

For itchy or watery eyes, your doctor may add **eyedrops**. There are many choices. Some, such as ketotifen (Zaditor), olopatadine (Patanol), and levocabastine (Livostin), contain antihistamines. Others, such as phenylephrine (Allergan Relief) and tetrahydrozoline (Murine Plus, Visine), include decongestants. Still others, such as loteprednol (Alrex, Lotemax), contain steroids. Some eyedrops, such as cromolyn (Opti-crom) and pemirolast (Alamast), contain mast cell-stablizers.

Finally, potent asthma drugs called **leukotriene antagonists** may relieve certain allergies. Montelukast (Singulair) helps reduce hay fever symptoms in children, and zafirlukast (Accolate) may help those allergic to cats.

Procedures

If your allergies are mild, a **nasal wash** can help clear mucus from your nose. Buy a saline solution at a drugstore or make your own (1 teaspoon of salt per pint of warm water). Bend over the sink, pour some solution into your palm, inhale it through one nostril, then let it out and blow your nose gently. Repeat with the other nostril.

If your symptoms persist or you have them all year despite medications, **allergy shots,** or immunotherapy, may be the best solution for you. Rather than just treating your symptoms, as many drugs do, this approach affects the underlying immune processes that trigger your allergies. You will need to go to the doctor's office for the shots, as often as twice a week initially, and then every 2 to 4 weeks. The shots contain tiny amounts of allergens: The dose is gradually increased, usually over the course of 2 to 3 years or longer. This allows your immune system to slowly become desensitized to a particular trigger, relieving your symptoms and lessening your need for medications.

Lifestyle Changes

Where allergies are concerned, prevention is still the best treatment. There's a lot you can do to help keep your symptoms at bay.
- **Stay indoors during peak pollen periods,** typically between 2 PM and 4 PM hot, dry, and windy weather spurs high counts. Levels tend to be lowest on rainy, cloudy, or windless days.
- **Avoid raking** grass or leaves, which can stir up molds and pollens.
- **Change clothes and shower** after being outdoors. Pollen collects on skin, hair, and garments. Don't hang clothes outdoors to dry.

Food Allergies and Intolerances

Certain foods—nuts, shellfish, and strawberries—seem to cause most acute reactions. If you're allergic, their effect usually is apparent within a short time of eating them. A scratchy throat, itchy mouth, vomiting, stomach cramps, hives, rash, and swelling of the face, hands, feet, or genitals may all be signs of an allergic reaction. If the reaction is severe, breathing difficulties and a systemic breakdown (called anaphylactic shock) can develop within minutes. This is a true medical emergency.

Food Allergies

If you're highly sensitive, even touching a surface containing trace amounts of the food can overwhelm your body, causing severe allergy symptoms. Peanuts are particularly lethal and the leading cause of food-allergy fatalities. Their effect is compounded because peanut proteins are found in unlikely places, such as potato chips, hot chocolate, spaghetti sauce, egg rolls, and ice cream.

Food Intolerances

A second form of food sensitivity is better termed a "food intolerance." No histamine is involved and antihistamines and allergy shots won't help. Intolerances produce a wide variety of symptoms, including fatigue, joint pain, congestion, bloating, and diarrhea. Because symptoms may appear as long as three days after eating the food, finding the culprits can be tough. The usual suspects are dairy, eggs, corn, gluten, and citrus.

A food elimination diet is a good way to ferret out trouble-makers. The process takes about three weeks and should always be supervised by a doctor. Begin by eliminating the following for a week: dairy products, egg, gluten (wheat, pasta, barley, oats, or rye), corn, and citrus. If you feel better and chronic symptoms improve, then you probably do have some food intolerances. Return one food group every three days, noting if symptoms reappear. At the end of the three-week reintroduction period, you should have a good idea of the dietary culprit (or culprits) behind your symptoms.

Treatments

The best treatment is prevention, so try to avoid foods that cause symptoms. Highly allergic people may take antihistamines as a preventive before dining out, for example, but this may dampen early warning signs of a bad reaction. If you are prone to severe reactions, such as from peanuts, you will need to carry epinephrine (adrenaline) with you and give yourself a shot at the first sign of trouble. The drug is sold by prescription as an EpiPen or Anapen. You should also have an antihistamine on hand. With severe reactions, every minute counts: You may not have time to wait for an ambulance.

- **Get a HEPA vacuum.** Studies show that vacuums equipped with HEPA (high-energy particulate air) filters remove allergens better than standard appliances. Carpets trap allergens, so vacuum often. Better yet, have hardwood or tile floors. Air cleaners may also help.
- **Forgo house plants.** They can trap mold and other allergens, so decorate with discretion.
- **Avoid feather pillows and down bedding.** Anti-allergen pillowcases and mattress covers may be best for you.

Natural Methods*

Instead of standard drugs, you might try supplements with **quercetin,** a plant pigment found in apples (500 mg two or three times a day). It can block allergic reactions to pollen and reduce inflammation in the airways. Naturally-oriented physicians also recommend **stinging nettle,** a native weed long used in folk medicine (250 mg three times a day). Look for capsules that contain the freeze-dried herb, or an extract standardized to contain 1% plant silica.

Natural methods are not subject to the same testing and regulation as prescription medications. Please seek your doctor's advice and use caution.

FINDING Support

- If you need an allergist, contact the American Academy of Allergy, Asthma & Immunology (1-800-822-2762 or www.aaaai.org).
- For local pollen counts, go to the National Allergy Bureau website at www.aaaai.org/nab, or call the Pfizer Pollen Count Line at 1-800-9-POLLEN.
- If you have food allergies, contact The Food Allergy & Anaphylaxis Network (1-800-929-4040 or www.foodallergy.org).

Alzheimer's disease

Scientists are continuing to unravel the mysteries of Alzheimer's disease, the much-feared, devastating brain malady that affects more than 4 million Americans. New treatments now slow the progression of symptoms and make home care easier.

LIKELY First Steps

- Begin **drug treatment** and **therapies** as early as possible.

- Consider **natural treatments** during early stages.

- **Treat any related conditions**. In the early stages, depression, anxiety, or irritability are common. Other symptoms, such as insomnia, delusions, or aggression may arise as the disease progresses.

- **Seek support** to help with transitions, decisions, and emotional upheaval.

- **Initiate discussion** about advanced directives and decisions while mental capacities are still intact.

QUESTIONS TO Ask

- Could it be something other than Alzheimer's? Could prescription medicines be causing these symptoms?

- Would it help to enter a clinical trial that's testing new drugs and treatments?

- Does Alzheimer's shorten a normal life span?

- Are there ways to avoid becoming a burden to others?

- What planning should be done for the later stages of the disease?

What is happening

Few ailments are as heartbreaking as Alzheimer's disease. Initially, the body remains vigorous, while the mind slowly and inexorably wastes away. Then mild disorientation and memory lapses give way to agitation, confusion, and helplessness. Eventually, what we know as the "self" disappears altogether.

Nobody knows what causes the mental wasting of Alzheimer's, although scientists have found that sticky protein plaques (called beta amyloids) and tangles of nerve cells progressively riddle the brains of people with the disease. Cells die off in large numbers, depleting brain chemicals that help us think and remember. The disease mostly strikes the elderly, and if someone in your immediate family has it, you may be more likely to get it. Having a stroke may play a role, as may head injuries, high cholesterol, slow-growing infections, declining estrogen levels, nutritional deficiencies, and other factors. If you go to your doctor about your forgetfulness, rest assured: The diagnosis is rarely Alzheimer's. In fact, people with the disease are sometimes unaware of their mental decline and deny it even exists.

Treatments

Doctors and psychologists can diagnose Alzheimer's with 80% to 90% certainty at an earlier stage, when people are most likely to benefit from drugs, counseling, and a broad range of therapies. While none cure Alzheimer's, these treatments can delay the disease's progression.

Most patients are advised to start on medication. Benefits may be modest, but drugs can temporarily reverse or stabilize progression of the illness, easing the burden on caregivers. Counseling and other lifestyle therapies can boost mood and enhance daily living skills.

Medications

The four Alzheimer's drugs currently available are called **cholinesterase inhibitors** and slow the breakdown of a memory-enhancing brain chemical called acetylcholine. Medications should be started as soon as possible, because they are most effective in the earlier stages of the illness.

Like all Alzheimer's drugs, **donepezil** (Aricept) and **rivastigmine** (Exelon) have only limited benefits for those with mild to moderate disease, but they may offer some aid for more advanced disease. Exelon may be the drug of choice for those with rapid progression of symptoms. Extracted from daffodil bulbs, **galantamine** (Reminyl)

Treatment options

Medications

Cholinesterase inhibitors	Most effective at early stage of disease.

Procedures

Psychotherapy	Helps patients cope with trauma and loss.
Physical therapies	Improve mobility, speech, daily function.

Natural methods

Herbs	Ginkgo biloba and huperzine A.
Vitamins	Antioxidants help protect brain cells.

has effects similar to Aricept and Exelon. One promising study indicates that this drug may have sustained effects that accumulate over time. These newer medications are generally preferred over **tacrine** (Cognex), the first Alzheimer's drug to become available. At high doses, tacrine can damage the liver.

Procedures

Psychotherapy can help Alzheimer's patients come to terms with what they are experiencing and aid them in coping with depression and anxiety. They may also benefit from **occupational therapy,** which provides tips and cues for remembering daily living skills like getting dressed and staying clean. **Physical therapy** helps patients stay mobile, and **speech therapy** improves communication. Medicare is now covering many of these costs.

Natural Methods*

Ginkgo biloba, derived from an ancient Chinese tree, may improve memory slightly by boosting blood flow to the brain and has few side effects, but may cause clotting problems and internal bleeding. Like **vitamins C and E,** the herb may also have antioxidant properties that protect brain cells. Long used in traditional Chinese medicine, the moss extract **huperzine A** is a cholinesterase inhibitor, similar to prescription drugs, and it appears to be as potent. However, combining this herb with a prescription drug could be risky. A potential drug overdose is possible.

Lifestyle Changes

- **Keep a notebook.** Include in it important information, like the names and birthdays of grandchildren.
- **Exercise.** A supervised walk several times a day can be calming and reduce the likelihood of wandering. One study showed it may also improve communication.
- **Limit caffeine.** Avoid coffee, tea, colas, and other caffeine-containing products (including some OTC medications). They can cause the jitters or sleeplessness.

TAKING Control

Tips for caregivers to help improve daily life include:

- **Simplify surroundings.** Excessive distractions can be stressful. Create soothing routines. And limit choices, such as what to eat or wear.

- **Redirect attention.** Don't argue if an Alzheimer's patient becomes irrational or upset. Share a chore, like folding napkins, or have a snack.

- **Install gates and safety locks.** They can prevent wandering and limit hazards.

- **Talk. Touch. Watch old home movies.** These activities are comforting for many people with Alzheimer's.

- **Communicate clearly.** Some people get confused because they don't recognize emotions. So be calm. Use short statements, and offer visual and verbal clues, varying your tone of voice and expressions.

▶ **NEW VACCINES SHOW PROMISE. One tested in mice, called m266, restored memory after a single shot. It's several years away from human testing.**

FINDING Support

- The Alzheimer's Association (1-800-272-3900 or www. alz.org) provides links to local chapters. ADEAR, the Alzheimer's Disease Education and Referral Center (1-800-438-4380 or www.alzheimers.org) gives updates on drugs and clinical trials. The U.S. Administration on Aging Eldercare Locator (1-800-677-1116 or www.eldercare.gov) offers referrals to home care.

Natural methods are not subject to the same testing and regulation as prescription medications. Please seek your doctor's advice and use caution.

Anxiety

We all need to be anxious sometimes. It's a normal, useful response to life's challenges and dangers. But for nearly 3% of us, occasional bouts of anxiety last weeks and even months. Then it's considered generalized anxiety disorder.

LIKELY First Steps

- **Counseling** with a psychotherapist to help look for the root of the problem.

- **Rapid-acting medications** to calm you down until **longer-acting antidepressant** drugs can take effect.

- **Lifestyle changes**, from meditation to proper diet and exercise, to help you deal with your anxiety on a daily basis.

QUESTIONS TO Ask

- Why are you giving me a drug for depression when I have anxiety?

- Are there any prescription or over-the-counter drugs that could be causing my anxiety?

- Is it okay to drink alcohol?

- Could a medical condition be contributing to my anxiety?

- Is there anything my family and friends can do to help me through this?

What is happening

Over countless millennia the human body has been conditioned to quickly respond to threats with fear and anxiety. This reaction, termed the "flight or fight response," primes the body to outrun, outthink, or outfight any opponent in sight. In fact, when you're moderately anxious, your ability to perform is greatly enhanced. That is why so many people think they actually do better when they're under stress.

When you have generalized anxiety disorder (GAD), your body fails to switch off that response when the threat is gone. Instead, it treats ordinary events as life-threatening. A bill is due, and the thought of it sends your heart racing. You sweat and fret at the thought of entering a room full of strangers. Sometimes your anxious feelings are just free-floating, with no discernible cause. Your brain profile begins to look like that of someone living in a war zone, with chemicals called neurotransmitters and a compound called gamma-aminobutyric acid (GABA) all out of whack. Bouts of misplaced anxiety can last from a few moments to years.

Classic symptoms of GAD include persistent dire feelings and unwanted thoughts, chest pains, an inability to properly concentrate, irritability, trembling, dry mouth, and hot flashes or chills. Studies of twins have found that in a third of cases, GAD has genetic causes. If a parent or sibling has it, you're more likely to show symptoms. The other two-thirds of the time, GAD comes from learned behaviors. Generally, it strikes children and teens.

Treatments

Here's the encouraging news: Half the people who receive proper treatment for GAD show improvement within three weeks. And 75% will feel a lot better within nine months.

The type of treatment regimen you need depends on the severity of your symptoms. If GAD isn't interfering with your life, you might begin with nonpharmaceutical options. Because many anxiety drugs have side effects that can make you dependent on them, it's often best to see them as a second choice. If GAD is making the simplest tasks impossible, you'll want to fight back with powerful medicines. Combining drugs and behavioral techniques can be even more effective. Whatever route you take, make sure you stick with it over the long haul: One study reported that two-thirds of those who were treated for GAD for only six weeks had symptoms return. Half required additional medications.

Treatment options

Procedures

Behavioral therapy	May be as effective as medication.
Insight therapy	Traditional talk-it-out approach.
Supportive psychotherapy	Positive, helpful advice.

Medications

Benzodiazepines	Good for acute attacks, quick-acting.
Tricyclics	Tried-and-true antidepressants.
SSRIs	Most popular long-term medications.
Newer antidepressants	Unique drugs with fewer side effects.

Lifestyle changes

Diet & exercise	Healthy choices can make a real difference.
Sleep	Getting enough is key for reducing anxiety.

Natural methods

Herbs	St. John's wort; take care with kava or valerian.
Alternative therapies	Meditation, acupuncture, stress reduction.

Procedures

When it comes to GAD, a psychotherapist's office is one of the best places to learn to cope with the outside world. **Cognitive-behavioral therapy** is especially useful if you have GAD. Two studies in the mid-1990s found that this technique caused the same beneficial brain changes as those found in people taking Prozac, a drug commonly prescribed for GAD. This therapy helps you make connections between the way you think and the way you feel. People who are chronically anxious often criticize themselves harshly, which can trigger even more anxiety. Cognitive therapy teaches you to substitute helpful thoughts for negative ones, develop coping strategies, and use imagery to ease your anxiety.

Insight therapy, also known as the "talking cure," was pioneered by Sigmund Freud. The technique involves intensive probing of the past and your mind's inner workings. The idea is to eventually produce that flash of understanding that leads you to the reason for your symptoms. Insight is accompanied by an emotional release that helps you heal. A doctor might also suggest **supportive psychotherapy.** You know how good it is to find an understanding and sympathetic ear, how calming it is to have someone you trust tell you that everything's going to be okay—that's the essence of supportive psychotherapy. An encouraging, positive psychiatrist or psychologist talks you through the tough spots and helps you to see that everything is going to work out.

TAKING Control

- **Breathe deeply.** Sit or lie with a pillow at the small of your back. Breathe in slowly and deeply so that your stomach moves out. Say the word "relax" to yourself just before exhaling. Exhale slowly, letting your stomach pull back in. Do this until you're calm.

- **You shall overcome.** Hold this thought in your mind. For most people, generalized anxiety disorder can be quelled within a few months with proper treatment.

- **Pay attention to your overall health.** Many people with GAD experience depression, which can be effectively treated. Chronic anxiety has also been linked to high blood pressure and an increased risk of heart attacks. Get checked out completely to be sure you're on a thorough treatment track.

▶ **THINK TWICE ABOUT KAVA.** This herb has been used by South Pacific islanders as a social lubricant for generations. It's now a favorite in this country for quieting mild anxiety symptoms, but several recent reports have linked kava to liver toxicity. If you try it, avoid alcohol and keep your dosage to no more than 120 mg of kavalactones (the active ingredient) a day. Don't use this herb for more than four weeks in a row.

▶**My anxiety seems to increase in the winter. Am I imagining it?**

There could be a very good reason for this. One of the symptoms of seasonal affective disorder (SAD) is anxiety. If you live in a temperate zone and find yourself irritable, depressed, or sleeping too much during winter months, have your doctor check you for SAD. To combat this problem, try getting out for early morning walks. A study in the British medical journal The Lancet *found that exposure to morning light (30 minutes at dawn) was an effective treatment for seasonal affective disorder. (For more on this ailment, see Depression, page 102.)*

Medications

Numerous drugs have been approved to treat anxiety. This is fortunate because some drugs have unacceptable side effects or just don't work for everyone. You won't know for sure how a particular medication will affect you until you start taking it, so if it's not right for you, ask your doctor to prescribe another.

If you're really handcuffed by anxiety, chances are you'll start with **benzodiazepines,** a group of fast-acting sedatives that includes stalwarts like diazepam (Valium), alprazolam (Xanax), and lorazepam (Ativan). Good for short-term relief, these drugs also have well-known side effects. Most notable is excessive sedation, which is eased when the dose is lowered. If taken regularly, they can be habit-forming. Some people report feeling out-of-focus, sometimes dangerously so. A Canadian study, for instance, found that those using benzodiazepines were 26% more likely to have a car accident.

Benzodiazepines work quickly—often within an hour. So they're useful until an antidepressant can kick in, which usually takes from two to five weeks. While older **tricyclics** can be effective, most doctors use the well-known **SSRIs (selective serotonin reuptake inhibitors),** such as paroxetine (Paxil) and venlafaxine (Effexor). **Newer antidepressants** like trazodone (Desyrel) and nefazodone (Serzone) help you get a better night's sleep; growing evidence shows that regular, good-quality sleep lessens anxiety. Another new drug, buspirone (BuSpar), has also gained wide acceptance because it has few side effects.

Even if antidepressants work, you'll want to keep the quicker-acting benzodiazepines around for the occasional times when things get overwhelming. A final word of advice on medications: Don't consider them a substitute for psychological counseling. Drugs are great at treating the symptoms, but they don't tackle the root cause.

Lifestyle Changes

Along with psychotherapy and medication, the bulwark of anxiety treatment, changes you make in your everyday life can help you deal with your problem on a very practical level. Try to:

Post-Traumatic Stress Disorder

Originally called shell shock by the combat veterans who experienced it, post-traumatic stress disorder (PTSD) is a severe form of long-term anxiety that can occur after extreme trauma. It can happen to both men and women who have been in a serious accident, seen unimaginable horrors, or been kidnapped, tortured, raped, or assaulted.

Symptoms include reliving the event through vivid memories or flashbacks, strong feelings of terror or helplessness, and behaving as if still in imminent danger, even though the event is long past. To be classified PTSD, symptoms must persist for more than a month. About 8% of Americans will experience PTSD at some time. It can even develop months or years after the triggering event took place.

Cognitive-behavioral therapy is effective for treating PTSD. So is the drug sertraline (Zoloft). A 2001 study in the *Archives of General Psychiatry* found that participants who received 50 to 200 mg of Zoloft a day for 12 weeks had significant improvement in their symptoms.

There are also encouraging reports about an innovative therapy for trauma called EMDR (Eye Movement Desensitization and Reprocessing), which uses visualization and self-hypnosis techniques to change brain connections and relieve PTSD.

Panic Attack

Take extreme, unshakable terror, pack it into 10 to 30 minutes, and you've got a panic attack. For that period of time, your breath is short, your heart is pounding, and you're probably thinking you're about to die. The symptoms are so awful that fear of having another panic attack is sometimes enough to set one off. For 1% to 2% of men and women, this becomes panic disorder—panic attacks that come from nowhere, rather than resulting from a scary encounter.

Treatment of panic disorder requires both therapy and drugs. You should always seek out a specially trained therapist skilled in handling panic disorders. Tricyclic and SSRI antidepressants, as well as medicines called MAO inhibitors, are very effective in blocking panic attacks, but they can take up to six weeks to start working. A sedative called alprazolam (Xanax) works more quickly and can be useful in the meantime.

- **Get moving.** Regular aerobic exercise (not strength or resistance training) has been shown to noticeably reduce anxiety. Jog, walk, swim, bike, even take yoga at least three times a week. Expect improvement in your mood (and waistline) in about three months.
- **Look in your fridge.** A healthful diet is important for lowering anxiety levels. Add as many vegetarian options as possible. A small study found considerably less anxiety among vegetarians. This may be because blood sugar levels are more stable in a vegetarian diet. Get rid of caffeine: It's a known contributor to anxiety. Sugar can also cause your body to mimic anxiety symptoms.
- **Develop good sleep habits.** Research shows that people with insomnia are at increased risk for developing anxiety. Avoid heavy meals before bedtime. Go to bed and get up close to the same time every day. Don't work out within three hours of bedtime, as it takes that long to cool all the way down.
- **Leave the booze in the bottle.** A few drinks may seem like a good way to calm down, but alcohol interferes with your sleep. It can also create an unhealthy dependence that may increase, not decrease, your anxiety over the long run.

Natural Methods*

The medicinal herb **valerian** is helpful as a mild sedative and sleep aid. Look for standardized capsules, tablets, or extracts, and follow the instructions on the label. Don't use valerian for more than two weeks in a row, however, and avoid sedatives (including alcohol) while taking it. **St. John's wort** can be useful for mild symptoms, but talk to your doctor first if you're taking a prescription medication. Relaxation techniques can also produce excellent results: **Meditation, acupuncture, massage,** and **stress-reduction audiotapes** are all fine ways to diffuse tension and anxiety.

Promising DEVELOPMENTS

- The mechanisms that underlie anxiety have long eluded researchers, but scientists at Columbia University in New York have made strides in solving that mystery. Their research, reported in the journal *Nature,* has shown that altering certain **receptors in the forebrain** of mice can both increase and decrease anxiety levels in the rodents. For the first time, this shows the exact location in the brain where anxious behavior originates, enabling future research to concentrate on that area.

FINDING Support

- For information on anxiety straight from the experts, contact the National Institute of Mental Health in Bethesda, MD (301-443-4513 or www.nimh.nih.gov).
- Check out Freedom from Fear, a New York-based national not-for-profit mental health advocacy association specializing in anxiety and depression (718-351-1717 or www.freedomfromfear.com).
- For more information about EMDR therapy for post-traumatic stress disorder, including studies that support its use and a list of clinicians who practice it, visit the website of the EMDR Institute at www.emdr.com.

*Natural methods are not subject to the same testing and regulation as prescription medications. Please seek your doctor's advice and use caution.

Arthritis

Three in seven Americans with arthritis know just how taxing simple actions, such as pulling up your socks or rising from a chair, can be. Finding the right treatment can make a dramatic difference in how those with arthritis feel every day.

LIKELY **First Steps**

- **Acetaminophen** for discomfort, OTC or prescription **NSAIDs** (including COX-2 inhibitors), or **opiates** for painful inflammation.

- Application of **topical liniments** and **heat or cold** for immediate relief.

- Strengthening **exercises** to enhance recovery.

- **Physical aids** such as shoe wedges, canes, and joint protectors (splints, braces) to ease joint stress.

- In time, **injections** or **surgery**, even a joint replacement, may be necessary.

QUESTIONS TO **Ask**

- Is there anything I can do to prevent my arthritis from getting worse?

- How likely is it that my other joints will start hurting?

- Should I stop playing golf? Tennis? Jogging?

- Am I a candidate for joint injections?

- How will I know if I need joint replacement surgery?

What is happening

Experts still aren't sure why cartilage, the shock-absorbing tissue that normally coats the ends of bones, sometimes breaks down. When it does, it causes those typical arthritis symptoms: stiffness and pain. Once the cartilage has worn down, your bones start to grate against each other. The roughened ends thicken and may develop knobby outgrowths called "spurs." Bits of cartilage break off in the joint space. After a while, the joint can look as if a dog has been gnawing at it. The breakdown of cartilage induces inflammation, which is enough to make your joint hurt. It's often associated with warmth, swelling, and stiffness that make symptoms worse. At first, you may feel pain only when you move the joint. Later it may hurt when you're not even moving. Some people notice cracking sounds of broken cartilage, so-called "joint mice," when they move a stiff joint.

Arthritis is a degenerative disease, and its causes are varied. Your family history may bear some responsibility: Your genes set the stage for a defect in the production of collagen, a protein crucial to cartilage. Perhaps you were injured (even decades ago), or you are overweight, or use a certain joint repetitively (maybe on the job).

Most people develop pain in just one or two joints, but any joint is vulnerable. Trouble spots include knees, hips, spine, and fingers. More than 100 conditions cause joint pain, so get a firm diagnosis before you label yours "arthritis." For information on related conditions, see rheumatoid arthritis (*page 272*), gout (*page 143*), lupus (*page 208*), fibromyalgia (*page 125*), and Lyme disease (*page 211*). The next few pages focus on osteoarthritis (OA), the most common form of arthritis.

Treatments

If you have arthritis, you probably have "good days" and "bad days." If it's a bad day, start by taking a painkiller (acetaminophen, an OTC NSAID, or a COX-2 inhibitor). You'll probably feel better in a couple of hours. Self-care remedies are also useful: Hot or cold packs, liniments, stretching, and natural methods of relaxing help control pain. The supplements glucosamine and chondroitin may prevent cartilage deterioration. It's important to know that you can control your situation by making changes in your lifestyle. You can prevent flare-ups, for example, by keeping your weight down, exercising regularly, and using doctor-recommended aids (shoe wedges, walking aids, braces). A physical therapist can provide specialized procedures. Ask your doctor for a referral so insurance will cover the cost.

Treatment options

Medications

Painkillers/NSAIDs	OTC and prescription, including COX-2s.
Topical liniments	Capsaicin and methyl salicylate can help.
Opioids	Tramadol or codeine for severe pain.

Lifestyle changes

Exercise	Stretching, resistance, low-impact aerobics.
Special aids	Joint protectors, footwear, pads, grippers.
Hot & cold treatments	Warm for stiffness; cool for inflammation.
Diet	Drop extra pounds; eat fish; get calcium.

Procedures

Injections	Steroids and hyaluronic acid help with pain.
Surgery	Arthroscopy and osteotomy for certain cases.
Joint replacement	Joint repair, scraping, or reshaping.

Natural methods

Supplements	Glucosamine/chondroitin for cartilage repair.
Relaxation techniques	Meditation, massage, biofeedback help pain.
Acupuncture	Ancient technique for pain relief.

Good medical options are also available. If swelling gets very bad, your doctor may use a syringe to drain fluid from around a joint, such as the knee. Steroid or hyaluronic acid injections can also bring relief. Overall, the odds are small that you'll need surgery to replace your affected joint, but it's reassuring that success rates for such procedures are very high. Surgeons often urge active people with arthritic knees to try low-impact aerobic activities—such as biking, walking, or using an elliptical trainer, rather than knee-stressing ones like running or skiing—before they consider joint replacement surgery.

Medications

No medicine can cure your arthritis, but many can ease pain and stiffness, making life comfortable again. Reach first for **acetaminophen** (Tylenol, Anacin-3, Panadol). If you're just a little achy and stiff, it might well do the trick, and it's very safe. Acetaminophen can't calm inflammation, if discomfort persists or there's actual swelling, add a nonsteroidal anti-inflammatory drug (**NSAID**), such as aspirin, ibuprofen (Motrin or Advil), or naproxen (Naprosyn). NSAIDs, available over the counter or by prescription in stronger versions (familiar brands include Voltaren, Arthrotec, Relafen, Feldene), block the body's creation of prostaglandins, substances that trigger

TAKING Control

- **Go to class.** Studies show that being actively involved in managing your own OA can dramatically lessen your pain. Check out the National Arthritis Foundation's Arthritis Self-Help Courses (ASHC). They're led by OA sufferers specially trained to share tips on treatments, exercise, and strategies for relaxation and coping.

- **Toss the heels.** Twice as many women as men suffer from knee OA, and Harvard researchers have a clue as to why. When walking in heels two inches or higher, the torque—the rotational force—applied around the inside of the knee is 23% greater than when barefoot. This is enough torque to destroy cartilage and cause arthritis. So opt for low-heeled or flat shoes, and keep the high heels for special occasions.

- **Get on the ball.** Try squeezing a tennis ball to relieve stiffness and strengthen your forearms and hands. Make a two- to three-inch cut in the ball for light resistance, and a one-inch cut to create moderate resistance.

- **Be hip on hips.** Don't just settle for a standard replacement hip. Ask your doctor about the procedure most appropriate for your age, condition, and lifestyle.

Tackling NSAID Troubles

NSAIDs taken more often or at higher doses than recommended can damage your stomach, kidneys, or liver. Stomach problems (nausea, heartburn, potentially serious bleeding ulcers) develop because NSAIDs knock out chemicals called prostaglandins that protect stomach tissues.

Alternatives

Ask your doctor about taking an NSAID with a **histamine blocker** (H₂ blocker) such as Tagamet, Zantac, Axid Pulvules, or Pepcid. These drugs suppress the production of damaging stomach acid. Another option is to add an anti-ulcer medication called a **proton pump inhibitor** (Prevacid or Prilosec). If you're already at risk for a stomach ulcer, your doctor might prescribe the **synthetic prostaglandin** Cytotec. This replenishes the prostaglandin supply, so ulcers heal and new ones are less likely to develop

Interactions

Other reasons to talk over your NSAID use with your doctor: Many of these drugs interact negatively with **common medications** such as anticoagulants, corticosteroids, diuretics, and ACE inhibitors. Be particularly cautious about taking an NSAID if you have a history of ulcers, stomach bleeding, asthma, hypertension, epilepsy, liver or kidney problems, or Parkinson's disease. **Age also matters:** If you're over age 60, you're four times more likely than younger adults to experience NSAID-related gastrointestinal bleeding or ulceration.

▶**Could I be doing something that's making my arthritis worse?**

First, make sure you truly have osteoarthritis. Lots of conditions can give you joint pain and stiffness (tendinitis, pinched nerve, lupus). So get a firm diagnosis before embarking on any treatment plan. The wrong exercise or a poorly fitting brace or other joint aid can cause more harm than good. Check with your doctor or physical therapist.

▶**Does it matter when or where I do my exercises?**

Yes, it does. Unless your joint inflammation is severe, do your exercises every day. Do them when your muscles are loose after a hot shower or bath and your medicine is at its peak. Try to exercise in a class setting rather than at home. Research from Britain indicates that because classes tend to be more rigorous and you have the support of others in the same situation, they are the best way to promote pain relief.

inflammation. If your arthritis is a constant problem, these drugs might cause some digestive side effects. Although generally quite safe, NSAIDs can irritate your stomach lining, causing queasiness, abdominal pain, and even bleeding (*see box above*). Along with NSAIDs, try a **liniment** (pain-relieving cream, rub, or spray). The popular ones (capsaicin cream and methyl salicylate products) must be applied four times a day for several days before you get results.

At one time, if you had side effects from NSAIDs or were at risk for an ulcer, your doctor might have suggested switching to prescription NSAIDs, also known as **COX-2 inhibitors,** introduced in the late 1990s. Celecoxib (Celebrex), rofecoxib (Vioxx), and valdecoxib (Bextra) once commanded 60% of the $6.6 billion arthritis-drug market. Recent studies, however, indicate that heart attack risk is four times greater than traditional pain relievers, and side effects as extreme as death have been linked to certain COX-2s. Vioxx was voluntarily pulled from the market by its drug manufacturer, but Celebrex, the more popular of the two, remains and is under FDA investigation. Clinical trials of Bextra indicate that a higher risk of stroke and heart attack can occur, especially in those with heart problems. Talk with your doctor if you are taking COX-2 inhibitors to discuss risks and alternatives to consider.

If your pain's severe, **opioids** such as tramadol (Ultram) or codeine are worth considering. Aim for the lowest effective dose so you can minimize the risk of becoming dependent (especially with codeine) or suffering side effects such as constipation, nausea, or drowsiness.

Lifestyle Changes

When your joints creak and ache, it seems counterintuitive to **exercise**, but exercise is one of the best arthritis remedies around. Done properly (good form is crucial), exercise can keep your pain and stiffness from veering out of control. You'll get the biggest payoff by doing **resistance training** with weights designed to strengthen and tone muscles. Such exercises stabilize joints and make them more flexible. Ask a physical therapist to show you exercises that will benefit your condition. Only after focusing on actions that build muscles should you add aerobics. **Low-impact aerobic exercises** (swimming, biking, walking) stimulate blood flow and ease joint stress by keeping your weight down. They also boost your mood. Working up a sweat can even make you feel less sensitive to pain. In time, tack on **stretching** and **range-of-motion exercises,** such as yoga and tai chi, to enhance flexibility and your sense of control over the pain.

You may be amazed at the strides you can make with exercise. An intriguing 2002 study found that knee OA patients who regularly lifted weights or exercised aerobically were much more likely to dress, bathe, and move from a bed to a chair independently than those who simply read information on disease management. While exercise is crucial, so is giving your joints a **rest.** Listen to your body. A little soreness the day after working out is normal, but if the pain keeps nagging you, ease up a bit.

Ask your doctor about **joint protectors** (splints, braces, neck collars, crutches, canes). They can support tender areas and are especially good for lightening the strain on lower body joints. Check out physical or occupational therapy catalogs or stores for supplies. For people with hand arthritis, special grip devices make opening jars easier. Foam pads attached to handles on garden and household tools also help. Pain in your knee or hip can be rectified with **orthopedic shoes** or footwear outfitted with shock-absorbing soles or wedge-shaped insoles. By distributing your weight evenly and correcting for improper alignment, such simple aids can make a big difference. For knee problems, try in-shoe heel wedges to lessen the lateral thrust on the joint. They allow many to postpone joint replacement surgery. Knee support with taping or a Velcro brace also helps.

For rapid relief from pain or stiffness without drugs, try **hot and cold treatments.** If there's no acute inflammation, apply warm compresses and heat lamps, or take hot showers or baths to ease stiffness. Hot wax or paraffin treatment kits do wonders for arthritic hands. When your joints are inflamed, ice is the way to go. A commercial cold pack or bag of frozen peas placed on the joint really works. You might want to alternate between hot and cold. Either way, 20 minutes will do it (less if your skin gets very red). Avoid direct skin contact by using a towel or other buffer.

Excess weight adds stress to your weight-bearing joints (knees, hips, feet). So diet and exercise to **drop any extra pounds** you may have gained over the years. A **healthy diet** also perks you up—chronic pain can wear out even the hardiest souls—and a high-fiber content can counter pain-medication–related constipation. Plan to eat lots of cold-water fish (salmon, herring, sardines), which are rich in **omega-3 fatty acids,** a natural anti-inflammatory. Or swallow a daily tablespoon of omega-3 fatty-acid-rich fish oil, evening primrose oil, or flaxseed oil. Getting lots of **calcium** and **vitamin D** will help keep your bones strong and better able to support your joints.

Watch Out for "Miracle Cures"

Given the millions of people with arthritis pain, it's no wonder that scams abound. Don't fall prey to hucksters: They get rich, and you're still in pain. Be wary of these "miracle cures":

- **Magnets.** While they won't hurt you, magnets probably won't help your pain much either. Best for the fridge, not for your arthritis.
- **Homeopathy.** Real evidence is hard to come by for this old-time approach, which involves minuscule doses of herbs and minerals.
- **Copper bracelets.** While some copper may be absorbed through your skin, there's no proof that such bracelets have any effect.
- **Bee stings.** Even folks with no known bee allergies can have fatal allergic reactions to this popular—and unproven—arthritis remedy.
- **Certain dietary supplements.** Products hyped as a "cure" should be eyed with suspicion. They may empty your wallet and interfere with other medications. Some are still under investigation, but may prove useful. The most promising ones for lessening inflammation and reducing pain include bromelain (from pineapple), MSM (an organic sulfur compound), and SAMe (a synthetic form of the amino acid methionine).

▶ **CONTRARY TO POPULAR THINKING, arthritis is not a normal part of aging. Half of all people with arthritis are under age 65.**

Promising
DEVELOPMENTS

- Pharmaceutical companies have **second-generation COX-2 inhibitors** in the pipeline. These new drugs may be even safer than current ones.

- Scientists have harvested and cultured **cartilage cells in vitro,** injected them into a diseased joint, and watched to see if they reproduce. So far, small bits have successfully formed cartilage to repair early OA damage.

- The NIH and four drug companies are looking for an **OA biomarker**—a chemical substance whose presence signals disease progression or the success of a treatment. This matters because OA pain is subjective and shifts without warning.

Procedures

If you have persistent pain, especially in the knee, a **steroid injection** may make you feel better. You can't have these shots more than once every three months, but you may enjoy about a three-week vacation from pain. Injections of a synthetic derivative of **hyaluronic acid** (Hyalgan or Synvisc) may give you longer-lasting relief. This gooey joint lubricant is a component of synovial fluid, which normally eases and cushions joints. Many people with OA have paltry amounts of it, and injections help replenish the supply. The FDA has approved once-a-week hyaluronic injections for knee OA in people who can't get relief from other treatments and aren't ready for surgery. After three to five weeks of injections, you may enjoy several months of pain-free movement. One study found it as potent as high-dose Tylenol. The series costs about $1,200. It's FDA-approved, and most insurance companies (and Medicare) will cover it. Immediate pain or swelling is unlikely, but long-term effects are not known.

If you still have pain and trouble moving, surgical joint repair using endoscopic techniques (called **arthroscopy**) is another option. After making two or three small incisions around the joint, the surgeon fishes out bits of bone and damaged cartilage. So-called "knee scraping" has gotten some negative press lately, however. In a widely

Total Joint Replacement Surgery

If you've exhausted other treatments, but joint pain and disability persist, a total joint replacement (arthroplasty) may be your best option. Thanks to advances in surgical techniques and construction of the artificial joint, many are happier—and living longer—after this surgery.

Hips and knees are the most commonly replaced joints. Ankles, feet, shoulders, elbows, and fingers can also be replaced. This surgery requires anesthesia. With the knee (*see illustration*), the surgeon removes the damaged ends of the bones and cartilage and inserts a metal-and-plastic substitute designed to restore normal knee movement. The joint surfaces are cemented or the bones are allowed to grow through mesh surfaces to the replacements. With hips, the surgeon replaces the damaged upper end of the femur—the ball—with a metal one and

attaches it to the rest of the leg bone. The damaged socket is replaced with a plastic one. Most replacement joints last 10 years. Some last as long as 20. Complications include infection, blood clots, and dislocation of the joint; discuss risks with your doctor.

Your orthopedic team will probably have you standing and walking the day after surgery. You'll probably use a walker or cane at first. Physical therapy will follow. You'll probably feel some pain for a while in the replaced joint, because your muscles will be weak from disuse. Exercise will help counteract this as well as speed your recovery. How much your new joint will improve your movement depends largely on how stiff you were before surgery. Although strenuous sports such as tennis aren't recommended, many people are thrilled to once again walk, dance, and play golf effortlessly and without pain.

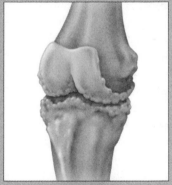

Arthritic knee joint, presurgery

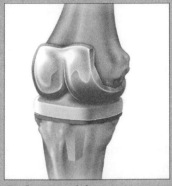

Replacement joint, postsurgery

reported 2002 study, patients were just as likely to say their knee felt better two years after sham surgery as they were after a pricey arthroscopic procedure. So talk it over with your doctor. **Osteotomy** may be an option if you have early-stage arthritis in one knee and no inflammation. By surgically reshaping the shinbone or thighbone, a surgeon can often improve the alignment, repositioning the joint so that your knee can once again move freely and carry your weight evenly. The knee won't look symmetrical, but it may not hurt as much. Osteotomy can also slow further joint deterioration.

Unicompartmental knee arthroplasty may also ease pain and delay total knee replacement. It works best if you're over age 60, are not obese, have no real inflammation, and the anterior cruciate ligament (ACL) at the back of your knee is intact. The surgeon removes diseased bone and puts in an implant. Joint motion and function are good because healthy parts of the knee are preserved. It's cheaper and less likely to cause complications than osteotomy, and recovery is short. As a last resort, if your pain's overwhelming and the joint is misshapen, consider a **total joint replacement (arthroplasty).** Success rates are high, and techniques improve all the time (*see box opposite*).

Natural Methods*

Certain alternative therapies can be quite helpful for arthritis, but every person is different. What works for your neighbor may not be good for you—and vice versa. You may also need to be patient. It may be several weeks before you feel any true benefit.

Many people report relief when they routinely take **glucosamine** and **chondroitin,** two dietary supplements widely advertised to help cartilage. Glucosamine sulfate is extracted from shellfish; chondroitin sulfate from cattle. Veterinarians have used these supplements to treat OA in animals, and European rheumatologists prescribe them routinely. After years of skepticism, American doctors are now guardedly optimistic. Data from trials is mixed, but a major NIH study is due by 2005. In the meantime, taking supplements may help you—and it probably won't hurt. Just don't buy the creams: They're useless.

An expert panel at the NIH recently approved **relaxation therapies** as a useful add-on treatment for arthritis. Stress and anxiety can tighten muscles around joints, worsening pain. Relaxation helps blunt this pain—and your perception of it—and enhances your capacity to cope. For **biofeedback** and **hypnosis,** an experienced therapist can show you several techniques to do on your own. **Deep breathing** relaxes you through the process of inhaling deeply and rhythmically. It's often taught in yoga classes. During **meditation,** you focus on awareness of what you feel, and what comes into your mind, at a given moment. The gentle kneading of **massage** can loosen and stretch tight muscles, improving your flexibility.

The NIH also supports use of **acupuncture** for pain relief. This ancient therapy has been practiced in China for 2,500 years. Western scientists think strategically inserted needles prompt the body to generate compounds that relieve pain and reduce inflammation. Just be sure your practitioner uses sterile, throwaway needles.

▶ **EVERY ADDITIONAL POUND OF BODY WEIGHT** places from two to four pounds of extra stress on the knees and hips during routine movement.

▶ **A KNEE INJURY BEFORE AGE 22** results in a threefold increase in the incidence of arthritis (in the same knee). The age at which the old injury typically strikes back as arthritis: the mid-50s.

▶ **IN RUSSIA, BLOOD-SUCKING LEECHES** are attached to pain trigger zones around joints to ease early-morning stiffness and muscle pain and increase range of motion. As the leeches suck blood through tiny incisions in their teeth, they also introduce saliva with analgesic and anesthetic compounds.

FINDING Support

■ The Arthritis Foundation in Atlanta, GA (1-800-283-7800) runs a friendly, hands-on website worth looking at. Log on to www.arthritis.org.

■ If you're interested in getting acupuncture for your OA, you can request a list of certified acupuncturists from the National Certification Commission for Acupuncture and Oriental Medicine (703-548-9004 or www.nccaom.org).

Natural methods are not subject to the same testing and regulation as prescription medications. Please seek your doctor's advice and use caution.

Asthma

This chronic respiratory disease affects more than 20 million Americans, including 9 million children. The good news is that self-monitoring, medications, and sensible lifestyle changes enable most people to lead active, healthy lives.

LIKELY **First Steps**

- An **inhaled bronchodilator** to open airways. Always keep one on hand in case of a severe attack.
- A **peak flow meter** to help you gauge when an attack is coming.
- **Preventive anti-inflammatory medications** to lessen the frequency and severity of attacks.
- **Knowledge of your triggers** enables you to avoid them.
- **Annual flu or pneumonia vaccine** to prevent respiratory infections.

QUESTIONS TO **Ask**

- Would you help me prepare an action plan?
- Should I bring my peak flow readings to my next appointment?
- Is it dangerous for me to exercise?
- Should I consider moving to a different climate?
- Will allergy shots help me?
- Should I see a specialist?

What is happening

The word *asthma* comes from the ancient Greek for "panting," but that tells only part of the story. No doubt it would have been unwieldy to also throw in the words for wheezing, shortness of breath, coughing, and tightness of the chest—the most common asthma symptoms. Exactly what causes this disease is unclear, but genetics, allergies, and environmental factors play key roles.

When you have asthma, your immune system overreacts to tiny substances in the environment—from pollen to dust mites—and treats these usually harmless materials as deadly invaders. This triggers a full-scale alarm in your respiratory system. Immune system defenders called mast cells, located in tiny passageways in your lungs, unleash a barrage of histamines and other chemicals. Your airways become inflamed and constricted, and your breathing tubes produce extra mucus. That makes it even more difficult for you to breathe.

An asthma attack can last for minutes or hours. It may come on gradually or suddenly, and it can strike at any time, day or night. About one-third of those with the disease have asthma in their family. About half of all cases start in children under age 10, but the disease can occur at any age. Patterns vary greatly from one person to the next, so it's important to learn what your triggers are and how your body reacts to them.

Treatments

There is no cure for asthma. It's important to understand that this is a chronic disease. Untreated, it can be fatal. Asthma claims about 5,000 lives in the United States annually, mainly among the elderly. You must be under a doctor's care for this condition. But most people with asthma can keep their symptoms in check with a combination of self-monitoring, inhalers, prescription drugs, and lifestyle changes and by avoiding common triggers.

Medications

If you have asthma, you will probably will need at least a couple of different prescription medications. Drugs such as bronchodilators relieve symptoms. Others, such as inhaled steroids, prevent new attacks. Knowing which drugs you're taking for what reasons—and how to take them properly—is absolutely crucial to managing asthma.

For immediate relief for an asthma attack, your best bet is a **bronchodilator inhaler,** which opens constricted airways. It includes short-acting beta2-agonists, such as albuterol, bitolterol, pirbuterol,

Treatment options

Medications

Bronchodilators	Open airways during asthma attack.
Corticosteroids	Oral or IV: short-term. Inhaled: long-term.
Leukotriene modifiers	Often combined with other medications.
Inhalers	Various types for different symptoms.

Lifestyle changes

Make a plan	Know your drugs, how to handle emergency.
Avoid triggers	Dander, pollen, cold air, dust, cockroaches.
Stop smoking	First- or secondhand smoke is dangerous.

Natural methods

Yoga	Defuses stress, an asthma trigger.
Nutrition	Apples, selenium, antioxidants: all helpful.

and terbutaline. An anticholinergic drug that relaxes lung muscle spasms, such as ipratropium bromide (Atrovent), may also be beneficial. For a severe attack, you may need **oral** or even **intravenous corticosteroids,** such as prednisone, prednisolone, or methylprednisolone to decrease the inflammation. Oral corticosteroids are typically prescribed for short-term use. They can cause side effects if taken at high doses for an extended period of time.

For long-term asthma management, the first line of defense is **inhaled corticosteroids,** which reduce inflammation in nasal passages and bronchial tissues. Familiar examples include fluticasone (Flovent), flunisolide (AeroBid), triamcinolone (Azmacort), and budesonide (Pulmicort). Inhaled corticosteroids are considered safe and rarely cause the more serious side effects reported with the oral forms. The new **leukotriene modifiers** also reduce bronchial inflammation. They work differently than inhaled corticosteroids, and many people find combining the two works better than either one alone. These drugs, including zafirlukast (Accolate), montelukast (Singulair), and zileuton (Zyflo), counteract leukotrienes—potent chemicals that constrict airways and increase mucus production. They can also soothe symptoms of nasal allergies.

Other useful asthma therapies include **sustained-release bronchodilators** such as salmeterol (Serevent); **combined medication inhalers,** like fluticasone/salmeterol (Advair Diskus) and ipratropium/albuterol (Combivent); **nonsteroidal inhalers** like cromolyn (Intal) and nedocromil (Tilade); and the **oral bronchodilator** theophylline. Just remember: Asthma medications affect people differently, so it's important to work with your doctor to find the right drug or drug combination for you. Also, because respiratory infections can trigger or worsen asthma, make sure you get an annual flu shot and are vaccinated against pneumonia.

TAKING Control

■ **Perform at your peak.**
A peak flow meter can help you head off an asthma attack before it becomes serious. This simple and inexpensive plastic gadget measures how fast you can exhale air from your lungs. People with untreated asthma have low "peak flow," which increases (often dramatically) a few minutes after they take medication. Measure your peak flow twice a day when your asthma is under control. You'll know what's normal for you. When these baseline readings begin to fall, you'll know you might be about to have an attack.

■ **Give yourself a spacer.**
A metered-dose inhaler lets out a burst of medication when you press down on it, but this most common type of inhaler can be tricky to time correctly. A special device called a spacer may help. This long plastic tube attaches to one end of the inhaler. The other end goes into your mouth. Once the inhaler is activated, the medication remains in the spacer until you inhale it. With some of these inhalers, like Advair Diskus, the metered dose is released only when you breathe in.

■ **Clean house.** Up to 90% of people with asthma react badly to dust mites. These tiny insects cling to carpets, mattresses, bedding, upholstered furniture, and even clothing. Solutions include banishing carpets, dusting religiously with a wet or oiled cloth, and using a vacuum with a microfiltration bag. Wash all bedding in hot water (130°F or higher) once a week, and consider replacing dust-catching blinds or curtains with shades.

Promising DEVELOPMENTS

A genetically engineered antibody may hold the key to a new class of drugs that can block the immune system overreaction that causes asthma attacks. **Omalizumab (Xolair)** targets immunoglobulin E (IgE), the antibody that causes mast cells to unleash histamine and other chemical weapons against allergens. The drug short-circuits the allergic reaction, by taking IgE out of circulation. Asthma patients who received Xolair by injection had less wheezing and coughing, and significantly fewer attacks that required hospitalization. The drug, being developed by Genentech and Novartis Pharmaceuticals, has recently been approved for moderate to severe symptoms in patients over the age of 12.

Lifestyle Changes

Though you will probably need prescription medications to help manage your asthma, there's a lot you can do to help yourself.

■ **Have a plan.** Develop an asthma action plan with your doctor. Make sure you share the information with your family. List the drugs you take for maintenance and prevention, those you'll take for specific symptoms, how you'll handle an attack, when to call the doctor, and where to go during a serious episode.

■ **Identify your triggers.** Keep a diary of attacks, noting what seems to cause them. Besides animal dander (particularly that of cats), pollen, cold air, exercise, dust mites, and cockroach droppings, other common triggers include aspirin, chocolate, milk, nuts, and fish. One study found that the diesel exhaust particles you'd breathe in just two days in Los Angeles can worsen asthma symptoms.

■ **Slim down.** Obese women, defined as those with a Body Mass Index of 30 or higher (*see page 355*), have almost double the risk of developing asthma as other women, according to one Canadian study. Another study that tracked a group of nurses found that those who gained more than 55 pounds after age 18 were almost five times as likely to develop asthma as those who kept their weight down. Obesity in men does not present as great a risk.

■ **Drink lots of water.** Here's another reason to down at least eight glasses of water daily: It loosens mucus to keep airways clearer.

■ **Keep indoor air dry.** Reduce humidity below 50%. Using a dehumidifier or air conditioner also keeps the dust mite population down. Be sure to change or clean filters often.

■ **Don't smoke.** And stay away from people who do. Secondhand smoke can trigger asthma attacks. It also increases the risk of *getting* asthma. One Swedish study of 8,000 adults found asthma in 7.6%

The Exercise Paradox

If you have asthma, exercise can help, however, up to 90% of people with asthma experience what's called exercise-induced asthma. That means strenuous activity can trigger an attack. Some people (including top international athletes) have *only* exercise-induced asthma. They never have symptoms unless they're exercising.

If you have exercise-induced asthma, you'll probably have symptoms within 5 to 20 minutes of starting vigorous exercise. You may have difficulty breathing, or experience cough-

ing, and tightness in your chest. Sometimes symptoms don't appear until after the workout.

Does this mean you shouldn't exercise if you have asthma? Certainly not. Doctors agree that sensible exercise can be beneficial for people with asthma (just check with your doctor first). A few tips:

● **Choose the right activity.** Swimming and water aerobics are excellent. Walking, hiking, bicycling, and downhill skiing are unlikely to trigger exercise-induced asthma.

● **Warm up and cool down.** If you plan vigorous activities, warm up thoroughly and take

time to cool down. This helps prevent sudden changes in the temperature and humidity of the air you're inhaling. Especially in cold weather, breathing through your mouth speeds cold, dry air to your lower airways that can trigger an attack.

● **Medicate before exercising.** Inhaling a short-acting beta2-agonist bronchodilator spray 15 minutes before exercise can usually prevent attacks. Some may need to use longer-acting anti-inflammatory medications.

Childhood Asthma

Between 1980 and 2001, asthma rates in children more than doubled. An estimated nine million children under 18 now have it, making asthma the most common chronic illness in kids. Four-fifths of them develop it before they're 5 years old. So be on the lookout for the following warning signs especially if you, your spouse, or both of you have asthma (remember, there's a strong genetic link here):

- **Coughing.** Could be constant, sporadic, or recurring.
- **Wheezing.** A whistling sound as your child exhales.
- **Shortness of breath.** After playing, does your child seem more out of breath than the other kids?

of those exposed to secondhand smoke as children, compared to 5.9% of those who grew up smoke-free.

■ **Bundle up.** Wintry air can trigger asthma. So cover your nose and mouth with a scarf. It'll help warm the air you're breathing.

Natural Methods*

Stress and extreme emotions can trigger asthma, so it's important to find ways to remain calm. One interesting study suggested that **yoga meditation** may help the effectiveness of asthma drugs. A group of people with asthma, who continued to experience symptoms while taking preventive medication, improved after practicing Sahaja yoga for four months. This form of Indian meditation teaches practitioners to attain "mental silence," a state of being alert without specific, focused thoughts. Lung tests showed that the yoga students were less susceptible to asthma triggers than those who practiced other relaxation techniques. Two months after they stopped practicing yoga, the benefits disappeared. **Acupuncture** may help improve short-term lung function, although the scientific evidence is less than conclusive. In one controlled study, nearly 50% of the asthma patients who practiced **guided imagery** were able to decrease, or even discontinue, their medication, compared to just 18% of the control group.

Certain foods can help you control your asthma. Researchers in the UK found that people who ate at least **two apples a week** had up to a 32% lower asthma risk than those who ate fewer. They also discovered that those who had at least 55 mcg of the mineral **selenium** each day—the daily value—were about half as likely to have asthma as those who consumed only 30 mcg or less. Selenium is found in such foods as Brazil nuts, fish, oysters, and sunflower seeds. Researchers believe that **antioxidants** like vitamin C boost lung health and may help lower the risk for asthma.

*Natural methods are not subject to the same testing and regulation as prescription medications. Please seek your doctor's advice and use caution.

An Eggs-citing Discovery

A 20-year-old woman in Spain was hospitalized with a nasty rash and asthma. Tests showed that she was allergic to grass pollen, cat dander, bird feathers, and eggs. Especially eggs. She was treated, put on an egg-free diet, and sent home, with her symptoms greatly improved. But 15 months later, she was back with a severe asthma attack brought on after she inhaled dust from the restoration of a 16th-century cathedral across the street from her home.

The paste used to protect the stone centuries ago contained egg, and some allergenic egg protein had survived in the patina of the cathedral wall. Researchers took an extract of the dust and tested it on the woman and 19 others, who served as controls. Five people in the control group were sensitized to egg, and all five of them had positive skin-prick tests to the extract.

FINDING Support

- The American Academy of Allergy, Asthma & Immunology has an excellent website at www.aaaai.org.

- The National Institute of Allergy and Infectious Diseases offers a Focus on Asthma section at www. niaid.nih.gov that includes highlights on the latest asthma research.

- For children with asthma, there's the AsthmaBusters club at www.asthmabusters.org.

Atrial fibrillation

This common heart rhythm disorder affects about 2 million Americans. Today, thanks to highly effective treatments, most people with A-Fib are able to get their heart beating regularly and drastically reduce the risk of developing serious complications.

LIKELY First Steps

- **Proper evaluation** of your symptoms by a cardiologist to get your treatment regimen off on the right foot.

- **Anticoagulant** drug therapy to prevent stroke.

- **Medications** to restore normal heart rate and rhythm.

- For some, a brief **electric shock** to jolt the heart back into its normal rhythm (called cardioversion).

QUESTIONS TO Ask

- Are there certain activities (e.g., sports or sex) I should avoid? For how long?

- Are there other changes I should be making in my lifestyle?

- Should I take an anticoagulant?

- Will I need a pacemaker?

What is happening

Like a car engine that runs smoothly only when its spark plugs are calibrated to fire in proper sequence, your heart depends on a regular, well-coordinated discharge of electrical impulses to beat properly. When its natural electrical conduction system is disrupted for any reason, you may experience an irregular heartbeat, or cardiac arrhythmia. One of the most common is atrial fibrillation, also known as A-Fib or AF.

This problem occurs in the atria, the two upper (and smaller) chambers of the heart. When your heart is functioning properly, the atria empty blood into the lower chambers (the ventricles) by a forceful pumping contraction (your heartbeat), triggered by a single electrical impulse. If the impulses are too small and weak, the result is a series of rapid, uneven contractions not strong enough to pump the blood forward. This is called atrial fibrillation, and can be constant or can occur in episodes that alternate with normal heart rhythm.

Although AF is not particularly dangerous, it can cause unpleasant symptoms and lead to serious complications. During an AF episode, the contractions of your atria are so rapid and chaotic that the atrial walls quiver (fibrillate), rather than pump, so your heart's upper chambers are only partially emptied of blood. That prevents the lower ventricles from filling properly. When that happens, your heart cannot keep up with your body's demand for blood. You may feel weak, dizzy, or short of breath. (You may even faint.) You may also experience heart palpitations or chest pains.

The real danger from atrial fibrillation is that stagnant blood left in the partially emptied atria can form a clot. If the clot breaks loose and enters your bloodstream, it could travel to your brain, causing a stroke. Such a dire event is largely avoidable when you take a blood thinner to prevent clots from forming in the atria.

Treatments

No special treatment may be required for an occasional episode of AF. Normal heart rhythm returns spontaneously in about half of all people after a brief, single episode of AF, especially in those with no underlying heart disease. But if you have recurrent or severe symptoms—or if age, general health, or other preexisting medical conditions (such as heart disease, high blood pressure, diabetes, or heart valve problems) place you at high risk for more serious com-

Treatment options

Medications

Anticoagulants/aspirin	Reduce risk of a clot-induced stroke.
Beta-blockers	Slow heart rate and make rhythm regular.
Calcium channel blockers	Alternative to beta-blockers.
Anti-arrhythmics	Restore normal heart rhythm.

Procedures

Electrical cardioversion	External or internal shock to regulate heart.
Catheter ablation	Destroys AV node; implants pacemaker.
Maze procedure	Effective, but aggressive, surgery.

Lifestyle changes

Exercise & diet	Smart daily regimens promote heart health.
Avoid alcohol & caffeine	Both can cause rhythm irregularities.

plications—you definitely need treatment. The initial priority is to prevent clots from forming and to prevent stroke. The long-term goal of AF therapy is to restore and maintain your normal heart rate and rhythm—a process doctors call cardioversion.

Medications

Your doctor may first have you take warfarin (Coumadin) or **aspirin,** to prevent blood clots and reduce stroke risk. The **anticoagulant** used will depend on your age and how many stroke risk factors you have (such as heart valve disease, high blood pressure, and a prior stroke). If your doctor recommends warfarin, you will be carefully monitored and your dose may be adjusted. Too much of this drug can cause uncontrolled bleeding. Xime lagatran (Exantra) may replace warfarin as the anticoagulant of choice for many patients. This new drug works well. It acts faster than warfarin. Unlike warfarin, it doesn't interact with food or medications, and one dose fits all, so there's no need for monitoring blood levels. It could be on the market later this year.

After you've taken anticoagulants for a month or so, your doctor will move to the next phase—medications to restore your heart's normal rate and rhythm. (This treatment is usually delayed until the blood thinner has taken effect: Abrupt normalization of the heart's rhythm can release a blood clot that may have begun to form.) **Beta-blockers,** such as atenolol (Tenormin), metoprolol (Lopressor), propranolol (Inderal), or sotalol (Betapace), and **calcium channel blockers,** such as verapamil (Isoptin) or diltiazem (Cardizem) are generally used to slow heart rate. Beta-blockers also regulate heart rhythm. An older medication, digoxin (Lanoxin), was once commonly used to slow the heart. New drugs have generally replaced it.

TAKING Control

- **Avoid caffeine and alcohol.** Either can trigger an episode of AF in otherwise healthy people. Binge drinking of alcohol is especially risky— which is why AF is sometimes referred to as "holiday heart." If you drink, don't exceed two drinks a day.

- **Quit smoking.** Nicotine is a drug. It can trigger abnormal heart rhythms.

- **Discuss anticoagulants.** Ask your doctor if taking an anticoagulant would be good for you, especially if you are an older woman with AF. According to a study in the journal *Circulation*, women age 75 and older with newly diagnosed AF were half as likely as their male counterparts to receive a prescription for the anticoagulant warfarin (Coumadin).

- **Take special care with herbal remedies.** Many formulations can interact dangerously with warfarin and other drugs you may need. In particular, avoid ginkgo biloba or garlic extract (these can cause hemorrhaging when taken with warfarin).

- **Just say "no" to street drugs** like cocaine, amphetamines, and other "uppers" or stimulants. They can cause the heart to race at a potentially deadly rate.

Pacemakers: Keeping a Steady Beat

A pacemaker is a battery-driven unit about the size of a matchbox. It's designed to provide regular electrical stimuli to control your heart rate. It consists of an impulse generator implanted just under the skin in your upper chest, and pacing lead wires that descend through a vein into the heart muscle (*see illustration at right*). The implantation requires minor surgery under local anesthesia and then a day or two of recovery time in the hospital. You can usually return to your normal activities within two weeks.

The unit will need to be tested and calibrated on a regular basis. Sometimes that can be done over the phone lines. The battery must be replaced every so often. Your doctor will check to see how much life it has left during your follow-up exams. Receiving a pacemaker may allow you to quit taking anti-arrhythmics and other drugs, freeing you from their side effects.

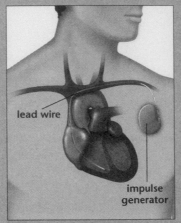

lead wire

impulse generator

Pacemaker precautions
You should be monitored regularly, wear a medical identification tag, and register with the manufacturer of your unit. Because pacemakers can be affected by strong electromagnetic fields (EMFs), you should avoid magnetic resonance imaging (MRI).

You can safely use common household items that produce EMFs (microwave ovens, cellular phones), but you should hold your cell phone at least a foot from your chest. Security devices pose no known threat, but try to move quickly through them.

Additional safety tips
- Be sure to tell surgeons or dentists that you wear a pacemaker, so they don't use an electrocauterization device to control bleeding. It can alter pacemaker settings.
- Before having any medically invasive procedure, ask your doctor about taking antibiotics to prevent infections that may affect the pacemaker.
- Avoid blows to the body near the site of your pacemaker. See your doctor if you receive such a blow.
- Check your pulse regularly to be sure your pacemaker is operating at the intended rate.
- Report any unusual symptoms to your cardiologist right away.

Promising
DEVELOPMENTS

- Researchers at the University of Buffalo have isolated a specific protein in the venom of **Chilean tarantulas**. It shows promise as the basis for a new class of drugs that could be used to block the aberrant electrical impulses causing atrial fibrillation.

- A study from Turkey revealed that **magnesium** can reduce the incidence of AF among patients undergoing bypass surgery. Only 2% of those who received magnesium supplementation experienced postoperative AF, compared with 21% of those who did not get the mineral.

Anti-arrhythmic drugs are used to regulate the heart's rhythm. These include amiodarone (Cordarone), flecainide (Tambocor), propafenone (Rhythmol), and disopyramide (Norpace). The best drug or drug combination often depends on whether you have underlying heart disease or high blood pressure. Recent studies suggest 200 mg of amiodarone a day is the most effective regimen for maintaining regular heart rhythm.

Procedures

If your AF persists despite the drugs, a number of different medical procedures might help. The least invasive is **external electrical cardioversion**, which can usually restore the heart's normal rate and rhythm. Performed under light sedation, this procedure involves delivering a high-energy electrical shock through two external paddles. The jolt briefly disrupts your heart's electrical activity and lets your normal heartbeat re-emerge.

For about 10% of AF patients, episodes continue despite these treatments. For them, surgery may be the next best option. The most common procedure is called a **catheter ablation.** Here doctors thread a tiny electrical wire (electrode) into your heart and destroy a tiny piece of heart muscle called the atrioventricular (or AV) node. This bundle of cells allows electrical impulses to pass from the atria down to the ventricles. If the hundreds of chaotic impulses from the fibrillating atria are blocked at the AV node, the heart rate slows down. Unfortunately, without any electrical impulses from the atria, the ventricles start pumping on their own, but at a rate too slow to sustain life. At the same time the AV node is destroyed, the surgeon inserts a permanent pacemaker. It keeps your heart pumping at a steady rhythm for the rest of your life (*see box opposite*).

A minimally invasive procedure known as **radiofrequency catheter ablation (RCA),** can permanently cure cardiac arrhythmias in some patients. Still in its infancy as a treatment for AF, RCA has a lower success rate than other ablation procedures (about 50% at best). RCA is often effective in people whose AF is triggered by extra heart-beats that arise within the pulmonary veins that return blood from the lungs to the left atrium.

Another choice is an **internal electrical cardioversion.** This is similar to the external variety, but instead of using paddles to give the shock, doctors insert a catheter through a vein and thread it into your heart where it delivers the shock. In some cases, this method has proven to be more effective than the external procedure.

A new, more aggressive approach called a **maze procedure.** To perform it, the surgeon makes a series of maze-like cuts in the walls of your atria, and then sews the incisions back together. When they heal, they form scar tissue that blocks the transmission of faulty electrical impulses, thus thwarting AF. After this invasive surgery, AF is unlikely to recur, but you will probably need a pacemaker and sometimes drugs to maintain a normal heart rate and rhythm. The maze procedure requires traditional open chest surgery, but mini-mally invasive techniques (going in via catheter, for example) are now under investigation.

When other heart problems are the underlying cause of AF, sur-gery to replace a damaged heart valve or to bypass blocked coronary arteries may clear up the atrial fibrillation as well.

Lifestyle Changes

There are a number of practical, everyday strategies to make your heart healthier.

- **Adjust your diet.** Reduce the amount of saturated fats, choles-terol, and trans fatty acids that you eat. Concentrate on fruits, vegetables, legumes, and whole grains; they should make up 60% of your diet.
- **Reduce your sodium intake.** Salt can often raise your blood pres-sure, compounding any AF problem you might have.
- **Control your weight.** Excess pounds tax the heart.
- **Exercise vigorously.** Try it for 30 minutes a day, three to four times a week, to keep your heart healthy and your blood pressure down.
- **De-stress.** Adopt some relaxation exercises or stress management techniques, such as yoga, tai chi, or meditation.

▶ **Does an episode of atrial fibrillation mean I have heart disease?**
Probably not. In many cases, an isolated instance of AF is trig-gered by something unrelated to your heart (binge drinking, for example). When that problem is treated or corrected, the fibrilla-tion goes away. A full diagnostic workup, including an ECG (electrocardiogram) by a cardiol-ogist, is always warranted to rule out underlying coronary heart disease, a heart valve problem, or other heart-related conditions.

▶ **Will I have to take heart rhythm medications for the rest of my life?**
Not necessarily. If doctors can restore a normal heartbeat and your heart rhythm stabilizes, you may be able to stop taking med-ication and see what happens. If episodes of AF continue to occur, you'll probably need long-term medication.

FINDING Support

The following organizations have excellent information about atrial fibrillation and other heart diseases:

- American College of Cardiol-ogy (1-800-253-4636 or www.acc.org).
- American Heart Association (1-800-242-8721 or www.americanheart.org).
- If you're looking for a support group to join, consult Mended Hearts, a Dallas-based organization (1-888-HEART99 or www.mendedhearts.org).

Back pain

Despite all the fancy surgeries and medications available these days, it's often basic remedies like ice packs and simple stretches that do the trick for an aching back. After the pain goes away, other sensible lifestyle changes may keep it from returning.

LIKELY **First Steps**

For acute low back pain:

- Alternate applications of **cold pack** and **heat.**

- Take **OTC pain medications,** or **prescription drugs** if the pain is severe. Try **medications,** including acetaminophen, NSAIDs, antidepressants, antispasmodics, and opioids.

- **Return to normal activities** as rapidly as possible.

For chronic back pain:

- **Visit a doctor or chiropractor** to assess the nature, degree, and cause of the pain.

- Pursue daily stretching and strengthening **exercises.**

QUESTIONS TO **Ask**

- When will my back stop hurting? Is there something I can do to hasten the process?

- Should I get a back x-ray? An MRI?

- Could another medical condition be causing my back pain?

- What do I need to know before I undergo surgery?

What is happening

The human back consists of a column of separate but intricately connected bones called vertebrae. A complicated lacing of ligaments, tendons, and muscles holds the vertebrae together in a flexible chain. Rubbery disks between them act as shock absorbers. The spinal cord, essentially a continuation of the brain itself, tunnels through the vertebrae, and a vast network of nerves emerges from the cord. Day and night, this mechanical wonder is subjected to pressure, twisting, and bending. It's no wonder things occasionally go awry. Back pain is the inevitable result—from ligaments that sprain, muscles that strain, disks that rupture, nerves that get pinched, or joints that get irritated.

More than 70% of Americans seek help for back pain at some point in their lives. You're more likely to experience back pain if your posture is poor, you're overweight, or the psychological stress in your life veers out of control. Illnesses such as weakened bones (osteoporosis), arthritis, and even metastatic cancer increase your risk too.

Back pain is labeled "acute" if it's intense and comes on suddenly. Pain that doesn't subside with standard treatments and lasts six months or more is considered "chronic." Back pain can affect every aspect of your life, from how you move around your house to how well you do your job. Because of it, you may feel sleep-deprived, physically and emotionally off balance, and even depressed. To make matters worse, even the best diagnostic test might not be able to pinpoint a cause.

Treatments

What helps one person's back pain doesn't necessarily work for the next. Your best bet with an acute episode is a day or two (at most) of bed rest if you think you need it, and over-the-counter medications to blunt discomfort and reduce inflammation. Muscle relaxants can ease painful spasms. Apply cold packs on and off for 48 hours, then heat. As soon as you can, get up and move around. Intense pain usually lets up in the first few hours, and there'll be steady improvement within the first two weeks. Most back problems resolve in six weeks, although sprained ligaments or muscle strains can take up to 12 weeks to fully heal. Once the pain has passed, avoid heavy chores and vigorous sports for at least two more weeks.

If your back continues to hurt, see your doctor. (Go sooner if you have numbness, weakness in your foot, a tingling sensation that

Treatment options

Lifestyle changes

Cold/heat treatments	First cold pack; then heat after 48 hours.
Exercise	Get out of bed and gradually get moving.

Medications

Analgesics	Tylenol; OTC and prescription NSAIDs.
Muscle relaxants	For spasms; short-term use only.
Opiates	For severe pain; short-term use only.
Antidepressants	Can relieve back pain.

Procedures

Spinal manipulation	By chiropractor, osteopath, physical therapist.
Injections	Anesthetic, nerve block, or steroids.
Surgery	Needed only rarely for structural problems.

Natural methods

Acupuncture/acupressure	To stimulate pain-blocking endorphins.
Massage/relaxation	To break chronic pain pattern; relieve stress.
Psychotherapy	Cognitive-behavioral therapy for emotions.

radiates into the buttocks or legs, or trouble passing urine or bowel movements—all signs of sciatica.) To treat chronic back pain, your doctor may prescribe a powerful NSAID or an opiate like Vicodin or suggest physical therapy. Rare cases may require surgery. Most important, you'll need to be a proactive patient, exploring lifestyle measures that ease your particular problem. Many experts stress the importance of breaking the vicious cycle of chronic back pain: injury leads to pain that leads to muscle tension. Then negative emotions (fear, anxiety, irritation) are followed by negative thoughts (worries, pessimism). This "emotional guarding" and subsequent restriction of physical activity causes muscles to lose strength and flexibility. At some point, even the most minor injury can start the cycle all over again.

Lifestyle Changes

With a wrenched back, your instinct is probably to get horizontal. Try tucking your body into a fetal position with a pillow between your knees, or lie on your back with your knees flexed, using two pillows to support your legs. As soon as you can, try to get out of bed and move around. Activity keeps your muscles strong and flexible. While bed rest was once the standard recommendation for back pain, doctors now think it can prolong recovery. Only people with a definite disk problem should spend more than a few days in bed.

After an injury, apply a **cold pack** every two hours while you are awake. Cold temporarily blocks pain signals to the brain, and slows

TAKING Control

- **Try alternating drugs.** Since acetaminophen and NSAIDs work differently, you can safely combine the two for more complete pain coverage. A long-acting NSAID such as Aleve is a good choice to take along with the shorter-acting Tylenol.

- **Consider a back brace.** If you have to stand or sit much of the time—or lift heavy objects—try a back brace. Properly fit and correctly worn, it can comfort and support you, but don't overdo it: A back brace limits normal movement, detracts from muscle conditioning, and reinforces the notion that your back needs protection.

- **Deal with your anxiety.** This can make back pain worse—and even perpetuate the problem. Anti-anxiety drugs (benzodiazepines are the classic choice) can blunt the jitters, although becoming dependent on them (physically and psychologically) is a risk. SSRI antidepressants also lessen anxiety but aren't habit-forming.

- **Try the Alexander technique.** Trainers of this mind-body re-education method use verbal instruction and gentle touch to teach proper alignment of the head, neck, and spine. The goal is to replace bad postural habits with good ones. Dozens of websites describe the technique and list practitioners.

- **Watch out for "miracle cures."** There aren't any. Back pain is simply too varied and complex. On the list: spinal traction, permanent bipolar magnets, and facet injections (steroids or anesthetics injected into connections between adjoining vertebrae).

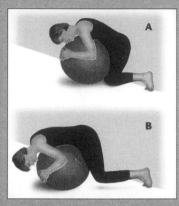
▶ **What's the Sarno approach, and does it work?**
Physician-author John E. Sarno, M.D., at the Rusk Institute of Rehabilitation Medicine in New York, contends that the intense emotional and psychological stress that results in muscle tension, not a physical abnormality, is to blame for most cases of chronic back pain. His treatment approach, outlined in his 1998 book, The Mindbody Prescription: Healing the Body, Healing the Pain, aims to resolve back pain (as well as pain in the neck, shoulders, limbs, and other areas) by addressing the key psychological factor: repressed rage. Stress reduction and psychotherapy are often the golden tickets for "thinking psychologically, not physically" when the pain occurs.

blood flow to lessen internal bleeding and swelling. Use a commercial cold pack, a bag of frozen vegetables, or ice in a dampened towel, to prevent muscle spasms, or apply an ice cube to the injured area. Limit cold pack treatments to 10 or 15 minutes at a time.

Heat relieves pain better than ice once 48 hours have passed (or if the pain is chronic). Heat lessens pain and boosts healing by stimulating blood flow. Try a hot water bottle, hot pack, heating pad (on moderate setting), a hot shower, or a soak in a hot tub. Repeat this up to four times a day, for no more than 30 minutes each time.

When you feel a bit better, **exercise** is essential. Within two weeks of the injury, start easy aerobics such as walking or bicycling. Gradually add exercises to strengthen your back and abdominal muscles, and gentle stretches to lengthen the spine and relieve compression of the vertebrae. Avoid jerking, bouncing, or movements that increase your pain. A daily regimen of stretches and exercises can make a huge difference if your pain becomes chronic (*see box above*).

Medications

One of the first drugs that you should reach for is **acetaminophen** (Tylenol). It's safe and it can quell mild to moderate pain. But if inflammation is causing your discomfort, **NSAIDs** may give you more relief: They calm inflammation and inhibit pain receptors. Good choices include aspirin, ibuprofen (Advil, Motrin), naproxen (Aleve, Naprosyn), and ketoprofen (Orudis). You might find that one works particularly well, while another doesn't seem to help at all. Be prepared for some trial and error.

NSAIDs can irritate your gastrointestinal (GI) tract, and long-term use may cause stomach bleeding. Enteric-coated forms seem to have fewer side effects. The risk varies, so be sure to tell your doctor about problems that develop with one NSAID. You may be able to switch to another. A new class of more GI-friendly NSAIDs called **COX-2 inhibitors** (Celebrex, Bextra, Vioxx) may be an option. The final verdict on their long-term safety is still out, however, and GI bleeding can (and does) occur. These prescription drugs are also expensive, typically costing about $250 for 100 pills.

If your back muscles are in spasm, **muscle relaxants** can help. They depress the nervous system, making muscles relax. Some doctors are loathe to use these drugs, which interrupt a key defense mechanism: the tensing of back muscles, which protects damaged disks or vertebrae. Take muscle relaxants, such as cyclobenzaprine (Flexeril), diazepam (Valium), carisoprodol (Soma), and methocarbomol (Robaxin), for a few days at most. Related reactions—drowsiness, dizziness, and dry mouth—can develop with them all.

Consider **opiates** for only the initial painful stages of acute back pain. They work by reducing the brain's response to pain, but they can be habit-forming. Common opiates include codeine, hydrocodone (Vicodin), oxycodone plus acetaminophen (Percocet), and oxycodone plus aspirin (Percodan). Many people, particularly those who have chronic pain, prefer the **longer-acting opioids,** such as controlled-release oxycodone (OxyContin) and controlled-release morphine (MS Contin), which need to be taken only once every 12 hours. Some doctors criticize the use of opiates for back pain, because these drugs can make you listless precisely when you should be up and about. Drowsiness, headache, constipation, and nausea are a few of the common side effects.

Don't be surprised if your doctor recommends **antidepressants** for chronic back pain, even if you don't think you have the blues. Some people get as much pain relief from antidepressants as they do from traditional painkillers. Low doses of a tricyclic antidepressant (Elavil, Endep, Norpramin) probably work best, although side effects (dizziness, drowsiness, dry mouth) can be irritating. The newer SSRI antidepressants (Prozac, Zoloft, Paxil) cause fewer side effects but may not do as much for your pain.

Procedures

About 30% of those with low back pain undergo chiropractic or osteopathic **spinal manipulation** in their search for relief. Studies show that this helps acute low back pain—especially within a few weeks of an injury. One review found that spinal manipulation with a **chiropractor** or **osteopath** increased the chances of recovering from acute low back pain within two to three weeks by nearly 20%. Some **physical therapists** do spinal manipulation as well. The goal of this procedure is to help build strength and flexibility, and eventually enable you to become aerobically fit.

Smart Moves

There's a lot you can do to recover from back pain—and to prevent future episodes. Here are some self-care measures that help:

● **When sitting,** keep your spine straight against the back of the chair. A good backrest can help support your lower back and encourage good posture. Cylindrical foam pillows called lumbar rolls will help keep you aligned (position them crosswise in the small of your back). Foam seat wedges can keep you from sinking down—and sacrificing your posture—on a squishy chair. Orthopedic neck pillows support the natural curve of the neck, keeping the spine aligned.

● **When standing,** avoid slumping. Set your head squarely above your shoulders, keeping your chin parallel to the floor and your neck straight. And most important: Try to keep your abdominal muscles tight.

● **To sleep better,** invest in a supportive mattress, or get a bed board to firm up a sagging one. Bed wedges are good for reading or watching TV in bed. Use them to elevate your knees and ease pressure on your back. Experiment with various pillows (or pillow combinations) to make sure your neck remains straight as you sleep. Before bed, ease your muscles with a warm bath.

● **To improve daily activities,** wear loose clothing for easy movement. Tight pants and girdles can weaken abdominals. Flat (or low-heeled) shoes won't increase the curvature of your back.

spinal cord

vertebra

chymopapain

normal disk

herniated disk

nerve root

1) Chemonucleolysis

needle

2) Percutaneous diskectomy

probe

3) Laser diskectomy

laser

Pain occurs when a herniated disk presses on a nerve root.

A spinal disk is said to herniate, or "rupture," when gristle-like tissue bulges into the spinal canal (*left*), due to excessive strain or age-related deterioration of supporting ligaments. Cross-sections of a herniated disk (*above*) show several minimally invasive surgeries. **1)** Chemonucleolysis, in which a needle injects an enzyme, chymopapain, into the bulging disk to dissolve portions of it. **2)** Percutaneous (through the skin) diskectomy, in which a probe removes part of the damaged disk through a small incision in the back. **3)** Laser diskectomy, in which a laser vaporizes part of the disk.

▶**I keep hearing about back therapies called TENS and PENS. What are they? Do they work?**

Whether TENS (transcutaneous electrical nerve stimulation) or the related technique PENS (percutaneous electrical nerve stimulation) can provide lasting benefit for chronic low back pain is unclear, but they can direct your attention away from the painful sensations and provide some short-term relief. TENS involves delivering mild electric pulses from electrodes on your skin. PENS runs the current through thin acupuncture needles, causing the sensation of gentle raindrops or tapping. Even though long-term benefits are still being studied, neither therapy can cause you harm.

Because chiropractors focus almost solely on the back, they are often the best choice for back pain. At your first visit, you will be thoroughly examined. You may have an x-ray or an MRI, if a herniated disk (sometimes called a slipped disk) is suspected. Chiropractors know that spinal manipulation can do more harm than good if your pain stems from a disorder such as osteoporosis, a herniated disk, a vertebral fracture, or a spine infection or tumor. You'll need to give chiropractic treatment about four weeks to work. If you don't feel a difference by then, it's unlikely it will help you.

To relieve symptoms and break a cycle of pain, some doctors recommend **injections** of anesthetics, nerve blocks, or steroids into "trigger" points along the spine. Experiments have tested injections of salt water and botulinum toxin (Botox), but its lasting benefits are still unclear. Many find relief for chronic pain from a failed back surgery or for severe leg pain (sciatica) with a **spinal cord stimulation device.** It blocks pain signals by stimulating the spinal cord with electrical pulses from a surgically implanted pulse generator. You control the pain by directing the outside generator to prompt the electrical pulsing.

When pain persists, many people think **back surgery.** This is not a good choice for most, however, and is less commonly recommended than it once was. Fewer than 5% of back pain sufferers—typically, only those with herniated disks, spinal stenosis (narrowing), sciatica, or other structural problem—are good candidates for surgery. It may relieve pain; but long-term results are about the same as with nonsurgical treatments. Be sure to get two or three opinions from qualified surgeons before agreeing to a surgical procedure.

If your herniated disk is causing nerve damage, you may need a **diskectomy.** The surgeon relieves pressure on the pinched nerve by making an incision in the outer layers of the disk and removing the gel-like center. Part of the vertebra may have to be removed (**laminectomy**). Problems can develop following diskectomy, due to the added strain on the other disks and the shift in the overall structure of the spine.

Several **techniques** less invasive than major back surgery have also been developed (*see illustration opposite*). In one, an enzyme called chymopapain, derived from papaya, is injected into a herniated disk to break it down. Chymopapain treatment is effective about 70% of the time, but is considered risky because of bad reactions (including severe allergic ones) to the enzyme; it's more commonly done abroad. In another, a probe is inserted through a tiny incision to remove part of a damaged disk. A third less invasive—but controversial—technique uses lasers to burn out the disk. Success rates vary widely.

Natural Methods*

If you're like most Americans with back pain, you've probably considered checking out a "natural" alternative—nearly 60% of us do. **Acupuncture** is a popular choice. Based on the ancient Asian theory that pain occurs when the body's natural flow of energy (*qi*) is off balance, acupuncture involves a practitioner inserting 10 to 15 hair-thin needles in the back and other parts of the body to balance *qi*. How actual pain relief occurs is a mystery. Conventional doctors believe the needles prompt nerves to emit natural, pain-blocking chemicals (endorphins). Many people get real—if transient—pain relief. To enhance the effect, the needles may be charged with electricity, heated, or periodically rotated. In a related therapy called **acupressure,** three to five minutes of continuous pressure and massage applied to an acupuncture point stimulates *qi*.

With straightforward **therapeutic massage,** back tension can melt away as the muscles are manipulated. The muscle movement overwhelms pain signals—at least temporarily. In 2001, Seattle researchers reported that therapeutic massage provided long-lasting benefits in reducing chronic low back pain and disability. Always use a massage therapist who's professionally trained and licensed.

To break a pattern that seems to be leading to chronic back pain, try learning **relaxation techniques,** such as yoga, tai chi, guided imagery, and meditation. Your metabolic response to meditation—the opposite of its response to stress—is believed to unravel the ravages of stress on your body. **Biofeedback** can help you become aware of how you can relax your body most effectively. Electronic sensors measure different bodily functions—such as muscle tension, pulse rate, and breathing pattern—while you practice various relaxation methods. In time, you'll learn to consciously regulate your body's stress levels without the sensors. **Cognitive-behavioral therapy** has proved quite useful for chronic back pain. This approach helps you gain insight into your emotions and provides tools for managing stress and effectively dealing with feelings of helplessness and depression.

Natural methods are not subject to the same testing and regulation as prescription medications. Please seek your doctor's advice and use caution.

▶ **IT'S A BIG AND VERY COSTLY PROBLEM:** More than $50 billion is spent each year on the diagnosis and treatment of back pain in the United States, according to the prestigious *Journal of the American Medical Association (JAMA).*

FINDING Support

- To find a pain treatment facility near you, contact the Commission on Accreditation of Rehabilitation Facilities (520-325-1044 or www.carf.org), which will provide a list of accredited programs. For information about local pain centers, try the American Pain Society (847-375-4715 or www. ampainsoc.org).

- For information on back surgery, call the American Academy of Orthopaedic Surgeons in Rosemont, IL (1-800-346-2267 or www. aaos.org). Helpful descriptions of back procedures can be found at www.spine-surgery.com and www. yoursurgery.com.

- To find a physical therapist, contact the American Physical Therapy Association in Alexandria, VA (1-800-999-2782 or www.apta.org). They can also refer you to "back schools," which are often less expensive than pain treatment facilities.

- To find a reputable acupuncture practitioner, contact the National Certification Commission for Acupuncture and Oriental Medicine in Alexandria, VA (703-548-9004 or www.nccaom.org).

Brain tumor

A diagnosis of a brain tumor is frightening news for anyone. But, cutting-edge research and treatment breakthroughs now mean many people with this condition are enjoying longer and more productive lives. And an increasing number are even cured.

LIKELY First Steps

- For most tumors, **surgery** to determine type and treatment, reduce their size, or remove them entirely.
- **Radiation therapy** to shrink tumors. Usually after surgery but sometimes as a stand-alone treatment.
- In some cases, **chemotherapy** to shrink tumors.
- **Investigative therapies** for problems that don't respond to standard treatment.

QUESTIONS TO Ask

- What type of brain tumor do I have? What does that mean?
- What are my chances for long-term survival?
- Are there risks in removing this tumor?
- What signs may mean my tumor is getting better or worse?
- Are there therapies I might try in other cities or even other countries?
- Where would you send a member of your family for the best treatment for this illness?

What is happening

The hard shell of your skull is a boon to your brain when it comes to protecting it from injury, but it's a disadvantage if you have a brain tumor. There's so little room for growth within the skull, a tumor can damage nerve tissue or dangerously increase pressure on your brain. This is why many benign (noncancerous) tumors can be serious, even though they contain normal-looking cells, grow slowly, and don't spread outside the brain. Malignant (cancerous) brain tumors cause even more problems: They grow faster and can destroy neighboring tissue. When these tumors originate in your brain, they're called primary tumors. If they spread from elsewhere, they're known as secondary tumors. Secondary (metastatic) malignant brain tumors are far more common than primary ones. They most often spread from breast or lung cancers, from melanoma (a type of skin cancer), or from blood cell cancers such as leukemia. Secondary tumors usually appear in more than one area of your brain.

A primary malignant brain tumor is classified based on the type of brain cell it came from and where in the brain it's located. About half are called gliomas, which grow from supporting cells of the nerve tissue. Gliomas can range from slow-growing to very aggressive cancers. (Generally, the more slowly a tumor grows, the better your prognosis.) Malignant brain tumors are "graded" according to their tendency to grow and spread: Grade I is the least dangerous. Grade IV is the most aggressive and fastest-growing.

Symptoms of a brain tumor vary greatly, depending on its size and location and the rate at which it's growing. The first symptom is usually recurring headaches from pressure building up inside your skull (although the vast majority of headaches aren't caused by brain tumors). A brain tumor can also affect your balance and cause dizziness, nausea and vomiting, gradual loss of movement in an arm or leg, seizures, hearing or vision problems, and personality changes. With so many types of tumors, it's important not to leap to conclusions. Studies that show people who survive for two years after being diagnosed with a brain tumor have a 70% chance of surviving for five years or more.

Treatments

The most effective therapy for you will be based on the type of tumor you have, how large it is, and where it's located. It also depends on your general health, age, and medical history. If you have

Treatment options

Procedures

Biopsy	Determines treatment for inoperable tumors.
Craniotomy	Provides surgical access to brain tumor.
Laser microsurgery	Pinpoints and destroys tumors.
Radiation therapy	Shrinks tumors; kills remaining cancer cells.
Brachytherapy	Implants radioactive "seeds" in brain.

Medications

Chemotherapy	Alone or in combination with other therapies.
Corticosterlods	Can reduce swelling within the brain.
Anticonvulsants	Help if seizures are a problem.

Lifestyle changes

Eat well	To stay strong for treatment.
See a therapist	For physical and psychological help.

a benign or low-grade tumor, your doctor may simply want to keep an eye on it but not actively treat it until it shows signs of growth. If you have any other kind of tumor, your medical team's immediate goal will be to reduce its size as much as possible (sometimes by removing it altogether). Various approaches may be used in this assault: including surgery, radiation therapy, chemotherapy, or new investigative procedures. While sometimes used alone, these techniques are most often deployed in combinations, and they are dictated by a specific situation.

Procedures

You'll probably start with surgery. That's standard operating procedure. It may be all you need for some benign and Grade I tumors. In most cases, though, surgery can't completely remove the tumor without doing unacceptable levels of damage to your healthy brain tissue. But it can reduce the tumor's size, alleviate your symptoms, and make other therapies more effective.

If your tumor is too deep or intertwined with healthy brain tissue to be removed, the surgeon may take a sample of it for a **biopsy**—an examination under a microscope. This reveals what type of tumor you have and helps your medical team determine which other treatments will be most effective.

Neurosurgeons have a number of techniques in their surgical arsenal. If the tumor is close to the surface of your brain and you're in good health, you'll probably have a **craniotomy.** Your surgeon will remove a piece of skull over the part of your brain near the tumor, remove the tumor as completely as possible, and replace the bone. If your tumor is in an area of your brain that controls motor function

Promising
DEVELOPMENTS

- A new type of treatment called **photodynamic therapy (PDT)** may reduce recurrences of certain types of brain tumors. Before surgery to remove the tumor, a patient is given a light-activated drug (Photofrin), which is absorbed by the tumor and makes the cancer cells fluorescent. During surgery, the surgeon directs a laser at the tumor cells, which activates the drug, killing the cells.

- **Monoclonal antibodies (MAbs)** are a particularly promising new treatment possibility. These genetically engineered antibodies are bound with radioactive iodine and put into a brain tumor. The antibodies lock onto certain tumor cells, and the iodine destroys them without the tissue damage caused by standard radiation treatment. In one study of people with high-grade gliomas, this treatment more than doubled the average survival time, from 11 months to 23 months.

- Someday a **vaccine** may be available for brain tumors. Researchers are currently working on it by taking tumor cells from a patient, inactivating them, then putting them back in the patient. The cells are harmless, but they prompt the immune system to attack the tumor as if it were an invader.

- Scientists are studying interleukin and interferon, two natural proteins that are toxic to many tumor cells. To date, a treatment called **IL-4 toxin** therapy, which combines interleukin with a cancer fighter derived from bacteria, has made tumors shrink in preliminary animal studies.

or speech, your doctor may perform surgery under local anesthesia to better measure your nerve response during the operation.

If the tumor can't be reached easily, another option is **laser microsurgery:** It vaporizes cancer cells with a specific type of laser beam. Your doctor may use it as a single procedure or following a craniotomy to eliminate any abnormal tissue still left. For this surgery, the surgeon may use a guidance system called **stereotactic localization** (stereotaxy). A rigid frame is screwed into the head. An attached scanning device displays a three-dimensional map of the brain, pinpointing the tumor's exact location. A frameless stereotaxy has also been developed.

After surgery, you'll probably have **radiation therapy,** even if it looks as if your entire tumor has been excised. (This is to eradicate microscopic cancer cells left behind in surrounding brain tissue.) Radiation is also used to shrink any part of the tumor that remains, or tumors that are out of reach or inoperable. If you have a metastatic malignant tumor, radiation is the mainstay therapy. It's typically directed at the whole brain to root out unseen problems. For some benign tumors, radiation is the only treatment needed. Radiation can have serious side effects, including temporary hair loss, nausea, and fatigue, as well as destruction of healthy tissue near the tumor (radiation necrosis). But studies show that for people with certain malignant brain tumors, it can significantly prolong life.

New techniques are used to protect unaffected brain tissue from large amounts of radiation while delivering high doses to a tumor. Refinements to **external-beam radiation,** which directs radiation from outside the body, have made it a precise and popular technique. Your medical team will recommend this if you have a large tumor or a high-grade tumor that has infiltrated surrounding areas. It can also prevent a recurrence of a benign tumor after surgery. Radiation is usually delivered five days a week for several weeks.

Stereotactic radiosurgery (which doesn't involve surgery) directs intense beams of radiation at the tumor alone An example is single-treatment gamma knife radiation, which uses several gamma rays that converge at one point on the tumor. Stereotactic radiosurgery is often used to treat a tumor deep in the brain, or in an area where surgical removal is dangerous. If your tumor is accessible, you could be a candidate for **brachytherapy,** in which radioactive "seeds" are implanted (sometimes permanently) into the tumor site. This is often used for tumors that recurred after being treated by external-beam radiation. It affects only the tumor, with fewer side effects than standard radiation.

Medications

Some types of brain tumors respond well to **chemotherapy** (one or a combination of anticancer drugs). Certain tumors can be treated by chemotherapy alone. For others, especially high-grade tumors, chemotherapy can enhance the effect of radiation. To get past the blood-brain barrier, which protects brain tissues from toxins, these drugs must be given in very high doses or in novel ways.

One solution is drug-soaked wafers, implanted during surgery into the tumor site, which slowly deliver chemotherapy. If you have a high-grade cancer, your doctor may use the drugs temozolomide (Temodal), thalidomide, or carmustine (BCNU). For many common brain tumors, a drug regimen called PCV (procarbazine, CCNU or lomustine, and vincristine) can be effective. If you have chemotherapy, you're likely to experience temporary nausea and vomiting, fatigue, and hair loss.

If you have a type of brain tumor that can't yet be cured, consider **investigative therapies.** The best (and sometimes only) way to benefit from new approaches is to enroll in a clinical trial, an experiment of new treatments. Promising research is being done on immunotherapy, gene therapy, drugs called **angiogenesis inhibitors,** which block the growth of blood vessels in the tumor, vitamins, toxins, stem cell transplantation, and more. Talk with your doctor about finding a well-designed trial with the greatest potential benefit for you.

Depending on your symptoms, your doctor may also prescribe other medications. If a tumor is increasing pressure on your brain, you'll likely be given **corticosteroids** to reduce swelling. Seizures can be controlled with **anticonvulsant drugs.** If you need them, ask your doctor for prescription **pain relievers.**

Lifestyle Changes

Being treated for a brain tumor is likely to sap your strength and energy. You can help yourself by **eating well.** Try to have a small meal high in protein and calories every few hours. Be sure to **take time for naps:** Medications and other treatments can be very fatiguing. If the tumor or your treatment has caused a physical impairment, **get physical therapy.** You'll learn techniques that make it easier to go about your daily activities. Dealing with any type of cancer is an emotional challenge, so don't be hesitant to ask for help. **Seeing a psychotherapist** can give you the support you need to cope more successfully with this difficult period in your life.

▶ **CELL PHONES AND BRAIN TUMORS don't appear to be connected. In fact, researchers found more cases of brain cancer only in people age 70 and older—the group least likely to use cell phones. Experts attribute rising numbers to better diagnostic techniques and to medical advances that allow people to live long enough to develop relatively rare diseases like brain cancer.**

FINDING Support

- The American Brain Tumor Association is an excellent source of patient information. It also lists clinical trials. Contact the ABTA in Des Plaines, IL (1-800-886-2282 or www.abta.org).

- To find a local neurosurgeon, contact the American Association of Neurological Surgeons in Rolling Meadows, IL (1-888-566-AANS or www.neurosurgery.org).

Breast cancer

If you're among the 200,000-plus women diagnosed with breast cancer this year, you have a good chance of beating this disease—much better than just a decade ago. The tough part may be sorting through all the options now available.

LIKELY First Steps

- Seek a **second (or third) opinion.**
- **Surgery** to remove the cancerous growth, sometimes followed by **chemotherapy** or **hormonal therapy.**
- **Radiation** to shrink the tumor and kill remaining cancer cells.

QUESTIONS TO Ask

- What are my chances of surviving this?
- What side effects can I anticipate from this treatment?
- Will my figure ever recover? What about reconstruction?
- Does this mean I'm at greater risk for other cancers?
- What experience do you have with breast cancer? What's your patients' survival rate?

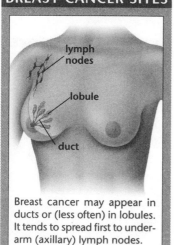

BREAST CANCER SITES

lymph nodes

lobule

duct

Breast cancer may appear in ducts or (less often) in lobules. It tends to spread first to underarm (axillary) lymph nodes.

What is happening

Surveys consistently show that breast cancer is the disease that women fear most, which makes an actual diagnosis all the more scary. While this reaction is understandable, it's important to realize that the outlook for women with breast cancer is steadily improving, with development of more sophisticated screening tools, earlier diagnosis, and more effective treatments.

A few basic facts: Breast cancer begins when abnormal cells start to grow and eventually form a tiny mass (tumor) in the breast. About 90% of the time, this malignancy occurs in the milk ducts (called ductal carcinoma), or in the milk glands (called lobular carcinoma). Sometimes, an overgrowth of abnormal cells along the lining of a milk duct stays confined to one spot, or in situ, a condition known as ductal carcinoma in situ, or DCIS (*see box, page 61*). Only rarely, however, does a tumor develop in the connective tissue or fat that makes up the rest of the breast.

At diagnosis, a breast cancer tumor is classified by stage—from 0 for the smallest to IV for the most serious—to indicate a tumor's size and whether malignant cells have spread elsewhere in the body. You may already know the stage of your disease. This is important because it helps clarify the best treatment options for your particular case (*see table, page 60*). Another important factor determined at diagnosis is whether the tumor is hormone receptor-positive (hormone sensitive). Anti-estrogen therapy and removal of your estrogen-producing ovaries are much more likely to work if it is.

For most breast cancers, it's good news if the lymph nodes (called axillary nodes) in the armpit closest to the affected breast (*see illustration at left*) are cancer-free, or "node-negative." This means it's unlikely the cancer has spread, or metastasized, through your lymphatic system to other sites in the body, and even if you're "node-positive," an excellent array of effective treatments is at your doctor's disposal.

Treatments

No single treatment strategy works for everyone. What's recommended for you may not be what's best for another woman. In general, key factors in determining the best treatment will be the tumor's size, aggressiveness, and location. The earlier the stage and the smaller the tumor, the more likely that surgery can remove it all and offer a total cure. There are also good options for more advanced stages, where the cancer has spread beyond the breast. In

Treatment options

Procedures

Surgery	Lumpectomy or mastectomy variations.
Radiation therapy	Whole-breast external beam most common; internal radiation, or brachytherapy with radioactive "seeds," for a lumpectomy.

Medications

Chemotherapy	For long-term, relapse-free survival.
Hormonal therapy	SERMs, like tamoxifen aromatase inhibitors.
Biological agents	Herceptin (monoclonal antibody).

Lifestyle changes

Get support	Soothes emotions; provides advice.
Make healthy choices	Nutritious diet, exercise, and weight control.
Reduce stress	Meditation, yoga, and massage can help.

designing a treatment, your doctor will also consider your age and general health, the size of your breasts, and whether or not you've gone through menopause. The strategy you're ultimately given will probably feature a mix-and-match of surgery, chemotherapy or hormone-blockers, and radiation.

Deciding which approach will be most successful for you can be tricky. It's normal to feel scared and overwhelmed by all the information and differing opinions you are offered. The appeal of one treatment over another can be frustratingly small. The most difficult program may not necessarily be the best: Some arduous regimens increase success rates by as little as 1%. On the bright side, unless the cancer is advanced, you have at least several weeks to research various options before starting treatment. See other doctors to confirm your diagnosis and discuss the treatment plan recommended for you. If you get two different opinions, see a third or fourth doctor.

Try to find experts you feel comfortable talking with about your fears—being anesthetized for surgery, losing part of your femininity, having cancer develop elsewhere in your body. Good doctors are familiar with such concerns and can give you insightful ideas for handling them. The decision is then up to you; many women find that writing in a journal and talking with friends and family leads them to a decision that they feel comfortable with.

Procedures

The first step in breast cancer treatment is **surgery** to determine, among other factors, exactly what kind of tumor it is and whether it contains hormone receptors. A surgeon or radiologist performs this initial procedure, called a biopsy. The next step for most women is to have the cancer excised. This is your best shot at a cure, at stopping

TAKING Control

■ **Bring a friend along.** When discussing treatment options with your doctor, have an advocate in the room to take notes and pose questions you can't ask. Even better: tape record the appointment. You can later review what was said at your leisure.

■ **Pose key questions to yourself.** Feeling comfortable with a treatment choice is critical, because there's often no "right" choice. Ask yourself: What feels best for me? Can I manage the side effects? What kind of support can I expect from family or friends?

■ **Sign up for a clinical trial.** This can put you in the hands of highly experienced doctors. The Physician Data Query system produced by the NIH's National Cancer Institute (www.cancer.gov/cancer_information/pdq) lists breast cancer trials.

■ **Plan for a wig.** Before you lose your hair from chemo, visit a wigmaker to choose a style and color that match your own. A hairdresser can add finishing touches. With a doctor's prescription, insurance companies will cover the expense.

Handling Chemo

See about getting anti-nausea drugs. And try to:
● **Eat five or six small meals** instead of three large ones.
● **Sip clear fluids** or suck on popsicles, ice chips, or Jell-O.
● **Avoid favorite foods,** so you won't dislike them later.
● **Rest quietly** after meals.
● **Pursue what relaxes you:** reading, soothing music.
● **Explore acupuncture,** especially for nausea.

▶**With breast cancer, can I safely eat soy foods or take soy supplements for my menopausal symptoms?**

Soy drinks and supplements have been touted as alternatives to hormone replacement therapy (HRT) because they contain chemicals with estrogen-like effects (phytoestrogens). Try them, and judge for yourself whether hot flashes and other menopausal symptoms ease. Women participating in trials haven't found soy foods to be any better than a placebo. There are also some concerns that, as a phytoestrogen, soy may induce breast cancers to grow when taken in concentrated supplement form.

▶**What is a sentinel node biopsy? Why is it done?**

In the last few years, sentinel node biopsy during surgery has begun to replace axillary (underarm) node removal as a method of analyzing those nodes for cancer. The lymph node that drains the cancer-containing part of the breast, called the sentinel node, is identified and removed. If no cancer cells are found, it is unlikely that the remaining axillary nodes contain cancer. This means further surgery isn't needed.

▶**My breast cancer has spread to my bones. Are there drugs that can help?**

Bisphosphonate drugs (clodronate, pamidronate) have been shown to slow cancer growth, reduce bone pain, and possibly prevent fractures due to weakened bones. Although expensive and given intravenously, the bisphosphonates do provide an important treatment option for women with metastasis to bone.

STAGES OF BREAST CANCER

Stage	Spread	Options
0	Abnormal cells present in breast ducts or lobules.	Monitoring, and/or tamoxifen or SERMs, or lumpectomy or total mastectomy.
I & II	**I** Tumor 2 cm in size, confined to breast. **II** Tumor 2 cm or less with spread to axillary node; tumor 2 cm to 5 cm with or without axillary node spread; tumor greater than 5 cm but hasn't spread to axillary nodes.	Breast-conserving surgery; lymph node sampling; radiation therapy; or modified or radical mastectomy; removal or radiation of lymph nodes. Plus: Chemo for hormone-negative tumors; hormone therapy (possibly with chemo) for hormone-positive tumors.
III	Tumor greater than 5 cm with spread to axillary or other nodes or tissues near breast.	Mastectomy with radiation therapy and chemo, hormone therapy, or both.
IV	Cancer has spread to other parts of the body.	Surgery or radiation for breast cancer. Plus: Chemo, hormone therapy, radiation to shrink tumors and ease symptoms.

the cancer from getting any bigger or spreading. If retaining the natural shape of your breasts is important to you, discuss different reconstruction options with a plastic surgeon (*see box, page 63*).

For tumor removal, there are also a number of options (*see illustrations opposite*).

- **If your tumor is stage I or II,** your surgeon should be able to remove the cancer completely, keeping your breast largely intact. Procedures called a **lumpectomy** or a **partial mastectomy** are used. You'll then need six or seven weeks of radiation to the breast to destroy any leftover cancer cells. Thousands of women now choose one of these breast-conserving approaches. The latest major research trials indicate your chance for long-term survival is the same with a lumpectomy as with partial or even radical mastectomy.

- **If your tumor is stage III or at an early stage but you have small breasts,** you may be better off having the entire breast removed with a procedure called a mastectomy. There are several variations. Most women have an operation called a **modified radical mastectomy,** which removes breast tissue, chest muscle lining, and axillary nodes. Only if the cancer has spread to muscles in the chest will a surgeon recommend a **radical mastectomy,** in which the breast, nodes, and muscles beneath the breast are removed. Sometimes presurgery chemotherapy shrinks a tumor sufficiently to make lumpectomy possible. Finally, a **total mastectomy** is a treatment option for DCIS (*see box opposite*).

After surgery, many women pursue **radiation therapy,** or radiotherapy, to destroy any wayward cancer cells in the breast, chest wall, or underarm area. (Sometimes radiation is recommended before surgery to shrink a tumor.) Sometimes key to surviving breast cancer, radiation is often worth the discomfort of fatigue, red or blistered skin, skin color changes, and other possible side effects. On a positive note, technical innovations in radiation have reduced the risk of such side effects.

Widely recommended **external beam radiation,** focuses two opposing beams of high-energy x-rays on the breast, angling them away from vital organs. The procedure is done five days a week, for about five weeks. Additional, even more precisely focused radiation is often given for another one to two weeks.

If you've had a lumpectomy for a small, early tumor, and are postmenopausal, you may be a candidate for a promising new radiation approach called **internal radiation therapy,** or brachytherapy. In this procedure, radioactive "seeds" (the size of rice grains) are implanted directly into the site of the excised tumor, where cancer is most likely to recur. You only need twice a day treatments for four or five days, and side effects appear to be mild. Much about this new technique remains unknown, but early results indicate that for some women, brachytherapy is as effective as standard radiation at preventing recurrence of breast cancer.

The latest findings show that combining radiation with breast-conserving surgery for stage I or II breast cancer offers the same odds for long-term survival as mastectomy. But without the post-surgery radiation, the risk of recurrence at or near the original tumor site is much higher. So if you're slated for a mastectomy, your doctor will likely recommend radiation therapy, especially if your tumor is large or many lymph nodes (usually four or more) are involved. It's less certain that radiation will benefit you if fewer (one to three) lymph nodes are involved.

Treating DCIS

Before an actual cancer develops, a woman may have stage 0, ductal carcinoma in situ (DCIS). Researchers call these preinvasive lesions, meaning they are cancerous cells gathered in a milk duct, about the size of a pinpoint, that haven't traveled beyond it. They may never develop into an actual tumor. Over time, however, untreated DCIS lesions often invade the milk duct wall, posing a risk they'll enter a blood vessel and spread elsewhere.

There's no set way to handle a DCIS. After the lesion is removed, some women opt to simply get frequent screenings. Others choose tamoxifen or similar drugs. Many get radiation treatment. Still others choose mastectomy. In deciding what to do, considerations will include your age and the DCIS's size, grade, and growth pattern.

OPTIONS FOR BREAST CANCER TUMOR REMOVAL

1) Lumpectomy

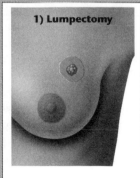

2) Partial mastectomy

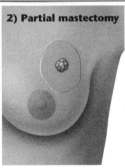

3) Total mastectomy

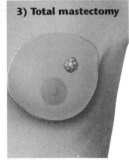

4) Modified radical mastectomy

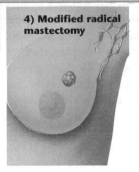

During a lumpectomy **(1),** the tumor is removed along with a margin of surrounding normal tissue (pink area). New minimalist surgical techniques involve taking out far less fat and surrounding tissue than was once done, reducing the risk of dented and otherwise misshapen breasts. Also breast-conserving is a partial mastectomy **(2),** in which slightly more surrounding tissue is removed.

Sometimes women with ductal carcinoma in situ (DCIS) undergo total mastectomy **(3).** All the breast tissue is removed, but underlying muscles and axillary nodes are left intact, along with enough skin to make the most of reconstruction options. More complete is a modified radical mastectomy **(4),** in which all breast tissue, chest muscle lining, and selected nodes are removed.

Treatments of Tomorrow

Dramatic advances are in the wings. Breakthrough surgical techniques can now destroy tumors while sparing considerable breast tissue. In **tumor ablation,** a probe inserted though a tiny incision delivers painless radio frequency energy to vaporize tumor cells. An **endoscopy** enables surgeons to examine (and possibly treat) tumors with a miniature fiber-optic camera inserted through the nipple. The **"smart" drugs** can block or bind to cancer-causing proteins or receptors. With **molecular forecasting,** doctors pluck and study strands of tumor DNA to predict which tumors are likely to spread—and which drugs might work. Experimental **biological agents** such as vaccines boost the ability of the immune system to fight the cancer. Even **bone marrow transplants** are being explored.

▶ **THE SURGEON'S GENDER MATTERS. The medical care surgeons provide may be similar, but the advice they give is slanted differently. Surveys show that female surgeons typically base their recommendations on what they feel is the woman's need for security and beating the odds. Male surgeons, on other hand, focus more on what they perceive as the woman's feelings about the importance of her breasts to her sense of femininity.**

Medications

After surgery for a stage I, II, or III cancer, you and your doctor make a decision about using anticancer drugs. Both chemotherapy and hormone therapy can be enlisted to patrol the whole body and destroy wayward cancer cells. This is often referred to as **systemic therapy.**

The heavyweight here is **chemotherapy,** which benefits most women with breast cancer. Whether you're pre- or postmenopausal, whether lymph nodes are involved or not, you're more likely to enjoy a long-term, relapse-free recovery if you undergo chemotherapy. Chemotherapy destroys normal healthy cells, as well as cancerous ones. So while it reduces the risk of cancer in another part of your body, your doctor won't recommend it if it poses more of a health risk than cancer. Chemotherapy probably won't be suggested if you have a cancer unlikely to spread, are over age 70, or are otherwise quite ill.

Most women start chemotherapy after surgery and continue treatments for about three months. If you have a relatively large tumor (more than 5 centimeters), your doctor may suggest presurgery chemotherapy with six months or so of additional chemo after surgical recovery. Good results have been seen by prolonging chemotherapy in women with lymph node involvement.

Chemotherapy agents all work a little differently. Some are taken orally, others by IV or injection. Side effects vary as well: If your reactions are very severe *(see box, page 59)*, talk with your doctor about switching drugs. Most regimens are given in cycles. Combinations such as **CMF** (cyclophosphamide, methotrexate, and 5-fluorouracil) or **CA** (cyclophosphamide and Adriamycin) are common. The hormone-receptor status of the tumor is also a factor in choosing chemotherapy. For example, adding **paclitaxel** (Taxol, derived from the Pacific yew tree) after CA further lowers the risk of recurrence with a hormone-receptor negative tumor.

If the tumor is hormone-positive, you will receive **hormonal therapy** (anti-estrogen treatment) following surgery—regardless of your age, menopausal status, lymph node involvement, or the tumor size. Anti-estrogen therapy is helpful even if only a tiny amount of hormone action is present: It can prevent your own estrogen hormones from stimulating cancer cells and growing new tumors.

The most common form of anti-estrogen therapy is a class of medications called **selective estrogen receptor-modulators (SERMs).** Most widely used is **tamoxifen** (Nolvadex), which blocks estrogen from latching onto breast cell receptors through trickery: Because tamoxifen closely resembles estrogen, breast cancer cells accept it instead. This prevents your own estrogen from delivering its "growth" (and cancer-stimulating) signal. It also prompts the cancer cells to die. Tamoxifen cuts the risk of a new cancer in the other breast by 50% and reduces the risk of cancer elsewhere in the body. Studies show that taking it for five years is better than for one to two; hot flashes and vaginal discharge are common side effects. If you have the BRCA1 gene (a genetic mutation linked to an inherited form of breast cancer), tamoxifen probably won't help prevent a new cancer, but it might fight breast cancer that's already there. Tamoxifen also lowers the risk for cancer if you have BRCA2, another gene variation.

New hormone therapy agents called **aromatase inhibitors** target estrogen—by blocking the action of an enzyme (aromatase) crucial to estrogen production. These drugs won't help if you're premenopausal, because they can't keep up with your ovaries' prodigious natural estrogen output. You can benefit, however, if you're postmenopausal and your cancer is advanced. The new drug **anastrazole** (Arimidex) appears to be at least as effective as tamoxifen.

Another treatment option for premenopausal women with hormone-positive tumors is medical or surgical removal of the ovaries. This halts production of estrogen, which fuels breast cancer growth, but it also ends fertility and can be emotionally taxing. If a breast cancer is very aggressive and has spread, the doctor may recommend a **biological agent**, the monoclonal antibody drug **trastuzumab** (Herceptin). It blocks the growth of cancer cells in about 30% of cases by targeting a protein (HER2) abundant in some tumors.

Lifestyle Changes

A good treatment strategy considers your emotions as well as your body. Here are a few things you can do:

- **Join a support group.** This can be tremendously important in helping you deal with fear, anger, loneliness, betrayal by your body, despair, and other feelings. There are groups to help your kids and other family members cope as well.
- **Exercise regularly.** Many women report exercise helps them tolerate therapy better. Ask about special arm and shoulder exercises if you've had lymph node surgery.
- **Eat a balanced and nutritious diet.** Good eating can bolster your body's drive to stay healthy and fight the cancer.
- **Keep weight under control.** Excess pounds may lower your odds or raise the risk of a cancer recurrence.
- **Concentrate on de-stressing.** Get plenty of rest; then explore techniques such as biofeedback, massage, and meditation.

FINDING Support

- Try the hotline of the National Cancer Institute (1-800-4-CANCER) for answers about diagnosis and treatment. Or log on to their website (www.cancer.gov).

- A unique resource called DIPEx (Database of Individual Patient Experiences) contains interviews with women who have had breast cancer, as well as news about treatment and complementary therapies (www.DIPEx.org).

- The nonprofit support group SHARE has helped millions of families cope with cancer (1-866-891-2392).

- The American Cancer Society's Reach to Recovery hotline lets you share your fears with a breast cancer survivor (1-800-ACS-2345).

- The Y-ME National Breast Cancer Organization has a 24-hour hotline and sponsors a monthly one-hour teleconference with a cancer specialist (1-800-221-2141 or www.y-me.org/english.htm).

- The Susan G. Komen Breast Cancer Foundation has a toll-free breast-care helpline (1-800-IM-AWARE).

Bronchitis

Each winter some 12 million people seek a doctor's care for bronchitis, a respiratory infection with a nonstop, body-racking cough. All they may really need to feel better, however, is good-quality rest, lots of fluids, and the right OTC drugs.

LIKELY First Steps

- **Analgesics** to relieve body aches, sore throat, and fever.
- **OTC cough medicines** with expectorants to ease continuous coughing and loosen phlegm, then suppressants to quiet a lingering, nagging hack.
- **Plenty of rest** to help your body fight off the infection.
- **Lots of fluids** to hydrate mucous membranes.
- For serious cases, a **bronchodilator** to help you breathe more easily.

QUESTIONS TO Ask

- Am I contagious?
- Does my overall health make me more prone to a bacterial infection?
- Should I stay home from work? For how long?
- When can I return to my fitness routine?

What is happening

Defined as an inflammation of the bronchial tubes, bronchitis is nearly always caused by a virus. You develop this respiratory infection when the virus enters your body through your nose or mouth. First it causes cold- or flulike symptoms in your nasal passages and throat. Then it migrates down your windpipe to your bronchial tubes, the doorways to your lungs. To prevent the virus from entering these vital organs, the tubes swell and their linings become inflamed. This protective inflammation results in a lot of mucus production in your bronchial tubes, and your body tries to expel it by coughing. As the virus replicates, the bronchial tubes become even more inflamed, causing the raw, painful cough so characteristic of this condition.

At first your cough is dry, or nonproductive (meaning nothing is being expelled from your lungs); this is largely due to bronchial irritation. As mucus production increases and your antibodies attack the invading organisms, you'll develop a wet, or productive, cough. When you cough, you'll bring up white, yellow, or green sputum (phlegm)—a mixture of mucus, dead viruses, and infection-fighting white blood cells.

There are two types of bronchitis. With **acute bronchitis,** severe symptoms usually ease up in two or three days. But a lingering, milder cough may hang on for several weeks. **Chronic bronchitis** is a different condition altogether. Primarily affecting smokers, it's said to be present when you have a mucus-producing cough on most days during a three-month period for two years in a row. Although long-term exposure to environmental irritants (dust, air pollution) can make you more prone to chronic bronchitis, smoking is by far the most common cause of this condition. If you keep smoking, repeated attacks of chronic bronchitis can eventually lead to serious lung damage (*see COPD, page 121*).

Treatments

The viruses that cause bronchitis do not respond to antibiotics—even though you may think you're sick enough to need them. Most cases of acute bronchitis clear up on their own within about two weeks, as long as you give your body what it needs most: plenty of rest and lots of fluids. You can treat a productive cough with over-the-counter expectorants and a lingering cough with suppressants. Bring down any fever with analgesics. Inhaling warm, moist air will also help clear your bronchial tubes.

Treatment options

Medications

OTC analgesics	Reduce fever and achiness.
Expectorants	Make it easier to bring up mucus.
Cough suppressants	For nagging but nonproductive cough.
Antibiotics	Needed only if secondary infection develops.
Bronchodilators	Open breathing tubes and ease coughing.

Lifestyle changes

Rest	What your body needs most.
Hydrate breathing tubes	Inhale steam or use a humidifier at night.
Keep air clean	Use an air purifier or AC with filter.

Natural methods

Fruits & vegetables	Vitamin C and flavonoids protect health.
Herbs	Soothe symptoms and build immunity.

For severe or persistent symptoms, your doctor may prescribe a bronchodilator medication so you can breathe more easily. You should you be treated with antibiotics only if you develop a secondary infection.

Medications

Start with over-the-counter medications. For fever or pain, an **analgesic** such as aspirin or acetaminophen (Tylenol) is a good choice. After that, what you take should be tailored to your symptoms.

- **If you have a wet cough,** your body is ridding itself of infected sputum. Let it. You need to use an **expectorant** containing guaifenesin (found in Robitussin and Sinumist-SR), which will help you bring up more sputum with every cough. Take a cough suppressant only at night, to help you sleep.
- **If you have a dry, hacking cough,** try a **cough suppressant** that contains the ingredient dextromethorphan (such as Sucrets 4-Hour or Vicks 44). The name of the cough medicine will end with "DM." If you're still coughing up sputum, a suppressant may make your symptoms worse or prolong your illness.
- **If you have dark yellowish-brown, thick sputum,** you may have developed a secondary infection. Especially if you have a high fever. Such an infection—more common in children, the elderly, and people with compromised immunity—can be treated with an **antibiotic** such as amoxicillin. Be sure to take the full course of the drug (usually 10 to 14 days), or your infection may return.
- **If you're constantly coughing or short of breath,** talk with your doctor about trying a **bronchodilator.** Also used to treat asthma, these inhalers contain short-acting beta2-agonists, with

TAKING Control

- **Get an annual pneumonia and flu vaccine. One pneumonia vaccination may last a lifetime, but you should probably get a flu shot every year.** Especially if you are over 65 or have chronic lung, heart, or kidney disease. It'll bolster your defenses against the viruses that cause bronchitis.

- **Avoid respiratory irritants.** Paint, dust, industrial fumes, and smoke can aggravate the lining of your bronchial tubes, making your cough worse. Consider using an air purifier or air conditioner to filter out such irritants.

- **Don't count on antibiotics if you smoke.** Recent research from Massachusetts General Hospital has found that antibiotics may be even less effective for smokers than for nonsmokers.

- **Don't smoke.** Just one puff of a cigarette can paralyze the cilia in your bronchial tubes. That can cause your current attack to last longer and make future attacks more likely.

▶**EVEN THOUGH ANTIBIOTICS ARE INEFFECTIVE against bronchitis-related viruses, a recent survey showed that 70% of patients with bronchitis symptoms asked for these medicines—and most doctors complied. This unfortunate practice needlessly exposes people to drugs they don't need (and to their side effects). It also promotes the growth of antibiotic-resistant bacteria. Always be certain that you have a bacterial infection before you ask for or take an antibiotic.**

Help from Herbs*

Certain herbs, long used in folk medicine, can bolster your immunity, soothe your cough, and loosen mucus.

For acute bronchitis
The following herbs are helpful for easing a bronchial cough:
- **Horehound** makes your cough more productive. You can fix horehound tea, or stir ½ to 1 teaspoon of liquid extract into a cup of hot water. Add honey to taste. Drink two or three cups of the tea every day until you start to feel better.

- **Slippery elm** coats your irritated throat with a gel-like substance. You can make a cup of slippery elm tea, or mix ½ to 1 teaspoon of liquid extract into a cup of hot water. Drink two or three cups a day until symptoms subside.

For chronic bronchitis
This group of herbs helps strengthen your immune system, enabling you to fight off recurrent problems. Their effectiveness diminishes with use, so rotate them over the course of a month.

- **Echinacea** helps cells produce a natural virus-fighter called interferon. At the first sign of bronchitis, start taking 200 mg of echinacea twice a day.
- **Astragalus** is used in Chinese traditional medicine to build stamina and vitality. Take 200 mg twice a day.
- **Pau d'arco** bolsters the body's defense against viral infections. Take 250 mg twice a day.
- **Medicinal mushrooms** (reishi or maitake) help ward off disease. Take 400 to 700 mg of either daily.

*Natural methods are not subject to the same testing and regulation as prescription medications. Please seek your doctor's advice and use caution.

▶ Am I at risk for contracting pneumonia?

In rare cases, germs can migrate from your bronchial tubes into your lungs, causing pneumonia. This usually affects children, the elderly, and people with weakened immune systems. Warning signals include a high fever (102° to 104°F), shaking chills, rust-colored sputum, and chest pain. If you have any of these symptoms call your doctor.

FINDING Support

- The National Jewish Medical and Research Center in Denver, CO, provides free information to help you quit smoking, clean your humidifier properly, and manage acute and chronic bronchitis and other respiratory diseases. You can call 1-800-222-5864 to speak with a nurse about your condition, or log on to their website at www.njc.org.

ingredients such as albuterol (Proventil, Ventolin) and salmeterol (Serevent). Inhalers relax the muscles around bronchial tubes, helping you breathe more easily.

Lifestyle Changes

In addition to taking medications, you can do a number of things to speed your recovery.
- **Rest.** Your body needs to recuperate, so call your boss and say you'll be taking a few days off. Now's a good time to catch up on sleep and open those books you've been meaning to read. (Besides, if you don't take it easy, you're likely to feel sick even longer.)
- **Drink plenty of fluids.** This will keep your mucous membranes moist, helping you to cough up sputum. Drink at least eight glasses of water or other clear liquids every day.
- **Keep nasal passages moist and clean.** Any type of moist air will help loosen sputum. Run a humidifier or vaporizer in your bedroom at night (clean your unit frequently with bleach to kill germs). Use an air purifier or air conditioner (with a clean filter) to remove dust, pollen, and other nasal irritants from the air.

Natural Methods*

Consuming the recommended five to nine daily servings of **fruits and vegetables** may prevent a future bronchitis attack. Both fruits and vegetables contain substances called flavonoids, which help protect cells throughout your body—including those in your bronchial tubes and lungs—from disease. Research in the Netherlands has found that eating plenty of foods rich in these substances can protect against chronic bronchitis. In addition, fruits and vegetables are excellent sources of vitamin C and beta-carotene, which bolster immunity. You can also turn to **herbal teas** and **immune-boosting herbs** (*see box above*).

Bursitis

It comes on as a dull ache and swelling in or around a joint. It usually follows strenuous activity. Bursitis can get pretty painful, but the basic treatment is fairly simple: Rest the sore joint and take an anti-inflammatory medication.

What is happening

Bursitis can hurt every bit as much as arthritis, although it isn't a joint disease. Instead, it affects fluid-filled sacs near joints, called bursae, that normally reduce friction between muscles and tendons and bones. When bursae become irritated, they fill with excess fluid. The pressure brings on a dull, persistent ache and a swelling in the joint that feels even worse when you move it.

Although bursitis can strike anyone, it develops most frequently in athletes, people who do manual labor, and couch potatoes who start to work out and overdo it. That's because overuse or injury is the most common cause of this condition. Bursitis typically affects the shoulder, but can also crop up in the elbow, hip, knee, or heel (or in any of the 150 bursae in the body). Bunions at the base of the big toe, for instance, are frequent triggers for bursitis.

Bursitis can be acute, or active for only a few days. It can be chronic, which means it lasts several weeks and recurs. If bacteria invade a bursa, they can cause septic bursitis (most common in the elbow). This infection can spread and become life threatening, so it must be treated right away. Most cases of bursitis are not serious and, if cared for, clear up in a week or two.

LIKELY First Steps

- **Rest and ice** the affected area. After swelling goes down, **apply heat**.
- **Anti-inflammatory medications** to reduce pain and swelling.
- **Stretching and strengthening exercises** once pain and swelling are gone.

QUESTIONS TO Ask

- If I have cortisone injections, will they ultimately damage my joint?
- Is there an underlying medical condition that might be responsible for my bursitis?
- When should I get either an x-ray or an MRI?

SHOULDER BURSITIS

inflamed shoulder bursa

clavicle

shoulder joint

deltoid muscle

The shoulder is one of the most common sites for bursitis, which occurs when the fluid-filled sac known as the bursa becomes irritated and fills with excess fluid. The swelling and pain that result can often be successfully treated with self-care measures and anti-inflammatory drugs.

- **Don't treat pain lightly.** If OTC painkillers haven't done much after a week, call your doctor about stronger prescription medications. Untreated pain can seriously impair your quality of life.

- **Try a low-impact sport while you're healing.** Switch to an exercise that won't bother your joint as you recover. Consider aquatic exercise, biking, and walking.

- **Don't stress your joints.** Don't rest your elbows on hard surfaces such as desks, and always use a cushioned pad if you kneel. Shoes that fit right will help prevent bunions that can trigger bursitis of the heel.

▶**What's the difference between arthritis and bursitis symptoms?**
Bursitis generally starts more abruptly than arthritis, and usually causes tenderness and swelling in one specific spot rather than all around the affected joint. Bursitis also typically allows much better range of motion than arthritis does. Be aware, though, that bursitis can be a sign that you're developing arthritis.

▶**I love tennis but have developed bursitis in my elbow. How can I ensure that it doesn't return?**
Warm up before you play and stretch afterward. Look into switching to a lighter racket, and make sure whatever racket you use has the right size grip for you. Invest in some tennis lessons or clinics to make sure you're using the proper technique.

Treatment options

Lifestyle changes

Rest	Allows injured bursa to heal.
Ice/heat	Ice to reduce swelling, then heat for stiffness.
Exercise	Start slowly; always stretch first.

Medications

NSAIDs	OTC or, if needed, prescription painkillers.
Corticosteroid injections	Relieve persistent, inflammatory pain.

Procedures

Diathermy/ultrasound	Improves blood flow around the area.
Bursa drainage	Relieves painful pressure.

Natural methods

Alternative therapies	Acupuncture and chiropractic ease pain.

Treatments

The main goal in treating bursitis is to ease pain and swelling until the condition resolves itself. In many cases, the inflammation will clear up with simple steps you can take at home and with OTC painkillers. But if the pain lingers for more than a week or so or recurs, make an appointment with your doctor. You may need prescription anti-inflammatory medications or other therapies.

Lifestyle Changes

When bursitis flares up, the following self-care tips can help:

- **Rest the part of your body that hurts.** Stop whatever activity caused the problem until you're pain-free. You can protect the area with an elastic bandage, sling, brace, or splint.
- **Use ice until the swelling goes down.** Apply it for 20 minutes, three to four times a day, until the sore spot is no longer warm to the touch.
- **Use heat to reduce joint stiffness** once the area isn't warm or red. Try a heat pack or heating pad, sit in a whirlpool, or soak in a warm bath. But if swelling reappears, go back to ice.
- **Stretch before and after doing anything strenuous.** Start any activity slowly, use proper technique, and don't push too hard.
- **Avoid repetitive movements.** If that's not possible, take frequent breaks to rest your joints and stretch your muscles.
- **When you feel better, lose extra weight.** Carrying excess pounds only puts extra pressure on susceptible joints.

Medications

You'll want to relieve pain and swelling as quickly as possible, for example, by using an **NSAID (nonsteroidal anti-inflammatory**

drug). The most commonly used are OTC drugs such as aspirin, ibuprofen (Advil, Motrin), and naproxen (Aleve), and, if pain is more severe, prescription NSAIDs, such as diclofenac (Voltaren), ketoprofen (Orudis), or nabumetone (Relafen). If you find that these are not strong enough, talk to your doctor about **COX-2 inhibitors,** such as celecoxib (Celebrex) or rofecoxib (Vioxx).

If your pain and swelling persist, you may need an injection of a **corticosteroid,** such as methylprednisolone (Depo-Medrol) or betamethasone (Celestone). Your doctor will probably inject a **local anesthetic,** such as lidocaine, directly into the bursa at the same time. The injection decreases inflammation so you can participate in rehab and resume your normal activities. You should be pain-free when you leave your doctor's office. For full relief, you may need to repeat the injection, but there's a limit to how many shots you can have: Steroids can weaken nearby cartilage or tendons.

An infection that develops in a bursa is treated with an **oral antibiotic** such as fluoroquinolone (Cipro), cephalexin (Cefanex), or amoxicillin/clauvulanate (Augmentin).

Procedures

Your doctor or physical therapist may want to try **deep heat therapy** (called diathermy) or **ultrasound,** which emits gentle sound-wave vibrations, to warm tissues and improve blood flow around the area affected by your bursitis. If your bursa is chronically infected, you may need a surgical procedure called an **incision and drainage** (known as an I and D). The doctor numbs your skin, opens the bursa, and drains the infected fluid. If, as rarely happens, bursitis doesn't clear up after 6 to 12 months, surgery may be needed to repair damage and relieve pressure in the bursa. This may be conventional surgery (called **open release surgery**) or less-invasive **arthroscopic capsular release surgery.**

Untreated, bursitis (especially in the shoulder) can lead to calcium deposits in the bursa that can cause a permanent lack of mobility and flexibility in the joint (frozen shoulder). In extreme cases, if a bursa has become stiff and hardened with calcification, the calcium deposit may have to be **surgically removed,** so resist the temptation to "tough out" the pain of bursitis without treating it.

Natural Methods*

The traditional Chinese healing technique **acupuncture** can ease bursitis pain. Acupuncture needles seem to trigger the release of endorphins and monoamines, chemicals that block pain signals in the spinal cord and brain. Seeing a **chiropractor** may help too. A spinal adjustment may free restricted movement of bones and release painful muscle tension. There is some disagreement about whether **massage** on or near a bursitis site is wise. Massage of surrounding muscles by a skilled therapist, however, can stimulate circulation to speed healing. Rubbing in **capsaicin cream,** made from the ingredient that gives chili peppers their heat, can encourage blood flow to the area, promoting relaxation and bringing pain relief.

Promising
DEVELOPMENTS

■ If you need surgery to relieve your bursitis, there's something new on the horizon to help you deal with postoperative pain. A recent study looked at the placement of a catheter for direct delivery of the **nerve block drug bupivacaine** into the joint following arthroscopic surgery. All patients with the catheter were able to perform range-of-motion exercises virtually pain-free. Consequently, 95% of them had near-complete restoration of range of motion without pain once the catheter was removed.

FINDING **Support**

■ The National Institute of Arthritis and Musculoskeletal and Skin Diseases Information Clearinghouse provides information about bone, muscle, and skin diseases, as well as various forms of arthritis and rheumatic disease (1-877-22-NIAMS or www.niams.nih.gov).

■ The American College of Rheumatology, in Atlanta, GA, is a national professional organization. It can help you with a referral to a rheumatologist or to another health specialist, such as a physical therapist. Fact sheets as well as lists of specialists by geographic area are available on the website at www. rheumatology.org, or call 404-633-3777.

*Natural methods are not subject to the same testing and regulation as prescription medications. Please seek your doctor's advice and use caution.

Carpal tunnel syndrome

In most cases the treatment for this painful condition is literally in your own hands. And if you act quickly at the first hint of symptoms, you can probably head off a full-blown flare-up, avoid costly trips to the doctor—and even prevent surgery.

LIKELY First Steps

- **Rest** the affected area to reduce swelling.
- **Take medications** to ease pain and inflammation.
- **Wear a wrist splint** to provide support.
- **Do exercises** to strengthen muscles and ligaments and prevent recurrences.

QUESTIONS TO Ask

- Is it possible that my CTS is due to another, undiagnosed medical condition?
- How long will it take until these treatments start to work?
- Do I need to switch careers or give up my hobby?
- How likely is it that I will need to undergo surgery?

What is happening

Carpal tunnel syndrome (CTS) usually begins gradually, with a numbness and tingling in your thumb, index, and middle fingers. It may come and go at this level for years, but sooner or later, your whole hand and wrist may begin to hurt much of the time. You may even have trouble doing simple things like picking up your coffee cup or twisting a doorknob. In especially severe cases, pain may spread up your arm to your shoulder. It could get so bad that it jolts you awake at night.

The cause of this wide range of symptoms is inflamed tendons or ligaments. They put pressure on the median nerve that runs through a narrow "tunnel" of wrist bones (carpals) and under the carpal ligament at the base of your palm. There can be many reasons for this inflammation. The most common culprit is forceful and repetitive hand movements. And while you may be quick to cite your computer as the source of the problem, this is far from established. In fact, a 2001 study reported in the journal *Neurology* found that regular computer users developed carpal tunnel syndrome at about the same rate as those who worked on them only occasionally.

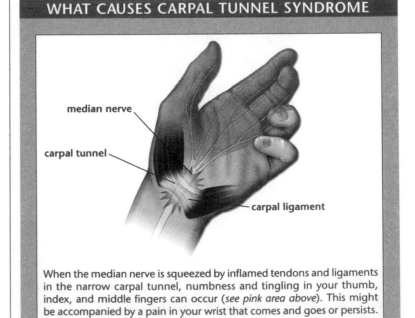

WHAT CAUSES CARPAL TUNNEL SYNDROME

median nerve

carpal tunnel

carpal ligament

When the median nerve is squeezed by inflamed tendons and ligaments in the narrow carpal tunnel, numbness and tingling in your thumb, index, and middle fingers can occur (*see pink area above*). This might be accompanied by a pain in your wrist that comes and goes or persists.

Treatment options

Lifestyle changes

Rest hand & wrist	Use a wrist splint until pain subsides.
Exercise	To improve function and reduce weight.
Limit activities	Avoid tasks involving repetitive movements.

Medications

NSAIDs	OTC or prescription to reduce inflammation.
Diuretics	Decrease fluids in the body.
Corticosteriod shots	For swelling, if NSAIDs/diuretics don't work.

Procedures

Surgery	A last resort, but often effective.

Natural methods

Acupuncture	Helps relieve pain.
Chiropractic	To release pressure on nerve.

Computer user or not, if you're a woman between the ages of 30 and 60, you're more susceptible to carpal tunnel syndrome. No one is sure quite why. It may have something to do with oral contraceptives or hormonal changes that accompany pregnancy and menopause. CTS is also more likely to develop if you have another underlying medical condition, such as an underactive thyroid, diabetes, or rheumatoid arthritis.

Hobbies and leisure activities can also contribute to CTS. If you're an overly aggressive knitter, fanatical garden-weeder, or gung-ho guitarist, you could be a candidate. And being overweight or a smoker will definitely increase your risk.

Treatments

Remedying CTS starts with four important Rs: rest, relief of pain and inflammation, rebuilding your muscles, and retraining yourself to perform daily activities differently. Add light exercise and visits to a physical therapist and you're likely to feel as good as new. Only a small percentage of cases ever need surgery.

But even when you're symptom-free, you're not off the hook. You'll need to keep CTS from recurring by tackling whatever caused it in the first place. This might mean losing some weight, treating an underlying medical condition, quitting smoking, or making your work area more user-friendly.

Lifestyle Changes

Many CTS treatment options involve things you can easily do on your own. Your doctor will tell you to **rest your affected hand and wrist** for at least two weeks so the inflammation can subside. This

TAKING Control

- **Keep your hands warm.** Working in a cold environment can contribute to hand pain. If it's not possible to turn up the heat, wear fingerless gloves.

- **Try voice recognition software.** If it's painful to use a keyboard, there are a variety of software packages available (ViaVoice, Nuance) that allow you to use a computer virtually hands-free.

- **Eat more apples and more onions.** Both of these foods are major sources of quercetin, a particularly powerful member of a group of plant pigments called flavonoids. With its proven anti-inflammatory properties, quercetin can help reduce inflammation in your joints and muscles.

▶ **SUPPLEMENTING YOUR DIET** with vitamin B_6 (pyridoxine) could help decrease the inflammation that produces CTS symptoms, and it may also improve your circulation. Another theory is that B_6 boosts the output of GABA (gamma-aminobutyric acid), a neurotransmitter that helps to control pain. If your discomfort is particularly severe, look for capsules or tablets containing pyridoxal-5-phosphate (P-5-P), the biologically active form of B_6, and take 50 mg three times a day. You can also get vitamin B_6 from fish, chickpeas, avocados, and bananas.

Exercises to Keep You CTS-Free

Performing a few stretches and gentle exercises every day can help relieve pain and gradually improve function in your hands and wrists. These movements double as preventive exercises, since toning and stretching muscles and ligaments guards them against future injury.

You can do these exercises in any order you wish, and repeat each one as many times as you like. Do them once a day, or even every hour, if necessary, for quick relief.

1. Lift your arms above your head and rotate them inward and outward.

2. Extend your arms in front of you and circle your hands at the wrists. Circle them first one way, then the other.

3. Hold your hands, palms up, in front of you. Close your fingers into your palms. Open your fingers as far as is comfortable, feeling the gentle stretch for a few seconds, then close them again.

4. Position your hands with your palms facing each other. Press your fingertips together. Hold for a few seconds, then release.

5. Wrap a rubber band around the fingers of one hand, so it reaches from your thumb to your pinkie. Spread your fingers. Hold for a few seconds, then release. Do the same using your other hand.

Promising
DEVELOPMENTS

■ Someday, when surgery is required, a technique called **percutaneous balloon carpal tunnel-plasty** may be able to relieve carpal tunnel syndrome without cutting the carpal ligament. The surgeon will insert a balloon under the ligament through a tiny incision in the palm, and inflate the balloon with saline solution. That stretches the ligament and takes pressure off the nerve. In one small study, every patient who had this procedure experienced relief from symptoms with no complications.

means temporarily staying away from any activity—whether it's cooking or caulking—that forces you to bend your wrist all the way up or down or puts pressure on the median nerve.

You can work on reducing the pain at the same time. To do this, **apply cold compresses** to the painful area for 15 minutes at a time, several times a day. This will also help bring down swelling. And while any form of exercise may seem too painful to think about, studies have shown that **yoga** can be beneficial for CTS. Not only do yoga postures stretch and strengthen the muscles of your upper body, they also promote the release of endorphins, the body's natural painkillers. Do some **stretching and strengthening exercises** daily to relieve pain and prevent recurrence (*see box above*).

It's just as important to **take a good look at your activities** and change any bad habits. To start:

■ **Take breaks from repetitive tasks.** If you're practicing the piano, for instance, take a 5-minute break every 15 minutes.

■ **Practice good posture,** and adapt it to the job you're performing. If you sit at a desk, for example, make sure your shoulders don't slump forward (this puts pressure on nerves in your back and arms).

■ **Modify your workspace.** If possible, choose ergonomically sound devices, such as a chair with a supportive backrest, an adjustable keyboard table, and a wrist rest (found at most office supply stores).

Once you've dealt with the pain, consider some larger lifestyle issues in order to keep CTS from recurring. **Losing weight** may be one of them. Obesity has been frequently linked to carpal tunnel syndrome. Extra tissue appears to put undue pressure on nerves in the hand and wrist, and obese people are predisposed to diabetes, which can be an underlying cause of CTS. **If you smoke, stop.** Smoking can aggravate CTS by restricting blood flow to the small blood vessels of the hand.

Medications

To relieve pain and swelling, your doctor will likely start with over-the-counter **nonsteroidal anti-inflammatory drugs** (NSAIDs), such as aspirin, ibuprofen (Advil), or naproxen (Aleve). If inflammation and pain persist, you may need a more powerful prescription NSAID, such as the COX-2 inhibitors celecoxib (Celebrex), rofecoxib (Vioxx), and valdecoxib (Bextra). A **diuretic** such as trichlormethiazide (Naqua) may also be beneficial.

If none of these drugs work, you may require an injection of a **corticosteroid medication** (such as Depo-Medrol) directly into your carpal tunnel. This can reduce the inflammation for at least a month. To protect your tendon from lasting damage, don't have more than three injections altogether.

If a medical condition (such as an underactive thyroid) is contributing to your CTS, your doctor will advise you about medications for the underlying disorder.

Procedures

Once your pain is under control, your best bet is to set up regular visits with a physical therapist for supervised **hand-and-wrist strengthening exercises.** You'll probably have to stick with this program for at least two months to see improvement.

Your doctor may suggest that you wear a **wrist splint** to keep your wrist from bending. You'll mainly wear the splint at night: As you sleep, you may unconsciously bend your wrist forward or back, aggravating the problem. You can wear it during the day if the pain bothers you. Your best bet is to continue using the splint until you're pain-free for at least two weeks. If your problem perseveres, your doctor may want to completely immobilize your wrist and forearm in a **plaster cast.**

If pain persists—even when you've followed your doctor's instructions to the letter—**surgery** may be required to cut the carpal ligament and relieve pressure from the median nerve. The most common procedure is **open carpal tunnel release (OCTR).** It requires a small incision in your palm and wrist. Results are generally good, especially if you have physical therapy after the scar heals. A new outpatient procedure called **endoscopic carpal tunnel release (ECTR)** has received a lot of buzz. Only two tiny incisions are made—one in your palm and one in your wrist. A telescope-like device called an endoscope is then inserted, allowing the surgeon to see inside the carpal tunnel at the point of pressure and make the cut. Recovery is often quicker with ECTR, but the jury is still out on recurrence rates after the surgery.

Natural Methods*

Before resorting to surgery, you might consider two other less conventional therapies. One is **acupuncture,** a centuries-old Chinese technique in which thin needles are inserted into key points on your body to relieve pain. The other involves a visit to your local **chiropractor.** In addition to manipulating your spine, the chiropractor can release pressure on the median nerve.

▶ **How can I tell for certain that my problem is carpal tunnel syndrome?**
Most doctors rely on your symptoms and their physical examination to diagnose CTS. If there is any doubt, your doctor will probably perform the "gold standard" diagnostic tests: electromyography (EMG) locates the nerve compression, and the nerve conduction velocity (NCV) test measures any motor delay in your nerve fibers. The doctor may also order magnetic resonance imaging (MRI) to show the area of compression.

▶ **If my carpal tunnel syndrome developed at work, is it covered under workers' compensation?**
It may be if your doctor is willing to state a belief that your condition is related to the work you do. To make a convincing case, your doctor will first have to rule out other causes, such as obesity, smoking, hormonal changes, genetic factors, and a wide array of medical conditions. These include diabetes, rheumatoid arthritis, lupus, hypothyroidism, chronic kidney disease, hepatitis C, and any condition that damages the muscles and bones.

FINDING Support

■ For up-to-date information on repetitive stress injuries and access to support groups for people with CTS, contact the Cumulative Trauma Disorders (CTD) Resource Network in Los Banos, CA (209-826-8443 or www.ctdrn.org).

Natural methods are not subject to the same testing and regulation as prescription medications. Please seek your doctor's advice and use caution.

Cataracts

Vision fuzzy? Feel like your glasses always need cleaning? You may be among the 1.5 million Americans slated for cataract surgery this year. Thanks to new surgical procedures, it's likely your eyesight will soon be as good as new.

LIKELY **First Steps**

- **A specialized eye examination** by an ophthalmologist to determine where the cataracts are located, if they're in one or both eyes, and how far the condition has advanced.

- **An assessment of your vision impairment** to find out whether you need surgery soon, just a follow-up appointment.

- Discussion with your doctor about possible procedures for **eye surgery** and how much time you should reserve for recovery.

QUESTIONS TO **Ask**

- Are there ways I can protect my eyes so my cataracts won't get worse?

- Will my other eye problems affect the outcome of my cataract surgery?

- Will I go blind if I don't have surgery?

- Will I need glasses or contacts even though I've had a lens implant?

- Will my children develop cataracts because I have them?

What is happening

Hanging suspended in a transparent capsule, just behind the pupil of your eye, is a clear lens. Its function is to make your vision sharp. But just about the time you cross the midpoint of life and head for your 60s and 70s, the lens often starts to become unreliable. Its protein fibers gradually begin to clump together, like sugar congealing in a container of maple syrup that causes a cloudiness that's known as a **cataract**.

When you look at something, light rays reflected from the object enter your eye through the cornea and the lens. The lens focuses the light onto the retina at the back of your eye, and it sends the image to your brain. When a cataract develops, the light rays are no longer precisely focused. They scatter before reaching the retina. Most people who get cataracts get them on the lens of both eyes, but not necessarily at the same time. In its earliest stages, a cataract may not cause a vision problem. But as the protein fibers begin to clump further and then break down, images dim. Colors fade and distinctions between light and dark turn fuzzy. Double vision may occur.

How much and how fast your vision is impaired depends not only on the size and density of the cataract but also on what type it is. There are several variations, and more than one type can develop in the same eye. Most common is a **nuclear cataract,** which occurs inside the core, or nucleus, of the lens. If it forms on the rear of the lens capsule, it's a **posterior subcapsular cataract.** When it affects the outer part of the lens, nearest the dome of the cornea, doctors call it a **cortical cataract.** A cataract on the edge of the cornea has little effect on vision. That's because it doesn't interfere with the passage of light through the center of the lens. A dense nuclear cataract causes severe blurring.

Although cataracts can form at any age—babies are occasionally born with them—most occur in later life. In fact, by the time you reach age 75 or so, your risk of having a cataract is equivalent to coming up "tails" with the flip of a coin—about 1 in 2. A number of factors increase that risk even more: smoking, lots of exposure to bright sunlight, and long-term oral corticosteroid use (especially at high doses). You are more likely to develop cataracts if you have a related health problem, such as glaucoma, diabetes, high blood pressure (hypertension), or an immune-system disease like rheumatoid arthritis. Genetics, too, can play a role. Far and away, the most dominant risk factor is aging.

Treatment options

Procedures

Phacoemulsification	Most common surgery; no sutures needed.
ECCE	Same success as phaco; sutures needed.
ICCE	Done very rarely, for special situations.

Lifestyle changes

Quit smoking	Reduces incidence; may improve sight.
Avoid too much sun	More than doubles cataract risk; harms lens.
Improve lighting	To reduce glare when doing close work.
Antioxidant foods	Fresh fruits and vegetables protect lens.

Treatments

Cataracts don't clear up on their own and no current medications, supplements, or eye exercises can reverse their development. The only way to restore your sight is to surgically remove the original lens before the problem gets worse. That said, if a cataract is at an early stage and not interfering with your vision, your eye doctor (ophthalmologist) will probably suggest you come in for a second checkup after six months. The presence of a cataract may even cause your close-up eyesight to improve temporarily (a phenomenon called "second sight"). You might be able to wait a while before getting any treatment. Cataracts can stop getting worse after a certain point. That's rare, but many people successfully delay cataract surgery for years.

Newer surgical techniques have eliminated the need to wait for a cataract to "ripen" (become totally opaque) before removal. Once you feel that the cataract is interfering with your everyday activities, it's time to proceed. In most surgeries, a synthetic UV-protective intraocular lens (IOL) is implanted to restore clear sight. In the small number of cases in which a lens can't be implanted, contact lenses or special cataract glasses with very powerful magnification are used. Don't postpone surgery indefinitely. Failing to fix your cataract when you need to could eventually lead to blindness.

Procedures

Even if your doctor says you are developing cataracts in both eyes, only one eye is treated at a time. Before scheduling surgery, an ultrasound evaluation measures the length of your eyeball. If you are having an artificial intraocular lens implanted, the doctor uses the results to select a lens with the appropriate curvature and power. This enables your vision to return to "normal" after surgery (though you may still need to wear prescription eyeglasses).

TAKING Control

■ **If you smoke, give it up.** Smoking doesn't cause cataracts, but research shows that this eye condition develops much more rapidly and more frequently in those who smoke. In fact, some of the damage caused by smoking may be reversed if you stop right away.

■ **Shield your eyes from bright sunlight.** A mild cataract condition is likely to get worse if your eyes are exposed to ultraviolet (UV) rays. Wear a wide-brimmed hat and sunglasses to protect your eyes from both UVA and UVB rays.

■ **Ask someone to help you after surgery.** Although the outpatient cataract procedure is simple and painless, you will need someone to drive you home from the clinic or hospital afterward. For the next few days, while your eyes are adjusting, you will need someone to drive for you and help you with household chores, especially those that require exertion.

■ **If a second eye needs surgery, don't wait too long.** In a study of cataract patients in England, doctors found the best results among those who had the second eye treated within six months. Those who waited 7 to 12 months often reported difficulties with depth perception, especially when walking and driving. Discuss your particular situation with your doctor.

►Will I need to repeat cataract surgery?

It is very rare to need a second operation, unless some adjustment needs to be made in the placement of the lens. About one in three people who has the surgery later develops another condition known as a secondary cataract. It may require a laser treatment.

The problem occurs when the remaining membrane of the lens capsule gradually becomes cloudy and begins to interfere with your vision the same way the original cataract did. The routine treatment is called YAG laser capsulotomy (YAG stands for yttrium aluminum garnet). Painless applications of this ultra-high-powered light open a tiny hole in the lens membrane. Once light can pierce this newly created opening, clear sight is restored.

►Can other vision problems be corrected during cataract surgery?

If what's called a single-focus intraocular lens is being implanted, your doctor may be able to adjust it to correct nearsightedness (myopia) or farsightedness (presbyopia). Other intraocular lenses, which have bifocal or multifocal capabilities, are also now being used. These work like bifocal glasses, allowing you to focus up close on a page if you're reading or far away if you're walking or driving. A new toric lens can be implanted to correct for astigmatism—a lens-shape irregularity that distorts vision.

Surgery for cataracts is safe and reliable: The success rate for all procedures is greater than 98%. No matter which one you have, it won't take more than an hour. Then you'll be allowed to go home. Some precautions are necessary during recuperation (*see box opposite*), but most people can resume normal activities within a couple of weeks.

Several kinds of surgery are recommended. With each, you follow a similar routine. You'll probably be given a sedative and a local anesthetic, but will be awake during the operation. If the doctor thinks you might be overly anxious, or if you're allergic to local anesthetics, you might be given general anesthesia.

■ **Phacoemulsification (phaco)** is the most common procedure for removing cataracts. To begin, the cataract is emulsified (or shattered) by ultrasound, which reduces the protein in the lens to small extractable pieces (*see illustration below*). The same ultrasound probe is used to suction out the particles. The surgeon then inserts a quarter-inch plastic or silicone intraocular lens through the original incision. Once the lens is in place and the tube is removed, the tiny slit is stitched closed or allowed to seal itself. You may need to wear an eye shield, mainly during sleep, for a few weeks after the procedure.

■ **Extracapsular cataract extraction (ECCE)** is an older and equally effective procedure some doctors continue to use. Rather than shatter the cataract into tiny bits, the surgeon cuts an exit just wide enough to inject a small quantity of clear gel to keep the space from collapsing. A needle is then inserted into the incision and through the pupil to open the front portion of the lens capsule, and the cataract is slipped out with tiny forceps. A lens is usually implanted at the same time, and the incision is closed with several sutures.

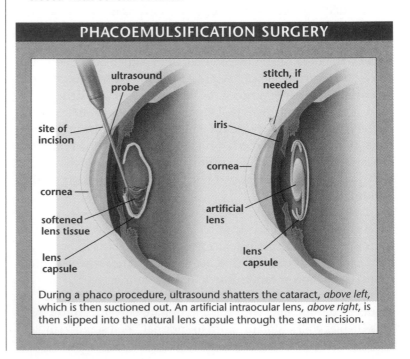

PHACOEMULSIFICATION SURGERY

ultrasound probe

stitch, if needed

site of incision

iris

cornea

cornea

softened lens tissue

artificial lens

lens capsule

lens capsule

During a phaco procedure, ultrasound shatters the cataract, *above left*, which is then suctioned out. An artificial intraocular lens, *above right*, is then slipped into the natural lens capsule through the same incision.

To make sure you don't injure the repaired eye or create complications that could harm your sight, this is what many doctors recommend for the days and weeks following cataract surgery:

- Avoid touching or rubbing your eye.
- Apply eyedrops to promote the healing process. You may not be required to wear an eye shield to protect your eye from injury. Many doctors don't use them anymore.
- Take ibuprofen (Advil) or acetaminophen (Tylenol) to relieve discomfort. Avoid taking aspirin: It can promote bleeding.
- Don't drive for at least three days. Before you get behind the wheel again, make sure you are comfortable with your distance vision and not distracted by sun glare or brightness.
- Wear dark glasses until you adjust to vision changes, especially if bright lights or full sunlight bother you.
- Sleep on your back in the weeks after the operation or turn the untreated side of your head toward the pillow. This prevents a buildup of pressure in the treated eye.
- Avoid lifting heavy objects or taking part in strenuous exercise. These activities can also increase pressure in the eye.

- **Intracapsular cataract extraction (ICCE),** performed in less than 1% of cases, removes the entire lens and its supporting structure. A special lens can be implanted, or you may be given eyeglasses or contact lenses. ICCE is usually recommended for someone who is extremely nearsighted or who has another eye disorder, such as glaucoma (*see page 139*).

After surgery, your doctor may prescribe antibiotic eyedrops to help prevent infection, steroid drops for inflammation, and an OTC pain reliever for discomfort. If you have excessive pain or inflammation, contact your doctor right away.

Most doctors schedule a follow-up examination the day after surgery. After that, you may not need to see the doctor for another month. As soon as your vision stabilizes, you can have it tested. You may need prescription glasses or contacts to improve upon the capabilities of the artificial lens. After a few months you may need to have the prescription changed.

Lifestyle Changes

You can't reverse cataracts, but making a few lifestyle changes can help you cope with vision problems and maybe slow their progress. **Quitting smoking** and **avoiding too much sun** (*see "Taking Control," page 75*) are two immediate steps you can take. Using a **reading light** the right way can make a difference. If glare gives you trouble, try sitting as close as possible to your reading lamp with the light shining over one shoulder. Try a 50-watt incandescent flood (not spot) if standard 60- to 100-watt bulbs cause a problem.

You may also be able to retard the development of cataracts by **eating plenty of nutrient-rich fruits and vegetables.** High in vitamins C and E and beta-carotene, these antioxidant compounds (also available in supplement form) help squelch free radicals—the unstable oxygen molecules that can weaken the delicate cell structure in the lens of the eye.

Promising
DEVELOPMENTS

- An experimental technique using a **laser device** may prove to be the most effective way to break cataracts into tiny particles needed for a phaco procedure (*see illustration opposite*). Research suggests this laser technique is gentler than the routinely used ultrasound and less likely to contribute to other eye problems. A number of eye centers in the United States are currently participating in clinical trials. Ask your doctor if such a center is located near you.

FINDING Support

- For the latest information on vision disorders and current clinical trials, contact the National Eye Institute in Bethesda, MD (301-496-5248 or www.nei.nih.gov).

Chronic fatigue syndrome

The origin of this elusive, debilitating illness remains unclear, even though half a million Americans suffer from its aches, pains, and persistent tiredness. A multifaceted approach may be the best way to boost your vitality and ease symptoms.

LIKELY First Steps

- Begin medical treatments, such as **pain relievers** for muscle aches and **sleep aids** for insomnia.
- Consider **antidepressants** or **anxiety relievers.** Depression or anxiety may be making you feel worse.
- Ease gradually into a regular **exercise program.** Pace yourself as you go.
- Find a counselor trained in **cognitive-behavioral therapy.**

QUESTIONS TO Ask

- Could an underactive thyroid be causing or worsening my fatigue? Can you test for this?
- Could I have Lyme disease?
- What can I do to improve my focus and concentration?
- Will I be tired for the rest of my life? How can I deal with that?
- Why do some doctors doubt that CFS exists?

What is happening

Doctors aren't sure why chronic fatigue syndrome (CFS) develops, although you may remember having had a bad cold or flu before coming down with this malady. Its lingering exhaustion, sore throat, problems with memory and concentration, muscle and joint pain, headaches, depression, and myriad other symptoms can make it difficult to work, sleep, or go about your daily activities.

It's hard to know why CFS produces such a wide variety of problems, because little is known about the basic illness and how it affects your body. One theory is that CFS is due to an overactive or underactive immune system, so you may hear it referred to as chronic fatigue immune dysfunction syndrome (CFIDS). Another theory is that a virus or other germs may be to blame, even though no single infection has been pinpointed. Imbalances in stress hormones and brain chemicals and abnormally low blood pressure have been noted in some people with CFS. That suggests that nervous system abnormalities play a role. In Europe, CFS is often referred to as myalgic encephalomyelitis (ME), which means brain and muscle inflammation. Researchers still cannot find any consistent patterns to explain the far-flung symptoms. It may well be that CFS results from a combination of factors.

CFS is a relatively new disease—it was first reported in medical journals in the 1980s, though earlier case histories suggest that it has probably been around much longer—and many disagree sharply about its definition and causes. Therefore it may be difficult to find a doctor who knows how to treat it properly. Some physicians dismiss it as being psychosomatic, or "all in your head." Given the scope of the problem, however, an increasing number of healthcare professionals are becoming versed in the care and management of chronic fatigue syndrome.

Treatments

Even though CFS has no known cause or cure, treating your symptoms will make you feel much better. A variety of therapies can help you improve enough to eventually resume all or most of the activities you enjoyed before becoming ill. You will most likely benefit from what's called a "multidisciplinary" approach, which combines conventional medicines with lifestyle changes, an exercise program, and counseling. Self-care is very important. A healthy eating program, scaling back on activities, getting plenty of rest, reducing stress, and

Treatment options

Medications

NSAIDs	For related muscle aches and pains.
Antidepressants	Promote sleep and help outlook.

Lifestyle changes

Moderate exercise	Start slow and build up.
Energy diary	Helps you plan for energy highs and lows.
Good diet	Provides nutritious underpinning.
Improve sleep habits	Important to combat fatigue.

Procedures

Psychotherapy	Cognitive-behavioral therapy for stress.

Natural methods

Relaxation techniques	Reduce stress and increase sense of control.
Acupuncture	Decreases pain and increases energy for some.
Nutritional supplements	Selected herbs and vitamins can help.

learning to accept your symptoms and limitations will go a long way toward getting you on the road to recovery. You may also find relief in various alternative therapies, such as acupuncture and relaxation techniques. An increasing number of mainstream physicians now take these approaches seriously.

Medications

No medicines will "cure" CFS, but some may relieve specific symptoms. For sore muscles and other aches, acetaminophen (Tylenol) or **NSAIDs** (nonsteroidal anti-inflammatory drugs) may bring relief. The latter include pain and inflammation relievers, such as aspirin or ibuprofen (Advil): Use them with care because NSAIDs may cause gastrointestinal bleeding and other side effects. Newer prescription anti-inflammatories **(COX-2 inhibitors)** such as celecoxib (Celebrex) may be safer. Long-term studies are continuing.

   Antidepressant drugs may also help relieve symptoms and treat underlying depression. The older tricyclic drugs, which include amitriptyline (Elavil) and doxepin (Sinequan), may be more effective than newer ones, such as the SSRIs fluoxetine (Prozac) and nefazodone (Serzone). Recent studies suggest tricyclics promote deep sleep and impede nerve pathways that transmit pain. Other treatments may improve sleep (*see Insomnia, page 188*), relieve digestive problems (*see Heartburn, page 161*), or alleviate additional CFS symptoms.

Lifestyle Changes

Adjustments to your daily routines can pay big dividends in how you feel. Here are some suggestions:

TAKING Control

■ **Choose a doctor** who is knowledgeable about chronic fatigue syndrome. Many physicians are unfamiliar with this illness. Some are even dismissive of it. Patient associations and support groups may help you find a good practitioner (*see "Finding Support," page 81*). Doctors and therapists trained in pain management or headaches may also have skills for treating your symptoms.

■ **Take it easy.** It's important to set limits and realistic goals. You may have to forego many of the activities you enjoyed before becoming ill, at least for a time. Find new interests or hobbies that work better with your restricted schedule.

■ **Deal with your feelings.** Helplessness and depression are common with CFS, but new classes of drugs can really help. Your goal is to feel better. Don't be embarrassed about taking drugs or seeking out a professional psychotherapist.

▶ **When can I expect to start feeling better?**
If you start a program outlined by a doctor familiar with chronic fatigue syndrome, you will begin to feel considerably better in as little as two or three weeks. That's because your physician will be selecting medications aimed at your most troubling symptoms, such as poor sleep or persistent muscle aches. When your symptoms diminish, your overall energy will improve considerably.

Promising
DEVELOPMENTS

- A nutritional supplement called **ENADA** may aid some men and women with chronic fatigue syndrome, according to results from a small pilot study at Georgetown University Medical Center in Washington, D.C. The supplement contains an active ingredient called NADH, which is related to the B vitamin niacin. Patients took 10 mg of ENADA on an empty stomach every morning for four weeks. Symptoms eased in 8 of 26 people who took the supplement, compared to only two people on a dummy pill. The researchers are expanding the study to evaluate more test subjects.

*Natural methods are not subject to the same testing and regulation as prescription medications. Please seek your doctor's advice and use caution.

- **Do some moderate exercise** if you can, but don't be overly ambitious. Exercising too strenuously can cause extreme fatigue or a relapse. A limited exercise program, supervised by a doctor or physical therapist, may be the best approach. The key is to take it slow. Very gradually increase your level of exertion, stopping before you become tired. Start with stretching exercises (one or two minutes a day), modest aerobic activities (such as walking 10 minutes three times a week, climbing the stairs in your home, or lifting groceries). Add some light weights (two pounds), with only a few repetitions, several times a day. Two 10-minute sessions on a treadmill may be better than a single 20-minute workout. Try to breathe deeply, using the muscles of your diaphragm rather than the upper lungs. Deep breathing improves exercise tolerance and it promotes relaxation.
- **Keep an energy diary** to record your ebbs and flows during the day. Schedule activities for times when you tend to have the most stamina. An occupational therapist can help you maximize your endurance at work and at home.
- **Eat a well-balanced diet** rich in fruits and vegetables to make sure you get the nutrients you need.
- **Practice good "sleep hygiene."** Choose a regular bedtime. Stay away from caffeine or exertion several hours before sleep. Use your bed for sleeping or sex, not reading or watching television. If you awaken during the night, don't toss and turn. Get up and read for a few minutes before going back to bed.

Procedures

A number of studies have shown that a type of short-term psychological counseling called **cognitive-behavioral therapy** can ease your distress, boost confidence, and help you better manage the stresses that you are experiencing. This approach can also help you set limits, meet challenges, and attain goals. A skilled cognitive-behavioral therapist will introduce you to new ways of thinking about your illness, so you can overcome pessimistic thoughts and reactions and regain a sense of control.

Rather than thinking you'll never again be able to play with your kids, for example, the therapist might help you focus on treatments that help you move ahead one step at a time. A study at London's King's College Hospital found that after six months, 70% of people with CFS who had cognitive-behavioral therapy felt better. That was true of only 16% of patients who practiced relaxation techniques but didn't have therapy. At follow-up interviews five years later, the researchers found that many patients still felt better and opted to continue this therapy on their own.

Natural Methods*

A number of mind-body techniques, as well as certain herbs and vitamins, can be useful in easing specific CFS symptoms.
- **Relaxation techniques,** such as yoga or meditation, can reduce stress levels and help regain a sense of control over your illness.

A Case of Mistaken Identity: Mononucleosis and CFS

Chronic fatigue syndrome came into its own as an illness in the 1980s. Doctors thought that it might be a lingering form of infectious mononucleosis, the infamous "kissing disease" that spreads among teenagers. The two maladies share many symptoms: muscle aches, headaches, swollen glands, sore throat, extreme exhaustion. Many CFS sufferers were infected with the Epstein-Barr virus, which causes mono, before developing CFS. Later studies found that many healthy people had also been infected with the Epstein-Barr virus, with no long-term effects. There is no evidence the two diseases are linked.

Some people with mononucleosis, including children and adolescents, do develop CFS. Scientists suspect that the incapacitation of mononucleosis keeps people bedridden and inactive, further weakening muscles and setting off a destructive cycle that can lead to chronic fatigue. British researchers report in the prestigious journal *The Lancet* that if you do get mono, a simple exercise program may help. After seven months, people with mono who began a gradual exercise program after recovering from mono were much less likely to develop CFS than those who remained inactive. The results are consistent with studies of people with chronic fatigue syndrome: Three-fourths of those who engage in exercise, particularly aerobic exercise, report feeling less fatigued and more fit a year later.

Relaxation also reduces muscle soreness. Tai chi, a Chinese exercise that combines movement, breathing, and mental concentration, may also be beneficial. Biofeedback, which uses a special machine to train your body to control heart rate and other involuntary responses, can also help you manage recurring pain.

- **Acupuncture,** in which very thin needles are inserted at specific points on the body, benefits some patients. Practitioners of this ancient Chinese therapy believe that it helps "unblock" the flow of the body's natural energy. Four or five sessions may be needed before you notice results. If you don't feel better after this time, acupuncture may not be right for you.
- **Nutritional supplements** such as melatonin (1 to 3 mg before bedtime) or the herb valerian (250 to 500 mg at bedtime) may help reset your body's natural circadian rhythms and improve sleep patterns. Some CFS patients have also reported benefits using **herbal products:** the antidepressant herb St. John's wort (300 mg three times a day), the aspirin-like herb white willow bark (1 or 2 pills three times a day), the pineapple-derived anti-inflammatory bromelain (500 mg three times a day), or capsaicin cream (apply to painful areas three times daily). A **high-potency multivitamin,** including vitamin C (1,000 mg) and vitamin E (400 IU), can also help to ensure you're getting a good daily balance of nutrients.

Outlook

While researchers struggle to find a cause and a cure for CFS, you can get considerable relief with a combination of therapies used under the supervision of a knowledgeable physician and skilled practitioners. People with CFS often feel they've turned a corner after several months, but temporary setbacks should be expected. In one study, nearly all patients who used a variety of treatments improved significantly. Most felt better for at least a year afterward.

FINDING Support

- Doctors still know little about chronic fatigue syndrome, and patients are often at the forefront of new breakthroughs and developments. The more you can learn about this disease from associations and support groups, the better prepared you (and your family and friends) will be to cope with your illness. The Chronic Fatigue and Immune Dysfunction Syndrome Association of America, a patient advocacy group, provides a wealth of information for those with CFS (1-800-44-CFIDS or www.cfids.org).

- Some people with CFS find it helpful to join a support group to swap stories and learn about new therapies. The Centers for Disease Control and Prevention in Atlanta (1-800-311-3435) has a useful state-by-state listing of support groups, plus international groups, on the Web at www.cdc.gov/ncidod/diseases/cfs/support/supus.htm.

Colds

There's a good reason this ailment is often called the common cold: It's estimated that Americans catch a stunning 1 billion colds each year. With the right remedies, however, you can get faster relief and maybe even shorten your cold's stay.

LIKELY First Steps

- **Rest** and **drink plenty of fluids** to ease your symptoms.
- **OTC medications** for your specific complaints (analgesics, decongestants, cough suppressants).
- **Vitamin C** or **herbal remedies** to shorten the cold's duration.

QUESTIONS TO Ask

- How many days should I stay home from work?
- Should I stop exercising temporarily?
- I've noticed the mucus I'm coughing up has turned yellowish-green. Does that mean I need an antibiotic?

What is happening

You don't catch a cold from being out in the cold. You don't catch a cold by going outside with wet hair. And despite what many people think, bacteria do not cause colds, viruses do—some 200 different strains of them. Rhinoviruses, which produce an estimated 30% to 40% of colds, are most active in spring, summer, and early fall. Coronaviruses are responsible for most colds in winter and early spring.

Any virus you're exposed to spreads the same way—by direct contact. If someone sneezes or coughs in your direction, you can breathe in the virus. It can also survive outside the body for up to three hours—on telephones, cups, kitchen counters, hands, and other surfaces you're likely to touch. If you pick up the virus and rub your eyes or nose before you wash your hands, you've given the bug a free ride to your mucous membranes. It'll start replicating with a vengeance.

In an effort to evict the unwanted guest, your immune system unleashes a counterattack that you recognize as the classic cold symptoms: runny nose, sneezing, and coughing. Most colds clear up within a week. Particularly stubborn strains can hang around for twice as long, and the severity of symptoms varies greatly from person to person. Unlike most illnesses, though, colds become less likely to bother you as you age. The average child gets six to eight colds a year. The average adult has two to four. By the time you're over age 60, you're likely to get less than one cold a year.

Treatments

The common cold is like the summertime blues: There ain't no cure—mostly because there aren't drugs (yet) that kill a wide range of viruses. For now, the best you can do is to make yourself more comfortable and try to help your immune system send your cold packing a day or so early. Getting rest and plenty of fluids is still a sound strategy. A number of simple steps—from keeping a positive attitude and taking the right over-the-counter medication to choosing immune-boosting foods and vitamins—will help you feel better faster. If your cold seems to worsen after a week or so, or if symptoms develop in your lungs or sinuses, consider a visit to your doctor.

If you have asthma, emphysema, or chronic bronchitis, see a doctor sooner: Cold symptoms can worsen the underlying condition.

Treatment options

Lifestyle changes

Fluids & rest	Cornerstones of successful recovery.
Good hygiene	Wash your hands often to keep the virus from spreading to others.
Stress reduction	Staying positive builds immunity.

Medications

Analgesics	Aspirin or acetaminophen relieves aches and lowers fever.
Decongestants	Help clear a stuffy nose.
Cough suppressants	Aid sleep at night; look for DM on label.

Natural methods

Vitamin C	May cut duration of a cold.
Zinc	Nasal zinc gluconate gel may be your best bet.

Lifestyle Changes

You can ease the misery of a cold with:

- **Rest.** Getting needed rest is probably the single most important thing you can do to help your body fight the infection.
- **Drink fluids.** Water is best, and steaming liquids or herbal tea can help clear your nose and soothe your throat. Science now supports what your grandma always told you: Chicken soup will fight your cold. Avoid alcohol and coffee while you're sick: They dehydrate you.
- **Use a humidifier.** Inhaling moist air will open your airways and help you breathe more easily.
- **Gargle with warm salt water.** This takes the "ouch" out of sore throats caused by colds. Do it several times a day.
- **Try nasal strips.** A nasal strip will open your nostrils, and may make breathing less of a chore despite your congestion.
- **Keep it clean.** If anyone in your family has a cold, use a virus-killing disinfectant to wipe kitchen counters and other surfaces you're apt to touch. You can make your own disinfectant by mixing one part bleach with 10 parts water.

When it comes to preventing future colds, your daily habits are very important. Here's how to keep viruses away in the first place:

- **Wash your hands.** Odds of catching a cold are in your own hands. "Operation Stop Cough," a campaign to get recruits to wash their hands at least five times a day, cut the rate of colds and other respiratory illnesses at a naval facility almost in half. Wash your hands often, especially before every meal.
- **Eat breakfast.** A study of 498 healthy individuals in Cardiff, Wales, found that those who started their day with breakfast got fewer and less severe colds than those who skipped their morning

TAKING Control

- **Don't accept antibiotics.** They're useless for viruses. However, a survey in the late 1990s found that doctors prescribed antibiotics to an astounding 60% of patients who came to them with colds.

- **Check OTC drugs for PPA.** If your nasal decongestant has been around for a while, check the label. In 2000, the FDA banned phenyl-propanolamine (PPA) in decongestants and appetite suppressants after a study found those who used products containing it had an increased risk for stroke.

- **Try steam inhalation.** Breathing in warm, moist air can loosen impacted mucus and help you decongest without a lot of drugs. (For other ways to clear your lungs, see page 254.)

Promising DEVELOPMENTS

- A weakened cold virus may be the key to shrinking tumors and even extending the lives of colon cancer patients for whom other treatments have failed, so says a preliminary study. The drug, called **Onyx-015,** is being developed by Onyx Pharmaceuticals. In a Stanford University study, the cold virus was injected into 35 people whose cancer had progressed to the liver. For some, the tumors disappeared within a few months: In others, tumors shrank. Larger studies are needed to confirm these promising preliminary results.

Tips on Blowing

How you blow your nose depends on what you want to blow out. For the thin, watery discharge of an early cold or an allergy attack, compress one nostril and gently blow out of the other. A vigorous honk is not any more effective, and all that energy can cause big trouble by sending infected mucus into your sinuses or middle ear.

Clearing out the thick, sticky mucus at a cold's end or from a bout of sinusitis is more difficult because your nasal passages are swollen. Try inhaling some steam before blowing or using an OTC nasal spray (Afrin or Dristan) to reduce swelling. Use the spray for only a couple of days: It can have a rebound effect, causing even more swelling. If you're still having trouble blowing, try a saline irrigation spray. It thins mucus and you can use it as long as you like.

meal. Many cereals are fortified with vitamins and other nutrients, and protein, which helps create antibodies that fight infections. That's two more reasons why breakfast is the most important meal of the day.

- **Think positive.** That same study found that those who approached life in a negative mood were more likely to get a cold or other illness. This supports what doctors have long known: Stress weakens your immune system.
- **Make friends.** At first glance, this notion may seem contradictory. You might think that the more people you hang out with, the more you'll be exposed to the viruses that cause colds. However, research has shown that having a large circle of family and friends may offer protection against colds. The reason: The more you're around those who care about you and support you, the better you're able to handle stress. That boosts your immune system, making it tougher for cold viruses to gain a foothold.

Medications

Choose products that target only the symptoms you have. There's no sense in taking a multisymptom medication unless you have everything it treats. It's a waste of money and it exposes you needlessly to potential side effects. For headaches, muscle aches, and fever, you can take **aspirin** or **acetaminophen.** One caution: Don't give aspirin products—the label may say salicylate or salicylic acid—to children who are under age 16. They could develop Reye's syndrome, a rare but potentially fatal disorder.

If you have a stuffy nose, decongestants come in two forms: nasal and oral. **Nasal decongestants** (drops, sprays, and inhalers) work fast, but they must be used frequently, and overuse can make your

IS IT A COLD OR THE FLU?

How can you tell what you're coming down with? Colds and flus are different illnesses and knowing what you have will make your treatment choices clearer. Check your symptoms against those below:

Symptoms	Cold	Flu
Fever	Usually not	101° to 103°F temperature for 3 to 4 days
Headache	Usually not	Very common
Body aches	Slight	Usual, often severe
Fatigue	Very mild	Can linger for 2 to 3 weeks
Total exhaustion	No	Develops early on
Stuffy nose	Usual	Occasionally
Sneezing	Usual	Occasionally
Sore throat	Usual	Occasionally
Cough	Mild to moderate	Usual, can become severe

Cold-Fighting Foods

Relief may be as close as your kitchen. You can speed your recovery with the following foods:

- **Broccoli:** A potent source of vitamin C, it can help send your cold packing. To soothe irritating coughs, sauté broccoli with fresh ginger.
- **Sweet potato:** It's high in beta-carotene, a powerful antioxidant that your body converts into virus-fighting vitamin A.
- **Chili peppers:** They get their heat from capsaicin, which breaks up mucus to make breathing easier. Use them in a fiery salsa.
- **Garlic:** It contains allicin, which can relieve congestion by regulating mucus flow. Cook it with onions to help shrink swollen airways.
- **Grapefruit:** Pink in particular is loaded with flavonoids to fight infections and increase immunity. Drizzle with honey if you have a sore throat.
- **Horseradish:** The allyl isothiocyanate in it makes your eyes water and helps thin mucus.
- **Oysters:** A great source of zinc, these immunity boosters may lessen a cold's severity and duration.
- **Tea:** They contain tannin flavonoids, which ease breathing by expanding bronchial passages. Brew your tea strong, inhale steam while it's hot, then drink a cup or two after it cools down.
- **Chicken Soup:** Homemade or store-bought, chicken soup lessens inflammation and relieves cold symptoms.

nose even stuffier. This rebound effect is exactly what you don't want. **Oral decongestants** have more side effects than drops and sprays: insomnia, a sense of anxiety, a rapid heart rate, and urinary retention in men with prostate problems. Antihistamines don't help: They dry up runny noses only in people with allergies, not those with colds.

If you have a dry, nagging cough, try a **cough suppressant** with DM (for dextromethorphan) on the label. A suppressant is especially good at bedtime to help you sleep without coughing. Though it may be unpleasant, your cough helps clear mucus from your throat. Use an expectorant if your cold develops into a more serious bronchial infection, usually characterized by a yellowish or greenish mucus, as opposed to the clear mucus that comes with a cold. **Saline nose drops or nasal wash** also can offer relief from congestion.

Natural Methods*

Vitamin C, a potent immunity-booster, may help cut your cold short and relieve symptoms. At the first sign of a cold, take 1,000 mg of vitamin C daily. Be aware that high doses can cause diarrhea in some people. When introduced in the mid-1990s, **zinc gluconate lozenges** were touted as being able to cut a cold's duration in half, but results of more recent studies have been mixed. **Nasal zinc gluconate gel** (Zicam) may be a better choice because the zinc stays in the nasal passages long enough to affect the virus. Some studies show that **echinacea** helps shorten a cold's duration and eases symptoms in some people. For best results, take the herb at the first sign of symptoms.

Natural methods are not subject to the same testing and regulation as prescription medications. Please seek your doctor's advice and use caution.

▶ **I've heard there's a new drug out that "cures" colds. Does it work?**
A new medication actually attacks a virus that causes colds. In clinical trials, pleconaril (brand name Picovir) cleared up cold symptoms a day earlier, on average, than a placebo. However, concerns were raised that the drug may spark new germ-resistant strains of cold viruses. There were also safety issues regarding whether it reduces the effectiveness of oral contraceptives. For now, the U.S. Food and Drug Administration has put the drug on hold.

FINDING Support

■ For detailed information on the latest research and trials regarding the common cold, visit the website of the Common Cold Centre at Cardiff University in Cardiff, Wales (www.cf.ac.uk/biosi/associates/cold/).

Colon cancer

Few things are as scary as learning you have cancer, a challenge that more than 130,000 Americans with colon cancer will face this year alone. But, more and more people are surviving this disease, many with complete recovery and cure.

LIKELY First Steps

- **Colonoscopy, blood tests, and radiological scans** to help determine if your cancer has spread and what your best treatment options are.

- **Surgery** to remove the tumor and surrounding tissue.

- In certain cases, **cancer drugs** (chemotherapy) may be given after surgery.

- In certain cases, **radiation** treatments may be needed before or after surgery.

QUESTIONS TO Ask

- What stage is my cancer? Where is it? How far has it spread?

- What surgery will I require?

- Will I need chemotherapy? Can I do it at home, rather than coming in to a clinic?

- Do I need radiation?

- Is there a clinical trial that would be right for me?

- Am I at risk for other cancers?

- Are my family members at risk? If they are, what should they do about it?

What is happening

Colon cancer occurs when abnormal cells grow out of control and form a mass, or tumor, in your large intestine. Doctors often refer to it as "colorectal cancer" because a malignancy can arise in either the colon or the rectum. The colon is in your abdomen. It leads to the rectum, which is just above the anus (*see illustration, page 88*). Cancer of the colon and rectum is the second leading cause of cancer deaths in the United States.

Usually slow-growing, colorectal cancers often originate in a cell with genetic mutations. Some people inherit genes that allow cells causing colon cancer to develop. More often, the abnormalities arise for unknown reasons, though diet appears to play an important role. Many colorectal cancers begin in a polyp that eventually forms a tumor. Left untreated, the tumor can bleed, obstruct your intestines, or break through your bowel wall. In time, cancer cells may spread to lymph nodes or to other organs, such as the liver or lungs.

When diagnosed, colon cancers are graded to indicate how aggressive they are. Tests determine whether the cancer has spread (metastasized) into lymph nodes or other tissues. Each cancer is ranked according to a four-stage scale, often expressed as I through

THE STAGES OF COLON CANCER

Stage	Spread	Outlook
I	Tumor has not gone beyond the inner lining of the digestive tract.	Five-year survival is 90% to 100%.
II	Tumor has broken through the muscular wall of the intestine but has not invaded any lymph nodes.	Five-year survival is 70% to 85%.
III	Cancer has spread to one or more lymph nodes.	Five-year survival is 40% to 65%.
IV	Tumor has spread to distant organs, often the liver.	Survival is 20% to less than 5%. This cancer is generally considered incurable.

Treatment options

Procedures

Surgical resection	Removal of tumor, lymph nodes, metastases.
Radiation therapy	Kills remaining cells; shrinks tumors presurgery.
Stent	Tube through tumor to prevent obstruction.
Laser ablation	Helps prevent obstruction, stop bleeding.
Colostomy	External opening for waste; often temporary.

Medications

Chemotherapy drugs	Kill cancer cells; often used in combination.

IV, to determine therapy and prognosis (*see table opposite*). People with stage I cancer, confined to the lining of the colon, have the best outlook. More than 9 of 10 patients with early-stage tumors will be alive five years after diagnosis—a figure specialists call "five-year survival." If cancer has not reappeared during this time, they're considered cured. Those with higher-stage tumors generally do not do as well, though most with stage II or III cancers can be effectively treated.

Treatments

Cancer of the colon and rectum is one of the most curable of all cancers. The choice of treatments usually depends on the stage of the disease. Patients of all ages, including the very old, can benefit. For most people, **surgery** to remove the tumor is the first step. Depending on the degree of spread and the location of the tumor, cancer-fighting **chemotherapy drugs** as well as **radiation therapy** may also be used to increase your chances of complete cure. Doctors who specialize in cancer care (oncologists) refer to drugs used after surgery to kill any remaining microscopic cancer cells as "adjuvant chemotherapy." Your treatment will be keyed to the stage of your cancer:

- **Stage I colon or rectal cancer:** Both can usually be cured by surgery alone. You probably will not need additional treatments.
- **Stage II colon cancer:** This may be treated with surgery alone. If your cancer has spread to the outermost colon wall, some doctors recommend chemotherapy to kill microscopic cancer cells that may remain after surgery (a regimen now under debate).
- **Stage II rectal cancer:** Radiation and chemotherapy is standard.
- **Stage III colon cancer:** Chemotherapy after surgery is standard.
- **Stage III rectal cancer:** Doctors prescribe chemotherapy after surgery. They often recommend radition before or after surgery.
- **Stage IV colon or rectal cancer:** Surgery may remove tumors in the intestine or in distant organs, such as the liver or lungs. This can produce good results if there aren't too many metastases. Chemotherapy and/or radiation may also help shrink the tumors.

TAKING Control

- **Stay positive.** A diagnosis of cancer is often overwhelming. Marshal your energies to gather information and resources. A close network of family and friends is vital. Support groups and counseling may improve coping skills.

- **Choose a hospital and surgeon** with a long track record. One study found that the more often colon cancer operations are performed in a given medical center, the less likely complications from surgery will be.

- **De-stress before surgery.** Music and relaxation tapes used before, sometimes during, and after surgery often help allay anxiety. Meditation, exercise, yoga, biofeedback, massage, and breathing exercises may also be useful.

- **Try ginger if nausea is a problem** because of chemotherapy. A cup of ginger tea or the powdered herb (100 to 200 mg) every four hours may quell symptoms. Take it with food to avoid stomach irritation. Let your doctor know if you are trying ginger or other remedies. Some vitamins, herbs, and nutritional supplements can interfere with surgery or medications.

- **Get regular follow-up tests.** Blood and stool should be tested on a regular schedule to help detect any recurrence. You'll need a colonoscopy after surgery and every few years (*see page 360*). This allows the doctor to remove precancerous growths called polyps and very early-stage cancers. If discovered a second time, cancer can often be completely cured with an additional round of treatment.

Promising
DEVELOPMENTS

- A new generation of drugs is being designed to attack cancer cells alone. One promising type blocks a protein called EGFR, or epidermal growth factor receptor, which is abundant on the surface of cancer cells. In preliminary studies, giving an **EGFR blocker** with standard chemotherapy prolonged survival in people with advanced colon cancer. Researchers speculate that these agents, which include such drugs as Erbitux and Iressa, might one day help to turn cancer into a chronic and manageable disease, much like diabetes.

- Investigators at Stanford University School of Medicine report that a genetically altered cold virus called **Onyx-015** has potential use against advanced colon cancer. The virus is injected into the hepatic artery, the main blood vessel that leads to the liver. It infects and multiplies in tumor cells, but leaves healthy cells alone. In a small pilot study, it shrank tumors that had spread to the liver.

- Popular arthritis pain relievers are emerging as weapons in the fight against colon cancer. The drugs, known as **COX-2 inhibitors,** relieve inflammation and may fight some of the cell changes that give rise to tumors. One such drug, celecoxib (Celebrex), has been approved to prevent an inherited form of colon cancer called familial adenomatous polyposis (FAP). Scientists are also testing these medications in combination with chemotherapy drugs to treat tumors that have already developed.

Procedures

Most people with colon cancer can benefit from **surgical resection,** the medical term for removal of their tumor (*see illustration below*). The operation, called a **partial colectomy,** involves cutting away a piece of the colon along with some surrounding normal tissue and nearby lymph nodes in case the cancer has spread. The colon is then reconnected. The procedure may take several hours and requires general anesthesia. Your doctor will probably do various preoperative blood tests and scans to help determine the degree of spread and prepare you for the operation. If cancer occurs in the rectum, the surgery may be more complicated: Many muscles and nerves that control sexual, bowel, and urinary functions cross through this area. Aftereffects may include poor bowel or bladder control and sexual problems, but these are often reversible.

Radiation therapy may be performed after rectal surgery to help kill tumor cells left behind and decrease the risk of recurrence. You'll probably need regular radiation treatments, five days a week, for five or six weeks. During the treatments, doctors aim high doses of x-rays at the tumor, often from different directions. The best results are obtained when a chemotherapy drug such as 5-FU is given orally or by IV infusion during the radiation. Increasingly, doctors use preoperative radiation to help shrink large tumors and make the operation easier. It may also eliminate the need for a colostomy. Radiation can be used to relieve pain and other symptoms when the tumor cannot be surgically removed or in cases of bowel obstruction.

Doctors may also insert a metal tube-like device called a **stent**, to reinforce the intestinal wall or keep the intestine open, or use a technique called **laser ablation,** which destroys cancerous tissue with

PARTICAL COLECTOMY

transverse colon
descending colon
cutter/stapler
small intestine
sigmoid colon
rectum
diseased colon
ascending colon
anus

In this common procedure, the surgeon cuts out the cancerous part of the colon (*at right above*), then staples together the remaining segments. About 75% of colon cancers occur in the sigmoid colon or rectum.

high-energy light beams, to keep the intestine open or stop bleeding. This is especially useful for those unable to tolerate surgery.

If a tumor is obstructing the bowel or the cancer has spread through the rectal muscles or into the anus, you may need a **colostomy.** This procedure creates an opening from the colon through the abdominal wall and allows wastes to leave the body and collect in an outside pouch. Most colon cancer operations do not require a colostomy. When one is performed, it is often temporary and can be reversed with a second operation. In addition, many appliances and techniques are available to keep bowel movements under control and help you stay clean and odor-free.

Medications

While **chemotherapy drugs** are designed to kill cancer cells, they are double-edged weapons: Because they attack healthy as well as cancerous cells, they can cause nausea and vomiting, diarrhea, hair loss, fatigue, mouth sores, and other reactions. On a positive note, because the dosages can be adjusted, and medications can minimize side effects, chemotherapy patients often miss only a couple of days of work.

For several decades now, **5-fluorouracil,** or 5-FU, has been the standard chemotherapy drug for colon cancer. To counter the toxic side effects of 5-FU, doctors usually give it with other drugs. The most common is **leucovorin,** a form of the B vitamin folic acid. These drugs are given intravenously in various combinations and schedules, so you may need to make daily or weekly visits to your treatment center over the course of several months. Doctors also implant pumps in the abdomen that continually dispense the drug. If you have metastatic disease that has spread to distant organs, 5-FU and leucovorin are usually combined with **irinotecan** (Camptosar), which boosts their cancer-killing effects and prolongs survival. The more you take, the greater the likelihood of side effects, so your doctor will keep a close eye on your progress.

Different medications and medication combinations are continually tested in clinical trials. Of particular note is **capecitabine** (Xeloda), the first oral colon cancer drug. It appears to be as effective as 5-FU for treating metastatic disease; tests are assessing its value for adjuvant chemotherapy. Other drugs, such as **oxaliplatin** and **raltitrexed,** may prolong survival and also reduce the likelihood of side effects.

Outlook

Treatment cures most people with colon cancer. It is important to have a doctor's exam every three to six months for the first three years after surgery. Your doctor will perform additional tests to be sure the cancer has not recurred. If it does recur, a second round of treatment is often successful. For end-stage disease, hospice care is a compassionate choice.

▶**When do you think I can expect to feel better?**
Because many people who have colon cancer don't have any symptoms, you may not notice any dramatic changes even after the surgeon has removed your cancer. Like many people, you may have become very weak and tired in the months before your diagnosis because your tumor was bleeding and made you anemic. Once the tumor is removed, you'll have much more energy. You may also have had constipation, diarrhea, or other bowel changes because of your cancer. These symptoms, too, will disappear in a few weeks. Many people are basically back to normal in two or three weeks after surgery. If chemotherapy or radiation is required, side effects may slow recovery. Side effects can usually be so well controlled that you may miss only one or two days of work during treatment sessions.

FINDING Support

- Some people with cancer benefit greatly from support groups, and they may even prolong survival. Contact the American Cancer Society to find a chapter in your area (1-800-ACS-2345 or www.cancer.org).

- The National Cancer Institute has a free helpline (1-800-4-CANCER) to answer your questions. You can also get information on the web at www.nci.nih.gov, including information on clinical trials for new drugs and treatments (www.clinicaltrials.gov).

Congestive heart failure

An increasing number (about 5 million Americans at last count) now live with congestive heart failure. This serious condition requires long-term treatment. Medical research is now keeping pace with a steady supply of new treatment breakthroughs.

LIKELY **First Steps**

- **Diuretic drugs** to reduce fluid buildup in conjunction with **ACE inhibitors** to open blood vessels.

- Other medications may be added, too, including **beta-blockers** to ease the heart's pumping action.

- Medical management of **related underlying problems,** such as coronary heart disease, high blood pressure, or anemia.

- Heart-healthy **lifestyle changes,** to maximize the effects of medications and other treatments.

QUESTIONS TO **Ask**

- What was the actual cause of my heart failure? Is there anything I can do to keep it from getting worse?

- What damage has been done to my heart? How long will I need to stay on medications?

- Would a pacemaker help my condition?

- Am I a good candidate for a heart transplant?

What is happening

When you have congestive heart failure (CHF), often called just "heart failure," your heart is no longer pumping in an efficient manner. Instead, blood and other fluids back up into your lungs and other tissues. Eventually this buildup, or congestion (hence the name "congestive" heart failure), prevents your body from getting enough of the oxygen-rich blood and nutrients it needs to thrive. You may notice you tire easily and are often short of breath. You may have developed a hacking cough or swelling (edema) in your ankles and legs. Simple tasks like climbing stairs or even working around the house may take more out of you. If other vital body systems are affected, you may have additional complications.

The good news is that unlike having a heart attack—a life-threatening emergency in which the heart suddenly "fails" (stops beating)—given good care, you'll probably be able to live with CHF for many years. You may have sudden flare-ups that require visits to the hospital. Your condition may worsen over time, but successful long-term management is the rule, not the exception.

Treatments

As frightening as the phrase "heart failure" might sound, restoring the heart's ability to pump efficiently is a fairly simple process. Once you are feeling better, the main task will be to determine why your heart started to perform poorly in the first place. The cause may have nothing to do with your heart: It may be the result of another ailment (such as diabetes, emphysema, thyroid disease, alcohol abuse, sleep apnea, anemia) or the use of certain medications (including muscle-enhancing steroids).

But if your episode of heart failure is like most people's—a consequence of an existing cardiac condition—you'll need to work with your doctor to deal with the underlying ailment. The ultimate goal is to allow you to resume your normal activities while preventing a heart attack, stroke, or other complication down the road. (For more specific treatments for common underlying conditions, see Atrial Fibrillation, Coronary Heart Disease, Heart Attack, and High Blood Pressure.)

To treat congestive heart failure, your doctor will probably begin by prescribing medicines to expel fluids from your tissues, open your blood vessels, and strengthen your heart. The earlier you start such a regimen, the better your long-term outlook. Portable pumps

Treatment options

Medications

Diuretics	Essential to relieve fluid buildup.
ACE inhibitors	Dilate vessels; used with diuretics.
Beta-blockers	Slow heart down, making pumping easier.
Digitalis drugs	Alternative if other drugs can't be used.

Procedures

Heart transplant	Reserved for most severe cases.
Heart-stabilizing devices	LVAD: Assists left ventricle pumping. Pacemaker: Steadies heartbeat. Defibrillator: Treats rhythm problems.

Lifestyle changes

Diet & exercise	Keep salt low, become moderately active.
Stress reduction	Proven benefits for heart disease.

Natural methods

Supplements	Consider amino acids and coenzyme Q_{10}.

and other technological advances are revolutionizing treatment for CHF. Such devices can ease your symptoms and they may reverse some of the damage to your heart, forestalling the need for a heart transplant. Lifestyle measures, from relaxation to exercise, are also important for anyone with CHF.

Medications

If you've been diagnosed with congestive heart failure, your doctor will probably prescribe a host of medicines to get the condition under control. These drugs are often remarkably effective in making you feel better quickly and can reduce your risk of complications if taken long-term. You may not have to be on medications forever: That depends on how well you respond and how reversible your heart damage is.

First on the list is a broad group of drugs known as **diuretics.** Commonly called "water pills," they help your body get rid of excess fluids that can build up in your legs, lungs, and belly during heart failure. That relieves such symptoms as cough, swelling, and shortness of breath. Less fluid allows your heart to pump more easily. You may receive one or more of these drugs: spironolactone (Aldactone), hydrochlorothiazide (HydroDiuril), and/or the extra-potent furosemide (Lasix). Your doctor will gradually adjust your dose to promote optimal fluid loss and periodically monitor you for such side effects as fatigue or irregular heart rhythms.

Diuretics are usually used along with **angiotensin-converting enzyme (ACE) inhibitors,** such as captopril (Capoten), ramipril (Altace), or lisinopril (Privinil, Zestril). By opening up blood vessels,

TAKING Control

- **See a heart specialist (cardiologist).** Nonspecialist doctors are less likely to prescribe ACE inhibitors and other useful medicines, possibly because of misplaced concerns about side effects.

- **Weigh yourself daily.** Gaining more than three pounds in a week may mean you're retaining fluids; your doctor may need to change your medications or up your dose. Rapid weight loss (10 to 15 pounds over six months) may signal a serious problem.

- **Be careful of NSAIDs,** such as aspirin, ibuprofen (Advil), and naproxen (Aleve). If you have CHF, these common pain relievers may increase the risk for relapse. Check with your doctor before using these over-the-counter drugs.

- **Watch it in the winter.** Surveys show that people with heart failure show up in emergency rooms more often during the winter months. That's probably a result of strenuous activities like shoveling snow. Other bad times: Mondays or any day between 8 AM to 3 PM.

- **Avoid overheating.** Warm baths (up to 106°F) and saunas (up to 140°F), once considered taboo for those with heart failure, may actually offer benefits. Provided you limit your exposure to 10 minutes or so. Check with your doctor. Never soak or sit in a sauna without letting someone know.

- **Monitor your symptoms.** If your skin suddenly becomes clammy and pale, your breathing is labored, or your symptoms rapidly worsen, go to an emergency room immediately.

Promising
DEVELOPMENTS

■ The first self-contained **artificial heart** gained worldwide prominence in 2001, when doctors at Jewish Hospital in Louisville, Kentucky, implanted it into 59-year-old Robert Tools. The yo-yo shaped two-pound device, called the AbioCor, is battery powered, quiet, and grapefruit-sized. Tools and a handful of others who received the device outlived all expectations. It's still a last-line option for the sickest patients, but these encouraging results have paved the way for larger clinical trials.

■ The FDA has approved eplerenone (Inspra) for treatment of heart failure in patients who have had a heart attack. According to the National Heart, Lung, and Blood Institute, this new drug significantly reduces mortality in patients with heart failure.

▶ **THE BATISTA PROCEDURE, is an innovative technique named for the Brazilian surgeon who pioneered it. This highly experimental surgery involves cutting away a living, golf-ball-sized portion of the failing heart. In early tests, reducing the heart's size in this way produced dramatic benefits for some patients. More recently, surgeons have questioned its effectiveness.**

these drugs lower your blood pressure and reduce strain on your heart. Unfortunately, studies show, ACE inhibitors are underprescribed. That's partly due to worries about side effects, including a persistent dry hack that's the infamous ACE inhibitor cough. If you can't tolerate ACE inhibitors, you may get similar benefits from the more expensive angiotensin-receptor blockers, such as losartan (Cozaar, Hyzaar) and valsartan (Diovan), which have fewer side effects, or from vasodilators such as hydralazine or nitrates.

Once you're stabilized on diuretics and ACE inhibitors, **beta-blockers,** which slow the heart down and make the pumping action easier, may prove a useful addition to the mix. Researchers are finding that beta-blockers, which also lower blood pressure and normalize rhythm, can be quite beneficial in strengthening the heart, as they lessen symptoms and help prolong survival in people with heart failure. Studies show these drugs reduce the chance of rehospitalization and even death due to heart failure. Commonly prescribed beta-blockers include carvedilol (Coreg) and metoprolol (Lopressor, Toprol). Your doctor will have to monitor you closely at first: In rare cases, these drugs worsen heart failure or nightmares, depression, fatigue, or cause other annoying side effects. Interestingly, beta-blockers may work better for whites than for African-Americans.

Digitalis drugs such as digoxin (Lanoxin), might be useful for those who don't respond to other medications. Also called glycosides, these drugs strengthen the heartbeat and increase blood flow to the kidneys, promoting fluid removal. Your doctor will check regularly for irregular heartbeats, digestive upset, visual disturbances, and other harmful side effects.

Other drugs used for heart failure include injectable vasodilators for emergency situations, amiodarone (Cardarone) for irregular heartbeats, and lung-strengthening asthma drugs. Many more drugs are currently under investigation.

Procedures

If your CHF worsens and medications no longer relieve your symptoms, a heart transplant or other procedure may be in order.

Heart transplants are usually reserved for those with severe disease marked by discomfort with *any* physical exertion and overt symptoms even at rest. A candidate for a transplant should generally have no other major illness and be younger than age 60 (although success has been achieved in older persons). With surgical advances, 85% of transplant recipients are now alive after one year, and 65% survive more than five years.

Due to a shortage of organs, many very sick patients must wait months for a suitable donor heart. However, a growing array of heart-stabilizing devices has proven useful as a "bridge to transplant" in these people. A **left-ventricular assist device (LVAD),** for example, is implanted in the chest or abdomen to take over the action of the left ventricle, the heart's main pumping chamber. (Some examples of these devices include the HeartMate, Thoratec, and Novacor.) Sometimes an LVAD allows the failing heart to recover, improving symptoms so much that a transplant is no longer necessary.

Another type of device, the **biventricular pacemaker** (such as the InSync system), is designed for the up to 50% or so of CHF sufferers whose left and right ventricles don't work together. This small device is implanted under the shoulder, with wire leads that deliver electrical signals to both sides of the heart. Patients who receive one generally show improved quality of life, are able to walk longer distances, and spend half as many days in the hospital as those without a pacemaker. There is also growing interest in the **implantable cardioverter-defibrillator (ICD)**—the pacemaker-like device that Vice President Cheney received—as a treatment for potentially fatal heart rhythms in those with heart failure.

Despite bleeding, blood clots, infections, and other complications, these and related devices are increasingly becoming end treatments in themselves, eliminating the need for a transplant. According to a study supported by National Heart, Lung, and Blood Institute, it significantly reduces deaths in patients with heart failure.

Lifestyle Changes

Simple changes can improve your quality of life and help you stay out of the hospital.

- **Go easy on the salt.** Aim for 2,000 mg or less of sodium a day. Too much salt makes the body retain fluids, and that raises your blood pressure. Salt also causes small blood vessels to constrict.
- **Exercise.** Once actively discouraged for those with heart failure, a moderate exercise program has proven beneficial for many with CHF. A few minutes of walking or light weights, two to five times a week, may be all it takes. Be sure to consult your doctor before starting any type of exercise program.
- **Seek support.** People who are married or who have a strong social network generally fare much better than those who go it alone. Try to cultivate friendships and join a local support group (see "Finding Support" at right).
- **Practice stress-reduction techniques.** Yoga, progressive muscle relaxation, or meditation have all proven effective. They lower blood pressure and provide other cardiac benefits, too.

Natural Methods*

A few small studies indicate that the amino acids **taurine** (500 mg L-taurine twice a day) or **arginine** (1,000 mg twice a day) may offer some therapeutic benefits for those with heart failure. Along with **coenzyme Q$_{10}$** (100 mg twice a day) other supplements have been proposed for treatment. Large studies of these substances are lacking, however, and none can cure heart failure. A healthy diet, rich in whole grains, fish, olive oil, and fresh fruits and vegetables, is always a good strategy.

Natural methods are not subject to the same testing and regulation as prescription medications. Please seek your doctor's advice and use caution.

▶ **How do I know if my CHF drugs are working?**
You'll start feeling better in a matter of hours. Diuretics ("water pills") quickly channel excess fluid through your kidneys—so expect a lot of visits to the bathroom in the first 24 hours. You'll also soon notice that your breathing is easier. Within a few days, the swelling in your feet should be nearly gone. Other medications, such as ACE inhibitors and digoxin, take a little longer to achieve their maximum benefit.

▶ **Can I still have sex?**
Certainly. Though you'll need to slow down if you develop chest pain (due to underlying coronary heart disease) or other troubling symptoms. If you are a man who takes Viagra, you shouldn't continue to use it while taking nitroglycerin or other nitrates for your heart condition. Even though the topic of sex may embarrass you, it's still a good idea to discuss it openly with your doctor.

FINDING Support

- The American Heart Association (1-800-242-8721 or www.americanheart.org) offers free brochures about heart failure and other heart ailments, including diet information. The association can put you in touch with local chapters offering advice and support groups.
- Is an organ transplant in your future? Visit the National Transplant Society (847-283-9333 or www.organdonor.org) for more information on this complex procedure.

Coronary heart disease

While it's true that more Americans die of coronary heart disease (CHD) than any other illness, things are changing. You're now far less likely to succumb to a fatal CHD-related heart attack, thanks to better medicines and real surgical innovations.

LIKELY **First Steps**

- **Lifestyle changes** (low-fat diet, exercise, weight loss, smoking cessation, stress reduction) to naturally halt or even reverse the disease.

- In tandem with lifestyle measures, **medications** (such as antiplatelets, beta-blockers, cholesterol drugs) to slow the disease, prevent complications, and control angina.

- For more severe disease, **surgery** (coronary artery bypass, angioplasty) to relieve symptoms and prevent impending heart attack or stroke.

QUESTIONS TO **Ask**

- Am I in good enough shape to start exercising right away?

- Which of my coronary arteries is blocked? Will my treatment change if it's the left anterior descending artery—which supplies up to 80% of the heart's blood?

- What type of blockage do I have (small and soft? large and close to a bend in the artery? long and hardened?) and how does this alter my treatment plan?

- Is it safe for me to have sex? Can I still take Viagra?

What is happening

Your heart is a giant muscle that needs lots of fuel (oxygen and various nutrients) to operate. A web of blood vessels called coronary arteries surround it just to provide this vital service. In a healthy heart, freshly oxygenated, nutrient-rich blood flows freely through smooth, flexible arteries. A diagnosis of coronary heart disease (CHD) means that the insides of the vessels have become clogged with fatty streaks called plaque. Blood can no longer flow effortlessly.

Sometimes, arteries get so plaque-riddled and narrowed that your heart doesn't receive enough oxygen-rich blood. Exert yourself—shovel snow, mow the lawn, climb onto the treadmill your kids gave you on your last birthday—and your heart may nearly scream for more oxygen. Below your breastbone, deep in your chest, come warning signs: an uncomfortable tightness and the sense that an elephant is standing on your chest. This wave of crushing pain that may spread down your arms and up to your jaw is angina (*see box, page 96*). And if one of the coronary arteries has become completely blocked, that part of your heart will get no oxygen at all. This is a heart attack.

Luckily, there are many things you can do to stop—and even reverse—this alarming progression of events. In taking charge of your CHD, you'll not only be able to prevent a heart attack but also reduce your chances of developing congestive heart failure (*see page 90*), heart rhythm disturbances like atrial fibrillation (*see page 44*), and other conditions associated with heart disease.

Treatments

The way you live your life—eating properly, exercising, not smoking, controlling your weight, reducing your stress—will be the determining factor when it comes to preventing and even reversing CHD. If you make (and stick to) the necessary lifestyle changes, the odds are that you'll lead a normal life.

Depending on what's causing your CHD (atherosclerosis, the accumulation of plaque on arterial walls, is the most common culprit), certain medications can help. For milder cases, a daily aspirin or stronger prescription medications can lower your risk of stroke or heart attack. For severe cases, surgery can be a lifesaving option. None of these will cure you of CHD. But the right procedure, an angioplasty or a bypass, can give you enormous relief from pain and discomfort and significantly prolong your life.

Treatment options

Lifestyle changes

Diet	Heart-healthy eating makes a big difference.
Exercise	Regular, raise-a-sweat activities are the goal.
Lose weight	Helps lower cholesterol and blood pressure.
Stop smoking	Risk of CHD drops dramatically in three years.
Stress reduction	May actually reverse CHD damage.

Medications

Antiplatelet agents	Daily low-dose aspirin or clopidogrel.
Beta-blockers	Significantly reduce risk of dying from CHD.
Calcium channel blockers	Open heart vessels and help angina.
Cholesterol-lowering drugs	Prevent heart attacks in CHD patients.
ACE inhibitors	Good for someone who's had a heart attack.

Procedures

Coronary artery bypass	Open heart surgery creates new pathways.
Angioplasty	Balloon-tipped catheter compresses plaque.

Lifestyle Changes

The greatest challenge facing you after a diagnosis of CHD may be simply changing your daily habits. This is much harder than it seems. It will require commitment and persistence on your part.

Start by reassessing what you eat and making some smart **dietary changes.** Your goal is to replace artery-clogging fare (foods high in saturated fat, total fat, and cholesterol) with a healthy variety of fruits, vegetables, grains, and low-fat dairy products. The likely result will be lower levels of both total and "bad" cholesterol. (*For more specifics, see High Cholesterol, page 176.*)

Your next order of business is to get some **regular exercise.** Walk. Run. Cycle. Swim. Burning at least 250 calories a day through exercise (the equivalent of about 45 minutes of brisk walking or 25 minutes of jogging) confers the greatest protection against CHD. Vigorous exercise not only works your heart muscle—encouraging blood flow through clogged vessels and making them more flexible—it helps by raising "good" cholesterol levels. Don't be intimidated by the need to work up a sweat. A well-known Harvard study of 40,000 female health professionals found that walking just one hour a week, at any pace, reduces the risk of CHD.

Exercising will also help you take off extra pounds. **Losing excess weight** has long been known to improve cholesterol levels, lower your high blood pressure, and reduce your risk of CHD. With less weight on your frame, your heart won't have to work as hard to

TAKING Control

- **Insist on a bypass surgeon with experience.** You'll want a veteran who performs more than 100 bypasses a year. University medical school hospitals and major medical centers are good places to look.

- **Ask about your odds** (for a longer life, a stroke, a fatal complication) before committing to bypass surgery or angioplasty. Many people never bother to check.

- **Eat more fish.** Recent trials show that people with CHD can dramatically lower their risk of dying by regularly eating fish (such as salmon) rich in omega-3 fatty acids.

- **Be cautious about supplements.** Popular herbs and vitamins, such as ginkgo biloba, garlic, vitamin E, fish oil, and coenzyme Q_{10}, can thin blood. If you're taking a heart drug that does the same thing—aspirin, warfarin (Coumadin), clopidogrel (Plavix)—serious bleeding problems could develop. Ask your doctor about interactions.

- **Don't forget your daily aspirin.** Do as your doctor orders. If you don't, you are twice as likely to die from CHD. A 1999 Duke University study found that one in five people with CHD fails to take aspirin regularly. If aspirin upsets your stomach, discuss effective alternatives with your doctor.

- **Deal with marital stress.** A 2000 study found that tension with a spouse hurts women's hearts in particular (men react more to work stress). If you've got problems at home, share them with a confidante.

About Angina

Angina (*angina pectoris*) is the intense chest pain that occurs when the heart muscle isn't getting enough oxygen. The harder the heart works—whether due to physical exertion or strong emotions—the more oxygen it needs. To control angina, educate yourself about why it happens and how aspirin and anti-anginal drugs can help.

Prevention (healthy diet, blood pressure control, no smoking) is critical, but **nitrates** are the pharmaceutical cornerstone of angina treatment. Nitrates release nitric oxide, relaxing key blood vessels. Forms include under-the-tongue tablets and sprays, ointments, and patches. **Rapidly acting nitrates** (such as nitroglycerin) dilate blood vessels and relieve or prevent symptoms. Preserve nitroglycerin potency by storing no more than 100 tablets at once (in the original container). Screw the cap on tightly after each use. **Longer-acting nitrates** (like isosorbide dinitrate) are used to dilate blood vessels and relieve or prevent symptoms. Surgical options for severe angina are limited. **Myocardial laser revascularization,** for example, involves aiming laser energy at blocked areas. It's very risky, but can bring relief in some cases.

If you've been treated for angina and develop heart attack symptoms, take nitroglycerin (under the tongue or in spray form). Take a dose every five minutes until pain subsides. Don't take more than three doses. Call 911. Chew an aspirin.

keep blood circulating. Another vital move is to **stop smoking.** One out of five CHD deaths can be traced directly to a tobacco habit. Smoking not only lowers "good" HDL cholesterol, it sabotages the elasticity of the aorta and ups your risk of a blood clot. In just three years of cigarette-free living, you may well wipe out a lifetime of cumulative heart damage.

All your good habits could be in vain if you can't work **stress reduction** into the mix. Chemicals released during stress can raise your blood pressure and trigger heart rhythm disturbances. Feeling stressed may put you off exercise or prompt you to eat fat-jammed junk foods. Whatever your stress triggers—job demands, family relationships, commuting—it's time to get your priorities straight and look at things differently. Try juggling your schedule to ease work overload. Explore meditation, yoga, or tai chi, ancient stress-busters that have endured because they work. Studies indicate that lowering stress may reopen clogged arteries, reducing angina and lessening your risk for a heart attack.

Medications

Even with lifestyle changes, many people require drugs to control the progression of the disease and its symptoms. If you have CHD (mild or advanced) or stable (predictable) angina, you'll probably be told to take a daily **low-dose aspirin.** This blood thinner is an antiplatelet agent: It inhibits tiny disk-shaped particles in your blood (platelets) from clumping together and blocking an artery.

If your CHD is deemed severe, the doctor may recommend the **antiplatelet drug** clopidogrel (Plavix) rather than aspirin. In a major 2001 study, the number of heart attacks, strokes, and deaths from heart disease in patients on clopidogrel was much lower than in those on aspirin. It's also better than aspirin or ticlopidine (Ticlid)—another antiplatelet agent—at reducing heart attack after angioplasty.

To lighten the demands on your heart, your doctor may prescribe a **beta-blocker,** such as propranolol (Inderal), metoprolol (Lopressor, Toprol-XL), or carvedilol (Coreg). These slow the heart rate and lower blood pressure. There's overwhelming evidence that beta-blockers can reduce the risk of dying from CHD. They're particularly valuable if you have silent cardiac ischemia, which reduces oxygen to your heart but doesn't cause chest pain (angina). If you have angina, the beta-blocker may lessen the need for pain-relieving nitrates. (Just remember, beta-blockers don't stop angina pain once it's started. Nitroglycerin is best for that.)

If beta-blockers or nitrates don't relieve your angina, your doctor may recommend a **calcium channel blocker.** By reducing the heart's oxygen demands and dilating its blood vessels, these drugs can give you enormous relief. Such benefits have made newer calcium channel blockers such as amlodipine (Norvasc) and nicardipine (Cardene), as well as long-acting nifedipine (Adalat, Procardia) popular for CHD.

If your cholesterol is high and a heart-healthy diet isn't doing the trick, **cholesterol-lowering drugs** like the statins can make a big difference. Lovastatin (Mevacor), pravastatin (Pravachol), and

Promising
DEVELOPMENTS

■ About 85% of angioplasty patients get stents, which reduce the need for follow-up procedures by about 33%. But complications such as blood clots and vessel scarring persist. The FDA recently approved medication-coated stents expected to reduce the likelihood of stent blockage and repeat heart attacks.

▶**A PHENOMENON KNOWN AS "ASPIRIN RESISTANCE" has doctors perplexed. In some people, aspirin doesn't adequately block thromboxane, the chemical that cues platelets to form life-threatening blood clots. If this phenomenon is evident in you, you may need a prescription antiplatelet medication like clopidogrel (Plavix).**

ANGIOPLASTY: THE ANSWER FOR A BLOCKED ARTERY

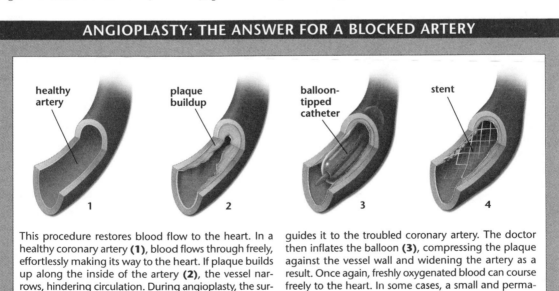

healthy artery

plaque buildup

balloon-tipped catheter

stent

1   2   3   4

This procedure restores blood flow to the heart. In a healthy coronary artery **(1)**, blood flows through freely, effortlessly making its way to the heart. If plaque builds up along the inside of the artery **(2)**, the vessel narrows, hindering circulation. During angioplasty, the surgeon inserts a balloon-tipped catheter into an artery through a small incision (usually in the groin), and guides it to the troubled coronary artery. The doctor then inflates the balloon **(3)**, compressing the plaque against the vessel wall and widening the artery as a result. Once again, freshly oxygenated blood can course freely to the heart. In some cases, a small and permanent metal mesh tube called a stent **(4)** is inserted to stabilize and literally prop open the artery.

simvastatin (Zocor) can prevent heart attacks and deaths due to CHD. Researchers hope that the newer statins—fluvastatin (Lescol), atorvastatin (Lipitor)—will be even better LDL-lowerers.

Sometimes doctors recommend **ACE (angiotensin-converting enzyme) inhibitors,** especially for those who have CHD-associated heart failure or who've had a heart attack. Ramipril (Altace) is particularly good at dilating blood vessels and lowering blood pressure.

Procedures

If your CHD becomes severe or your angina comes and goes or lasts for more than 20 minutes, your cardiologist may recommend surgery. The two standard procedures are bypass surgery (*see illustration, page 250*) and angioplasty (*see illustration, page 97*). There are pros and cons to each and the choice may not be easy to make. For a **coronary bypass,** formally known as a coronary artery bypass graft (CABG), the surgeon opens your chest wall to expose your beating heart. After connecting you to an external pump that acts like a heart, the team temporarily stops your heart. The surgeon stitches a healthy, plaque-free section of vessel (from your leg or chest) next to the problem artery, creating a new route for blood to flow freely. If more than one artery is congested, the surgeon may place several grafts. About 500,000 bypasses are performed each year.

- **Pros of bypass:** It maintains blood flow in the affected artery for a longer time than can be expected with angioplasty. A repeat procedure is not usually necessary (at least not for many years).
- **Cons of bypass:** This major open heart surgery requires general anesthesia and several days in the hospital, followed by weeks of home recuperation. Complications can include heart attack, infection, postoperative confusion and thinking problems, or even a stroke from tiny clumps of plaque that can be stirred up by the procedure and caught in a narrowed brain artery.

With an **angioplasty,** your cardiologist restores blood flow to the heart by inflating a balloon inside the artery to compress plaque against vessel walls. This revolutionary technique began two decades ago and, with 900,000 angioplasties performed each year, is now more popular than bypass surgery.

- **Pros of angioplasty:** It takes about one hour, requires only local anesthesia and one night in the hospital, and recovery is relatively rapid.
- **Cons of angioplasty:** There's a 20% to 30% chance the artery will block up again (restenosis), making a second procedure necessary. Other potential risks: blood clots, artery spasms, or a heart attack due to coronary artery injury. The use of stents has considerably reduced concern about restenosis.

Outlook

You'll know you're getting better when you have less chest pain and more energy. As you make a serious commitment to the positive changes that reverse heart disease, you may mark the diagnosis of CHD as a positive wake-up call to a long and vigorous life.

Depression

Everyone gets sad sometimes. It's all part of being human, but if you're one of the 19 million Americans with true depression, you know the difference. Today, promising treatments are revolutionizing the course of this potentially devastating illness.

What is happening

For generations, depression was stigmatized as a personal weakness. Even friends would exhort the sufferer to "snap out of it." Then, in the 1980s, scientists started using cutting-edge imaging techniques to take a closer look at what happens in the brain when a person feels depressed. They found that the condition has a lot more to do with brain chemistry and genetics than it does with willpower.

When you're fine with the world and not feeling depressed, plentiful stores of chemical messengers called neurotransmitters zip effortlessly around your brain. They literally leap critical gaps between the brain's millions of nerve cells, called neurons, and keep communication flowing. When you're depressed, this easy interchange breaks down. The key mood neurotransmitters—chemicals such as serotonin, norepinephrine, and dopamine—become unbalanced. Then neurons have problems conducting impulses back and forth.

Depression can take many forms. Its causes are complex. Underlying brain chemistry is all-important in some people. In others, a single upsetting event can trigger a downward spiral. In most people, a complex interaction of internal chemical imbalances and external factors (*see box at right*) is involved. Most of the time, depression is formally diagnosed after at least two consecutive weeks of sadness, sleeplessness, poor appetite and concentration, or loss of interest in normally pleasurable activities. More severe forms of clinical depression can be acutely distressing and debilitating. Their symptoms can last for months or years.

Treatments

No two cases of depression are alike. You may need to combine several therapeutic approaches to find the mix that's best for you. Medications, psychotherapy—or both—are the first step for most people with milder depression. The newer antidepressants (SSRIs particularly) adjust chemical imbalances and have transformed many lives. When an SSRI works, you'll likely feel a bit better within a week, although its full effect will take several weeks. If it doesn't work, your doctor may switch you to another SSRI or different antidepressant. These drugs aren't addictive. You can safely take them for a long time.

Psychotherapy often works as well as medication for mild to moderate symptoms of some types of depression. However, your best chance to feel better, and even banish the depression altogether, is to pursue drugs and therapy simultaneously. If you start

LIKELY **First Steps**

- **Antidepressants** to correct imbalances in brain chemistry and improve mood.
- **Psychotherapy** to unveil sources of depression and help you cope with them.
- For severe depression, **shock therapy (ECT)** to dramatically reset brain function.

QUESTIONS TO **Ask**

- Will I have to take this medicine for the rest of my life?
- Am I going to gain weight while I'm on this antidepressant?
- How likely is it that my depression will get worse?
- Will this happen to my kids?

Why You? Why Now?

Depression can result from a single underlying cause or from numerous factors working simultaneously—from an emotional upset or traumatic loss to a genetic predisposition. Implicated as well are health problems (heart disease, hypothyroidism), medicines (beta-blockers, corticosteroids), hormonal shifts (menopause), and lifestyle (alcohol habits, lack of exercise, poor diet).

TAKING Control

- **Steel yourself for a search.** The odds that the first antidepressant you take will lift your depression are only 65%. So don't be surprised if you have to try a few before settling on one (or a combo). The good news: Increasingly sophisticated antidepressants are becoming available.

- **Investigate what's worked for family members.** If a certain antidepressant relieves symptoms for a parent or other close relative, mention this to your doctor. The same drug may work best for you, too.

- **Tell your doctor about herbs you take.** Many herbs and supplements interact with prescription antidepressants, blunting their action or causing serious reactions.

- **Stick with it.** The longer you stay in treatment—medications or therapy—the less likely you are to have another depressive episode.

- **Ignore drug company ads.** Try as they might to convince you otherwise, there's no good evidence that one SSRI antidepressant (Paxil, Prozac, or Zoloft) is superior to another. So says a 2001 research study.

- **Write a list of questions for a prospective therapist.** What kind of experience do you have? How will you treat me? What will this approach do to help me? Are there any risks?

- **Take suicidal feelings seriously.** This is an emergency. Talk with someone. Call your doctor. Go to the hospital. Sign a contract promising not to hurt yourself. Have guns removed from your home, and don't drive.

Treatment options

Medications

SSRIs	First-line drugs; correct chemical imbalances.
Heterocyclics	Formerly tricyclics; long history of use.
Newer antidepressants	Unique drugs with fewer side effects.
MAO inhibitors	Older drugs; often interact with other meds.

Procedures

Psychotherapy	Talking can be as effective as medication.
Behavioral therapy	Good for clearly defined problems.
ECT	Electroconvulsive therapy for severe cases.

Lifestyle changes

Diet & exercise	Provide physical support, emotional lift.
Sleep	Getting the right amount is critical.
Stay connected	To friends, family, and spiritual beliefs.

with psychotherapy and don't feel any relief within 6 weeks or feel only somewhat better by the 12-week mark, adding antidepressants is a smart move. In fact, antidepressants are a good first step, even for severe, debilitating depression. After that, ECT (electroconvulsive therapy) may be your next logical option.

Along with these medical approaches, you'll need to develop smart lifestyle strategies. Focus on communicating openly with your doctor, exercising regularly, and maintaining a healthy diet. Most people eventually find a balanced approach that makes them feel much better and helps them deal with their depression. Concentrate on finding the combination that works best for you. If your depression doesn't lift completely during the first intensive phase of treatment, the risk for relapse is high. Enlist those who care for you to help you get on the road to recovery as quickly as possible.

Medications

When selecting an antidepressant, your doctor will consider many factors, ranging from your other medical conditions and medications to the nature of your depression—mild or severe, brief or long-term, with or without psychotic features. This decision is often far more complex than it seems. And the more severe or complicated your depression, the more likely that your family physician will refer you to the care of an expert; probably a psychiatrist who is well-versed in the actions, benefits, and drawbacks of the dozens of antidepressants available today.

Many patients with mild depression are now started on **selective serotonin reuptake inhibitors (SSRIs),** such as Prozac, Luvox, Paxil, and Zoloft. (Prozac was the first SSRI. Its introduction in the late 1980s was a milestone in depression treatment: It offered an alternative to cruder, less-precise drugs.) SSRIs are relatively safe to use if you have another illness, even a psychiatric one like obsessive-compulsive disorder, panic disorder, social phobia, or bulimia. In fact, these conditions often improve with the addition of SSRIs. Easy to manage and taken only once a day, SSRIs are less likely than older drugs to cause annoying reactions that might tempt you to stop taking them. Their side effects (mild nausea, headache, diarrhea) also tend to fade once your body adjusts. For some, the worst drawback is loss of interest in sex.

Once a treatment of choice, **heterocyclic antidepressants** (originally called **tricyclics**) still have a special place in the panoply of drug options, with names such as Elavil, Tofranil, and Pamelor. On the plus side, they're proven entities. Psychiatrists know what to expect when prescribing them, and they can offer significant relief from depression. On the downside, side effects (drowsiness, dry mouth, blurry vision, and weight gain) have now relegated these drugs to second-choice status. However, if insomnia accompanies depression, doctors may take advantage of the drowsiness side effect and prescribe a small dose of a heterocyclic at bedtime.

Each of five **newer antidepressants** has a unique mechanism of action and isn't classified in any of the preceding groups. Exactly how buproprion (Wellbutrin) works is not known, but it seems to affect serotonin and a second neurotransmitter called dopamine. (A side effect causes smokers to lose interest in cigarettes, so it's also marketed under the name Zyban.) Venlafaxine (Effexor), nefazodone (Serzone), trazodone (Desyrel), and mirtazapine (Remeron) also have this dual neurotransmitter action, changing brain levels

HOW SSRI MEDICATIONS WORK

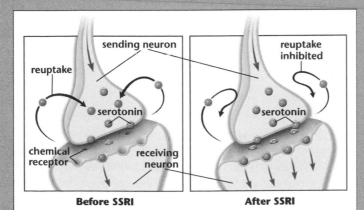

Before SSRI   **After SSRI**

Some types of depression appear to be related to low levels of the brain neurotransmitter serotonin. This is because neurons sending the serotonin reabsorb, or reuptake, too much of the chemical (*above left*). Antidepressant drugs called selective serotonin reuptake inhibitors (SSRIs) work by preventing this reuptake (*above right*), allowing more serotonin to be delivered to the receiving neuron—and to the brain in general.

Alternative Remedies

Despite enthusiasm for them, few herbs or other natural methods have proved effective for depression. This includes megavitamins, acupuncture, and electro-sleep therapies. Popular herbs like valerian, ginseng, St. John's wort, and the supplement SAMe continue to be dogged by questions over purity, dosage, safety, and lack of evidence (there are few well-designed studies).

Recent research has only increased concerns. A 2002 *JAMA (Journal of the American Medical Association)* study found the oldest and most popular herbal antidepressant —St. John's wort—ineffective for 340 people who were moderately to severely depressed. Mild depression wasn't studied, though, and many herbalists were quick to point out that the herb was never meant to treat major depression.

St. John's wort contains at least 10 pharmacological compounds, so ask your doctor. Recent findings indicate it can alter the effectiveness of other drugs, including blood thinners, oral contraceptives, AIDS/HIV drugs, and even other antidepressants.

▶ANTIDEPRESSANT DRUGS have a powerful appeal: Among Americans treated for depression in 1987, just 37% took antidepressants. By 1997, nearly 75% did. Conversely, about 71% underwent psychotherapy in 1987. Only about 60% did by 1997.

SAD No More: Beating the Wintertime Blues

Diminishing levels of sunlight are thought to affect the body's production of serotonin, a hormone that seems to promote a positive mood. So if your sadness, fatigue, sugar cravings, or excessive sleepiness sets in each fall and continues through the winter, when the hours of sunlight dwindle, you may have **seasonal affective disorder (SAD)**. If you do, make a conscientious effort to go outside frequently. Take a daily walk. Lunch al fresco.

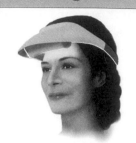

Battery-powered light visor

Researchers report that more intense treatment with bright light—via a full-spectrum lightbox that you use for 30 to 60 minutes on a regular basis—can fully ease symptoms in 50% of SAD sufferers. Investigators are also looking into supplementation with vitamin D, a nutrient the body produces in response to sunlight, to improve mood and outlook.

Various other light devices can be purchased. Battery-powered light visors (*left*), for example, are effective and convenient. They let you move around while you're getting your daily light dose. One cautionary note: Indoor tanning lights don't work for SAD.

▶Help! I've lost interest in sex since filling my antidepressant prescription.

Many antidepressants—SSRIs, tricyclics, MAO inhibitors—cause lack of interest in sex, as well as difficulties with erections and orgasm. Some 80% of SSRI users struggle with these issues. Things might perk up as your body adjusts to the drug. Ask your doctor about lowering your dosage or skipping it occasionally. Certain antidepressants (Remeron, Serzone, Wellbutrin) are less likely to cause sexual problems.

▶Do "mood foods" work?

Proof is sparse, but many contend that packing your diet with certain foods makes you feel better due to increased levels of serotonin, the brain's mood-controlling compound. Often suggested are complex carbohydrates (rice, potatoes) or foods rich in the amino acid tryptophan (turkey, salmon, milk). The best evidence is for omega-3 fatty acids, essential for brain function. Good sources include salmon, anchovies, and caviar.

of both serotonin and norepinephrine. If serotonin is affected more than norepinephrine, as with Serzone and Desyrel, the effect is sedation. If the reverse, as with Effexor or Remeron, you may feel stimulated or unable to sleep. Let a clinician familiar with these medications select what's best for you.

Lastly, over past decades, countless people have found relief with **monoamine oxidase inhibitors (MAO inhibitors),** such as Nardil, Marplan, and Parnate. These drugs are prescribed primarily by psychiatrists with extensive experience and knowledge about how they work, who will benefit from them, and what side effects might result. MAOs can cause serious interactions if combined with certain antidepressants, vasoconstrictors, and decongestants. Also, they can produce problems when taken along with tyramine-rich foods, such as dark chocolate, aged cheeses, and certain red wines.

If an antidepressant isn't making you feel better, your doctor may add a mood stabilizer like lithium or a thyroid hormone to your regimen. In many cases, one of these can make all the difference.

Procedures

Psychotherapy may be the place to start, especially if you're only mildly depressed. This type of verbal (and nonverbal) exchange can sometimes work as effectively as drugs. Side effects are less of an issue, and you don't have to worry about interactions with other medicines (this can be particularly important for older people who are taking lots of pills). There are drawbacks, however. Psychotherapy alone is not effective for severe depression; this give-and-take process can take longer than drugs to work (results in six to eight weeks or more versus four to six weeks with medication) and it can be expensive.

A skilled therapist will often mix and match therapeutic approaches based on what you're going through. **Psychodynamic therapy,** for example, looks to past experiences to shed light on why you're feeling what you're feeling now. **Interpersonal therapy,** or crisis intervention, works especially well when an immediate problem—a child leaving home, a spouse dying—is causing you to feel low.

Behavioral therapy attempts to change destructive patterns of acting or thinking by honing social skills, self-control, and problem-solving strategies. It works best when the problem can be clearly defined and "good behavior" rewarded. It's often blended with **cognitive therapy,** which boosts confidence and counters your fear of failure by showing you how competent you can be. In **group therapy,** you're given a chance to share your feelings (and solutions) with others.

If your depression is severe and psychotherapy combined with medications hasn't improved how you feel, your doctor may recommend **electroconvulsive therapy (ECT),** which shocks the nervous system and resets the brain's chemistry. It may be an option if you're losing touch with reality (psychosis), or threatening suicide.

Experts aren't sure exactly why ECT works. Electrodes are placed on the head and an electric current causes a brief convulsion. General anesthesia prevents pain from muscle contractions. Most patients are treated every other day for five to seven sessions. Headache and memory loss sometimes occur, but are almost always temporary. Despite its Hollywood image as being barbaric, ECT is quite safe: One study showed that treatments relieved symptoms in 80% of patients with severe depression.

Lifestyle Changes

Swim, bike, walk. **Get regular exercise.** You'll feel better in part because you took charge. You may also have a surge of "feel-good" (and pain-relieving) substances called endorphins. Countless studies reinforce the emotional lift of exercise. Stress and anxiety drop. Blood gets flowing. Blood pressure falls. Negative emotions—helplessness, anxiety, hostility—diminish. Even a simple 15-minute walk can enhance your mood. A small Johns Hopkins study found that adults who were fitter and relatively lean were more likely to feel happier, but the benefits won't last unless you keep at it.

Exercise also improves **sleep,** another key factor in improving mood. The right amount of sleep is critical. Seven to eight hours a night is ideal. Avoid napping, and get up at the same time every morning. (*For advice on good sleep habits, see Insomnia, page 188.*) Aim for a **healthy diet,** too. Poor eating can increase fatigue and feelings of unease.

You might also explore your **spiritual side,** whether religion or other beliefs, for answers to meaning in life. Meditation and yoga are risk-free ways to get a valuable perspective on your daily troubles. **Stay connected** socially in any way you can. Adopt a pet. Take a class. Or join a club related to something you're interested in (maybe bridge, chess, gardening, or walking). If you find yourself turning to alcohol or drugs, ask your doctor about a support group that can help you reduce your intake: Both alcohol and drugs can trigger and intensify depression.

Promising DEVELOPMENTS

■ Exciting research from the University of Illinois indicates that a new technique—**repetitive transcranial magnetic stimulation (rTMS)**—may ease severe depression. A handheld wire coil placed over the brain's left prefrontal cortex often shows abnormal electrical activity and decreased blood flow in people who are depressed. A focused, rapidly fluctuating magnetic field is administered. Unlike ECT, sedation is not necessary and memory problems aren't a risk.

FINDING Support

■ Friends, family, or your primary care doctor may be able to recommend a good therapist. Or contact the American Psychological Association in Washington, D.C., for information on state psychological associations (1-800-964-2000 or www.apa.org). The American Medical Association's website can also lead you to a local psychiatrist (www.ama-assn.org).

■ For additional information, try Mental Help Net (www.mentalhelp.net), the Mental Health InfoSource (www.mhsource.com), Psychology.com (www.psychology.com), or the Depression and Bipolar Support Alliance (the former National Depressive and Manic-Depressive Association) at 1-800-82NDMDA or www.NDMDA.org.

Diabetes type 1

Refinements in the care of this serious, lifelong disease have improved—from the development of new forms of medication to pumps that continuously deliver insulin to the blood. Managing this complex condition is easier now than ever before.

LIKELY First Steps

- **Daily insulin injections** to replace the hormone no longer produced naturally.
- Careful **glucose testing** to monitor blood sugar levels.
- A special **diabetes diet** tailored to you, and **regular exercise** for general health and improved blood sugar control.

QUESTIONS TO Ask

- Would any of the new insulin forms be good for me?
- Given my medical history, are there steps I need to take to avoid diabetic complications?
- What kind of exercise is best?
- Should I try an insulin pump?

Emergency! Diabetic Ketoacidosis

When you lack the insulin needed to process glucose, your whole metabolism shifts as your body turns to fat stores for energy. This creates waste products called ketones. Too many of them can lead to coma or even death. Get help immediately if you feel mentally clouded, or have a dry mouth, extreme thirst, or nausea and vomiting.

What is happening

A healthy pancreas contains cells that produce insulin, a hormone that transports a form of sugar called glucose from the bloodstream into all your cells. It's an important job: Sugar is the body's fuel. When you develop type 1 diabetes, however, your immune system gets confused and destroys the insulin-producing cells in the pancreas. Because the insulin supply then dwindles, your cells are deprived of glucose, which builds up in your bloodstream. Your body then tries to get rid of this excess glucose through your kidneys, its normal filtration system. That can make you feel weak and hungry, need to urinate frequently, and be intensely thirsty. If you don't drink a lot of water, you may even get dehydrated.

Such high blood glucose is known as hyperglycemia. It can cause serious health problems. Blood vessels and nerves can become damaged, leading to kidney failure, blindness, heart disease, and other complications. In fact, diabetes is one of the leading causes of death and disability in America. There are three variations: Type 1, once known as "juvenile" diabetes, usually appears before age 30. It accounts for about 5–10% of all cases and its onset may be sudden. Most people who have diabetes have type 2, or "adult-onset" diabetes (*see page 107*). The third form, gestational diabetes, develops only during pregnancy.

Treatments

To deal with this chronic, potentially damaging disease, you'll need long-term specialized medical care. Your caregivers will help you learn how to keep your blood sugar levels in normal ranges, and how to give yourself daily insulin injections. To determine how much insulin you need, you'll have to test your blood sugar levels several times a day. If they're too high, you inject insulin. If they're too low (a condition called hypoglycemia), you eat a sugar-containing food such as orange juice or candy. In the long run, a balanced diet and regular exercise will go a long way toward regulating your blood sugar levels.

There's no cure for diabetes, but by monitoring your blood sugar levels and maintaining meticulous control, you can dramatically reduce your risk for damage to your eyes, nerves, kidneys, and blood vessels, as well as other complications (*see box, page 109*). The good news is that once you start treating diabetes, you'll rapidly feel better, and you'll find there's practically no limit to your daily activities.

Treatment options

Procedures

Glucose testing	Do this often to determine insulin needs.
Insulin pump	Implanted for continuous monitoring.

Medications

Fast-acting insulin	Works in 15 minutes; good before meals.
Intermediate-acting insulin	Peaks in 2 to 4 hours.
Longer-acting insulin	Can last 10 to 20 hours.

Lifestyle changes

Diet	Aim to keep weight in check.
Exercise	Regular activity aids glucose regulation.

Procedures

The goal of successful diabetes management is to get just enough insulin to keep glucose levels neither too high nor too low. This can be a delicate balance to maintain: You'll need to do regular **glucose testing,** from one to four times a day. Aim for pre-meal levels of 90 to 130 milligrams per deciliter (mg/dL), and bedtime levels of 100 to 140 mg/dL.

To test glucose levels, most people use a device that makes a tiny jab in their fingertip. Then they place a drop of blood on a specially treated test strip, and insert the strip into a glucose meter for a reading. Microneedle devices are so tiny you can barely feel the pinprick. Ask your doctor about the possibility of using an **insulin pump.** Worn on your body (*see illustration, page 106*), this amazing device is programmed to silently inject insulin all the time.

Rarely, for people with very severe diabetes, a **transplant** of the pancreas or a double pancreas/kidney transplant may be needed.

Medications

To keep your blood sugar levels within normal limits, you'll need insulin therapy, in amounts determined by your weight, diet, activity level, overall health, and other factors. Insulin is destroyed by digestive juices, so you can't take it by mouth. It must be injected through the skin.

Various forms of insulin are used for different situations. **Fast-acting insulin** (Humalog, Novolog) enters the blood in 15 minutes. It can be valuable before eating and for tight glucose control. **Intermediate-** and **longer-acting insulins** are active for more than 24 hours. The relatively new Glargine (rDNA origin) is particularly valuable because insulin levels remain nearly constant throughout the period. Your doctor will help design a program using one or more types of insulin to optimize your blood sugar

TAKING Control

- **Wear medical identification** (a bracelet or medallion) saying you have diabetes. If you're unconscious in an emergency, a medical team will need this information.

- **Get a good health-care team.** Count on seeing your doctors, nurses, and dietitians every one to three months. Ask your local hospital if a Certified Diabetes Instructor is on staff.

- **Make a smart plan.** Educate yourself about the disease—and let others help you devise a strategy for dealing with glucose testing, insulin shots, exercise, and diet.

- **Overwhelmed? Start by visiting an outpatient diabetes clinic** every day until you and your family feel confident and comfortable. What now seems so new (and maybe frightening) will soon become second nature and little more than a minor inconvenience.

- **Improve the accuracy of your home glucose monitor** by taking these simple measures. Keep the monitor clean. Test it once a month. Recalibrate it whenever starting a new packet of strips. Use fresh strips. Periodically, compare your results with those from a laboratory.

- **Take care if you get sick.** You're especially susceptible to diabetic ketoacidosis (*see box opposite*) if you develop the flu or a urinary tract infection. Never stop your insulin during an illness. Check your urine for ketones every six hours. If your condition is worsening, let your doctor know right away.

► **Does it really matter where on my body I inject the insulin?**

Yes. The injection location will affect your blood glucose levels. Insulin enters the bloodstream fastest when you inject it into the abdomen. It takes a little longer if you inject it into the upper arm, and even more time when injected in the thigh and buttocks (often best for a bedtime insulin shot). Shift your exact injection site regularly to avoid developing hard lumps or extra fatty deposits at that spot.

FINDING Support

■ The American Diabetes Association can provide a wealth of information (1-800-DIABETES or www.diabetes.org). The National Institute of Diabetes & Digestive & Kidney Diseases (NIDDK) supports a very proactive website with tips on managing your disease (www.ndep.nih.gov).

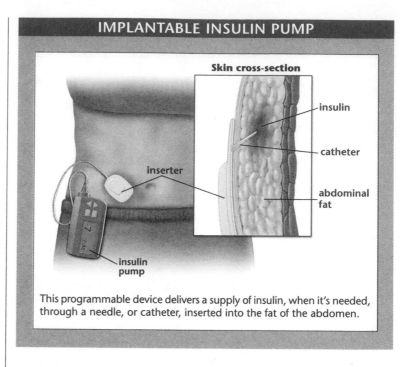

IMPLANTABLE INSULIN PUMP

Skin cross-section

insulin

catheter

abdominal fat

inserter

insulin pump

This programmable device delivers a supply of insulin, when it's needed, through a needle, or catheter, inserted into the fat of the abdomen.

control. A common regimen includes a short-acting insulin before you eat, and a longer-acting one for coverage between meals or at night.

Most people admit that insulin injection is far simpler than they thought it would be. After a couple of meetings with an instructor (often a nurse), you'll feel comfortable drawing insulin into a syringe, cleaning your skin with alcohol, and administering a virtually pain-free shot. Prefilled insulin "pens" are convenient. Jet injectors use a high-pressure stream of air to send a fine flow of insulin through the skin. They're bulky, expensive, and not pain-free, but they're a good choice if you're afraid of needles. Battery-operated insulin pumps can achieve tighter glucose control.

Lifestyle Changes

Stick to a strict timetable for injections, glucose testing, meals, and exercise. A chart or a portable journal can be very helpful. **Wise diet choices** will make a huge difference in how you feel (*see Diabetes Type 2, page 108*). Some people with type 1 diabetes gain weight when they start insulin because their cells have been "starved" for sugar, but, unlike type 2 diabetes, obesity is rare.

The best way to control your weight is through **exercise,** which can even lessen your insulin needs. When your body is active, its demand for glucose increases—and the glucose in your bloodstream is used up first. Time your injections to avoid working out when insulin is peaking. (If you don't, you risk a dangerous drop in blood sugar.) A few other tips: Avoid exercise if your glucose is above 300 mg/dl or under 100 mg/dl. Inject in sites far from the muscles you exercise most intensely. Eat a snack (bread, pasta, or potato) 30 minutes before you work out.

Diabetes type 2

The key to dealing with this disease, which affects about 15 million Americans, is to feel a sense of control. After all, most diabetes problems can be prevented or delayed with smart living, a measure of diligence, and the right medications.

What is happening

The type of diabetes that develops slowly during adulthood—and is generally manageable with diet, weight reduction, and medication—is called type 2. With this form of the disease, you aren't producing enough insulin, and your cells are no longer responding to the insulin you do produce. The pancreas, an organ tucked against the back of your abdomen, produces insulin, a hormone that enables your body to use sugar (glucose). Without enough insulin, glucose builds up in your blood instead of entering your cells, which need it to function. This causes high blood sugar, the source of many complications. If you don't treat it, it can eventually damage your eyes, kidneys, nerves, and blood vessels (*see box, page 109*).

Generally, diabetes occurs for two reasons—it may run in your family, making you genetically susceptible, or you may have taxed your body's glucose-balancing system from poor eating habits and excess weight gain. Type 2 accounts for about 90–95% of diabetes cases. Most of the remainder, termed type 1, are found before age 30. They occur when the immune system attacks insulin-producing cells in the pancreas (*see page 104*). A third type (gestational) occurs only during pregnancy. It clears up after childbirth.

Treatments

Type 2 diabetes is a serious disease, and there's a big payoff if you become proactive about managing it. You can learn how to minimize or even eliminate the need for drugs, and dramatically postpone complications. Keeping your blood glucose in the normal range and improving your body's use of insulin are daily goals. Many people aim for "tight glucose control," taking all the steps necessary (diet, drugs, frequent self-testing) to avoid marked fluctuations in their glucose levels. With type 2 diabetes, lifestyle changes (meal planning, regular exercise, weight loss) can be very effective. In time, you may need to take oral diabetes drugs. About 40% of those with type 2 diabetes eventually need insulin injections.

It's important to see your doctor regularly (at least four times a year, plus specialist visits) and to develop a healthcare team to answer questions that help you implement an overall plan. Diabetes affects your entire body, so it's critical to watch for complications and take preventive measures. To lessen certain health risks, you may need heart, blood pressure, or cholesterol-lowering drugs, and your eyes, kidneys, nerves, and feet may need special care.

LIKELY **First Steps**

- **Lifestyle changes** (healthy diet, regular exercise) to lower blood sugar and enhance overall health.
- **Weight reduction** to prevent worsening of disease and reduce risk of complications.
- **Oral medications** to stave off initiating **insulin injections**.

QUESTIONS TO **Ask**

- Will I ever need insulin?
- How can I tell if I'm developing complications?
- Should I aim for very tight blood glucose control?
- How often do I need a hemoglobin A1c test done?

▶ **Are sweets safe or not?**
It's really not a question of "safety," but concentrated sweets are extremely caloric and use up your allotment of carbohydrates (and fats) for that day. If you simply must have a chocolate chip cookie, deduct its carbohydrate and fat amounts from your next meal. When you discover your portions have been reduced by a third, you may think twice about the same cookie next time. Choose low-fat sweets, such as fig bars or graham crackers, instead of ice cream.

TAKING Control

- **Expand your annual check-up.** Be sure to add an eye exam by an eye specialist (ophthalmologist) and foot exam by a podiatrist. Don't forget a flu shot and ask your doctor if you need another pneumonia vaccination.

- **Have a hemoglobin A1c test.** At first, your doctor will check your long-term glucose control every two to three months with this blood test, also known as HbA1c. A score higher than 8 means you need more control. Below 7 is ideal. If your doctor hasn't done this test, consider finding a more knowledgeable doctor.

- **Avoid foot problems.** Give your feet the best possible care. Wear shoes that fit. With a doctor's prescription, some expenses related to footwear can be defrayed by Medicare.

- **Eat at regular times.** Many foods are converted to glucose, and you need to hold those levels steady. Schedule meals and snacks for about the same time every day. Try to eat consistent amounts— and don't skip meals.

Promising
DEVELOPMENTS

- Three new combinations of oral agents have recently been approved. Glipizide/metformin (Metaglip) and glyburide/metformin (Glucovance) contain sulfonylureas. Like the other two, rosiglitazone/metformin (Avandamet) contains metformin.

- Look to the news for more on an experimental treatment (**protein GLP-1**) for type 2 disease. It not only helps with glucose control, but may make you slimmer.

Treatment options

Lifestyle changes

Diet/weight control	Essential for good diabetes management.
Exercise	Makes cells more insulin-sensitive.

Medications

Sulfonylureas	First-line drugs; promote insulin production.
Biguanide	Most popular oral diabetes medication.
Meglitinides	Fast and flexible; good before meals.
Alpha-glucosidase inhibitors	Delay complex carbohydrate digestion.
Thiazolidinediones	Decrease insulin resistance.
D-phenylalanine derivative	New drug to treat post-meal glucose spikes.

Lifestyle Changes

Achieving a healthy lifestyle is critical for keeping diabetes under control. A **good diet** and weight reduction, if needed, are the first goals— and the most challenging. Anyone can swallow pills, but it takes real willpower to change long-established patterns of poor eating. A dietitian with training in diabetic meal planning can help formulate a program well suited to your needs. Sadly, more than half of all people with diabetes abandon their diet therapy. Relying on luck and medications, they risk serious problems down the line.

The basics of a diabetes diet are the principles of healthy eating, with calorie restrictions. When you start getting 50% of your daily calories from carbohydrates, 30% from fats, and 20% from protein, you'll realize that if everyone ate like this, less obesity as well as diabetes would persist. Such an eating plan also reduces your chances of developing heart disease and cancer. The real challenge is portion control.

If you're overweight, **shedding a few pounds** will improve your blood glucose levels: Losing just 10% of your body weight can slow the progression of diabetes. If weight is an issue for you, consider a support group, like Weight Watchers, and ask your doctor about one of the new drugs for weight control, like Meridia or Xenical (*see Obesity, page 238*). **Regular exercise** combined with calorie restriction will speed your weight loss. When you have diabetes, exercise has an added benefit: It increases your cells' sensitivity to insulin and enables them to use glucose more efficiently. Exercising as little as 30 minutes, three times a week can help, but engaging in something vigorous every day is best. Choose activities that are aerobic: bicycling, swimming, or walking, as opposed to resistance exercises, like weight lifting. **Kick the smoking habit!** The double damage inflicted on your circulation by diabetes and smoking can eventually result in amputation of your toes or feet. Diabetes greatly increases the risk of hardening of the arteries (artherosclerosis), which leads to heart attacks, stroke, and narrowing of the arteries that supply blood to the lungs. These problems are the major cause of death in diabetics. They may be prevented by smoking cessation, and through cholesterol and blood pressure control.

Medications

The six main classes of oral diabetes drugs act on different sites in the body and employ different mechanisms, but they all have one goal: to control blood sugar levels. They'll work only if your pancreas still produces some insulin. The drugs can be used alone, in combination, or with insulin. Your doctor will recommend insulin injections only when oral medications are losing their effect.

For over 30 years, **sulfonylureas** (Glucotrol, DiaBeta, and others) have been the first-line drugs for diabetes, lowering blood sugar by prompting the body to increase insulin production. Low blood sugar (hypoglycemia) is a common and serious side effect of these medications. Over time, a sulfonylurea drug may stop lowering your blood sugar sufficiently, so you'll need to try something else.

To increase your body's sensitivity to insulin (your own or injected forms), the oral medication **metformin** (Glucophage) is valuable. It reduces the liver's production and release of glucose, and increases glucose uptake into muscle cells. This drug can be used alone before a sulfonylurea is tried, or with a sulfonylurea to boost its glucose-lowering effect. With Glucophage, hypoglycemia isn't a problem: You may lose weight due to diminished appetite. Diarrhea can occur but may disappear over time.

Like the sulfonylureas, a group of drugs called **meglitinides,** such as Prandin, stimulate the pancreas to produce insulin. They work quickly and act for only a short time, so you need to take them before every meal. Because meglitinides lower blood sugar, their main side effect is hypoglycemia. Other drugs are taken with meals. The **alpha-glucosidase inhibitors** (Precose, Glyset) will delay the digestion of complex carbohydrates and table sugar. Their purpose is to blunt the increase in blood sugar that normally occurs after eating. Because these drugs interfere with digestion, some people experience mild gas and bloating, but these side effects often subside with long-term use.

Relatively new and quite pricey, **thiazolidinediones (TZDs),** or glitazones, decrease muscle-cell resistance to insulin by activating certain genes involved in fat synthesis and metabolism. Obese people resistant to insulin often take TZDs; Avandia and Actos are currently approved by the FDA. Rezulin, another one of these drugs, caused liver problems and was withdrawn from the market. Avandia and Actos do not appear to cause liver problems, but your doctor will probably want to check your liver enzymes anyway.

The new drug Starlix, a **D-phenylalanine derivative,** lowers glucose levels by stimulating the pancreas to release insulin. It works quickly and acts to prevent the blood glucose increase that occurs after eating. The risk for hypoglycemia is low. (*If you need insulin injections, refer to Diabetes Type 1, page 104.*)

Diabetes Complications

Diabetes affects various body systems.

Eyes: Jeopardizing delicate blood vessels in the eye, diabetic retinopathy is the leading cause of blindness in U.S. adults. When caught early, problems can be treated with laser surgery. Tight glucose control lessens retinopathy risk.

Kidneys: Nephropathy, or damage to the small vessels within the kidneys, is the leading cause of kidney failure. Tight glucose control and treatment with ACE inhibitors often prevents problems, but dialysis or a kidney transplant is sometimes needed.

Nerves: Diabetic neuropathy occurs when nerves—usually in the legs and the feet—have been damaged by diabetes. Medications used to control neuropathy include antidepressants (Effexor, Serzone, Wellbutrin, Zoloft), the anti-seizure drug Neurontin, and the painkiller Ultram.

Feet: Infections, injuries, and even gangrene (which necessitates amputation) can develop in your feet as a result of poor circulation. Don't treat such problems yourself; see a podiatrist. Impaired vision and nerves mask pain, so people with diabetes often don't detect sores developing on their feet.

FINDING Support

■ To find a dietitian in your area and more information on diabetes, contact the American Dietetic Association in Alexandria, VA (1-800-877-1600 or www.eatright.org).

Diverticulitis

This painful intestinal condition is widely believed to be the unhappy result of too little fiber in your diet. Most cases can be treated with medication and rest, and future incidences prevented by making healthier lifestyle choices.

LIKELY First Steps

- **Antibiotics** to battle inflammation and infection.

- **Analgesics for pain** and **bed rest** until symptoms ease.

- **Liquid diet** to let colon heal, then **increased fiber** to prevent recurrences.

- If necessary, **surgery** to deal with complications.

QUESTIONS TO Ask

- How long before I can resume my normal activities?

- What are the chances that I'll need surgery?

- If I can't tolerate a high-fiber diet, are there other ways to help my digestive tract?

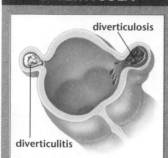

DIVERTICULA

diverticulosis

diverticulitis

When diverticula, the little pouches on the walls of the colon (*see cross-section above*) bulge, the result is a typically benign condition called diverticulosis. If they're inflamed, or infected and pus-filled, it's called diverticulitis. Quick treatment prevents complications.

What is happening

If your diet is heavy on highly refined processed foods and light in fruits, veggies, and whole grains, you're missing a vital ingredient for a healthy colon: fiber. Without fiber—a natural stool softener—constipation is often the order of the day, causing pressure to build up inside your colon (large intestine). Over time, the colon walls weaken and a lot of little pouches, called diverticula, start bulging out like weak spots in an inner tube (*see illustration*). This is called **diverticulosis:** It's quite common. About a third of Americans over age 45 have it, so do 50% of those between ages 60 and 80, and nearly two-thirds of everyone older than that. Diverticulosis rarely causes problems. Most people don't even know they have it unless it's discovered during testing for another ailment.

Diverticulosis can become serious, however, if food particles get trapped in the pouches and bacteria builds up. The resulting inflammation and infection is the basis of a condition called **diverticulitis.** Characterized by intense abdominal pain that's hard to ignore, diverticulitis often comes on suddenly, producing a tenderness in your lower left abdomen. The infection may also give you fever, chills, vomiting, cramping, and constipation.

Although diverticulitis is simple to treat, in rare cases, people develop complications. In the most severe cases, diverticula become filled with pus and develop into abscesses. Sometimes these perforate, allowing infected pus to leak into your abdominal cavity. This is called peritonitis, a life-threatening condition requiring emergency surgery. An infection that spreads outside your colon can also lead to a fistula, which occurs when the tissue of one organ—in this instance, your colon—sticks to another organ, and the infection burrows into it. With diverticulitis, the other organ is often the bladder, and the result can be a severe urinary tract infection. Sometimes an infection can leave scarring, called adhesions, resulting in blockages of the intestine.

Treatments

If caught early, a mild case of diverticulitis often clears up after two or three days of oral antibiotics, bed rest, a clear liquid diet to allow your colon to heal, and an analgesic for discomfort. If you have severe pain or a serious infection, your doctor will probably want to hospitalize you so medications and fluids can be delivered intravenously. About 20% of those who suffer repeated diverticulitis

Treatment options

Medications

Antibiotics	Clear up inflammation and infection.
Analgesics	For pain; no NSAIDs if you have bleeding.

Lifestyle changes

Take it easy	Stay in bed if possible.
Watch diet	Avoid high-fiber foods at first; then eat more.
Exercise	Helps prevent constipation; stay hydrated.

Procedures

Colonoscopy	And/or x-rays to find source of bleeding.
Surgery	To remove abscess, fistula, or diseased colon.

flare-ups will require surgery to recover from intestinal complications. If you have any of the following symptoms, you should get emergency medical treatment right away: bloody stools, a persistent high fever, inability to have a bowel movement, or severe abdominal pain or tenderness.

Medications

If your symptoms are mild, your doctor will probably prescribe two **antibiotics:** metronidazole (Flagyl) and a second broad-spectrum antibiotic, such as ciprofloxacin (Cipro) or amoxicillin/clavulanate (Augmentin). You're likely to feel better in a few days, but stay on these drugs for the full course prescribed.

For pain, consult your doctor about taking an **analgesic.** If you have bleeding, avoid nonsteroidal anti-inflammatory drugs (NSAIDs), such as aspirin or ibuprofen: They can hinder blood clotting. It may be safest to take acetaminophen (Tylenol), but you may need something stronger, so ask your physician first.

If your symptoms are more severe, your doctor may hospitalize you to get **intravenous antibiotics, pain relievers,** and **fluids.** You may get intravenous nutrition, too, to give your inflamed colon a complete rest. For most people, this leads to a full recovery.

Lifestyle Changes

For a milder case, once you have your medications in hand, the best thing you can do is climb into bed and rest until you're feeling better. **Watch your diet,** too. Initially, you'll need to stay on liquids and soft foods. In a few days, your doctor will probably start you on a low-fiber diet.

After about a month, you're likely to get the go-ahead to begin introducing high-fiber foods and start **exercising.** Your doctor will probably want you to drink plenty of water throughout your recovery.

TAKING Control

- **See a gastroenterologist** instead of an internist or family physician. In a recent study by Loyola University Medical Center in Illinois, people with diverticulitis who were treated by gastroenterologists had a shorter hospital stay and were less likely to need re-admission.

- **Avoid enemas.** Even though they may seem like a good solution for a problem that results from constipation, they can aggravate diverticulitis symptoms.

▶ **THE SEED CONTROVERSY.** For years it's been standard medical wisdom that if you have diverticulitis, you should steer clear of nuts, seeds, and popcorn because they get trapped in diverticula and cause inflammation. It turns out, however, there is no scientific evidence to support this. Most doctors now tell their patients that they themselves should be the judge of what they can eat. So, if they don't bother you, enjoy strawberries, tomatoes, sunflower seeds, cashews, and all your favorite dishes that contain seeds and nuts.

Preventing Diverticular Attacks

If you have diverticulosis or you've recovered from a bout of diverticulitis, a trouble-free digestive tract should be a top priority. There's plenty you can do to keep your colon healthy:

● **Increase your fiber.** The American Dietetic Association recommends 20 to 35 grams of fiber daily. Replace white rice and breads with bran cereal, oatmeal, whole-grain breads, and brown rice. Put cooked dried beans or peas on the menu once a week. If you're not used to a high-fiber diet, add these gradually to avoid painful gas.

● **Eat your vegetables and fruits**—they're fiber-rich too. A good start is five daily servings of fruits and vegetables, cooked or raw, and preferably, unpeeled when possible.

● **Go when you need to.** When you feel the urge to move your bowels, head for the bathroom right away rather than waiting.

● **Drink lots of fluids,** at least eight glasses a day of water, juices, and soups. This helps move the added fiber through your digestive system.

● **Get regular exercise.** Three to five times a week go for a brisk walk, ride your bike, jog, swim, or dance around the house.

● **Use a bulk-forming laxative** for occasional constipation. Good choices are products containing psyllium (Metamucil) and calcium polycarbophil (FiberCon). Don't forget dried fruits: They're a natural laxative and good source of fiber.

▶**DIVERTICULITIS IS VIRTU-ALLY UNKNOWN in the less developed countries of Africa and Asia. That's because the diet in these countries is vegetable-based and high in fiber. When inhabitants of these nations immigrate to the United States and start eating the way many Americans do (lots of meat and pro-cessed high-fat foods), they tend to start devel-oping diverticulitis.**

FINDING Support

■ For the latest medical and nutritional treatments for diverticulitis, and ways to cope with digestive illness, contact the Intestinal Disease Foundation in Pittsburgh, PA (877-587-9606 or www.in-testinalfoundation.org).

■ To find a gastroenterologist in your area, use the Locator Service of the American Gas-troenterological Association (www.gastro.org).

Procedures

If your diverticulitis doesn't respond to medication, or you have frequent or severe attacks, your doctor may recommend surgery. (This is particularly true if you're under age 50 and have even one severe attack. Diverticulitis tends to be more aggressive and recur more often in younger people.) Although a small abscess can be drained with a relatively minor procedure, more invasive surgery may be needed to eliminate a large abscess, remove a fistula, or clear an obstruction in your intestine. If you develop perforations or peritonitis, you'll need emergency surgery.

The surgeon usually treats any complication by removing the diseased part of your colon and reattaching the cut ends in a **partial colectomy** (*see illustration, page 88*). If you have wide-spread inflammation, you may need two operations. First, the surgeon clears away the infection in your abdominal cavity, removes the affected part of your colon, and attaches the healthy colon to a temporary opening in your abdomen. This **colostomy** serves as an artificial anus. A bag, attached to the opening, receives stools and keeps them completely away from the infected area. Once the inflammation clears up, the surgeon performs a second operation to reattach the ends of your colon and close the hole in your abdomen. Your bowel movements will return to normal.

Diverticular bleeding normally stops by itself, but your doctor may still want to perform a **colonoscopy.** This examination of your colon uses a long, flexible scope to find the source of the bleeding (*see page 360*). If you have very heavy bleeding, the doctor may also take **specialized x-rays** to locate the problem. Bleeding that doesn't stop by itself can sometimes be controlled by injecting **vasopressin,** a drug that constricts your arteries. This effect can be dangerous, especially in older people, so your doctor may recom-mend a partial colectomy instead.

Ear infection

You don't have to be a kid to get an ear infection. Adults, too, are sometimes plagued by the nagging pain and pressure of an earache. But targeted medications can bring quick relief—and sometimes aching ears clear up on their own.

What is happening

Ear infections generally arise when bacteria, viruses, or fungi take hold in various parts of your ear, causing inflammation and pain. In adults, an earache most often signals **otitis externa**—an outer ear infection also known as swimmer's ear. This condition occurs in your ear canal, the passage through which sound travels to your eardrum. Constant moisture in the canal encourages bacteria and fungi to grow. It also softens the canal's lining, allowing the germs to invade more easily.

Swimmer's ear can strike landlubbers, too. Excessive earwax, exposure to harsh chemicals in products such as hair dyes, use of ear plugs or stereo headphones, excessive sweating from physical activity, chronic skin conditions such as eczema, psoriasis, or seborrhoea, or even wayward insects can trigger inflammation. Symptoms often begin with itching that gradually worsens into pain, especially if you frequently tug the earlobe. Your outer ear may be red, and the canal may look swollen. If it oozes yellowish fluid, call your doctor.

Otitis media affects the middle ear between the eardrum and inner ear. It most often strikes young children. By age 3, about 70% of kids have suffered at least one middle ear infection, but getting older doesn't grant you immunity. In both children and adults, viral and bacterial attacks—often resulting from a cold, flu, allergy, or sinus infection—can cause mucus and pus to collect in the eustachian tube that connects your middle ear with the back of your nose. This can provoke pain that is sharp and sudden or dull and throbbing, and often accompanied by fever and nasal congestion.

Treatments

Earaches can be excruciating, but the pain is usually short lived and complications are rare—if you get prompt treatment. A festering infection can muffle your hearing, or perforate your eardrum. It can spread to nearby bones and tissue, but rarely does. Most outer ear infections have the happy distinction of being among the most easily treated medical conditions. It often takes only a gentle wax removal or a dose or two of medicated eardrops. Many middle ear infections, especially in adults, clear up on their own.

Medications

An outer ear infection typically requires topical antibiotics. If your doctor suspects a bacterial infection, you may get a prescription for

TAKING Control

- **Take a drug-free approach to otitis media.** According to the U.S. Agency for Health-care Research and Quality Control, 80% of middle ear infections in children heal on their own. Many experts suggest giving mild cases a day or two before resorting to antibiotics.

- **Stay the course.** If you are prescribed antibiotics, be sure to take the full course even if you feel better in a day or two. If you don't, harmful germs may remain, rally, and strike again.

- **Give your hearing aid a rest.** Avoid using this device during treatment. When your ear is healthy, remove the hearing aid often to air out the ear canal.

- **Try herbal eardrops.*** You can relieve a mild earache caused by otitis externa in about 10 minutes with mullein flower eardrops, available at health-food stores. The drops reduce swelling and help fight infection-causing microbes. Avoid the drops if there's any chance of a ruptured eardrum. Symptoms include draining from the ear or intense pain.

*Natural methods are not subject to the same testing and regulation as prescription medications. Please seek your doctor's advice and use caution.

FINDING Support

- For details on the causes and treatment of outer and middle ear infections, check out www.medem.com, a website with information culled from leading medical societies, including the American Medical Association and the American Academy of Pediatrics.

Treatment options

Medications

Antibiotics	Eardrops or oral; corticosteroid if swelling.
Antifungals	When a fungus is the cause.
Anesthetic eardrops	To relieve pain while antibiotics take effect.
Analgesics/NSAIDs	In addition to antibiotics for pain.

Lifestyle changes

Good ear hygiene	Keep ear canal clean; remove wax properly.

antibiotic eardrops (ofloxacin otic, gentamicin, or tobramycin) with or without a **corticosteroid** such as ciprofloxacin hydrochloride plus hydrocortisone (Cipro HC) to reduce swelling. For a suspected fungus, **antifungal preparations**—cresyl acetate (Cresylate) and ketoconazole cream (Nizoral)—are effective. For a severe case, the doctor may add an **oral antibiotic** such as trimethoprim/sulfamethoxazole (Bactrim), cephalexin (Keflex), or levofloxacin (Levaquin) to the artillery.

Because of concerns about antibiotic-resistant bacteria, many experts advocate giving middle ear infections time to improve on their own. If your doctor thinks you need oral antibiotics, most adults and children receive amoxicillin (Amoxil, Larotid) or amoxicillin/clavulanate (Augmentin). **Anesthetic eardrops** containing benzocaine (Auralgan), available by prescription, provide quick relief even before antibiotics take effect.

Even if you're using a prescription antibiotic, you'll probably want to rein in pain with an **over-the-counter analgesic,** such as acetaminophen (Tylenol), or a **nonsteroidal anti-inflammatory drug (NSAID)** like ibuprofen (Advil) or naproxen (Aleve), which also reduces inflammation. For severe pain, you may require a powerful prescription painkiller such as codeine.

Lifestyle Changes

Medical treatment goes hand in hand with being good to your ears. Whether you have an infection or not, always **clean your ears with care.** Don't try to remove dirt with your fingernail, a hairpin, or even a cotton swab. Any of them can scratch the ear canal. Use damp cotton balls or a warm washcloth instead.

If you tend to accumulate **earwax,** place a drop or two of warm mineral oil or vegetable oil in your ear. Lie on your opposite side for about five minutes to let the oil penetrate, then flush out the loosened wax with a bulb syringe filled with warm water. You can try one of the commercially available earwax removal "systems," (Bausch & Lomb, Murine), which contain eardrops and a syringe. Follow the label directions carefully.

Eczema

New types of creams have revolutionized the treatment of eczema, an itchy, unsightly skin disorder also known as dermatitis. Altering your lifestyle, environment, and diet are often key to clearing up your patches of red, rough skin.

What is happening

Eczema can first appear as cradle cap in babies. It then disappears, and may recur elsewhere on the body later in childhood. Ultimately, most children outgrow it. When adults who have this disorder have irritation, the immune system mounts a defense reaction that includes initiating inflammation with the release of chemicals that cause red, itchy blotches. (Eczema means "to boil out" in Greek.) These lesions may appear on the scalp, wrists, and hands, as well as at the crease of the elbows, in back of the knees, and sometimes elsewhere on the body. Eczema has been dubbed "the itch that rashes" rather than the reverse, because discomfort to the skin occurs before a rash appears.

Several different types of eczema exist, but most are related to a personal or family history (*see box, page 117*). If your eczema flares after contact with certain foods, drugs, or animal dander, you have **atopic dermatitis**, a chronic form of the disorder. If handling certain metals, fragrances, or cleaning products triggers your eczema, the diagnosis is **contact dermatitis**, which usually stops once the offensive substance is removed. Emotional stress can also set off eczema **(neurodermatitis)**, as can poor circulation in the legs **(statis dermatitis)**, and extremes in weather and humidity.

Treatments

To control eczema, you need to identify and eliminate agents that trigger responses in your immune system by noting where the rash occurs. If it appears on your hands, for example, the culprit is likely to be something you're touching. You may also need to work with an allergist to determine which substances are problematic. It's also a good idea to undertake a food elimination diet with "controlled food challenges" (*see page 27*). Foods such as wheat, soy, eggs, milk, fish, and nuts are common culprits. Having an immunoglobulin E (IgE) blood test may also be useful.

Many cases of eczema respond to soothing creams, but stubborn outbreaks often require oral medication. Sometimes secondary bacterial infections develop on already irritated skin. Prescription antibiotics help with this malady.

Lifestyle Changes

Many self-care strategies will stop your eczema flares or reduce their frequency. Try the approaches on the following page:

LIKELY First Steps

■ **Identification and elimination** of eczema triggers.

■ OTC or prescription **creams and ointments** to control eczema.

■ **Oral medications** for hard-to-treat cases.

QUESTIONS TO Ask

■ Why does my eczema come back when I stop using a steroid cream?

■ Are medications that I take for other ailments aggravating my eczema?

■ Why undergo tests for allergies if my eczema has already been diagnosed?

TAKING **Control**

- **Use gloves.** Moisturize your hands well and don cotton gloves for any "dry" work around the house or on the job—especially when working with problematic substances. Wearing loose-fitting vinyl gloves over the cotton gloves will protect your hands when doing dishes and "wet" work.

- **Wash away irritants.** Use a liquid laundry detergent, rather than a powder, and wash new clothes before wearing them to rinse out fabric-sizing chemicals. Add extra rinse cycles, if necessary.

- **Don't put up with pain.** If any topical treatment you're using stings or is painful, stop using it, and tell your doctor. You can be switched to a different cream or ointment.

▶**TWO OF THE NEW EURO COINS**—the one-euro and the two-euro—have proved a real problem for some of the cashiers and shopkeepers in the European Economic Union. In the industrial world, about 15% of women and up to 5% of men are allergic to nickel content, according to a recent study. Some 30% to 40% of those with nickel sensitivity will develop hand eczema after contact with the coins.

Treatment options

Lifestyle changes	
Identify triggers	Foods, animal dander, chemicals, stress.
Skin care	Don't scratch; moisturize; watch cosmetics.
Medications	
Topical corticosteroids	OTC or prescription to clear up flares.
Oral corticosteroids	Only for severe cases.
Antihistamines	To control itching.
Topical immunomodulators	Nonsteroidal; for moderate to severe eczema.
Natural methods	
Key nutrients	Prevent dryness and boost immunity.
Licorice cream	Make sure it contains glycyrrhizin.
Procedures	
Phototherapy	Ultraviolet light/PUVA therapy.

- **Identify and avoid eczema triggers.** You may have an allergy to molds, dust mites, animal dander, chemicals, detergents, and metals (such as nickel or chrome). If dust mites aggravate your eczema, replace your bedding with hypoallergenic covers and do some ruthless housecleaning.

- **Don't scratch**, no matter how aggravating the itching. It can worsen the rash and cause infection. Put ointment in the refrigerator to chill before applying, for extra analgesic effect.

- **Bathe in lukewarm, not hot water** laced with bath oil, baking soda, or a commercial oatmeal bath (Aveeno). Use fragrance-free, nondrying soaps, such as Dove, Alpha Keri, or Eucerin, and cleansers such as Cetaphil, or baby shampoo. Pat rather than rub your body dry.

- **Keep your skin moist.** Dry skin is vulnerable, so routinely apply a nonirritating emollient moisturizer. Use it within three minutes of a bath or shower, and immediately after washing your hands. Good choices include petroleum jelly, Vanicream, and DML.

- **Stop using cosmetics and creams** if a rash appears on your face. After your rash clears up, add them back, one at a time, with a week between additions, until you identify the troublemaker.

- **Wear loose clothing.** Fabrics that "breathe" (cotton and other natural fibers) irritate less than woolens and acrylics.

- **Control your surroundings.** Your skin prefers the thermostat at 68°F with a comfortable humidity level. Use a humidifier in winter and a dehumidifier in summer.

- **Try to minimize stress,** a common eczema trigger. Practice deep breathing, walking, or dancing. Consider seeing a psychotherapist or joining a support group for people with eczema.

Medications

The outbreak's severity determines the medication you'll need. In general, oozing spots require a liquid or lotion, while rough, dry patches need an ointment or cream. Treat mild cases with a topical over-the-counter **1% hydrocortisone cream** (such as Cortaid), applied no more than twice a day after washing. If your eczema is more intractable, you may need a **prescription topical corticosteroid.** There are brands in a whole spectrum of strengths. Your doctor will decide which is right for you. Your doctor may suggest that you apply a moisturizer over it. Powerful **prescription oral corticosteroids** (prednisone, methylprednisolone) are used for severe cases and should be managed by a physician familiar with their specialized and limited use.

The annoying itching may be relieved with over-the-counter **oral antihistamines** such as diphenhydramine (Benadryl), chlorpheniramine (Chlor-Trimeton), or the prescription hydroxyzine (Atarax). These help quell the urge to scratch, but cause drowsiness. Ask your doctor about cetirizine (Zyrtec), a new, nondrowsy histamine blocker. If your skin is not acutely inflamed, your doctor may prescribe a shampoo or ointment containing coal tar (such as Tegrin Lotion or Denorex Medicated Shampoo) to reduce itching and inflammation.

The most promising development in the treatment of moderate to severe eczema is the new, nonsteroidal **topical immunomodulators** (TIMS) such as tacrolimus (Protopic) and pimecrolimus (Elidel). Unlike topical steroids, which can seep into the bloodstream and cause systemic problems if given in high doses, Elidel remains within the skin, and seems safe for long-term, intermittent use.

Natural Methods*

Getting **key nutrients** through foods and daily vitamin/mineral supplements can have numerous benefits. Foods rich in vitamin A, beta-carotene, and essential fatty acids may help to combat skin dryness. Foods high in zinc, the antioxidant vitamins C and E, and the flavonoid quercetin may quell inflammation. Apply a **licorice cream** that contains glycyrrhizin; as a natural anti-inflammatory, licorice may help relieve eczema on its own, or can be applied over a cortisone cream.

Procedures

Phototherapy using ultraviolet (UV) light is a treatment option if you have atopic dermatitis. In this procedure, you expose your skin to UV lamps at a prescribed wavelength. You may also find **PUVA therapy** beneficial. This procedure combines an agent (psoralen) that boosts the therapeutic effect of light with ultraviolet A (UVA) light. These treatments are expensive and increase the risk of skin cancer. Ask your doctor if either of these might benefit you.

Natural methods are not subject to the same testing and regulation as prescription medications. Please seek your doctor's advice and use caution.

Nothing to Sneeze At

If you have atopic eczema, you belong to a large, diverse family: Those who have hay fever (allergic rhinitis), asthma, and other kinds of allergies. It's common for eczema sufferers to come from clans where wheezing and sneezing is the norm, and sometimes to be doubly afflicted. Moreover, children with eczema may grow out of their itchy skin condition, only to develop hay fever or asthma later.

The mechanism that causes such allergic reactions appears genetic: Your body is programmed to react adversely to an antibody called immunoglobulin E, or IgE. This substance adheres to mast cells, which cause the swelling, redness, and itching of an allergic reaction. It's no surprise that allergy and eczema sufferers usually have high levels of IgE in their bloodstream.

FINDING Support

- For the latest information on eczema treatments, as well as listings of medical providers who specialize in dermatitis, visit the website of the National Eczema Association for Science and Education, www.nationaleczema.org, or call the NEA in Portland, OR, at 1-800-818-7546.

- The American Academy of Dermatology's website, www.aad.org, has helpful information about eczema and other skin ailments.

Emphysema

Every day the average person takes about 17,000 breaths. Emphysema can make each one a real struggle. If you have this problem, there are a number of positive steps you can take to breathe more easily and greatly improve your quality of life.

LIKELY **First Steps**

- **Smoking cessation** to slow progression of the disease.
- **Medications** to ease breathing and fight infections.
- **Avoidance of air pollutants** to protect against irritation.
- **Breathing techniques** to strengthen your breathing muscles.

QUESTIONS TO **Ask**

- Do I have the right inhaler? Am I using it correctly?
- Is it safe for me to fly?
- Would it help me significantly to move to a warmer, drier climate?
- Would I be a good candidate for a lung transplant?

What is happening

Your lungs are packed with tiny air sacs called alveoli, which are ringed by microscopic blood vessels (capillaries). In healthy lungs, air flows easily in and out. Oxygen passes efficiently into the capillaries while carbon dioxide, the waste product, returns to the lungs and is exhaled. Someone who has emphysema has fewer alveoli. The ones they have lose their elasticity, making breathing difficult (*see illustration below*).

A persistent, mucus-producing cough and shortness of breath are the first and most obvious symptoms of emphysema. They're probably what brought you to the doctor. Some people with emphysema describe the effort to draw enough air into their lungs as "trying to breathe through a pillow." As the disease progresses, so does breathing difficulty. In advanced stages, people often fight for air after just a few steps. Emphysema also taxes your heart by forcing it to work harder to circulate blood through the lungs.

Nearly 3 million Americans have emphysema. Some 90% of cases are triggered by long-term cigarette smoking. Irritants in the smoke inflame alveoli walls, which then lose their elasticity. About 3% of cases are the result of an inherited genetic abnormality called alpha-

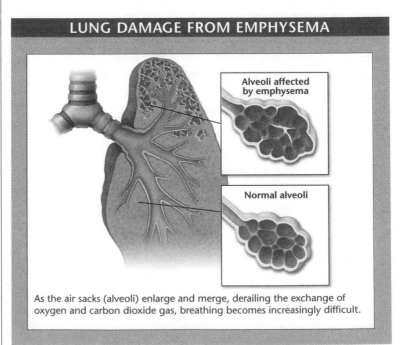

LUNG DAMAGE FROM EMPHYSEMA

Alveoli affected by emphysema

Normal alveoli

As the air sacs (alveoli) enlarge and merge, derailing the exchange of oxygen and carbon dioxide gas, breathing becomes increasingly difficult.

Treatment options

Lifestyle changes

Stop smoking	Essential for any improvement.
Learn better breathing	Special techniques strengthen muscles.
Avoid "bad" air	Especially smoke and very cold weather.

Medications

Bronchodilators	Relax breathing muscles, expand airways.
Corticosteroids	Ease inflamed respiratory system.
Antibiotics	Fight respiratory infections.
AAT supplement	Injections treat genetic emphysema.

Procedures

Supplemental oxygen	Improves stamina.
Surgery	Reduces or replaces diseased lungs.

1-antitrypsin (AAT) deficiency. Exposure to airborne irritants, such as coal dust, grain particles, smoke, or textile fibers, may also lead to emphysema. Emphysema is a serious, generally irreversible disease, but you have the power to minimize its impact on your life.

Treatments

The goal of emphysema treatment is to slow or even halt the disease's progression. There's no debate: **The single most important step you can take is to stop smoking.** To further ease your distress, your physician will prescribe medications that open your lungs, reduce airway irritation, and when the need arises, short-circuit potentially dangerous infections. You can help reduce your symptoms by taking certain precautions, starting an exercise program, and learning special breathing techniques.

Lifestyle Changes

If you smoke cigarettes, you must quit. Should you continue to smoke, your emphysema will become worse, regardless of the medical care you receive. If you **stop smoking,** you will vastly improve your life—not to mention prolong it—and be able to maintain your independence. Committing to this lifestyle change is difficult for many people, but it can be done. You don't have to do it alone: Various proven options can help you kick the habit, which include therapy, medications, and support groups (*see Tobacco Dependence, page 314*).

You can also benefit from learning new **breathing techniques,** either through a hospital program recommended by your doctor, or by doing pursed-lip breathing (*see box, page 120*) on your own.

TAKING Control

■ **Enroll in an outpatient rehab program.** Health professionals will guide you through aerobic exercise and breathing techniques, answer questions, provide education, and direct you to support groups for pulmonary patients. Such programs improve your ability to cope with emphysema.

■ **Plan before you fly.** Increase your mobility by ordering supplemental oxygen equipment before flying. Airlines will not allow you to bring your own oxygen unit on board the aircraft, but they'll supply it if you ask.

■ **Maintain your weight.** Emphysema makes it easy to lose weight. Labored breathing consumes a lot of calories and makes eating difficult. Eat several smaller meals of nutritionally rich foods each day, and take a high-potency vitamin and mineral supplement.

Promising DEVELOPMENTS

■ A University of Pittsburgh researcher is developing a device (the **Hattler Respiratory Catheter**) that can act as an artificial lung for someone with emphysema. Threaded into a major leg vein, the catheter provides about half of the oxygen an adult body needs. It can stay in place for as long as two weeks, making it potentially useful for emphysema patients who develop pneumonia or other respiratory complications and need extra help breathing while their lungs heal. The device is under review by the Food and Drug Administration.

Pursed-Lip Breathing

Help yourself breathe more easily with a 10-minute exercise called pursed-lip breathing. Here's how:
1. Just before beginning an activity, lie flat on a bed with your head on a pillow.
2. Inhale through your nose for about four seconds, consciously moving your abdominal muscles to fill your lungs with air.
3. Purse your lips and exhale through your mouth, making a hissing sound. The exhalation should last twice as long as the inhalation. You should feel pressure in your chest and windpipe.
4. Repeat the exercise a number of times. You can do pursed-lip breathing any time you need more air, even while standing.

▶**TO STRENGTHEN YOUR BREATHING MUSCLES,** try a hand-held device called an incentive spirometer. It contains a breathing gauge that measures how forcefully you exhale. Use it for 15 minutes, twice a day.

▶**COMMONLY USED FOR ASTHMA,** the oral bronchodilator theophylline (Theo-dur, Uniphyl) is occasionally prescribed for emphysema. Some experts question how helpful it is, but many people who've tried it report that they breathe more easily.

Many other actions will confer benefits as well. To get the best health payoff, try to incorporate the following into your lifestyle:

■ **Seek out "good" air.** Avoid smoke-filled rooms or places with high levels of particulates in the air. Stay indoors on cold days or when air quality is poor.

■ **Get plenty of fluids.** Drink water—at least eight glasses a day—to thin mucus secretions. Moisten indoor air with a cool-mist humidifier.

■ **Protect against infections.** Steer clear of people with colds or the flu: Emphysema lowers your resistance to infectious diseases, which can pose a serious threat. Wash your hands frequently to reduce the risk of contracting a respiratory infection. Get a flu shot every year and a pneumonia vaccination as recommended by your practitioner.

■ **Follow an exercise routine** set up with the help of your doctor. Mild to moderate exercise improves endurance and cardiovascular health, reduces breathlessness, and boosts your sense of well-being.

■ **Find out about postural drainage,** a way to drain mucus by hanging your head lower than your torso. Ask your doctor or physical therapist to teach you this technique.

■ **Avoid high altitutes** and extreme temperatures.

Medications

When you stop smoking, adding drug therapy will help you breathe more easily. Whether your disease stems from cigarettes or a genetic abnormality, your doctor will prescribe **bronchodilator drugs** to relax breathing muscles and expand constricted airways. Most bronchodilators are used with a portable device called a metered-dose inhaler. It allows the drug to enter deep into your lungs. When using an inhaler, be sure to follow the proper technique, which your doctor can explain, to ensure that you receive the maximum benefit from the medication. If you can't operate an inhaler—due to arthritis, or some other reason—a nebulizer can do all the work for you, but is not portable.

Among the bronchodilators, **anticholinergic drugs,** such as ipratropium (Atrovent), are often the first choice. They last for about six to eight hours and have few side effects. The other most commonly used bronchodilators are **beta2-agonists,** including albuterol (Proventil), metaproterenol (Alupent), and salmeterol (Serevent). Beta2-agonists act more quickly than anticholinergics, but last for only three to six hours. They are also more likely to cause anxiety, tremor, restlessness, headaches, and other side effects. Some physicians prefer the drug Combivent (a combination of ipratropium with albuterol). It's double-barreled assault that may be superior to taking either type of drug alone.

If your respiratory system is severely inflamed, you may receive **corticosteroids.** These drugs, taken through inhalers, include beclomethasone (Beclovent), budesonide (Pulmicort), and fluticasone (Flovent). The FDA recently approved tiotropium (Spiriva)

About COPD

Emphysema and chronic bronchitis are the two main respiratory conditions referred to as **chronic obstructive pulmonary disease (COPD).** Both typically owe their origin to smoking cigarettes, block air flow to your lungs, interfere with the exchange of oxygen and carbon dioxide in your bloodstream, and cause labored, and sometimes painful, breathing.

For each condition, the goal of treatment is to optimize your physical abilities and improve your airway function enough to allow you as normal and independent a life as possible. Medications for both conditions are generally the same, and both are incurable but often controllable—*if you stop smoking.*

for treatment of COPD. One inhalation treatment can control symptoms for up to 24 hours.

Emphysema makes you more vulnerable to upper respiratory infections, which can pose serious risks because they lead to bacterial infections. If you show signs of infection, your doctor will prescribe an **antibiotic,** such as cefuroxime (Ceftin) or levofloxacin (Levaquin). Antibiotics are useless against viral infections such as colds and the flu. Doctors frequently prescribe them to patients with emphysema whose risk of complications is so high.

For the small percentage of patients whose emphysema is caused by AAT deficiency, drug treatment involves weekly or bimonthly injections of a **purified form of human AAT.** This helps keep AAT levels within the normal range.

Procedures

If your lung function becomes very low, **supplemental oxygen** can bring relief and reduce risk of medical complications. Therapy may be continuous or noncontinuous. Oxygen units may be portable or stationary.

In severe emphysema, **surgery** may be an option. Lung-volume reduction surgery removes the most diseased parts of the lung, allowing remaining tissue and muscles to work better. Many people who undergo lung-reduction return to their daily activities without supplemental oxygen. According to a 2000 report, nearly 75% of patients who undergo this procedure are alive after five years. A 2003 report showed that it works best for patients with disease in their upper lungs.

If your emphysema is advanced or you have the inherited form of the disease, you could be a candidate for **lung transplantation.** One major transplant center reports that 83% of those who undergo this surgery survive at least one year, and 54% live at least five years. The best candidates for lung transplantation are under age 65 and in good health aside from lung disease.

Erectile dysfunction

All men experience erection problems on occasion, so don't panic when it happens to you. But if loss of potency occurs on a regular basis and it's upsetting your life, definitely talk with your doctor. Safe and effective remedies are available.

LIKELY **First Steps**

- **Consultation with your doctor** to determine the cause of your impotence.
- **Medications** (probably Viagra) may be prescribed.
- **Counseling** to ease depression or anxiety, which may be contributing to your problem.
- Lifestyle measures such as **relaxation techniques** to counter stress, and **exercise** to boost vascular health.

QUESTIONS TO **Ask**

- Could my ED be caused by medications I am taking?
- What do I do about my declining interest in sex?
- Could we discuss options with my partner?
- Will I have to use injections?
- Would surgery be a good choice for me?

Cyclist's Caveat

If bike riding is your passion, take heed. Studies have found that some bike seats press on pelvic artery nerves, putting male bicyclists who ride more than five hours a week at an increased risk for developing ED. Seats designed with special grooves are available to prevent this problem.

What is happening

Most men don't really think about how an erection happens until it doesn't. Deeply unsettling, erectile dysfunction (ED), or impotence, is actually quite common, affecting a quarter of men over age 65. Normally an erection occurs when a man becomes sexually aroused, setting off a cascade of chemical reactions in the nervous system. A key player is nitric oxide, which helps arteries widen and relax, increasing blood flow to the penis up to 30-fold and causing it to swell. Veins that normally draw blood away constrict, so blood is held there and the penis remains erect. After arousal, an enzyme called PDE5 helps reverse this process, returning the penis to a flaccid state.

Not so long ago, your doctor would probably have attributed erectile problems to stress or performance ("honeymoon") anxiety. Today, experts believe 80% of cases have medical roots. Anything that diminishes blood flow to the penis can contribute to ED. Atherosclerosis (or "hardening of the arteries" that leads to heart attack and stroke) and diabetes are common culprits. Drug side effects, particularly from blood pressure pills and antidepressants, can also reduce potency. Prostate surgery, radiation treatments for cancer, hormone imbalances, injuries, and nerve disorders such as Parkinson's disease are among the other conditions that may be involved.

Because this condition is fraught with emotional repercussions, it is not surprising that many men with ED become anxious or depressed, lending a psychological component to the condition.

Treatments

Until a few years ago, treatments for ED tended to be complex. Not many men talked about them. The fanfare over the drug Viagra changed all that. Generally safe, easy to use, and remarkably effective, it's now the treatment of choice for most impotent men. Various other treatments are also available: Some men may prefer injectable medications, vacuum devices, and implants. Counseling helps many men. Of course, everyone can benefit from measures such as relaxation and exercise, which help prevent ED problems from recurring or worsening.

Medications

Discovered by accident when researchers noticed erections as a side effect in men taking an experimental drug for heart disease, **Viagra** (sildenafil) has revolutionized the treatment of ED. The first truly successful pill for impotence, Viagra can help problems that stem

Treatment options

Medications

Viagra	Safe, widely used, very effective.
Hormones	Testosterone to increase sex drive.
Alprostadil	Delivered as shots or insertable pellets.
Yohimbine	Boosts blood flow to penis.

Procedures

Pump devices	Create vacuum, drawing blood to penis.
Implants	Semirigid or inflatable rods placed in penis.
Surgery	Good for correctable blood vessel problems.
Counseling	Complements medical treatment.

Natural methods

Supplements	Herbs and the amino acid arginine.
Relaxation techniques	De-stress with meditation, yoga, massage.
Diet & exercise	Relieve stress, aid vascular health.

from physical or psychological causes, or a combination of the two. In tests, two-thirds of men with ED who took the drug were able to have sexual intercourse. In real life, many doctors note, an even higher proportion of male patients may benefit.

Viagra blocks the PDE5 enzyme, keeping smooth muscles relaxed and enhancing blood flow to the penis. Because PDE5 and related enzymes are also present elsewhere in the body (the digestive tract and eyes), the pill can sometimes cause side effects, such as flushing, digestive upset, headaches, and nasal congestion. But even for most heart patients, Viagra is remarkably safe. The only individuals who cannot use the drug are those taking nitrate drugs, such as nitroglycerin, for heart disease. You may need to experiment to find the best dose; you'll know in an hour or less whether the drug will work for you. Absorption is slowed considerably when the pill is taken with a high-fat meal. Finally, you need to be sexually aroused for Viagra to work, so if you take it and change your mind, you can still leave the house without fear of embarrassment.

It's important to note that Viagra works on the mechanics of erections, not on your sexual interest. If you have little or no sex drive, hormone imbalances may be to blame. Rather than Viagra, your doctor may suggest the hormone **testosterone** via a patch, cream, or injections. If you don't respond to Viagra, you may benefit from a blood vessel-widening drug related to Viagra called **alprostadil** (Caverject), which is injected directly into the penis. It sounds painful, but many men become comfortable with the technique. In one study, almost a third of those who had successfully tried Viagra and injectable drugs opted for

TAKING Control

- **Talk with your doctor.** Don't be embarrassed. Medical help is available. Your primary care physician can refer you to a urologist, a specialist in problems of the urinary tract.

- **Share concerns and decisions with your partner.** Treatment for ED is often most successful when couples work at it together.

- **Stop smoking.** Smokers are nearly twice as likely to suffer from ED as nonsmokers. Smokers with high blood pressure are 26 times more likely to have the problem.

- **Drink in moderation.** Having an alcoholic drink can loosen inhibitions, but more than one can impair potency.

- **Exercise.** One report noted inactive men are more likely to have ED than those who exercise 30 minutes a day.

Promising DEVELOPMENTS

- New, more potent "sons of Viagra" may be on the way. **Cialis** (tadalafil) works in 15 to 30 minutes and lasts for 24 hours or more. (Viagra takes 30 to 60 minutes to take effect and lasts for 4 to 6 hours.) Another drug, **vardenafil,** may be effective for men with diabetes or who are recovering from prostate surgery.

- Alternative drugs are in the pipeline for men who don't respond to Viagra or who take nitrates for the heart. **Uprima** (apomorphine) increases levels of a brain chemical called dopamine. **Vasomax** (phentolamine) also targets the nervous system and has been approved for use in Mexico and Brazil.

▶ **TRY A BEDTIME "POSTAGE STAMP" TEST. Encircle your penis with stamps from a roll, gluing the ends. If nighttime erections occur, the stamps will be torn in the morning. That is a sign that problems are probably temporary.**

FINDING Support

■ The National Institute of Diabetes & Digestive & Kidney Diseases offers information and news updates on ED (301-654-4415 or www.niddk.nih.gov).

■ Diabetes is a common cause of erectile problems. The American Diabetes Association offers brochures and advice about men's sexual health (1-800-DIABETES or www.diabetes.org).

■ Counseling can allay anxiety and enhance treatment. The American Association of Sex Educators, Counselors and Therapists (www.aasect.org) offers online referrals for therapists in your area. You can also join an anonymous support group for those with ED at www.alt-support-impotence.org.

the latter because they preferred the quality of their erections. One rare but potentially dangerous side effect is priapism, a persistent, painful erection requiring emergency care. A system called **MUSE,** which inserts alprostadil pellets into the penis tip, is an effective alternative to injections. Finally, an older drug called **yohimbine,** derived from tropical tree bark, boosts blood flow to the penis, although less successfully than Viagra. Too much can cause a dangerous rise in blood pressure.

Procedures

Mechanical **pump devices** that create a vacuum around the penis, drawing blood into the organ, may be an effective option for achieving erection. An elastic band is placed around the base of the penis to maintain the erection. Surgical **implants** can restore erections by placing semirigid or inflatable rods into the penis. Although rarely used, **surgery** to correct blood vessel problems may be effective, especially for younger men who have had injuries to the penis.

Even if the cause of your ED is purely physical, you may benefit from **psychological counseling.** Seeing a counselor can enhance the effects of medical treatments and help you resolve work, family, or money issues that may be diminishing your sexual enjoyment. Engaging your partner in therapy sessions may also be beneficial. A sex therapist can address issues about performance or embarrassment.

Natural Methods*

Natural substances that enhance blood flow and protect blood vessels may also be helpful. Candidates include the herb **ginkgo biloba** (80 mg three times a day) or the nitric-oxide-enhancing amino acid **arginine** (500 mg L-arginine three times a day). Learning to relax is an effective and risk-free way to enhance your sex life. **Meditation, massage,** or **yoga** can all help you unwind. **Exercise** is also an excellent stress-reliever and, along with a **heart-healthy diet,** promotes blood vessel health. The same measures that protect the blood vessels to your heart also protect the vascular health of your sex organs.

Natural methods are not subject to the same testing and regulation as prescription medications. Please seek your doctor's advice and use caution.

Fibromyalgia

So many doctors are unfamiliar with the painful and confusing condition called fibromyalgia that just getting a diagnosis may be something of a relief. You can now begin an effective treatment program and quickly get on the road to recovery.

What is happening

Fibromyalgia, which means "pain in the muscles," is more a condition defined by symptoms than a specific ailment. Nobody is sure what causes it, although the widespread soreness, headaches, poor sleep, and myriad of other symptoms are very real, disrupting the lives of 5 percent of the U.S. population. Although you may feel extremely uncomfortable, there is no evidence of an actual disease occurring in your body, nor are there any lab tests to identify it (one reason why you may have gone to many doctors before it was finally identified).

Some experts believe fibromyalgia may originate in the brain, possibly due to low levels of a nervous system chemical called serotonin. Females have especially low levels of serotonin, which may explain why 9 out of 10 fibromyalgia cases occur in this sex. Women are also most often victims of migraines, irritable bowel syndrome, depression, anxiety, panic attacks, and other disorders that may be due to low serotonin levels. Serotonin seems to have been installed in humans as a buffer against the "fight or flight" response. Without enough serotonin, your body becomes more susceptible to stressful events. (Picture James Bond as the one person who has plenty of serotonin!) When you're constantly stressed, your muscles contract, setting off a destructive chain of events.

Serotonin is also important for assuring deep, restorative sleep, and disruptive sleep patterns have been blamed for bringing on fibromyalgia or making it worse. Because your muscle pain makes it hard to get a good night's rest, you get tired. Lack of sleep causes even more stress. You may also become anxious, forgetful, and depressed, which further contribute to the downward spiral of out-of-control stress that may ultimately lead to fibromyalgia. Other possible causes include injuries, infections, or hormonal disturbances, although these, too, remain uncertain.

Treatments

Even though fibromyalgia is poorly understood, effective therapies are at hand. Treatment usually follows four key steps. First, have your doctor prescribe a good pain medicine. Second, get something to help you sleep better, if necessary. Third, antidepressants will help raise your serotonin levels. Finally, but no less important, you'll need to address the sources of stress in your life and start making changes. Learning some relaxation techniques can help.

LIKELY First Steps

- **Pain-relieving medications** to reduce muscle aches and soreness.
- **Sleep aids** to restore healthy sleeping patterns.
- **Antidepressant medications** to boost serotonin levels in the brain.
- **Stress-relieving measures,** such as relaxation and cognitive-behavioral therapies.
- **Low-impact and stretching exercises** at first, with aerobics and strengthening added gradually.

QUESTIONS TO Ask

- Will my pain and fatigue keep getting worse?
- Why do all my tests and x-rays show there is nothing wrong with me?
- Why are you prescribing antidepressants when I'm not depressed?
- Are some of my other problems, like irritable bowel syndrome and PMS, related to my fibromyalgia?

TAKING Control

- **Choose a doctor who has experience** treating fibromyalgia, not someone who thinks it's "all in your head." A good choice may be a rheumatologist (a physician who specializes in diseases of the joints and muscles), a physiatrist (a doctor who is expert in physical medicine and rehabilitation), or a specialist in pain management. It may also be a good idea to see a physical or occupational therapist.

- **Use memory aids.** If you suffer from the bouts of forgetfulness and poor concentration commonly called "fibro fog," try some basic memory-rechargers. Repeat things to yourself, write items down, and make plenty of lists. Break complex tasks into smaller steps, and keep distractions like loud music to a minimum.

- **Keep a diary** of your pain and energy levels to record your best times of day. Use those periods to do important things like writing letters or paying bills. Many people with fibromyalgia say they function best early in the day.

- **Try heat.** A heating pad, electric blanket, or warm bath may bring relief.

▶ **DOCTORS DON'T KNOW WHY, but fibromyalgia sufferers tend to be especially sensitive to the side effects of drugs. If any of your medications are causing problems, ask your doctor about reducing the dose or splitting your pills into pieces.**

Treatment options

Medications

Pain relievers	Soothe sore and aching muscles.
Trigger-point injections	Quick relief: lidocaine into tender points.
Antidepressants	Increase serotonin levels and ease fatigue.
Sedatives	Very helpful as a sleep aid.
Muscle relaxants	Flexeril is a good option.

Procedures

Psychotherapy	Cognitive-behavioral therapy is quite effective.

Lifestyle changes

De-stress	Try meditation, yoga, or biofeedback.
Exercise	Start slow; stretching reduces muscle pain.
Rest	Devise a healthy sleep regimen.

Natural methods

Massage	Especially deep tissue (myofascial) therapy.
Asian medicine	Acupuncture and qigong may help.

Getting fibromyalgia out of your life is truly a matter of trial and error: A nightly hot bath with Epsom salts, an electric blanket, a weekly massage, acupuncture, low-impact aerobics, muscle relaxants, antidepressants—all have helped others. If you're in a stressful life situation and can't figure out how to solve it, consider visiting a therapist who has worked with other fibromyalgia patients. The sooner you begin treatment, the better. Someone who has been suffering from fibromyalgia for only a few months, for example, typically responds much better than someone who has endured the condition for more than a decade.

Medications

You may start feeling better after you start taking the right medications. Most doctors begin by treating different sets of symptoms with specific drugs. **Pain relievers,** for instance, may bring rapid relief to your sore and aching muscles. Acetaminophen (Tylenol) is often recommended, but stronger medications may be more appropriate. Opioids such as hydrocodone (Vicodin), available as a pill, or fentanyl (Duragesic), worn as a skin patch, act on the central nervous system and can be very effective for relieving pain. However, some physicians and patients worry about overdependence on these drugs. Tramadol (Ultram) or tramadol/acetaminophen (Ultracet) may be good alternatives, though they may cause dependence. Because fibromyalgia is not caused by inflammation, anti-inflammatory drugs (NSAIDs), such as aspirin, ibuprofen, and naproxen, won't provide any long-term benefit.

You can sometimes get dramatic pain relief in minutes with **trigger-point injections:** The anesthetic **lidocaine** is injected into the muscle "tender points" that are sensitive to touch in those with fibromyalgia. Such injections help break the pain cycle, and may provide lasting relief. A small pilot study from the United Kingdom found that giving lidocaine intravenously may also help relieve pain. In those who received the IV infusions, pain intensity dropped from 9 to 5 on an 11-point scale. Patients also felt less depressed, better able to cope, and reported improvements in their social and sex lives.

Taking low doses of an **antidepressant medication** can help treat any underlying sleep disorder and alleviate its accompanying pain and fatigue. These medicines are called antidepressants only because they were first used to treat depression, one of many ailments caused by a disturbance of serotonin. Because they work in different ways to increase levels of this chemical in the brain, "serotonin modulators" is probably a far better name for them. The older **tricyclic antidepressants,** such as amitriptyline (Elavil, Endep), may be particularly effective for relieving pain. The newer **SSRI antidepressants,** such as fluoxetine (Prozac), sertraline (Zoloft), and paroxetine (Paxil), may help lift depression. Low doses of both are sometimes prescribed together. A third type of antidepressant, trazodone (Desyrel), may also help relieve symptoms.

Because not getting a good night's sleep is probably contributing to your problem, a gentle **sedative sleep aid,** such as zolpidem (Ambien) or zaleplon (Sonata), may work wonders. They take effect within 30 minutes and you will wake up without the drug "hangover" so common with stronger sleeping pills. **Muscle relaxants,** such as cyclobenzaprine (Flexeril), may also be beneficial.

Procedures

A psychological counseling approach called **cognitive-behavioral therapy** may offer great benefits for those with fibromyalgia. The technique combines cognitive approaches, which help you address self-defeating thoughts that can aggravate pain, with behavioral therapies, which help you initiate changes that will relieve your symptoms. Unlike other types of psychotherapy, the course of treatment may be relatively brief, lasting from one to several months. If you feel that nothing can help you improve or you can't take the pain another day, cognitive-behavioral therapy may be a good step for you.

Lifestyle Changes

A number of strategies you can follow in your day-to-day life will make a real difference in how you feel.
- **Reduce stress.** Schedule a time each day to relax. Pace yourself, and don't overcommit.
- **Exercise regularly.** The key is to start slowly and not overdo it. Doing low-impact activities such as swimming or aqua aerobics a few days a week is an excellent way to start. You can graduate to other aerobic activities like walking, and work up to strength training using light hand weights or machines. Stretching the

Brain Surgery for Fibromyalgia?

When TV reports aired several years ago showed how skull surgery dramatically relieved symptoms in two women with a fibromyalgia-like illness, many people took notice. People with fibromyalgia and maladies such as chronic fatigue syndrome thought the four-hour, $30,000 operation might be a magic cure for their persistently aching muscles and disabling fatigue. Doctors worried it was a medical scam.

Pioneered by surgeon Michael J. Rosner of Park Ridge Hospital in Fletcher, North Carolina, the procedure involves removing a piece of the skull at the back of the head. Medical follow-up indicates that the brain surgery may be effective—but not for fibromyalgia.

Instead, this procedure may benefit those who have a rare skull abnormality called the Chiari malformation, a defect that squeezes the brain and causes severe pain, numbness, difficulty concentrating, and other complaints.

Surgery may also help those with a narrowed spinal canal. Some of these patients are mistakenly diagnosed with fibromyalgia—but their conditions are rare and can be diagnosed with scanning techniques. **The bottom line:** People with fibromyalgia will not benefit from such surgery.

▶**LEARN MORE ABOUT fibromyalgia and its treatments. You will probably have to "mix and match" therapies to arrive at a combination that's effective for you.**

FINDING Support

■ For news updates on fibromyalgia and a list of local chapters, contact the Arthritis Foundation (1-800-283-7800 or www.arthritis.org). You can also get information from the National Fibromyalgia Partnership (866-725-4404 or www.fmpartnership.org).

■ Interested in joining a study testing new treatments for fibromyalgia? Try the National Institutes of Health clinical trials site at www.clinicaltrials.gov.

■ Looking for a doctor experienced in treating fibromyalgia or for a pain clinic near you? The American College of Rheumatology has a state-by-state physician finder at www.rheumatology.org/directory. For a pain clinic check out www.pain.com.

muscles is also important for reconditioning them and reducing pain.

■ **Consider physical therapy,** which concentrates on different muscle groups. It's also a good complement to an exercise regimen.

■ **Get enough rest.** Try to follow a regular sleep schedule. Limit daytime napping, and use your bed only for sleeping or sex.

Natural Methods*

Relaxation techniques (meditation, yoga, hypnosis, biofeedback) can be beneficial for those with fibromyalgia. **Massage** may help to relieve stress and pain, so may a massage variant known as myofascial trigger point therapy, in which deep tissue around tender points is vigorously worked. **Chiropractic manipulation** of the back may ease soreness. Some sufferers find relief by applying **magnets** to painful areas, although this approach remains unproven.

Acupuncture, in which thin needles are placed at strategically situated points in the body, is a popular Chinese remedy for relieving the pain of fibromyalgia. The National Institutes of Health cites this technique as a possible treatment for the condition. You should begin to feel and sleep better within six to eight sessions. Another traditional Chinese treatment to bolster the body against stress is **qigong,** a 4,000-year-old healing art combining movement, focus, and controlled breathing. In a study at the University of Maryland, an eight-week program of qigong, combined with cognitive-behavioral therapy and meditation, effectively eased fibromyalgia symptoms.

Outlook

Try to stay upbeat. Although there is no cure for fibromyalgia, many people with this condition experience marked, almost complete pain relief after just a few weeks of specialized treatment.

Natural methods are not subject to the same testing and regulation as prescription medications. Please seek your doctor's advice and use caution.

Flu

We've known about the flu forever: Hippocrates first described this illness in 412 B.C. Only recently has science finally started to unlock the mysteries of influenza and develop medications that can get us back on our feet faster.

What is happening

Influenza—most of us are well enough acquainted with it to call it by its nickname, flu—is caused by one of three strains of viruses. The first flu virus (Type A) was identified in the 1930s. We now know it as the most common, as well as the most serious. Type B viruses generally produce a milder version of the flu than Type A. Type C rarely causes illness in humans.

Flu viruses are highly contagious, entering your body through your nose or mouth. You can inhale the virus when someone with the flu sneezes or coughs near you, or you can catch it by shaking hands or kissing someone who is still infectious. The virus can live up to three hours outside the body, so you also can pick it up from surfaces such as telephones, doorknobs, or shared cups. You become infected when your unwashed hands touch your nose or mouth.

The good news about the flu is that once you've had a particular strain of the virus, you're permanently immune to it. The not-so-good news is that the viruses constantly transform themselves, so new variations make the rounds every year. That's why new flu vaccines are developed for every flu season.

After the virus enters your body, it can take up to four days for flu symptoms to strike. They can be hard to distinguish from the common cold (*for differences, see the table, page 84*). You are most likely to spread the flu to others from the time you first encounter the virus—before you even have any symptoms—until three or four days after symptoms appear. The flu tends to arrive all at once, with a fever of 101° to 103°F that lasts for three to five days, headache, chills, dry cough, stuffy nose, sore throat, body aches, and loss of appetite. It generally takes most people about 10 days to recover.

The flu season usually runs from November to March, sometimes into April. An estimated 35 to 50 million Americans catch the flu each year, according to the Centers for Disease Control. Children are two to three times more likely to get it than adults.

Treatments

Prescription and over-the-counter medications can help you feel better faster and reduce the duration of the flu by a couple of days. That may not sound like much, but when you're down with the flu, two days can seem like forever. The cornerstone for recovery probably hasn't changed a great deal since Hippocrates: Get lots of

LIKELY **First Steps**

- **Antiviral medication** within 36 hours of symptom onset to shorten the duration of the infection.

- **Over-the-counter drugs** to ease symptoms.

- **Bed rest** to allow your body to recuperate from the stress of the infection.

- **Lots of fluids** to thin mucus.

QUESTIONS TO **Ask**

- Do you think one of the new prescription antiviral drugs would help me?

- I have asthma. Should I get the flu vaccine?

- How do I know when I've stopped being contagious?

- How can I keep from spreading the virus to my family?

- When can I go back to work?

- **Choose multivitamins carefully.** One study of 79 adults age 65 and older found that those who took a daily multivitamin with no trace minerals (tiny amounts of zinc, copper, iron, magnesium, or selenium) received less protection from their flu vaccine. In choosing a multivitamin, look for one that contains these trace minerals, which can help boost immunity. Talk with your doctor about which supplement is best for you.

- **Skip antibiotics.** These medications only work against bacteria, and virus causes the flu. However, if you develop a secondary bacterial infection as the result of the flu, you may need antibiotics after all.

Promising
DEVELOPMENTS

- **A 2003 U.S. study** found that in patients over 65, flu shots reduce risk of hospitalization for heart disease, stroke, pneumonia, or influenza, as well as the risk of death from all causes during flu season. These findings highlight the vaccine's benefit in non-respiratory illness.

Treatment options

Medications	
Antivirals	Can cut two days off your bout with the flu.
Decongestants	Clear a stuffy nose.
Cough medicines	Expectorants or suppressants, as needed.
Vaccine	Prevents most infections.
Lifestyle changes	
Rest	So your body can heal.
Humidifier and/or steam	Thins and "washes out" mucus.
Lots of fluids	To break up congestion.
Natural methods	
Zinc gluconate lozenges	May lessen duration of the flu.
Echinacea	Helpful immune-boosting herb.

rest and drink plenty of fluids. There are other steps you can take to get faster relief—from making sure you have warm, moist air to breathe to sucking on zinc lozenges.

While most people recover from the flu on their own, there can be serious complications. Pneumonia heads the list. At greatest risk are the elderly and those with chronic lung conditions. Pneumonia can be caused by a bacterial infection that strikes your flu-weakened lungs, or even by the flu virus itself. Call your doctor if you aren't feeling better after five days, or if, after you start feeling better, you have a sudden relapse.

Medications

To benefit from the latest flu-fighting drugs, call your doctor for a prescription at the first sign of symptoms. Two new **antiviral drugs**—oseltamivir (Tamiflu), taken orally, and zanamivir (Relenza), a nasal spray—have been proven to reduce the duration of the flu by two days, but only if you start them within 36 hours after symptoms appear. They work against Type A and B flu strains. Tamiflu has been approved by the FDA for treatment of uncomplicated flu for anyone over age 1, and for flu prevention in those age 13 and older. Relenza is approved for treatment for those age 7 and older. Be aware that these medicines are expensive, and not all health insurance plans cover them. Other medications treat specific symptoms:

- **If you have a stuffy nose,** your best OTC option is a **decongestant** containing pseudoephedrine (Sudafed, Drixoral).
- **If you have a cough,** try **cough suppressants** that contain dextromethorphan (Robitussin Maximum Strength, Drixoral Cough) to relieve a dry cough, and **expectorants** containing guaifenesin to loosen and get rid of thick mucus and sputum.

- **If you have a fever, headache, or muscle aches,** turn to OTC drugs like **aspirin** or **acetaminophen.** For children or adolescents, stick with acetaminophen (Tylenol) only.
- **If you have a sore throat,** pick up a **throat spray** containing phenol (such as Vicks Chloraseptic). This will soothe your aching throat quickly, if only temporarily.
- **If you want to avoid contracting the flu,** get the **influenza vaccine.** An annual flu shot will prevent infection in over 70% of healthy adults. The best time for the shot is between October and mid-November each year, to give your immune system one to two weeks to build immunity to the virus.

It's important that you be vaccinated if you're in one of the following categories: adults age 50 and older, especially those in nursing homes; pregnant women who will be in their second or third trimester during flu season; people with HIV or depressed immunity; those with chronic heart, kidney, or lung disease; and people with diabetes or blood disorders such as anemia. Don't delay. There isn't always enough flu vaccine to go around.

Lifestyle Changes

When the flu hits, doing some or all of the following will ease your symptoms and help you feel better:

- **Get bed rest,** preferably in a warm room with good ventilation. Your body needs rest to recover.
- **Use a humidifier** in your bedroom to help ease congestion. Change the water and filter regularly to prevent mold growth.
- **Take steamy showers,** and let the warm water stream down your face or boil a pot of water and inhale the steam. Just let the water cool a bit so it's not too hot to inhale.
- **Get enough fluids**—at least eight 8-ounce glasses a day—to help thin out mucus. Have some chicken soup. It can help provide needed nutrients, and the steam aids in clearing congestion.
- **Soothe your sore throat.** Try gargling with salt water (dissolve ½ teaspoon salt in ½ cup warm water) several times a day. For temporary relief, suck on hard candy or throat lozenges.
- **Wash your hands frequently** to keep from spreading the flu and its misery around. This is especially important after sneezing, blowing your nose, or touching your face.

Natural Methods*

The scientific jury is still out on **zinc gluconate lozenges,** but there is some evidence that they can relieve symptoms and help cut the duration of the flu. Suck on one lozenge every four hours. You'll know it's working for your particular virus if your sore throat feels better after your fourth tablet. The herb **echinacea** has long been considered an immune-booster, and many believe it can help shorten the duration of the flu. If you use an echinacea product (best taken as a liquid extract or standardized extract in pill form), start taking it at the first sign of the flu, and stop taking it once you feel better.

▶**I hate shots. How else can I take the vaccine?**
The FDA has approved FluMist, a nasal spray that uses live influenza virus as a vaccine for the prevention of influenza. It is indicated for healthy children and adolescents aged 5 to 17 years, and healthy adults aged 18 to 49 years. It should not be given to patients with underlying medical problems, asthma, or emphysema. You should consult your doctor to determine if this nasal vaccine is appropriate for you.

FINDING Support

- For current information on research into new treatments and vaccines, check out the National Institute of Allergy and Infectious Diseases' Focus on the Flu site at http://www.niaid.nih.gov/newsroom/focuson/flu00/default.htm.

- For a current map showing where flu outbreaks have been reported, go to the homepage of the National Flu Surveillance Network at http://www.fluwatch.com. You can even enter your ZIP code and find out if there have been reports of the flu in your town.

*Natural methods are not subject to the same testing and regulation as prescription medications. Please seek your doctor's advice and use caution.

Gallstones

If you have gallstones, you're in good company: About 20 million other Americans have them as well. Today, newer, less-invasive surgical techniques will help you banish gallstone pain and be back on your feet faster than ever before.

LIKELY **First Steps**

- For mild symptoms, **lifestyle changes** (low-fat diet, exercise, weight loss if needed) to control and even eliminate the disease.
- For acute gallstone attacks, **hospitalization** for treatment with IV antibiotics, painkillers, and fluids.
- If other treatments fail or complications develop, **surgery** to remove the gallbladder.

QUESTIONS TO **Ask**

- Is it possible that my abdominal pain is not from gallstones? Could it be caused by a peptic ulcer or pancreatitis?
- If I improve my diet, will the gallstones eventually dissolve on their own?
- Should I take a painkiller like aspirin or Tylenol when gallstone pain hits?

What is happening

Think of your gallbladder as a way station, a place where bile (a thick greenish-yellow digestive juice) from your liver is stored. When your body needs bile to help absorb fat, the gallbladder propels bile into your intestines. Bile contains a mix of cholesterol, calcium, and bilirubin, a waste product from old blood cells. If too much of one of these builds up, crystals form, clump together, and enlarge into gallstones. A stone can be as tiny as a grain of sand or as big as a golf ball.

Odds are, you won't have symptoms and will learn about your stones during another test (a chest x-ray often includes the gallbladder). Although these "silent gallstones" are generally harmless, they can create problems. If a stone tries to squeeze through the narrow duct from your gallbladder to your small intestine, you'll have severe pain until it passes. A more serious condition called acute cholecystitis occurs when the stone can't pass: This creates a blockage and sometimes even a potentially life-threatening infection in the gallbladder or the duct. Acute cholecystitis will respond to antibiotics once the stone passes or is removed.

If you have an infection or a blocked duct, you'll know it. Pain that starts in your upper right abdomen that may radiate to your back or right shoulder, and if you breathe deeply, it gets worse. Pain that comes in waves is called colic: Your duct is struggling to pass a stone. If the pain is more constant, and the areas are tender, acute cholecystitis may be the problem. Gallbladder flare-ups frequently occur after eating a large or fatty meal. Bloating, nausea, and vomiting may also be present. Warning signs of a prolonged blockage are a high fever, jaundice, and constant pain.

Just why some people develop gallstones is a mystery. Every medical student knows the profile of an at-risk person as the five "Fs": someone who is Fair (light complexion), Female (estrogen boosts cholesterol secretion), Fat (excess weight also ups cholesterol output), Fertile (previous pregnancies), and older than Forty. Other risks include a history of crash dieting, diabetes, or an inflammatory bowel condition.

Treatments

If you have gallstones but don't have symptoms, your doctor will probably recommend a wait-and-see approach. Most mild, intermittent symptoms respond to certain lifestyle changes: following a low-fat diet and losing some weight. If you've passed one gallstone

Treatment options

Lifestyle changes

Weight loss & diet	Trim extra pounds, excess sugar, and fat.
Stay regular	Constipation adds to gallstone risk.
Exercise	Can reduce risk of attack by one-third.

Medications

Painkiller	IV Demerol or Talwin for acute pain.
Antinausea drugs	IV drugs for vomiting in acute attack.
Antibiotics	IV drugs for infection.
Ursodiol	Slowly dissolves stones; rarely effective.

Procedures

Open cholecystectomy	Traditional abdominal surgery; rarely used.
Laparoscopic surgery	Accounts for 90% of gallbladder removals.
ERCP	Removal of duct stones via oral endoscope.

and x-rays show more are present, your doctor will likely suggest surgery. If you are having symptoms of acute cholecystitis, with constant pain and fever, your doctor will want you hospitalized for intravenous antibiotics and pain control. For recurring attacks, or after an episode of acute cholecystitis that has "cooled down" with antibiotics, your doctor may advise surgical removal of the gallbladder, a process greatly simplified by laparoscopic procedures.

Lifestyle Changes

The top priority of most people who've passed a gallstone is to keep it from happening again. You can reduce the number of repeat episodes (and maybe even prevent them) by doing the following:

- **Watch your weight.** An ideal body weight can help keep gallstones from forming. If you need to shed pounds, don't lose too much too fast: Rapid weight loss increases gallstone production.
- **Reduce dietary fat and sugar.** Both have been linked to an increased risk for gallstones. Instead, eat a diet rich in fruits and vegetables; vegetarians infrequently get gallstones.
- **Drink plenty of fluids.** At least six to eight glasses a day will help you maintain the right water content for bile.
- **Stay regular.** Eating fiber-rich foods is always helpful. For occasional constipation, use a bulk-forming laxative, such as psyllium (Metamucil) or calcium polycarbophil (FiberCon).
- **Exercise.** A study of 45,000 male health professionals found that moderate to vigorous exercise reduced the risk of gallstone attacks by one-third. Try to get 30 minutes of aerobic exercise—jogging, swimming, biking, playing tennis, brisk walking—at least three to five times a week.

TAKING Control

- **Keep moving** if you're having a gallstone attack. After you've called your doctor, you may be able to make yourself more comfortable by walking or lying on a bed and rolling from side to side.

- **Be alert for abdominal pain** even after your gallbladder is removed. Gallstones can still form in your bile ducts. If you feel pain in your upper abdomen, notify your doctor.

- **Shun the sun.** There may be a link between prolonged sun exposure and gallstone development. Avoid sunbathing if you are in any way at risk for developing gallstones.

Beware of the Liver "Flush"

A popular home remedy for gallstones, the liver "flush" is a drink made up of olive oil, lemon juice, and herbs. It's reputed to literally flush gallstones out of your gallbladder. Don't believe it. What comes out aren't really stones at all, but chunks of a soaplike material that's formed in the intestines by mixing the oil, the lemon juice, and certain minerals. Not only is this drink ineffective, the oil could make your gallbladder contract. That can shift a gallstone and induce a severe gallbladder attack as the stone moves down (or even blocks) your bile duct.

▶Why is my doctor going to take out my whole gallbladder rather than just my gallstones?

Removing your gallbladder is the only way to keep gallstones from coming back. If you've had gallstones, you're likely to continue to form them even if your existing ones are removed. A gallstone attack is painful and debilitating. While some people only experience one every few years, others have them with great frequency. This is why most people, told that after surgery they'll never pass another gallstone, ask, "Where do I sign?"

▶Don't I need my gallbladder to digest food?

Contrary to what you might think, removing your gallbladder doesn't interfere with digestion. Bile will simply pass from your liver right into your small intestine. You may experience some gas and bloating, but sticking to a low-fat diet will remedy those symptoms. Some people report that bowel movements are looser and more frequent after surgery, but this typically improves with time.

▶HEREDITY CAN PLAY A MAJOR ROLE in determining your risk for gallstones. Among the Pima Indians of Arizona, for example, nearly 70% of women develop gallstones by the time they reach age 30.

Gallbladder Disorders

Gallstones are the most common—but not the only—disease of the gallbladder. Others include:

- **Polyps in the gallbladder.** New ultrasound techniques can help determine when a polyp is benign, requiring no action, and when it's malignant, needing removal.
- **Acalculous cholecystitis.** This is a gallbladder inflammation without stones. The acute version usually strikes people in a weakened condition—from a serious illness, surgery, burns, or a systemic infection. The chronic version stems from anatomical defects. Treatment is surgical removal of the gallbladder.
- **Cancer of the gallbladder or bile ducts.** Very rare, it's usually found in people over age 70. If the cancer has not spread, your doctor will remove your gallbladder and bile ducts.

Medications

If you have intense pain in your upper abdomen, call your doctor right away or go to an emergency room. You'll probably be put on **intravenous (IV) medications,** which may include a **painkiller** such as meperidine (Demerol) or pentazocine (Talwin), **drugs to stop your vomiting,** and if you have signs of an infection, **antibiotics.** You'll get electrolytes and fluids by IV. If your pain clears up and lab tests don't reveal any complications, you're likely to be sent home with oral painkillers, and perhaps antibiotics. Schedule a conversation with your doctor regarding surgery.

There is medication to dissolve gallstones, ursodeoxycholic acid, or **ursodiol (Actigall).** It's not widely used, because it's expensive and effective in only about 10% of cases. If you really want to avoid surgery (or have serious health concerns that rule it out), your doctor may recommend this drug, which is taken orally and dissolves the stones over a period of one to two years. It works only if your stones are small and composed of cholesterol. A word of warning: Because there's about a 50% chance of recurrence within five years, you may need long-term, low-dose maintenance.

Procedures

For gallstones that cause problems, the most common treatment is surgery to remove the source—your gallbladder. Each year, over half a million Americans have this procedure, called a cholecystectomy. Until 1990, it was done via a long abdominal incision, in an operation called an **open cholecystectomy.** Today, some 90% of gallbladder removals are performed with a less invasive technique called a **laparoscopic cholecystectomy,** known as a "lap choly" (*see illustration opposite*). Four small incisions are made in the abdomen. Then the gallbladder is removed, using a tiny video camera and flexible surgical instruments. If problems occur, the surgeon can revert to a conventional open cholecystectomy.

With a lap choly, you'll need to stay in the hospital for only a day (sometimes even less if you have outpatient surgery), vs. five days after open surgery. Your recovery time should be short; many people are back at their regular activities within a week. (Traditional surgery has a four- to six-week recovery period.) Under most circumstances, surgery is elective, meaning you can decide when you want it done. But if you're hospitalized and tests indicate that you have a serious complication, such as an abscess or gallbladder perforation, you'll need surgery immediately.

If your doctor suspects that you have a gallstone stuck in a bile duct but no infection, he may recommend an **endoscopic retrograde cholangiopancreatography (ERCP).** In this procedure, a flexible viewing tube with surgical attachments is passed through your mouth, esophagus, and stomach to your small intestine and into the tiny opening where the bile duct enters. Your doctor can actually see the stone for himself, grasp it with surgical instruments, and remove it from the duct.

A small number of people may be able to treat their gallstones with procedures less invasive than surgery. One involves ultrasound waves (a process called **extracorporeal shock wave lithotripsy**) that pulverize gallstones, so they're small enough to pass through bile ducts or be dissolved with medication. To be a candidate, you must have only one small stone and a healthy gallbladder. Doctors recommend it only in rare cases, because stones have a 50% chance of recurring in five years. Another procedure, only for small gallstones, infuses a solvent directly into your gallbladder via a long, thin needle. The solvent, **methyl tert-butyl ether (MTBE),** dissolves cholesterol gallstones in a day or two. As with other nonsurgical remedies, recurrence is a possibility.

Promising DEVELOPMENTS

■ It may seem like science fiction, but it's real: The Food and Drug Administration has approved the first **robotic surgical device** for removing gallbladders and performing other abdominal operations.

Here's how it works: A robot is equipped with arms attached to a laparoscope and other surgical instruments. A surgeon sits nearby and directs the robot with foot pedals, hand grips, and voice commands. A computer translates them into digital impulses.

What's the advantage? With the robot, there are no extra hand movements or shaky instruments. Robot "wrists" are highly flexible, so they can reach through laparoscopy incisions too small for a surgeon's hands. The use of the computer allows for a 3-D image, which gives a better view than the two-dimensional image used in conventional laparoscopy.

So far, only a small number of major medical centers use robotic surgery, but its use is likely to spread. Eventually, it may even allow specialists to perform surgery on patients hundreds of miles away.

FINDING Support

■ For the latest information on preventing and treating gallbladder diseases, you can contact the National Digestive Diseases Information Clearinghouse in Bethesda, MD (www.niddk.nih.gov/health/digest/nddic.htm).

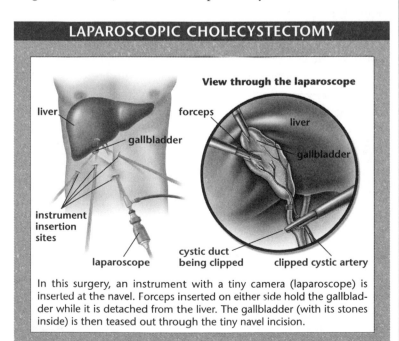

LAPAROSCOPIC CHOLECYSTECTOMY

View through the laparoscope

liver

forceps

gallbladder

liver

gallbladder

instrument insertion sites

cystic duct being clipped

laparoscope

clipped cystic artery

In this surgery, an instrument with a tiny camera (laparoscope) is inserted at the navel. Forceps inserted on either side hold the gallbladder while it is detached from the liver. The gallbladder (with its stones inside) is then teased out through the tiny navel incision.

Genital herpes

Some 20% of the American adult population is infected with herpes simplex virus, which causes genital herpes (and cold sores). Although there is no cure, effective medications—and a prudent lifestyle—can ease symptoms and keep outbreaks in check.

LIKELY **First Steps**

- **Pain relievers** to ease body aches and fever.
- **Topical anesthetics** for pain and itching.
- **Antiviral medications** to speed healing and prevent recurrent outbreaks.

QUESTIONS TO **Ask**

- Do I have to call the doctor for a prescription each time I sense a flare-up?
- How long do I need to abstain from sex?
- Does herpes increase my risk of getting other sexually transmitted diseases?

▶**HERPES SIMPLEX HAS TWO DIFFERENT FORMS: HSV-1 and HSV-2. Until recently it was assumed that HSV-1 infections produced only cold sores and fever blisters of the mouth, and did not attack the genital area as HSV-2 does. However, recent research shows that HSV-1 causes just as many new cases of genital herpes as HSV-2. Both types of HSV can be transmitted through vaginal, oral, or anal sex, as well as by kissing and other skin-to-skin contact.**

What is happening

Most likely, you contracted genital herpes through a mucous membrane or a small opening in your skin during unprotected sex with an infected partner. If you've just been diagnosed, you may feel a variety of emotions—fear, anger, betrayal, confusion—but don't panic. You are hardly alone. The herpes simplex virus (HSV), which causes the genital blisters and sores that typically mark this disease, is the most common viral infection in the United States today, striking men and women equally. It can be a frustrating and painful condition for some, but it is rarely dangerous.

Skin lesions typically begin 2 to 12 days after the virus enters your body. Your first episode (called primary herpes) is likely to be your most severe: An eruption of painful red blisters on your genitals or in the genital area; itching or burning; fever and body aches; and swollen glands, particularly in the lymph nodes near your groin. Herpes is most painful and contagious during the first 24 to 48 hours, when the sores are open and "weeping." Once the blisters burst, they crust over and turn into an itchy rash that may last for another week. After the primary outbreak, you may not have another episode for years, or you could have an attack as often as once a month. Some people continue to suffer extreme symptoms. Others have such mild symptoms they virtually go unnoticed. In fact, the virus is frequently transmitted by people who don't know they are infected or don't recognize that the virus is in an active phase (*see box, page 138*).

Once you are infected, the virus stays in your body for life, virtually sleeping in the roots of nerves next to your spinal cord. Each recurring attack is basically the same: The virus "awakens," travels down the nerves, and bursts through the skin. Common triggers include stress, fatigue, excessive exposure to cold or heat, or other infections such as a cold or the flu. In some women, PMS or menstruation may bring on a flare-up. As time goes by, the number of outbreaks tapers off and symptoms become less severe.

Treatments

There is no cure yet for herpes simplex, but a number of OTC and prescription drugs can relieve symptoms and shorten the duration of an outbreak. If you have mild symptoms or infrequent episodes, you may prefer to treat herpes on your own with self-care measures. You'll have to be careful about sex (*see box, page 138*), avoiding it altogether when you have an open sore.

Treatment options

Medications

OTC pain relievers	Aspirin, Advil, Tylenol, Viractin cream.
Antiviral drugs	Zovirax, Valtrex, Famvir for recurrent cases.

Lifestyle changes

Boost immunity	Through proper diet, sleep, and exercise.
Good hygiene	Bathe often; urinate with care to avoid pain.

Natural methods

Lysine	May reduce flare-ups and promote healing.
Melissa cream	Can help sores heal.
Echinacea extract	Apply often to reduce pain from open sores.

Medications

To relieve fever, headache, or achiness at the start of an episode, try an **OTC pain reliever,** such as acetaminophen (Tylenol), or a non-steroidal anti-inflammatory drug (NSAID), such as aspirin, ibuprofen (Advil), or naproxen (Aleve). Topical lidocaine jelly (5%) can be used for local pain related to blisters. Another topical OTC anesthetic, tetracaine (Viractin cream), has been found to relieve itching, but has little effect on other symptoms. None of these medicines will shorten the course of the outbreak.

If you're experiencing a primary episode or have more than six outbreaks a year, your doctor will probably recommend taking a prescription **antiviral medication.** It will block the reproduction of the virus, relieve your symptoms, and help you recover more quickly. Three prescription medicines are approved to date; all work similarly, are considered safe, and have virtually no side effects. **Acyclovir** (Zovirax) has been used since 1985 and is now available in generic form. It is most effective against an active infection if taken within 24 hours of the first symptoms and may reduce the frequency of viral shedding (*see box, page 138*). **Valacyclovir** (Valtrex) has acyclovir as its active ingredient, but is better absorbed by the body and can be taken less often. **Famciclovir** (Famvir) works much the same way as acyclovir, but it is better absorbed, and requires fewer doses. Both acyclovir and famciclovir are available as a cream, but the capsules and tablets are much more effective.

Antivirals are generally prescribed in two ways: **Episodic therapy** involves taking the medicine for three to five days during an outbreak. While this can shorten the duration by about two days, it does not affect the frequency of future attacks. The other method is **suppressive therapy,** in which you take one or two doses of medicine every day to prevent attacks. It works only as long as you take the drug, though some people find flare-ups are less frequent and less severe even after the drug is stopped (*see "Taking Control," above*).

TAKING Control

- **Know your body.** Take note of itching, tingling, and other sensations that precede your herpes attacks (this is called the "prodrome"). Staying alert makes early treatment possible and helps curb the spread of infection.

- **Reduce stress.** Cognitive-behavioral methods and other stress-reduction techniques have been found to be effective in reducing herpes-related depression. They may stimulate virus-fighting antibodies.

- **Take a break.** If you're on daily suppressive drug therapy, stop the pills for a short time each year to see if flare-ups continue to recur. You may find you no longer need the medication.

Promising DEVELOPMENTS

- A new class of drugs called **cdk-blocking agents,** if proven safe in humans, could keep HSV in permanent inactive state. The compounds stop an invading virus from using the human host's cdk, a substance that drives cell division.

- **Resiquimod,** a topical gel, shows promise in significantly delaying recurrent genital herpes outbreaks. It could provide an alternative to suppressive therapy.

- A long sought-after **herpes vaccine** has shown promise in mice. Scientists hope to develop a similar vaccine for humans that will prevent herpes in people unaffected by the disease and halt it in those already infected.

Frequently Asked Questions About Herpes

Getting herpes can be a troubling event that raises endless questions. The following are some of the more common queries about the virus that doctors answer daily.

Will herpes spread to other places on my body?

It's rare, but possible. Because herpes typically enters your body through a break in the skin, preventing self-infection is simple: Don't touch the sore—especially if it's your first outbreak, which is the most virulent. If you do, wash your hands as soon as possible. Soap and water kills the virus.

Can herpes be active without causing symptoms?

Yes, via a process called "viral shedding," in which the virus begins to multiply and becomes transmittable, but doesn't produce visible blisters or inflammation. In fact, studies show that nearly 90% of people infected with herpes don't recognize symptoms or else mistake them for something else. Women with HSV-2 are more likely to transmit the virus when they are asymptomatic.

How can I reduce the risk of transmitting herpes?

Inform your partner and abstain from sex when symptoms are present. Latex condoms offer some protection, but the virus can spread from uncovered lesions or in sweat or vaginal fluids to places the condom doesn't cover. (In addition, sex can irritate sores and slow the healing process.) Medicines may curb spreading: Early studies show that antiviral drugs reduce the shedding of the live virus from the sores, thus reducing the risk of transmission.

What if I have herpes when I'm pregnant?

Less than 0.1% of babies born to mothers with herpes contract the disease. Precautions are nevertheless advisable because HSV infection in a newborn is serious. It can be life-threatening. If you suspect you are having an outbreak during the late stages of pregnancy, your doctor will take a culture to be sure. A Cesarean section is required if lesions are visible when labor begins.

▶ **DON'T USE LUBRICANTS that are petroleum- or mineral-based (petroleum jelly, baby oil) with a latex condom. They can weaken the condom, causing it to break.**

FINDING Support

- The American Social Health Association (ASHA) sponsors the Herpes Resource Center, offering educational materials and a hotline that provides counseling and referrals to support groups (1-800-230-6039 or www.ashastd.org).

- The Centers for Disease Control and Prevention's STD Hotline provides material related to the diagnosis and treatment of herpes and other sexually transmitted diseases, as well as referrals (1-800-227-8922).

*Natural methods are not subject to the same testing and regulation as prescription medications. Please seek your doctor's advice and use caution.

Lifestyle Changes

Regardless of whether you use antiviral therapy, maintaining a **healthy diet** and getting plenty of **sleep** and **exercise** are important for helping your immune system defend against genital herpes. Here are some additional self-care measures you can try:

- **Apply ice.** An ice pack wrapped in a thin towel can temporarily relieve the pain of an open sore. Don't chill too long.
- **Bathe often.** Take lukewarm baths to soothe burning. To avoid irritation, dry off with a blow dryer on cool instead of a towel.
- **Urinate with care.** To prevent the pain caused by urine touching an open sore, urinate in the tub at the end of your bath or in a cool shower. Urinating through a small tube, such as a toilet paper roll, also protects sensitive surrounding tissue.

Natural Methods*

One of the more popular (and scientifically studied) alternative remedies for herpes simplex is the amino acid **lysine.** Many people have found it reduces flare-ups and quickens healing. A dose of 1,000 mg of L-lysine taken four times a day at the first sign of an outbreak has been shown to be safe and free of side effects. A cream made from **melissa**, an herb from the mint family, may also promote healing of herpes lesions. Look for a product, such as Herpalieve or Herpilyn, that contains a concentrated extract of the herb. A few drops of **echinacea extract** (Echinforce) applied gently to sores every few hours can help relieve pain.

Glaucoma

If you've actually been diagnosed with glaucoma—a condition that can lead to blindness—count yourself lucky: You can take action. With today's treatments, you need never miss a sunset, the smile on a child's face, or even your favorite TV show.

What is happening

If you have glaucoma, the fibers of your optic nerve are beginning to die off, probably due to excessive fluid pressure inside your eye. This problem, intraocular pressure (IOP), is caused by a buildup of a watery fluid (aqueous humor) that normally fills your eyeball and produces IOP, the same way that air from a pump creates pressure in a tire. To keep the pressure at a safe level, fluid constantly drains through a sievelike network of connective tissues called the trabecular meshwork (*see illustration*) or through an alternate drainage system called the uveoscleral pathway. It then empties into a drainage channel located where the iris and the cornea meet. This area of the eye is known as the drainage angle.

When anything prevents aqueous fluid from draining, pressure in your eye increases and eventually kills nerve cells. If the condition isn't treated with medication or surgery, your peripheral vision—your ability to see objects at the edge of your visual field—will begin to disappear. As more cells die, your central vision will go as well. The final result: total, irreversible blindness.

In the United States, the most common type of glaucoma (some 90% of cases) is **open-angle glaucoma,** which occurs when the trabecular meshwork becomes partially blocked for some reason (*see illustration*). Although the drainage angle remains open, the aqueous humor drains too slowly. Fluid backs up and slowly causes pressure. You can have this condition for years before you realize it.

A far less common variation is **closed-angle glaucoma** (*see box, page 142*). This condition, which causes intense pain and other symptoms, occurs suddenly. It is a medical emergency and requires immediate treatment.

Exactly which biological mechanism triggers glaucoma remains a mystery, but there are a few suspects. One is a natural body process called apoptosis, during which cells are programmed to commit suicide. It may contribute to the pressure in open-angle glaucoma by reducing the number and activity of the cells in the eye's drainage channel. Low blood pressure or other circulatory problems can cause this condition by reducing blood flow to the optic nerve.

Treatments

There is no need for anyone with glaucoma to go blind. The therapies available today are safe and very effective. However, they

LIKELY **First Steps**

- **Specialized tests** to determine the level of pressure in your eyes and indicate how far the disease has progressed.

- **Eyedrop medications** to bring pressure inside your eyes under control.

- **Surgery** only if medications cause problematic side effects or don't help.

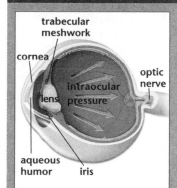

OPEN-ANGLE GLAUCOMA

trabecular meshwork
cornea
optic nerve
intraocular pressure
lens
aqueous humor
iris

Typically, open-angle glaucoma (the most common form of this ailment) occurs when the trabecular meshwork in your eye becomes partially blocked. The clear fluid known as aqueous humor (which normally drains from the eye into the bloodstream at the same rate that it's produced), begins to build up. This puts pressure on the optic nerve, causing gradual loss of vision that, if left untreated, can result in blindness.

QUESTIONS TO **Ask**

- Will treatment keep my vision from getting worse?

- How do I know my medications are working?

- Do you think I'm a candidate for surgery?

- Will the dosage of the beta-blockers I take for high blood pressure have to be adjusted if I use beta-blocker eyedrops?

- Could any of the other drugs I'm taking be aggravating my condition?

TAKING **Control**

- **Try vitamin E*.** There is no evidence to show that it works directly on glaucoma, but this nutrient is often recommended by doctors for its ability to clean up destructive oxygen molecules, known as free radicals, which roam through your circulatory system. Vitamin E may also help improve your visual field. The standard dosage, in capsule form, is 400 IU a day.

- **Sit still and relax.** Meditation, biofeedback, and other approaches to relaxation seem to have some therapeutic effects on glaucoma. No one knows why.

- **Keep your head up.** Anything that requires you to lower your head— such as bending over to tie your shoes or practicing certain yoga poses—may increase your IOP. Try not to let your forehead drop lower than your chin for any length of time.

*Natural methods are not subject to the same testing and regulation as prescription medications. Please seek your doctor's advice and use caution.

Treatment options

Medications	
Miotics	Old-line treatment to increase fluid outflow.
Beta-blockers	Usually the first choice for reducing IOP.
Carbonic anhydrase inhibitors	Reduce fluid in eye; topical or oral.
Alpha-2 adrenergic agonists	Brimonidine may replace some beta-blockers.
Prostaglandin agonists	Increase fluid outflow and blood flow to eye.
Procedures	
Filtration surgery	Drains fluid; medications may not be needed.
Laser trabeculoplasty	Very effective but eyedrops still needed.
Drainage tube	Best for rare glaucoma due to iris swelling.
Lifestyle changes	
Aerobic exercise	May lower IOP by up to 20%.
Care with liquids	Not too much coffee; regulate fluid intake.

control only the progress of the disease, they can't reverse damage that's already been done. Obviously, the sooner you see an eye doctor (ophthalmologist), the better. Treatment will include regular eye exams—perhaps as often as once every three months—along with medications and, if necessary, surgery.

Medications

Most medications used to treat glaucoma are eyedrops aimed at lowering IOP. These drugs can preserve vision, but they must be taken for life.

Until recently, **miotics** were most doctors' first choice for glaucoma. These drugs, which include pilocarpine (Pilocar) and carbachol (Isopto Carbachol) work well in reducing IOP. Some doctors still recommend them, but they must be taken several times a day. Some patients can have a hard time keeping up with the regimen. Many doctors have switched to newer classes of drugs. They are easier to use.

The most commonly prescribed of the new generation of glaucoma eyedrop medications are **beta-blockers.** They reduce the amount of fluid your eye produces. (If you have high blood pressure, you may already be familiar with beta-blockers. They're often taken orally to control hypertension.) The oldest and most prescribed beta-blocker eyedrop is timolol (Timoptic Ocumeter, Timoptic-XE). Newer ones such as betaxolol (Betoptic), levobunolol (Betagan), and carteolol (Ocupress) are just as effective.

If a beta-blocker fails to sufficiently lower your IOP, your doctor may add a **carbonic anhydrase inhibitor (CAI),** which reduces

Maximizing Your Eyedrops

The way you administer your eyedrops can make a big difference in how well they work. In fact, with the right technique you can actually increase the amount of medication you absorb by 50%. The best method is called tear duct occlusion. Here's how to do it:

- **Wash your hands** with soap and water. If you're using ointment and eyedrops, apply the ointment first.

- **Lie down.** Press the tip of your middle finger to the inside corner of your eye. Use your index finger to pull the lid down, forming a pouch.
- **Look up.** Release a drop of medication into the pouch (don't touch your eye with the dropper).
- **Close your eye** for a minute, maintaining pressure at the corner of your eye to prevent the drops from leaking into your nose. Wipe your

closed eyelid dry with a tissue. Wait about five minutes before administering a second drop.
- **Note:** Some eyedrops may cause burning or stinging. That is probably not due to the drug itself but to the antibacterial preservatives in the solution. The feeling can be used to your advantage: It lets you know that the drop actually got into your eye.

IOP by cutting down on fluid production. You'll probably be given eyedrops containing dorzolamide (Trusopt) and brinzolamide (Azopt) or an oral form such as acetazolamide (Diamox), methazolamide (Neptazane), or dichlorphenamide (Daranide).

Other doctors make **alpha-2 adrenergic agonists** their first choice or combine one with a beta-blocker. These drugs decrease fluid production, and also increase the fluid outflow through the uveoscleral drainage pathway. Research has shown that at least one of these drugs, brimonidine (Alphagan, Allergan), is more effective for regular use than certain beta-blockers. **Topical prostaglandin agonists** have proven extremely effective, reducing IOP (anywhere from 45% to 71% in one study). They not only increase fluid outflow but also improve blood flow to the eye. Among those available are latanoprost (Xalatan), unoprostone (Rescula), bimatoprost (Lumigan), and travoprost (Travatan).

Procedures

If medications don't control your glaucoma the way your doctor would like, or if side effects from the drugs are making your life difficult, you may need surgical procedures to get relief, but surgery doesn't cure glaucoma. More than 50% of surgical patients will have to start taking glaucoma medications within a couple of years of their procedure. The most common types of surgical interventions are:

- **Filtration surgery (trabeculectomy)** involves creating an opening with a flap in the sclera (the white of the eye). This allows aqueous humor to drain from the eye and be reabsorbed by the body. About half the patients who have this procedure no longer need glaucoma medication, and 40% of the remaining patients experience better control of their condition. For some reason, filtration seems to work better for Caucasians than other racial groups.
- **Laser trabeculoplasty** involves burning 80 to 100 little holes in the drainage area of the eye. It takes about 15 minutes, is performed

▶ **I've heard there's a connection between glaucoma and Alzheimer's. True?**
No one is sure exactly what causes glaucoma, but researchers have come across some tantalizing and fascinating clues. One is called beta amyloid buildup. Beta amyloid is a sticky protein that forms clumps or patches in the brains of victims of Alzheimer's disease, where it wreaks havoc on cells and contributes to memory loss, dementia, and other familiar symptoms of the disease. Researchers have found similar clumps in the retinas of rats with glaucoma. Could it be that beta amyloid also clogs the drainage vessels in the eyes of humans? The research did not show that glaucoma causes Alzheimer's, but the answer may prove helpful to people with Alzheimer's—and to those who have glaucoma.

Promising DEVELOPMENTS

- A new technique for treating glaucoma, **enzymatic sclerostomy,** may soon eliminate the need to cut the eye surface during surgery. The technique uses a "biological knife," an enzyme that can be selectively activated to make areas of your eyeball more porous and drain more fluid. Experimentally tried on 15 patients, it brought down their IOPs by an average of 43%. The technique is still too technically difficult to perform on large numbers of people, but researchers hope it will be part of your eye doctor's regular arsenal before long.

- Other new options to conventional glaucoma surgery also hold great promise. These include **goniocurettage,** the scraping away of portions of the blocked outflow tissues; **pneumatic trabeculoplasty,** which places a suction ring over the eye to lower IOP and improve drainage; and **trabecular aspiration,** in which a vacuum removes material that could be preventing outflow.

FINDING Support

- If you want more information on glaucoma, the best place to get it is the Glaucoma Research Foundation in San Francisco, CA (at 1-800-826-6693 or www.glaucoma.org).

- The American Academy of Ophthalmology in San Francisco, CA, provides referrals to ophthalmologists (1-800-222 EYES or www.aao.org).

Closed-Angle Glaucoma

Unlike the more common open-angle glaucoma, closed-angle glaucoma is a **true medical emergency**. How do you know if you might have it? Look for the following symptoms: severe, sudden pain (usually in one eye), nausea and/or vomiting, blurred vision, or rainbow-colored halos around lights.

Closed-angle glaucoma often begins as a structural deformity, which creates an unusually narrow drainage angle between the iris and the cornea. Anything that causes your pupil to suddenly dilate—including antihistamines and antidepressants, darkness, or emotional stress—can close off the angle and circulation of the aqueous humor. This causes intraocular pressure (IOP) to shoot up to dangerous levels. If something isn't done immediately to bring the pressure back down, you can lose your eyesight in as little as a few hours. Emergency room doctors will likely treat you with powerful **IOP-reducing drugs** and **laser iridotomy**, a procedure that makes a hole in the iris. You may need filtration surgery if permanent damage has occurred.

Unfortunately, closed-angle glaucoma is likely to be a twice-in-a-lifetime event. If you experience it in one eye, you're at high risk for having the same problem occur in the other eye within 10 years. So, if your doctor finds narrow angles, preventive laser iridotomies are in order.

on an outpatient basis, and causes little or no pain. It's very effective in lowering IOP, but you'll still need to use eyedrops (at lower doses) every day. You may need more surgery or new medications within two to five years.

- **Drainage tube implantation** involves placing silicone tubes (or shunts) in the eye to create an artificial drainage pathway. It works best for patients with glaucoma caused by swelling of the iris and for children born with abnormalities in the trabecular meshwork.

Lifestyle Changes

Although your eye doctor will be your guide, there are some lifestyle changes you can make to help manage your condition. One is **regular exercise.** Glaucoma patients who do aerobic exercise, such as brisk walking, three times a week have been found to lower their IOP by as much as 20%. But if you stop exercising, your IOP will rise again.

In addition, try to **limit coffee and other fluids.** Some studies have shown that caffeine can boost your IOP for several hours. Other studies have found that drinking a quart or more of liquid within about half an hour can raise IOP. Drink plenty of fluids to keep yourself hydrated, but do it by drinking small amounts throughout the day.

Gout

For years, this condition was mistakenly thought of as a "rich man's disease." But gout doesn't check your bank statement before it strikes. Potent medicines and lifestyle changes can now end the excruciating pain and get you back on your feet.

What is happening

An acute gout attack feels like shards of broken glass have been jammed into your big toe or one of your other joints. The "shards" are actually uric acid crystals, and the question is: How did they wind up in your toe (instep, ankle, knee, finger)? It all starts with purines, chemical compounds in your DNA. Humans are the only mammals that lack an enzyme to break down purines, so when they're metabolized by the body, they become uric acid. This seemingly useless substance is produced by the liver, released into the blood, and usually passes through the kidneys to be excreted.

For unknown reasons, some people accumulate uric acid. They either produce too much of it or excrete too little. Genetics seems to play some role: Up to 20% of people with gout have a family history of it. Lifestyle factors such as obesity, eating lots of animal protein, and drinking too much alcohol are also contributing risk factors. When too much uric acid builds up, it spills over into the fluid that cushions the spaces around your joints. Most of the time it stays harmlessly in this solution. Trouble starts when you get dehydrated for some reason: Your body pulls fluids from everywhere, including the joint fluid; causing the uric acid to crystallize into monosodium urate inside certain joints. Your immune system then leaps into action, inflaming the affected joint in an effort to expel the "foreign" crystals from your body.

Gout attacks usually occur in men over age 40 (it takes years for uric acid levels to build up). Less than 5% of gout patients are women: It's thought that estrogen helps move uric acid through the kidneys and out of the body. (This may be why women who get gout are usually postmenopausal.) About half the time, gout strikes the big toe. It often strikes late at night or early in the morning, causing inflammation and swelling: Even the weight of a bedsheet can be excruciating. Untreated, an attack will usually peak one to two days after symptoms first appear, and subside within a week, but it may last longer.

Treatments

To treat a gout attack, you must stop the immune reaction that is causing the pain and you need to dissolve the uric crystals by rehydrating your joint fluid. This means your essential first step is to drink lots of water. Then you'll need medication to reduce the inflammation around your joints. You may be lulled into a false sense of security when your joints go back to working just fine. One study found that 62% of patients with gout had another attack

LIKELY First Steps

- **Drink lots of water immediately** to lessen symptoms; keep drinking long term to help flush out the uric acid.
- **Take NSAIDs like Indocin** to relieve inflammation.
- **Use colchicine** to reduce your immune reaction.
- **Abstain from alcohol.** It dehydrates you, making a gout attack more likely.

QUESTIONS TO Ask

- Do I need a blood test to determine if I have gout?
- Could other medications I'm taking make my gout worse?
- Does being overweight contribute to my gout attacks?

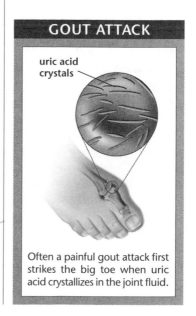

GOUT ATTACK

uric acid crystals

Often a painful gout attack first strikes the big toe when uric acid crystallizes in the joint fluid.

TAKING Control

- **Be a smart drinker.** If you want to have a beer, a glass of wine, or other alcohol, be sure to compensate by downing lots of water before you go to bed. This will keep you hydrated, which helps prevent a gout attack.

- **Try some fruit.** Although cherries are widely acclaimed as the most effective fruit for gout (*see box opposite*), strawberries and blueberries also seem to help keep it at bay. Interestingly, celery (and celery seed extract) has a similar effect.

- **Take care with diuretics.** If you're on a diuretic drug for high blood pressure or a heart problem, be aware that it could worsen your gout by making you excrete excess fluid. Check with your doctor.

- **Plan a gout-free vacation.** Travel can throw off your eating and drinking patterns. Before you go, talk with your doctor about preventive measures. Your physician may prescribe medication just in case a gout attack strikes while you're away.

►**MEAT, FISH, AND POULTRY have moderate levels of gout-related compounds called purines in their DNA. Certain foods contain particularly high amounts, especially liver, shrimp, and herring. In the past, only the better-off could afford to maintain a diet of such purine-rich foods. That led to the traditional nickname for gout: rich man's disease.**

Treatment options

Medications	
Indocin	Reduces inflammation and swelling.
Painkillers	Prescription NSAIDs, codeine, as needed.
Corticosteroids	If other drugs aren't tolerated.
Colchicine	Slows initial immune reaction.
Antigout drugs	Affect uric acid production and excretion.
Lifestyle changes	
Stay hydrated	Essential for forestalling acute attacks.
Dietary measures	Avoid purine-rich foods and alcohol.
Weight loss	Choose a low-fat diet, low in animal protein.
Natural methods	
Supplements	Bromelain, quercetin, fish oil, vitamin C.

within a year, and 78% within two years. By 10 years, nearly 93% had suffered a recurrence.

Untreated, gout can develop into a chronic disease with large, solid deposits of uric acid crystals called tophi that settle around joints and other areas. A buildup of uric acid can also cause painful kidney stones, but with proper treatment, gout rarely becomes chronic. Medications can blunt an acute attack and help prevent recurrences. Lifestyle changes, from losing weight to watching what you eat and drink, can make a big difference.

Medications

When acute gout strikes, you need relief—fast. The first choice is the prescription nonsteroidal anti-inflammatory drug (NSAID) **indomethacin (Indocin),** in doses of up to 200 mg a day. It knocks down inflammation and swelling caused by the immune reaction to the uric acid crystals. It usually starts to work within 24 hours, and often much sooner. For severe pain, your doctor may prescribe more powerful **painkillers,** such as codeine or meperidine. A prescription-strength version of a familiar NSAID such as ibuprofen (Motrin) may help. Your doctor may prescribe one of the newer COX-2 inhibitors, such as celecoxib (Celebrex), rofecoxib (Vioxx), or meloxicam (Mobic). These block inflammation, but tend to be gentler on the stomach than other NSAIDs. Another option, if you can't tolerate the preferred drugs or they don't relieve your symptoms, is **corticosteroids,** such as triamcinolone (administered by injection) and prednisone (taken orally).

To decrease your immune responsiveness, your doctor may prescribe the potent antigout drug **colchicine,** derived from the autumn crocus and used for centuries to combat gout. It's very effective, and usually taken every hour initially until the pain subsides (for severe attacks, it can be injected). By the tenth dose, most people experience improvement. But because colchicine comes with a slew of nasty side effects (nausea, vomiting, diarrhea, abdominal cramps) and most of which are dehydrating, the dose is usually limited to twice a day.

After the acute attack has passed, your doctor may prescribe other **antigout drugs.** Most often used for long-term treatment, **allopurinol** (Lopurin, Zyloprim) slows production of uric acid and helps prevent recurrences. Some doctors prescribe small doses of colchicine along with the allopurinol. Medications such as probenecid (Benemid, Parbenem, Probalan) and sulfinpyrazone (Anturane) help prevent gout by increasing excretion of uric acid in the urine. ColBenemid, a combination drug, teams probenecid with colchicine to reduce acidity in the urine. Some physicians prescribe probenecid and allopurinol together.

Lifestyle Changes

You can't prevent your first gout attack, but you can decrease the risk of recurrence. Here are a few of the most effective strategies:

- **Don't get dehydrated.** This is yet one more reason to drink at least eight glasses of liquids a day. Doing so helps keep your joint fluid intact and flushes uric acid out of your system.
- **Avoid purine-rich foods.** Watch out for organ meats (liver, kidneys, sweetbreads), anchovies, shrimp, sardines, fish roe, yeast, herring, and mackerel. Vegetables high in purines include: mushrooms, asparagus, cauliflower, and spinach.
- **Lose weight the smart way.** Obesity is a strong risk factor for gout, especially in men. If you want to lose weight, avoid a high-protein plan (Atkins, the Zone, Sugar Busters). Increasing your animal protein intake boosts purines and makes your gout worse.
- **Avoid alcohol.** It makes you urinate and can dehydrate you. Second, it inhibits the excretion of uric acid while it boosts uric acid production. So drink lots of water, and limit yourself to two drinks a day if you're a man, one drink if you're a woman. One study found alcohol to be the only significant risk factor for women with gout.

Natural Methods*

There are several good choices for gout in Mother Nature's storehouse. **Bromelain,** an enzyme found in pineapple, is believed to pack anti-inflammatory properties that can help cut a gout attack short. Take a bromelain supplement once every three hours to relieve pain, then twice a day to help prevent future attacks. **Quercetin,** a flavonoid found in plants, is believed to help lower uric acid levels. It's better absorbed when taken with bromelain.

Whether **fish oil** helps relieve gout pain is debatable, but it is an effective anti-inflammatory. **Vitamin C,** if taken in small doses throughout the day, is thought to help release uric acid from body tissues and speed it out of the body. Never take one large dose of this vitamin: It can increase the risk of freeing up too much uric acid all at once, which could cause a kidney stone.

*Natural methods are not subject to the same testing and regulation as prescription medications. Please seek your doctor's advice and use caution.

It's the Cherries

A half-pound of cherries a day keeps the gout away, or so goes the folk wisdom. While hard scientific evidence is lacking, lots of anecdotal evidence suggests (and many gout sufferers agree) that dark cherries can help prevent gout attacks.

Cherries are loaded with flavonoids, potent antioxidants known to have anti-inflammatory properties. Flavonoids help reduce uric acid levels and block the inflammation-causing substances that are released in the joint when crystals start building up.

If you want to give cherries a try, eat a half-pound of fresh or canned cherries a day. Or drink about 2 cups of real cherry juice. Many health-food stores carry cherry fruit extract capsules. For relief for a gout attack, take 2,000 mg (usually two capsules) three times a day. To help prevent future attacks, take 1,000 mg, (or one capsule), daily.

FINDING **Support**

- The Arthritis Foundation maintains an excellent website at www.arthritis.org, which offers background on gout and gout drugs, as well as physician referrals. Or you can call 1-800-283-7800.

- The National Institute of Arthritis and Musculoskeletal and Skin Diseases (NIAMS), part of the National Institutes of Health in Bethesda, MD, has detailed information about gout and current research efforts (toll free: 1-877-22-NIAMS or www.niams.nih.gov).

Gum disease

The bad news: At some point in your life, you'll probably have the red, swollen, and even bleeding gums that signify gum disease. The good news: Nearly all early cases can be reversed and then kept at bay with dental visits and proper oral hygiene.

LIKELY First Steps

- **Floss and brush regularly** to control gum redness, swelling, or tenderness.
- **Get your teeth cleaned twice a year**—more often for persistent gingivitis.
- **Have a deep cleaning,** if needed, to remove tartar and damaged tissue.
- **Undergo surgery** if your disease is advanced to reduce the size of pockets under the gums.

QUESTIONS TO Ask

- How much time should I spend flossing and brushing?
- How do I floss around my bridgework?
- Can I control my gum disease without medications?
- Do you think I should see a periodontist?

What is happening

About 75% of Americans age 35 and older have some degree of gum disease. Gum disease is also called gingivitis. Unlike many infections, it doesn't hurt at first. You may have it years before you know you have it. Over time, the bacteria causing the infection can seriously damage gum tissue and weaken the bones that hold your teeth in place.

Bacteria that live in the mouth normally produce a thin, sticky film called plaque. In small amounts, plaque is helpful. It provides a protective barrier against further bacterial incursions. When too much plaque accumulates, it clings to the teeth and gets beneath the gum line. If not removed promptly, it gradually hardens into a rock-hard layer called tartar. Tartar is impossible to remove with regular brushing. It irritates the gums and causes redness, tenderness, or bleeding—the first signs of gingivitis.

Most gingivitis occurs when people don't brush or floss their teeth often enough. Other risk factors are also involved. Up to 30% of Americans, for example, have a genetic susceptibility for developing gum disease. It's more common in women because increases in the hormone progesterone in the days prior to menstruation can increase inflammation and reduce the body's ability to repair gum damage. Gum disease can also be caused, or worsened, by smoking, uncontrolled diabetes, or the use of medications that reduce the flow of cleansing saliva.

You can almost always reverse mild gum disease by removing plaque before it turns into tartar, but you have to catch it early. If you don't, gingivitis can progress to a more serious condition called periodontitis, which destroys the bone and other tissues that hold the teeth in place. (*For treatment information for periodontitis, see Tooth Loss, page 318.*)

Treatments

Your dentist will know if you have gingivitis just by looking in your mouth. Your gums will be slightly swollen, they'll bleed easily, and they'll be deep red rather than healthy pink. To determine how serious the condition is, the dentist will use a small metal probe to measure the space between your teeth and gums. A groove deeper than about an eighth of an inch may may mean that gingivitis is damaging tissue and has created "pockets" that are vulnerable to continued infection.

Treatment options

Lifestyle changes

Brush & floss	Removes plaque before it causes problems.
Drink water	Increases saliva to wash away bacteria.
Eat well	More fruits and vegetables; avoid sugary foods.

Medications

Mouthwash	OTC or prescription; fights gum disease.

Procedures

Routine cleaning	Keeps your gums disease-free.
Full-mouth debridement	Removes tartar; smoothes and planes teeth.
Gum surgery	Deals with damaged tissue under the gums.

Natural methods

Natural products	Try those with bloodroot or coenzyme Q_{10}.

Early-stage gum disease will probably disappear once you have your teeth professionally cleaned. More serious cases will require more extensive treatments, but it needn't go that far. You can almost certainly put your gums back in the pink with some simple steps.

Lifestyle Changes

Good dental hygiene will reverse most cases of gingivitis. The most important thing is to **brush your teeth** at least twice a day to remove soft plaque before it hardens. Be sure to brush first thing in the morning, because the reduced flow of saliva at night gives bacteria a chance to multiply. To get the most out of brushing, start with a dry brush. One study found that dry brushing, followed by brushing with toothpaste, reduced plaque deposits by 67%. Old-fashioned toothbrushes work fine, but **electric toothbrushes** (such as Sonicare and Interplak) can be even more effective at removing plaque.

Use a **toothpaste approved** by the American Dental Association (ADA). The best ones contain fluoride, a mineral that inhibits bacteria and strengthens tooth enamel. The only toothpaste approved by the Food and Drug Administration for treating gum disease is **Colgate's Total.** Along with fluoride, it contains triclosan, a germ-killing compound that remains in the mouth after brushing.

Don't forget to **floss your teeth before brushing.** Flossing removes plaque between the teeth, where a brush can't reach. Waxed and unwaxed flosses are equally effective, but you'll want to avoid too-thin flosses: They can cut into the gums and cause bleeding. If the spaces between your teeth are too tight to admit regular floss, try **Gore-Tex floss.** It slips easily between the teeth and is unlikely to break or fray.

▶Is trench mouth the same thing as gingivitis?

Not quite. Despite its medical name—acute necrotizing ulcerative gingivitis—trench mouth has little in common with the gingivitis most of us get. Trench mouth is a serious gum infection that causes bleeding, painful sores, and a foul-smelling odor. It occurs mainly in adolescents and young adults, and it's frequently linked to stress, poor eating and oral hygiene habits, smoking, and too much alcohol. Trench mouth was common among soldiers in the trenches in World War I (hence its name). The rare cases that occur these days are treated by a series of visits to the dentist for thorough tooth and gum cleaning, antibiotics, and hydrogen peroxide rinses.

▶I'm thinking of getting my tongue pierced. Will it damage my teeth or gums?

It may. A study in the Journal of Periodontology, which looked at 52 young adults, found that 35% of those who had worn tongue jewelry for four or more years had receding gums. The bigger the jewelry, the bigger the problem: Large objects in the tongue are more likely to exert damaging pressure on the gums. Researchers also found that 47% of those with barbell-style tongue jewelry also had chipped teeth, probably because they tended to bite the metal. Because of these and other risks—infection and a loss of sensation—tongue-piercing isn't recommended. If you decide to get it done anyway, see your dentist regularly in order to identify and correct potential problems before they get more serious.

If regular brushing and flossing don't eliminate gum disease, your dentist may recommend **rinsing with an antibacterial mouthwash.** Listerine helps reduce plaque.

What you eat and drink also plays a role in controlling gum disease. **Drink at least eight glasses of water a day.** It increases saliva flow and reduces inflammation and plaque buildup. Eat a well-balanced diet—and be sure to **include plenty of fruits and vegetables.** They're rich in vitamin C, a nutrient that promotes gum health and healing. A report in the *Journal of Periodontology* found that people who don't get enough vitamin C are almost 1.5 times more likely to develop gum disease than those who get the recommended 75 to 90 mg daily. **Avoid sugary foods.** They make the mouth more acidic and promote bacterial growth.

Quit smoking, which increases gum inflammation by over-stimulating the immune system. One study found smokers 11 times more likely than nonsmokers to harbor harmful oral bacteria.

Medications

If your gums stay red and swollen after several weeks of good home care, your dentist might recommend that you use a **prescription mouthwash** that contains chlorhexidine gluconate (Peridex, PerioGard). It reduces plaque by 55% and gingivitis by 30% to 40%. It has an unpleasantly bitter taste, though, and it may stain your teeth or dental work. Therefore, it's only prescribed when basic oral hygiene doesn't do the trick.

Procedures

When you have gum disease, you'll need **regular cleanings** every three months by a dental hygienist or a dentist who specializes in

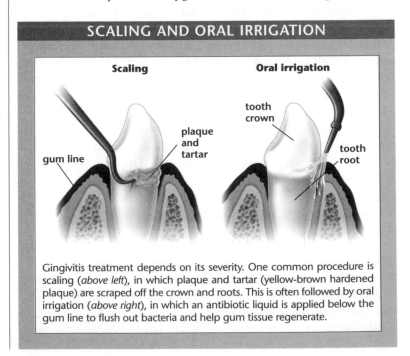

SCALING AND ORAL IRRIGATION

Gingivitis treatment depends on its severity. One common procedure is scaling (*above left*), in which plaque and tartar (yellow-brown hardened plaque) are scraped off the crown and roots. This is often followed by oral irrigation (*above right*), in which an antibiotic liquid is applied below the gum line to flush out bacteria and help gum tissue regenerate.

Preserve Your Gums, Protect Your Heart

You wouldn't think that what happens in your mouth could affect your heart, but studies have shown that it can. People with gum disease are more likely to develop heart disease or stroke than those with healthy gums.

Researchers now think that one of the organisms that causes gum disease, *P. gingivalis*, contributes to the formation of arterial plaques, fatty deposits in the arteries that can impede or block the flow of blood to the heart or brain. In a study in the journal *Circulation*, laboratory mice infected with this bacterium developed larger plaques than those that were germ-free.

It's not entirely clear how the germs that cause gum disease damage arteries. The bacteria may secrete poisons, called endotoxins, into the bloodstream. The toxins trigger inflammation in the blood vessels, which promotes the formation of plaques. Scientists believe these endotoxins travel from the mouth into the bloodstream.

But bacteria isn't the only culprit. In the animal studies, the only mice that developed arterial plaques after exposure to the germs were the ones fed a high-fat diet. These mice had a genetic mutation that's been linked to heart disease. Still, any degree of arterial inflammation is potentially serious.

Experts are beginning to realize that keeping your gums infection-free may be one more important way to protect your heart.

---

gum disease (a periodontist). If you've had gingivitis for years, your dentist may need to remove all of the accumulated plaque and tartar. Called **full-mouth debridement,** or scaling and root planing, this process is much more involved than a routine cleaning. Over a period of weeks, the dentist will use manual instruments as well as ultrasound to break down and remove tartar from your teeth. Damaged tissue will be removed. The surfaces of the teeth and the roots will be smoothed, making it harder for plaque to accumulate later on. Even if you don't need a full-mouth debridement, your dentist will probably apply an **antibiotic or dental rinse** under the gums to eliminate the possibility of infection (*see illustration opposite*).

If deep pockets remain underneath the gums even after extensive cleaning, you'll probably need **gum surgery** to reduce the size of the pockets and allow the dentist to thoroughly clean away accumulated tartar. The most common procedure, **open flap curettage,** involves cutting a small flap in the gum to expose the tooth and root. Damaged tissue is cleaned or removed, and the gum flap is replaced.

Natural Methods*

The herb **bloodroot** contains a chemical compound called sanguinarine, which has potent antibacterial properties. You can buy natural toothpaste and mouthwash containing this ingredient in health food stores.

Another way to reduce gingivitis is to paint **liquid folic acid** along the gum line with a cotton swab twice a day. Using a toothpaste that contains **coenzyme Q$_{10}$,** an antioxidant, may reduce gum inflammation. Yet another natural method is to massage your gums with **powdered vitamin C,** then rinse thoroughly with water. Repeat this treatment once or twice a day for best results.

Natural methods are not subject to the same testing and regulation as prescription medications. Please seek your doctor's advice and use caution.

▶ **Can gum disease ever be contagious?**

It could be. Researchers have found that the bacteria P. gingivalis can be transmitted from an infected person to another through intimate contact over a long period of time. If you are being treated for gum disease, restrict kisses to quick pecks until your dentist or periodontist gives you the all-clear.

FINDING Support

- For the latest information about the prevention and treatment of gum disease, or to find a dentist in your area, get in touch with the American Dental Association in Chicago, IL (312-440-2500 or www.ada.org).

- To get free brochures on periodontal disease and oral health, or to locate a periodontist in your area, contact the American Academy of Periodontology, in Chicago, IL (1-312-787-5518 or www.perio.org).

Hair loss

Since mankind first put chisel to tablet, humans have been fretting over the loss of their hair. Now, for the first time in history, a number of effective treatments can help you better determine the fate of your pate.

LIKELY First Steps

- **A physical exam** to rule out any underlying medical or psychological disorder.
- **Medications** to slow the rate of hair loss and, ideally, help hair grow back.
- **Lifestyle changes** to nourish your scalp and help you keep the hair you have left.
- **Hair transplants, weaves,** or **wigs** to achieve more immediate results.

QUESTIONS TO Ask

- Does it make a difference whether my hair is falling out or breaking off?
- Could any medications I'm taking be causing my hair loss?
- Do you think the hair loss could be the result of a hormone imbalance?
- Could there be long-term effects from taking hair loss medications every day?
- Could I be shampooing too often?

What is happening

Thinning hair has many causes. The most common is male- and female-pattern baldness, medically known as androgenetic alopecia, in which hair thins gradually. This affects about two-thirds of men to varying degrees, often starting in their 20s and continuing throughout life. About 40% of women are susceptible, though they generally lose far less hair than men. Pattern baldness is genetic, but it's a myth that you inherit it only from your mother's side.

You do inherit a sensitivity to dihydrotestosterone (DHT), a hormone produced when testosterone comes in contact with an enzyme in your hair follicle called 5-alpha reductase. If you're prone to this type of hair loss, DHT slowly strangles the hair follicles on the top of your head. For unknown reasons, the follicles on the sides and back of the head aren't affected by DHT. That's why men are often left with a fringe of hair.

Patchy baldness, or alopecia areata, is another common form of hair loss, affecting about 5 million people in the United States. This immune-system disorder causes coin-sized areas of your scalp to suddenly shed hair. When stress causes hair loss, it's called telogen effluvium. This can be brought on by illness, major surgery, a traumatic event, or even childbirth. Your hair may not start falling out until three to six months afterward, so you may not make the connection. It often grows back after just a few months.

There are some other, rarer reasons why you might be losing your hair. One condition, called trichotillomania, is an abnormal desire to tug and pull at your hair until it comes out. Traction alopecia comes from wearing ponytails or braids pulled so tight that the hair is tugged out by its roots. Ringworm is a fungal infection that causes your scalp to scale and flake and makes your hair break off. Poor nutrition can cause hair loss, so can certain medications and chemotherapy. Once these problems are addressed, your hair will grow back.

Treatments

Your doctor will begin with a physical exam to rule out any underlying health conditions, especially if your hair loss was sudden. If a medical problem is the cause, your hair will grow back after it's treated. For other types of hair loss, a host of treatment options are available. Pattern baldness often responds to topical and, in men, oral medication. If that doesn't produce the results you want, you

Treatment options

Medications

Topical minoxidil	Regrows top-of-head hair in 40% of people.
Finasteride	Quite effective; best used at early stage.
Cortisone	Treats patchy baldness (alopecia areata).
Drithocreme/PUVA	Topical cream plus ultraviolet A radiation.
Antifungals	Combat ringworm-related hair loss.
Antidepressants	Treat obsessive-compulsive behavior.

Procedures

Hair transplantation	Can produce healthy, growing hair.
Hair weaves	Make thinning hair look thicker.

Lifestyle changes

Don't smoke	Smoking is linked to hair loss.
Handle hair with care	Use mild shampoo; comb gently.

Natural methods

Aromatherapy	May help with alopecia areata.
Saw palmetto	A natural alternative to the drug finasteride.

can investigate hair replacement surgery. When ringworm is the cause, antifungal creams will clear it up. Patchy baldness can be treated to a large extent with cortisone creams and injections or oral cortisone. For immediate results, you can opt for a hair weave, wig, or hairpiece.

Medications

Two drugs are currently approved by the Food and Drug Administration to treat pattern baldness. The first is **topical minoxidil,** often sold under the brand name Rogaine. It's available without a prescription and can be used by both men and women. It comes in two strengths—a 2% and a 5% concentration (the 5% solution is said to grow more hair more quickly). Minoxidil does have its limitations: Only about 40% of people applying it twice a day for a year will have moderate to dense hair growth, and it works only on the top of the head. You also have to use it indefinitely; any new hair it produces usually falls out within three months of stopping the drug.

The second medication is **finasteride** (Propecia), a prescription pill for men only. (It doesn't help women and can cause birth defects.) This drug blocks development of DHT, and it's quite effective if taken daily. About 80% of men will slow their hair loss, and about 60% will see some new growth. It works best, though, in younger men who are just beginning to lose their hair. Some dermatologists suggest combining finasteride and minoxidil.

TAKING **Control**

- **Go for the bald and bold look.** Perhaps more than ever, a clean-shaven head is not only acceptable for men, but fashionable and attractive.

- **Consider camouflage.** A short haircut for women or one that's layered can hide thinning hair. If you're showing more scalp than you'd like, invest in a wig, or a hairpiece.

- **Think about joining a support group.** It can be a good way to meet others who are going through the same thing. Don't underestimate the psychological impact of losing your hair. It's tough for men, and can be devastating for women.

- **Get a yearly physical.** A number of studies have found that men who started losing their hair early in life are at greater risk for heart disease.

- **Shop around for a surgeon** if you're considering hair transplants. Ask to see at least a dozen different before-and-after photos. Find out if the surgeon will give you names and phone numbers of some patients he's worked on. Investigate his reputation with other doctors.

▶MALE PATTERN BALDNESS **is generally found only in men of European origin. By the age of 50, half these men will lose their hair. Asians, Native Americans, and most Africans and African-Americans will never go bald.**

▶How much hair loss is considered normal?

Here's an irony for you: Your hair is supposed to fall out. It is, after all, dead tissue, comprised of the same protein—called keratin— that makes up your fingernails and toenails.

About 90% of the healthy hair on your head right now is in a four- or five-year growth period. The other 10% is in a resting phase. That lasts a couple of months, then it falls out. Most people, shed 50 to 100 hairs a day. That may sound like a lot, until you consider that you had 100,000 hairs on your head in your youth.

Hair loss begins when the rate of shedding exceeds the rate of regrowth. It also happens when the new hair is thinner than the hair you just lost. Many balding people lose several hundred hairs a day. You'll know if you are keeping an eye on what's showing up in your hairbrush.

Patchy baldness sometimes responds to **cortisone creams, injections,** and **pills.** If they don't work, your doctor might want you to try **anthralin cream (Drithocreme)** and **5% minoxidil,** coupled with psoralen and ultraviolet A radiation **(PUVA therapy).** For hair loss due to ringworm, an **oral antifungal medication** like griseofulvin (Grisactin) or a **topical antifungal** may be prescribed. If trichotillomania is your diagnosis, you'll probably start on **an antidepressant,** such as Prozac or Zoloft, that fights obsessive-compulsive behavior, and be encouraged to seek counseling as well.

Procedures

Hair transplantation has been around in some form since the 1950s. It has come a long way since early attempts, where an unnatural hair-line and uneven growth often made people look like they had "doll hair." These days, surgeons take micrografts—tiny bits of scalp containing only a few hair follicles—and transplant them to the bare portions of your scalp. These donor hairs come from the sides and back of your head, where your hair remains full. Hair transplantation is an option for both men and women. The benefit is that this procedure produces healthy, growing hair. It's expensive, though—easily $10,000 for the initial sessions, with additional fees for touch-ups. You'll need one every year or two unless the cause of your hair loss is eliminated, because the original hair on the top of your head will continue to fall out, leaving bald patches around the transplanted hair.

Hair weaving—also called hair intensification or hair integration—is a nonsurgical option for people with thinning hair. It's done by weaving human or synthetic hair to existing locks. It has some drawbacks: It's expensive (up to $2,500), it makes it hard to keep hair and scalp clean, and it stresses the hair attached to the weaves, often making it fall out. That's why the American Hair Loss Council recommends that if you go this route, you should remove the weave after a few weeks.

Lifestyle Changes

Making lifestyle changes usually won't regrow hair you've already lost, but it can help you hang on to what you still have.

- **Don't smoke.** Smoking, associated with skin disorders, may cause early balding in some people. An Italian study in 2000 found that mice exposed to three months of cigarette smoke lost lots of hair and turned prematurely gray.
- **Wash hair with care.** Highly alkaline shampoos can make a mess of your scalp over time and may cause hair to thin. Try baby shampoo or a volumizing shampoo that adds protein to hair shafts, making them look thicker. Pat your hair dry afterward.
- **Treat hair tenderly.** Minimize bleaching, curling, and straightening, and stay away from tight ponytails and braids. Use a wide-tooth comb on your hair. Don't overbrush.
- **Avoid chlorinated pools.** Pool water can contain more alkaline than the harshest shampoo.
- **Eat a balanced diet.** Choose lots of fish, poultry, fruits, and vegetables. Avoid fatty foods and red meat. These can boost testosterone levels, making DHT levels jump.

Natural Methods*

Try **massaging your scalp** daily. It feels great, and it increases blood flow, speeding along nutrients and sloughing off biological waste products. Be careful not to rub roughly; knead gently but firmly with your fingertips. If you're into more experimental techniques, consider **aromatherapy.** One study showed it to be helpful for treating alopecia areata, or patchy hair loss. In 1998, clinicians reported in the *Archives of Dermatology* that 44% of study participants with alopecia areata experienced new hair growth after using an aromatherapy oil compound. The researchers used a base of jojoba and grapeseed oils, mixed in essential oils of lavender, cedarwood, thyme, and rosemary, and massaged it on participants' scalps once a day. If you're unsure how to make such a concoction, see an aromatherapist. **Saw palmetto,** an herbal remedy, has been said to affect men's conversion of testosterone to DHT, much like the drug finasteride. Look for a standardized extract with 90% essential fatty acids and sterols: Take 160 mg twice a day. Don't take it if you're also taking finasteride.

Outlook

There's never been a better time to be balding. It's taken researchers a while to understand some of the mechanisms at work in hereditary hair loss, but they're quickly cracking the code. New drugs are on the horizon, surgical techniques have been refined, and scientists are making great strides toward grasping the genetic workings of baldness. They're even delving into cloning healthy hair follicles! Not surprisingly, some researchers predict that treating hair loss will soon be as easy as a trip to the barber.

Natural methods are not subject to the same testing and regulation as prescription medications. Please seek your doctor's advice and use caution.

Promising DEVELOPMENTS

- The FDA recently approved a drug called **dutasteride** for the treatment of enlarged prostates. Some preliminary studies suggest that it might also be as good as, or better than, finasteride for treating male pattern baldness. It's in further trials now as a hair loss treatment.
- A drug that's long been used to reduce inflammation may have a new life as a treatment for patchy hair loss (alopecia areata). In a study published in the *Journal of the American Academy of Dermatology,* about half of the patients who took **sulfasalazine (Azulfidine)** experienced partial or total regrowth of their hair.

FINDING Support

- For more information on hair loss and its treatments, visit the American Hair Loss Council's website (www.ahlc.org).
- The American Academy of Dermatology posts the latest findings on treating hair loss on its website at www.aad.org. Or call 1-888-462-DERM.
- Many bald-is-beautiful Internet sites offer support and practical advice for men. Take a look at www.baldrus.com or www.headshaver.org.
- If you would like more information about alopecia areata, contact the National Alopecia Areata Foundation in San Rafael, CA (1-415-472-3780 or www.alopeciaareata.org).

Hearing loss

It's a natural sign of aging: One in three people over age 60 and half of those older than 85 have some hearing loss. But new sophisticated technological advances can dramatically improve your hearing, no matter how old you are.

LIKELY First Steps

- **A physical exam** to find the cause of hearing loss.
- **Avoiding loud noises** that can further damage hearing.
- **A hearing aid** to amplify sounds.
- **Medications** to treat any ailments that may be impairing your hearing.

QUESTIONS TO Ask

- Could any medications I take for other conditions cause hearing loss?
- Why do I have so much earwax?
- Is there a hearing aid that corrects only the pitch I can't hear?
- Would cochlear implant surgery correct my condition?

What is happening

The most common cause of hearing loss is a normal age-related condition called presbycusis, a word derived from the Greek for "old hearing." The ancient Greeks got it right: Hearing often degenerates with age. A major contributing factor can be exposure to loud noises at work (jackhammers, jet engines) or play (loud music, fireworks). Former President Bill Clinton (a saxophonist and rock-concert goer) began wearing hearing aids at age 51 after tests confirmed he had lost the ability to hear some high frequencies. But you don't have to attend noisy concerts or political rallies to lose your hearing. It can occur over time, when receptor cells in the inner ear wear out. Hearing loss also tends to run in families.

Brian Wilson and The Beach Boys summed it up pretty well: Hearing is all about "good vibrations." Sound waves are vibrations that move through the air. Once they enter the human ear, they pass through the eardrum, then the middle ear, where three tiny bones called ossicles act as an amplifier. Once ushered into the inner ear, the vibrations move through a fluid in the snail-shaped hearing center called the cochlea, which contains tiny, specialized hair cells. The fluid stimulates these hair cells, which produce nerve impulses that are sent to the brain. How the fluid moves the hair cells determines how correctly the brain is able to distinguish vowels from consonants, differentiate between a dog barking, a baby crying, or a spouse speaking.

As people age, hair cells can degenerate. The first sign of hearing loss is usually difficulty with high-frequency sounds like birds singing or children's voices. You also have problems understanding what someone is saying when there's a lot of background noise. Exposure to loud noises also can damage hair cells, causing hearing loss (*see box opposite*). A normal conversation registers at about 60 decibels. Prolonged exposure to decibel levels over 75 can damage hearing, and regular exposure of more than one minute to levels above 110 decibels can cause permanent hearing loss.

Treatments

Hearing loss could be masking another problem. There's little you can do about it on your own, so you should see a doctor. You need to be checked for conditions such as diabetes or high blood pressure, both associated with hearing problems. If you get a clean bill of health, you may be referred to an ear, nose, and throat doctor (otolaryng-

Treatment options

Lifestyle changes

Avoid loud noises	To preserve the hearing you have.
Exercise	Sedentary lifestyle is linked to hearing loss.
Turn off background sound	Makes it easier to hear.

Procedures

Hearing aids	For mild to profound hearing loss.
Cochlear implants	Help if hearing loss is profound.

Medications

Cerumenolytics	Dissolve earwax.
Antibiotics	Treat ear infections.

ologist) for specialized testing and a rundown of your treatment options. Your doctor may recommend a hearing specialist (audiologist), who will conduct a test to determine the type and degree of loss. An audiologist can fit you with a hearing aid. Although such devices are undeniably pricey, most people who opt for them are delighted as the world of sound is restored. In certain cases, surgery may be recommended.

Some causes of hearing loss can be corrected: Removing excess earwax (*see box, page 156*) can make a difference. The right medications restore hearing affected by a virus, bacteria, or allergies.

Lifestyle Changes

Although you may not be able to regain the hearing capacity you've lost, you can take steps to keep what you have and make the most of it. The following may be helpful:

- **Avoid loud noises.** If you go to a noisy concert or sporting event, use earplugs. They won't keep you from hearing what's going on, but they'll keep the dangerous decibel levels from damaging your ears. The same goes for any time you're around loud noises, such as construction and even traffic (*see box at right*).
- **Exercise.** Researchers from the University of Wisconsin looked at 1,600 people between ages 52 and 97. They found that those who exercised were 32% less likely to have impaired hearing than those who didn't work out. Those with cardiovascular disease (sometimes fueled by a sedentary lifestyle) were 54% more likely to have hearing loss.
- **Give up cigarettes.** A study in Japan of 1,554 men who worked at the same company found that those who smoked were more than twice as likely to have hearing loss as those who didn't.
- **Turn off background noise.** If you have trouble understanding what people are saying, get rid of distracting background sounds by turning off the TV, radio, or CD player, the dishwasher, or moving away from the commotion.

TAKING Control

- **Get a medical exam before you buy a hearing aid.** You'll need a written evaluation from your doctor to buy a hearing aid. People 18 and over can sign a waiver for this exam, but that may not be a good idea. Taking test results to a hearing aid dealer increases the odds that you'll get the hearing aid that's right for you.

- **Make hearing loss prevention your job.** An estimated 30 million American workers are exposed to dangerous noise levels on the job. If you work around loud noises, wear earplugs or earmuffs. The National Institute for Occupational Safety and Health (NIOSH), part of the Centers for Disease Control and Prevention, recommends a hearing-loss prevention program for all workplaces that have dangerous noise levels. For more information, contact NIOSH (1-800-35-NIOSH or www.cdc.gov/niosh).

Know Your Noises

Prolonged exposure to sound levels above 75 decibels is considered potentially harmful to your hearing. Compare these common decibel levels:

- Whisper: 20
- Refrigerator humming: 40
- Normal conversation: 60
- City traffic: 80
- Lawn mower, motorcycle: 90
- Wood shop noise: 100
- Chainsaw: 110
- Snowmobile: 120
- Rock concert: 140

The Facts About Earwax

Earwax gets a bum rap. We really should appreciate it more than we do. Glands near the outer ear canal form it to protect the ear canals and eardrums from water and infection. The wax traps dirt and dust particles, lubricates the skin in the ear canals, and even helps fight off fungus and various bacteria.

Earwax normally performs its thankless tasks, then migrates toward the outer ear, where it dries up and flakes away. Problems can arise when there's too much wax. A buildup can block the ear canal and cause temporary hearing loss. Consider the following solutions for dealing with earwax:

- **Use a warm, wet washcloth** to clean your outer ear whenever you shower or bathe.
- **Try using warm olive oil or baby oil** if you have earwax accumulation. Place the oil in an eyedropper and put one or two drops in your ear a couple of times a week.
- **Consider hydrogen peroxide**. This option softens earwax and helps it make its natural migration out of your ear. Use an eyedropper to place a couple of drops in your ears once a week.
- **See your doctor,** especially if the earwax has become impacted. A doctor can use prescription wax softeners, water jets, or special instruments to clear out problem wax.

■ **Teach your family and friends how to speak.** A few simple suggestions can help those who talk with you most communicate more clearly. They don't need to shout, but tell them to speak a little louder and enunciate well. Make sure they face you squarely and aren't eating or chewing gum while they talk.

Procedures

Many people with hearing loss are greatly helped by a **hearing aid.** These devices basically amplify sounds. A tiny microphone picks up sound waves and converts them to electrical signals, which are then sent through an amplifier to your ear. Although a hearing aid can't restore normal hearing, it can improve your hearing and your quality of life. One study of 2,300 hearing-impaired adults over age 50 found that those with untreated hearing loss were more likely to report depression, anxiety, and paranoia than those with hearing aids. The untreated group also felt more isolated and was less likely to take part in organized social activities. If your doctor or otolaryngologist recommends a hearing aid, heed the advice. (*For information about the types of hearing aids that are available, see the box opposite.*)

If you have lost most or all of your hearing, a **cochlear implant** may restore a sense of sound that can help you understand speech without lip reading or sign language. This complex electronic device intercepts useful sounds and sends electrical impulses to the brain via electrodes placed in the cochlea (*see illustration below*). It doesn't repair your body's natural hearing system, but

COCHLEAR IMPLANT

A cochlear implant is a wonder. Here's how it works: A mini-microphone behind the outer ear picks up sounds and sends them to a calculator-sized speech processor (often worn on a belt). The processor arranges the sounds and sends them to a transmitter implanted in the ear. The transmitter then converts the sounds to electrical impulses, sending them along an array of electrodes implanted in the cochlea. The electrodes stimulate the auditory nerve to deliver the impulses to the brain.

Buying a Hearing Aid: Know Your Options

If your doctor recommends a hearing aid, see an audiologist to determine which type best suits your needs. The one you get will be based on how much hearing you have, your daily activities, cosmetic concerns, and cost. Most dealers offer a free 30-day trial period for hearing aids, and you may require several adjustments before yours feels comfortable.

Types of hearing aids
The three main types of hearing aids are:
- **In-the-ear (ITE).** This model fits completely in the outer ear, and its components all fit in a hard plastic case. It can be used for mild to severe hearing loss.
- **Behind-the-ear (BTE).** The components are contained in a behind-the-ear case, connected to a plastic ear mold that fits inside the outer ear. A BTE hearing aid is for mild to profound hearing loss.
- **In-the-canal (ITC).** Customized to fit in the ear canal, this is almost invisible. It treats mild to moderately severe hearing impairment.

Types of circuitry
Three types of electronic circuitry are available:
- **Analog/adjustable.** This circuitry is built by a laboratory to specifications based on volume levels and other information your audiologist provides. Only slight adjustments can be made once the hearing aid is delivered. This is generally the least expensive mechanism.
- **Analog/programmable.** Programmed by a computer, this type can handle more than one program at a time. It lets the wearer change settings to reflect the listening environment, such as a walk in the country or a dinner in a noisy restaurant.
- **Digital/programmable.** Digital circuitry is programmed by a computer, and sound quality and response time can be calibrated for you. The digital microchip provides the most flexibility, so your audiologist can make individual adjustments. This is typically the most expensive circuitry.

compensates for it in a way that allows you to communicate in person and over the phone.

In about 2% to 3% of cases, hearing loss may be caused by otosclerosis. This hereditary disorder occurs when abnormal bone forms around the tiny bones in the ear known as ossicles. During **stapedectomy surgery,** one of the bones (the stapes) is replaced by a prosthesis made of plastic and wire. Such a procedure can be effective at restoring hearing.

Medications

For most cases of natural hearing loss due to age or exposure to loud noises, no medications can help. When hearing loss is caused by another problem, you may find relief in a bottle. **Cerumenolytics** (Debrox, Cerumenex) can help dissolve excess earwax and clear up the problem. **Antibiotics** combat ear infections (*see page 113*), and an **anticoagulant** can help if the loss of hearing is caused by a blood clot in an artery feeding the ear. For hearing loss related to various allergies (*see page 23*), **antihistamines** and **decongestants** may provide relief.

FINDING Support

- The National Institute on Deafness and Other Communication Disorders, part of the National Institutes of Health, has detailed information on hearing loss, including the latest research news, at www.nidcd.nih.gov.

- Hearing Center Online, a website sponsored by Audiotech Healthcare, has lots of fun stuff, including an interactive ear, an Earwax Museum that features histories of hearing aids and hearing devices, facts about famous folks with hearing problems, and even hearing-related games and crossword puzzles. Log on to www. hearingcenteronline.com.

Heart attack

Roughly 1.2 million Americans will have a heart attack this year—and about half of them will die from it. Thanks to improved emergency-care strategies, however, over 90% of those who make it to the hospital in time for treatment will survive.

A
B
C
D
E
F
G
H
I
J
K
L
M
N
O
P
Q
R
S
T
U
V
W
X
Y
Z

LIKELY **First Steps**

- **Call 911** immediately to get medical help and quick transport to the hospital emergency room.

- **Chew an aspirin** to reduce the severity of the attack; **take nitroglycerin** for chest pain (angina).

- ER doctors will administer **thrombolytic drugs** to dissolve artery-blocking clots and minimize tissue damage.

QUESTIONS TO **Ask**

- How badly has my heart been permanently damaged?

- Can my heart disease be reversed?

- Am I a good candidate for a cardiac rehabilitation program?

- When will I be able to return to work? Drive a car? Resume having sex?

▶ **HEART ATTACKS are three times more apt to occur between 5 AM and 9 AM. In northern climates, heart attacks tend to be more common during the winter. More than 70% of heart attacks happen at home.**

What is happening

Every muscle in your body needs a steady supply of blood to function properly. Your heart is no exception. Coronary arteries nourish your heart muscle with plenty of oxygen and nutrients to keep it pumping day and night. If one of these arteries becomes blocked—usually the result of a blood clot forming at a site where the artery has become narrowed by plaque—the heart muscle is deprived of blood and may begin to die. This tissue death is called a myocardial infarction (MI) or, more commonly, a heart attack.

Unless the blockage in your artery is cleared and blood flow is restored, your heart muscle usually cannot survive for more than three hours. After that, the affected section will die, becoming useless scar tissue and permanently impairing your heart's ability to pump effectively. Destruction of a large enough portion of the heart can be fatal. That's why it is crucial to get medical care as quickly as possible at the first sign of a heart attack. Every minute counts.

Most people are familiar with classic heart attack symptoms—crushing chest pain or shooting pains radiating along the upper left arm—but a heart attack can manifest itself in a variety of ways. Women tend to have more subtle symptoms, which may delay timely treatment. Be on the lookout for any of the following: uncomfortable pressure, pain, or tightness in the chest that lasts for more than 10 minutes; pain in the shoulders, jaw, neck, and arms (especially the left); chest pain (whether severe or mild) accompanied by light-headedness, cold sweat, shortness of breath, nausea, or unusual feelings of dread or impending doom.

Treatments

The key to surviving a heart attack is quick action. If you or someone you're with experiences any of the symptoms of a heart attack for more than 10 minutes, seek **emergency medical assistance.** Most people admitted to emergency rooms for a suspected heart attack turn out to be suffering from severe heartburn, a panic attack, or another problem. Still, it's better to err on the side of caution. Call 911 for emergency medical services (EMS).

At the first sign of symptoms, chew and swallow **an aspirin,** unless you suffer from gastrointestinal bleeding or have had major surgery during the previous week. A single (325 mg) aspirin can help the blood clot start to dissolve; chewing the tablet gets the

Treatment options

Medications

Aspirin/nitroglycerin	Chew aspirin right away; nitro for chest pain.
Thrombolytics	Dissolve clots; can stop attack in progress.
Anticoagulants	Prevent clots and another attack.
Narcotics	For intense chest pain.
Antihypertensives	Beta-blockers et al. to improve heart function.

Procedures

Emergency measures	Call 911; oxygen, CPR, defibrillator by EMS.
Angioplasty	Widens clogged artery; restores blood flow.
Bypass surgery	Only if drugs or angioplasty fail.

Lifestyle changes

Exercise	Start slowly, then follow doctor-directed plan.
Cardiac rehabilitation	For advice on diet, smoking cessation, stress.

medicine into your bloodstream more quickly. Just be sure to let emergency personnel know you've taken the aspirin.

Paramedics will administer **supplementary oxygen** through a mask or nasal tube in an effort to save oxygen-starved heart tissue. They may also perform **cardiopulmonary resuscitation (CPR)** or use an **electrical defibrillator** (a device that shocks the heart back to a proper rhythm) if your normal heartbeat is disrupted. Once you're in the hospital, the immediate goals of the emergency team will be to clear the blocked coronary artery and restore blood flow to your heart, as well as ease your pain and discomfort.

Medications

Relatively new medications known as **thrombolytics,** or "clot-busting" drugs, can virtually stop a heart attack in progress by dissolving the deadly blood clot. If one of these drugs is administered within the first half hour after onset, you may suffer little or no permanent damage to the affected heart muscle. These revolutionary drugs—including tissue plasminogen activator (t-PA), alteplase, streptokinase, urokinase, tenecteplase, and anistreplase—have dramatically boosted heart attack survival rates. Their benefits significantly diminish within two or three hours after the attack, but by that time, damage is irreparable, even if blood flow is restored.

You will also be given an **anticoagulant,** such as heparin, warfarin, or the newer drug tirofiban, to prevent new clots from forming and causing another heart attack. **Nitroglycerin** (in the form of tablets placed under the tongue or an injection) can alleviate pain by widening the vessels leading to the heart, and improving the delivery of oxygen. **Narcotics** like morphine or meperidine

TAKING Control

- **Act quickly.** Don't ignore your symptoms. About half of all heart attack patients wait too long—at least two hours—before getting help. Not waiting can make the difference between life and death.

- **Plan ahead.** Identify the hospitals or medical centers nearest your home or office best equipped to deal with cardiac emergencies. This is especially important if you are at high risk for a heart attack.

- **Plot the route** in advance. Make sure that you and your spouse (or someone close to you) know the fastest way to the best medical facility.

- **Quit smoking.** Cutting out tobacco, studies show, can reduce your risk of a heart attack by 50% to 70%.

- **Get moving.** Regular aerobic exercise nearly halves your risk of a heart attack (a 45% reduction), yet more than 60% of Americans are sedentary.

- **Ask your doctor** about getting your C-reactive protein (CRP) level measured as part of your routine blood work. Experts are finding that a high CRP indicates above-average inflammation, a scenario that raises your heart attack risk—even if your cholesterol is low. Statins, aspirin, and other anti-inflammatories can lower CRP. So can certain lifestyle measures.

Aspirin: The Wonder Drug

Studies show that taking one adult aspirin (325 mg) every other day or a baby aspirin (81 mg) every day can reduce the chances of heart attack by up to 40% in high-risk patients. Chewing an aspirin shortly after the onset of a heart attack reduces the risk of imminent death by 25%.

Many doctors already advise a daily low-dose aspirin for men over age 40 and women over 50 who have at least one heart disease risk factor. If your doctor thinks you are a good candidate for such therapy, be sure to take the aspirin with food to reduce the risk of gastrointestinal bleeding. Avoid alcohol, because it further promotes stomach upset and bleeding when taken with aspirin. If regular aspirin gives you heartburn, use a buffered, enteric-coated, or time-released formulation. Save money by buying a generic product.

FINDING Support

- Mended Hearts is a national support group for heart patients and their families. Contact them for information and referrals (1-888-HEART99 or www.mendedhearts.org).

- The American Heart Association provides information and public education programs on all aspects of heart disease. Check for local chapters in your area (1-800-242-8721 or www.americanheart.org).

(Demerol) may be used for more intense pain. **Tranquilizers** or **sedatives** may be used to help ease the terrible anxiety that can accompany a heart attack.

Once you're stabilized, your doctor may prescribe **antihypertensive drugs**—beta-blockers, angiotensin-converting enzyme (ACE) inhibitors, and diuretics—to reduce the rate and force of your contractions so your heart needs less oxygen. This helps minimize destruction of heart tissue. And when you leave the hospital, if you don't receive a prescription for long-term beta-blocker therapy, ask why. Studies show these drugs can dramatically reduce your risk of a second heart attack. Cholesterol-lowering statin drugs and daily low-dose aspirin therapy can significantly lower your risk as well.

Procedures

As an alternative to thrombolytic drugs, doctors may decide to give you an emergency **angioplasty** (percutaneous transluminal coronary angioplasty, or PTCA). This involves inflating a tiny balloon in the clogged artery to compress the blockage and restore the flow of blood through it (*see page 97*). Studies show that emergency PTCA is at least as effective as clot-busting drugs, especially for patients who develop very low blood pressure.

In very rare cases, coronary artery **bypass surgery** may be performed if thrombolytics or angioplasty don't work well enough after a heart attack. However, it is generally better to postpone this procedure for a few days until your condition stabilizes. Both surgical procedures require highly trained personnel who may not be available in all facilities. A **pacemaker** (*see page 46*) or implantable cardiac **defibrillator** may be warranted. You may need **surgery to repair injury** to the heart or blood vessels.

Lifestyle Changes

During your hospital stay, you should gradually increase your **physical activity** and start to regain your strength—the sooner, the better. If recovery is uneventful and surgery isn't needed, you will likely be discharged in about a week. Within about four to eight weeks, you may be able to resume normal activities (including work and sex), if you can handle moderate exertion such as walking up two flights of stairs without chest pain or shortness of breath.

Before leaving the hospital, you will probably undergo a modified exercise stress test to help your doctor devise an **individualized exercise plan** for you to follow in the ensuing weeks. Your doctor may also recommend a supervised outpatient **cardiac rehabilitation program,** involving low-intensity exercise to help you regain strength and endurance. A good program will also offer comprehensive personalized advice and support on diet, smoking cessation, and stress control, as well as emotional and psychological support for patients contending with anxiety, depression, and family or occupational problems. If possible, you should take part in a rehabilitation program for at least two months.

Heartburn

From a tiny twinge to a sensation like a blowtorch behind the breastbone, heart-burn intensities affect some 25 million Americans every day. Near-complete relief is possible with a combination of lifestyle changes and the right medications.

What is happening

Despite its name, heartburn has nothing to do with your heart: It's the result of a mechanical problem in your digestive tract. Gastro-esophageal reflux occurs when stomach acid splashes back and upward into your esophagus, the tube connecting the back of your throat to your stomach. Heartburn happens because a valve between your esophagus and stomach—the lower esophageal sphincter (LES)—which is normally clamped tight during digestion, has weak-ened (*see illustration below*). Frequent simple heartburn damages the lining of the esophagus. This condition is called gastroesophageal reflux disease, or GERD.

While your stomach is built to handle powerful digestive juices, your esophagus is not. Hence, the burning sensation in the center of your chest during heartburn is truly just that—an acid burn. You might also have a hot acidy taste, feel a lump in your throat, or have an asthma-like chronic cough when acid travels down your breathing tube. Over time, stomach acid can wear down your tooth enamel. The constant erosion of the internal lining of your esoph-agus can lead to a more serious disorder called Barrett's esophagus (*see page 163*).

LIKELY **First Steps**

- **Medications** to soothe the pain and discomfort of heartburn.

- **Lifestyle changes** to address the root of the problem.

- If all else fails, **surgery and other procedures** to correct the anatomical problems that lead to heartburn.

QUESTIONS TO **Ask**

- Does chronic heartburn increase my risk for cancer?

- Could my heartburn be caused by *H. pylori,* the bac-teria that can cause ulcers?

- Could my asthma be related to my heartburn?

- Might any of the medications or nutritional supplements I take be causing my heart-burn symptoms?

- Should I have an endoscopy?

THE MECHANICS OF HEARTBURN AND GERD

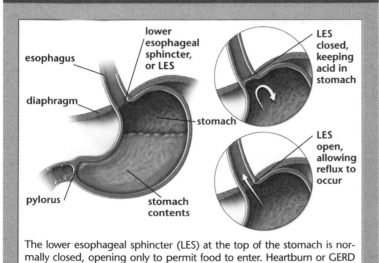

The lower esophageal sphincter (LES) at the top of the stomach is nor-mally closed, opening only to permit food to enter. Heartburn or GERD occurs when the LES spontaneously relaxes, allowing digestive acids, food, and liquids to flow backward (reflux) into the sensitive esophageal tissues.

TAKING Control

- **Drink a large glass of warm water.** This will wash the misplaced acid back down and ease your pain. If water isn't handy, chew a stick or two of gum to produce more saliva.

- **Get rid of the extra pillows.** While it's good to raise your whole upper body when lying down, elevating just your head worsens heartburn symptoms.

- **Avoid stooping or bending.** This bumps up the pressure in your gut, making heartburn worse. If you need to pick up something, crouch.

- **Keep a heartburn diary.** Record the time of each episode and what seemed to contribute to it. This will make it easier to determine which lifestyle changes and treatments will work for you.

▶ **SOME DOCTORS TREAT HEARTBURN** conservatively at first, especially in milder cases. They start with antacids, progress to H₂ blockers like Pepcid AC, and then finally to prescription drugs. Other experts are bucking this trend and moving directly to prescription proton pump inhibitors (drugs that slow your stomach's acid production) even for milder cases of GERD. Their reasoning is that these drugs are more effective, and need to be taken only once a day.

Treatment options

Medications

Antacids	For occasional heartburn relief.
H₂ blockers	Reduce stomach acid production.
Proton pump inhibitors	Improve GERD symptoms in 80% of sufferers.
Prokinetic agents	Speed food through the stomach.

Lifestyle changes

Diet	Eat small meals; avoid heartburn triggers.

Natural methods

Deglycyrrhizinated licorice	Reduces stomach acid.

Procedures

Endoscopic procedures	Stretch esophagus and/or tighten LES.
Fundoplication	Surgery to strengthen faulty LES valve.

You're more likely to have chronic heartburn if you're significantly overweight, smoke, take medications that make your lower esophageal sphincter relax, or have certain medical conditions (*see Hiatal Hernia, page 164*). At least 25% of pregnant women experience heartburn due to increased hormone levels that cause the LES to stretch farther open than usual.

Treatments

If you have heartburn or GERD, you have multitudes of treatment options. The right choice for you will depend on how often you experience symptoms and how seriously your esophagus has been damaged. Therapies range from simple diet "don'ts" and over-the-counter antacids and H₂ blockers to pricey prescription drugs that control esophageal movement or turn off production of stomach acid. In severe cases, surgery may be needed to get the LES to behave itself once and for all.

Medications

For relief of heartburn once or twice a month, nothing beats **antacids.** They neutralize the stomach acid that has splashed up into your esophagus. They're also cheap, effective, and remarkably fast-acting. You're undoubtedly familiar with brands that have become household words: TUMS, Alka-Seltzer, Maalox, Mylanta, and at least two dozen others—along with their generic equivalents. If you're taking prescription medication of any kind, check with your doctor or pharmacist before adding an antacid. An antacid can block the absorption of certain drugs.

Alginic acid (Gaviscon and other brands) is a unique antacid specifically designed for heartburn. This drug works by mixing with your saliva and gastric juices to form a foam that floats to the top of your stomach and up into your esophagus. While other antacids move forward into your small intestine, Gaviscon's backward foam can neutralize esophageal acid within minutes.

If you're experiencing heartburn throughout the day, the next step is OTC **histamine (H_2) blockers,** which reduce acid production. These drugs include cimetidine (Tagamet HB), famotidine (Pepcid AC), nizatidine (Axid AR), and ranitidine (Zantac 75). Although they take longer to kick in than antacids—up to 90 minutes—H_2 blockers compensate for the delay by lasting for about 12 hours. Many people need two doses a day, and it's usually best to take one of them at bedtime, when heartburn symptoms are most intense. You can also use H_2 blockers in combination with antacids, getting immediate relief from one while waiting for the longer-term effects of the other. Prescription-strength H_2 blockers are available.

Your doctor may suggest a **proton pump inhibitor** (also called an acid pump inhibitor), such as omeprazole (Prilosec), or lansoprazole (Prevacid) if OTC drugs aren't doing the trick. This type of drug works by inhibiting the mechanism, or "pump," your stomach uses to excrete acid, and has been shown to improve symptoms in up to 80% of those with GERD. Finally, if none of these drugs make you feel better, you may need a prescription **prokinetic agent,** such as metoclopramide (Reglan). It strengthens your struggling LES and helps move food through your stomach more quickly.

Lifestyle Changes

Doctors have found that lifestyle changes alone can reduce or eliminate GERD symptoms in about half of those who live with them. Once you get the pain and burning under control, set your sights on changing the habits that may have caused the problem in the first place. You can:

- **Quit smoking.** There are so many reasons to stop for good—and getting relief from heartburn is yet another. Smoking dries up your saliva, a natural lubricant your body uses to wash down gastric

▶ **What is Barrett's esophagus?**

This condition, named for British surgeon Norman Barrett, is a complication of GERD that appears in a small number of people. It occurs when the cells lining the esophagus are overexposed to gastric juices, become permanently damaged, and enter a precancerous state. Some people with Barrett's esophagus develop esophageal cancer. For that reason, it's a good idea to have an endoscopy if you've had heartburn for more than a few years. A doctor will slip a thin, lighted tube down your throat to check for any signs of cancer. One study from the University of California at San Francisco found that esophageal cancer caught early by endoscopy led to much higher survival rates over five years.

Promising
DEVELOPMENTS

- The gamma-amino butyric acid agonist **baclofen** is showing great promise as a weapon against GERD. In one study, it reduced the number of participants' reflux episodes by as much as 70%. It also helped prevent relaxation of the lower esophageal sphincter—the major cause of GERD.

Hiatal Hernia

If you were to check for a hernia, chances are you'd look around your abdomen or groin for the telltale bulge. But one type of hernia isn't so easy to spot—and some doctors think it may be a major reason we develop gastroesophageal reflux disease (GERD).

A hiatal hernia happens when a portion of the stomach protrudes through an opening in the diaphragm (the muscular wall separating the chest and the abdomen). The origin of a hiatal hernia isn't always known—it may be present at birth, or the result of trauma, such as a car accident. Whatever its cause, doctors surmise that it may weaken the sphincter that leads into the stomach and cause acid to back up into the esophagus, causing heartburn. Many people with hiatal hernia have no heartburn, and most people with heartburn do not have hiatal hernia.

More than 40% of us have a hiatal hernia, though few are aware of it. If you seem to be suffering from moderate to severe heartburn, make sure your doctor checks you for this type of hernia. In the worst cases, a surgeon can operate to reduce its size.

juices. The nicotine in cigarettes also relaxes the LES, making it even easier for acid to flow backward.

- **Shed extra pounds.** Studies have shown time and again that GERD accompanies girth. A potbelly often pushes upward against the stomach and forces acid into a weakened LES.
- **Take a walk after meals.** A leisurely stroll after dinner can encourage intestinal movement and reduce heartburn. The worst thing you can to do is lie down for a quick nap right after eating. All that food gets jammed up against the LES, making heartburn almost a certainty.
- **Loosen things up.** Tight underwear, pants, girdles, belts, and any other too-snug apparel increase abdominal pressure. Choose loose-fitting clothes and you'll feel more comfortable.
- **Stay regular.** When you're constipated, straining to have a bowel movement increases pressure in your abdomen. More pressure equals more stomach acid going up where it doesn't belong. To prevent constipation, be sure to exercise often, drink lots of water throughout the day, and eat plenty of dietary fiber. The simplest way to do that is to add ample fruits, vegetables, and whole grains to your diet.
- **Raise the head of your bed.** If heartburn keeps you awake at night, try raising the head of your bed with six- to eight-inch blocks. This keeps your stomach contents from pushing upward. Foam wedges you can sleep on do the same thing—look for them at better drugstores or in medical supply stores. Regardless of whether you raise the head of your bed, try to stay on your

left side as you slumber. Your stomach extends into the left side of your abdomen, so sleeping on this side keeps anything in your stomach and away from your LES.

Natural Methods*

People have been drinking milk to relieve heartburn for decades. Don't: This natural remedy doesn't work. In fact, milk stimulates acid production, making your heartburn worse. Instead, try the healing compound **deglycyrrhizinated licorice (DGL).** Take one or two lozenges after eating. Chew them slowly, so all the active compounds get put to work coating and repairing the stomach's mucous lining.

You might try a teaspoon of **baking soda** in a cup of warm water. This provides immediate relief if you don't have antacids close by. Be warned: You'll belch mightily, so be prepared. Sucking on **hard candies** produces extra saliva, washing acid away. Don't use peppermint. It can make heartburn worse.

Procedures

For the most severe cases of GERD, medication may not provide enough relief. Sometimes people just aren't able to make the necessary lifestyle changes. This is when you should probably talk to a surgeon. For about 5% of those with severe heartburn and GERD, surgery is the best option.

If chronic GERD has scarred your esophagus and narrowed the opening—you'll know, if you have difficulty swallowing food—your doctor may recommend **endoscopic dilation.** In this procedure, a balloonlike device is inserted into your esophagus and inflated, stretching the esophagus open. This outpatient procedure boasts a high rate of success.

Endoscopic suturing is an option for controlling heartburn. The surgeon places a couple of stitches near your weakened LES, helping knit it more tightly together. This procedure takes about an hour, and can be reversed if it doesn't work for you.

In the most complex surgery for GERD, called **Nissen fundoplication,** a surgeon wraps the upper part of your stomach around the LES and attaches it firmly in place. This creates a stronger valve and, for most people, eliminates GERD symptoms for at least 10 years. Fundoplication has traditionally required a large incision in the abdomen and a recovery period of four to six weeks.

Today, many surgeons are recommending **laparoscopic fundoplication.** This far less invasive procedure is performed through a few tiny incisions, using remotely guided instruments. With this approach, you're typically back to normal activities within a week. It's important to know, though, that the surgeon's skill makes all the difference. Be sure to pick a doctor who has performed laparoscopic fundoplication at least several dozen times a year for at least three years. Ask about the success rate, and if you don't like the answer, don't hesitate to find another surgeon.

*Natural methods are not subject to the same testing and regulation as prescription medications. Please seek your doctor's advice and use caution.

Heartburn or Heart Attack?

You get a sudden, severe attack of heartburn. You figure you'll brush it off with a couple of antacids. But before you do, remember that the pain of a heart attack can be almost indistinguishable from that of severe heartburn.

Call 911 if what you think is heartburn is accompanied by any of these symptoms, which can indicate a heart attack:

- Pain that radiates into your jaw or out your left arm.
- Tightness or pain in the center of your chest.
- Cold sweats, nausea, and vomiting.
- Dizziness and shortness of breath.
- Increased pain when you exert yourself.

FINDING Support

- Want to see how others deal with their heartburn pain? Contact the National Heartburn Alliance, a nonprofit organization in Chicago, IL, dedicated to sharing information about heartburn and its effects (1-877-471-2081 or www.heartburnalliance.org).

- You can also find good information at the websites of the American Gastroenterological Association (www. gastro.org/public.html) and the American College of Gastroenterology (www. acg.gi.org). Both sites have good doctor-locator tools to help you find a heartburn specialist in your area.

Hepatitis

While some types of hepatitis bring on a flu-like illness and disappear, others cause chronic liver disease that can lead to life-threatening complications. New therapies are proving effective for such stubborn infections, even offering a cure for some.

LIKELY First Steps

- If you have **acute hepatitis** (type A), ask your doctor if family members or close contacts should receive a gamma globulin shot.

- **Antiviral drugs** prescribed for chronic disease, including interferon-alpha (for hepatitis B), can also be combined with ribavirin (for hepatitis C).

- You may need a **liver biopsy** (a thin needle inserted to remove some tissue) to assess damage to that organ.

- Regular **follow-up visits** and **blood tests** to assess liver enzymes and the amount of virus in your body.

QUESTIONS TO Ask

- What type of hepatitis do I have—A, B, C, or another?

- If I've never had a transfusion, how did I get hepatitis?

- Am I contagious? Can I give this to my partner or kids? If I get pregnant, how can I protect the baby?

- Do you think my condition will get worse?

- How often will I need follow-up visits?

- What could happen if I decide not to have any treatment?

- Will I eventually need a liver transplant?

What is happening

Hepatitis means "inflammation of the liver," and is usually caused by an infection from one of the hepatitis viruses. These organisms zero in on your liver and multiply, inflaming the organ and causing potential damage. Other infections, medications, exposure to toxic chemicals, immune system disturbances, or years of alcohol abuse may also be responsible. Vital for cleansing your body of wastes and promoting digestion, your liver secretes a yellow fat-digesting substance called bile. If the liver becomes inflamed by hepatitis, bile backs up, giving your skin and eyes a yellowish tinge called jaundice. You may feel tired, feverish, nauseated, achy, or itchy, with nagging pain on the right side of your abdomen. That's where your liver is located.

Your disease may be short-lived (acute) or persistent (chronic). Acute hepatitis is usually caused by the type A hepatitis virus. It crops up in day-care centers and college dorms and in some exotic locales, where it spreads through tainted food or water. It can make you sick for several weeks, but usually goes away without causing complications. Chronic hepatitis, caused by hepatitis virus types B or C, may begin with a similar, acute flu-like illness, but lingers as the viruses slowly incubate in your liver. Hepatitis B and C are much harder to contract than type A. To acquire either, you need to have contact with infected blood such as through a bad transfusion, sexual contact, or sharing needles (possibly even those used for tattoos and body piercing).

More than 1 million Americans have chronic hepatitis B. More than 4 million have hepatitis C, and there are millions more sufferers throughout the world. Most people were infected years ago, before blood was carefully screened: You may have carried B or C around for decades without even knowing you were infected. Many chronic viral carriers never develop liver problems. Treatment is key to preventing severe and potentially fatal liver scarring (cirrhosis), cancer, or other lasting damage.

Treatments

Therapies for acute type A hepatitis are limited (*see box, page 169*). More and more people, however, are learning they have chronic hepatitis, especially type C, and effective virus-fighting drugs are available for treatment. Doctors generally recommend medications only if tests such as a liver biopsy show active disease that is damaging your liver. New drug combinations appear to be increasingly effec-

Treatment options

Medications

Antivirals	Interferon-alpha, ribavirin; ask about pegylated interferon-alpha shots.
Nucleoside analogue	Lamivudine to control hepatitis B.
Immunosuppressants	Indefinitely after liver transplant.

Procedures

Liver transplant	Viable option for advanced hepatitis C.

Natural methods

Herbs	Certain botanicals can strengthen the liver.

tive at warding off such conditions as cirrhosis and liver cancer, as well as other long-range complications.

Because the usual virus-fighting therapies can have unpleasant side effects, you may wonder if taking medicines is the right thing to do, particularly if you felt fine when you received your diagnosis. A number of patients drop out of therapy or refuse to begin it because of the troubling side effects. Whether this is wise is not yet known. On a positive note, newer drug combinations are less likely to cause unpleasant side effects, so if your doctor has suggested you start therapy (especially if your liver biopsy shows inflammation), you're better off going along with the drug program. Lifestyle choices can also contribute to—though not guarantee—a good outcome. A healthful diet, stress reduction, avoiding liver toxins such as alcohol, and getting plenty of rest all seem to be valuable for maintaining a healthy liver.

Medications

The mainstay of treatment for **hepatitis C** has long been a virus-fighting drug called **interferon-alpha.** The medication, a protein, is injected and fortifies your immune system to mount an attack against the virus. To boost effectiveness, interferon-alpha is often combined with a second antiviral called **ribavirin** (Rebetol), which may be mixed with it or given separately as a pill. Treatment may take six months to a year or longer.

A big problem with interferon-alpha is its unpleasant side effects: It can make you feel exhausted, forgetful, depressed, or like you have a bad case of the flu. Even worse, the form of interferon-alpha commonly used in the past successfully eradicated the virus in only 10% to 20% of people who endured the grueling regimen; about 40% when it was combined with ribavirin. Not surprisingly, the drug acquired a bad reputation. Many people opted to forego interferon-alpha treatments altogether.

A new, improved, and more easily tolerated form of this medication, **pegylated interferon-alpha** (PEG-Intron, Pegasys), is now available. The drug remains active in your bloodstream much longer,

TAKING Control

- **Refrain from alcohol,** which can tax your liver. If you have acute illness, give your liver a rest for at least a month after recovery. If you have chronic disease, avoid alcohol long term.

- **Don't smoke.** Researchers in Taiwan report that cigarettes can further damage your liver, especially if you drink.

- **Watch your drugs and medications.** They are processed through the liver and can tax an organ recovering from hepatitis. Even common pain relievers such as acetaminophen (Tylenol) can be potentially harmful. Check with your doctor about any drugs you're taking.

- **Get plenty of rest.** Set limits and adjust your schedule so you don't overdo it.

- **Relax.** Stress-relieving techniques like meditation, massage, or a hot bath can help you unwind.

Promising DEVELOPMENTS

- Drug "cocktails" in development may boost the effectiveness of existing drugs and enhance the likelihood of cure. One, called a **protease inhibitor,** blocks a protein hepatitis C viruses require to reproduce. That stops the virus dead in its tracks. Even more promising are **polymerase inhibitors,** such as adefovir dipivoxil, which prevent hepatitis B viruses from making copies of themselves. A third prospect, **ribozyme,** is an enzyme that acts like a microscopic pair of shears to snip the hepatitis B or C virus into inert pieces.

Considering the Gift of Love?

Most donor livers are obtained from cadavers, but more and more family members and friends are stepping up to donate part of their livers to loved ones in need. Half or more of a healthy organ may be removed, a feat made possible by the liver's amazing ability to regenerate rapidly. Several weeks after the operation, both donor and recipient can expect to have full-sized, fully functional livers. Some 1,000 of these living transplant operations have been performed in the last 10 years. The procedure is more complicated than related procedures (such as live kidney donations) and can take up to 18 hours. The vast majority of these operations are successful, one reason they are becoming increasingly commonplace.

▶ Should I be vaccinated against hepatitis?

There are safe and effective vaccines against hepatitis A and B, but they don't help if you're already sick. Hepatitis A vaccine is good for travelers to countries where the disease is common. Kids are routinely immunized for hepatitis B, and a combined A and B vaccine is available.

The chameleon-like hepatitis C has eight different virus forms. This has stymied attempts to develop a vaccine, although work on it is progressing. If you have hepatitis C, your doctor may vaccinate you against hepatitis A and B so you are not further jeopardized by those illnesses.

so you need only weekly shots; a welcome change from the older form's thrice-weekly regimen. About half of the people who take pegylated interferon-alpha are cured, and the success rate increases to about 60% with ribavirin. You may have more energy, less fatigue and pain, and fewer side effects with the newer drug, and making it easier to stick with the treatment. Fatigue that's a major problem may be due to anemia. A medication called erythropoietin alfa (Procrit) may help.

During your treatment, your doctor will likely perform regular blood tests to measure virus levels and liver enzymes in your blood, which indicate active inflammation. If you are responding well to therapy, your liver enzymes should begin to decrease within three months. You may also get a liver biopsy, in which a hollow needle is inserted through your ribs and into the liver to remove a small amount of liver tissue for analysis.

If the older form of interferon-alpha did not help you in the past, you might consider the newer form of the drug. About 20% of those who did not have success with the older drug are cured with the newer one. In some cases, a 6- to 12-month course of drug therapy appears to work, but the virus later rebounds in even higher numbers. In this situation, a second course of drug treatment may be called for. More than half of those who undergo a second course are cured. If you try interferon-alpha and the virus persists, the drug still helps protect your liver against inflammation. Some people with severely damaged livers stay on low doses of interferon-alpha permanently. It may slow progression of the disease and forestall the need for a liver transplant.

Interferon-alpha is also commonly prescribed for **hepatitis B.** People with this form of chronic hepatitis may also benefit from a **nucleoside analogue drug** called lamivudine (Epivir, 3TC, Zeffix). Originally designed to combat HIV (the AIDS virus), lamivudine has been found to prevent the hepatitis B virus from reproducing, though it rarely eliminates it entirely. It also suppresses liver inflammation and induces remissions in more than half of those who try it. The drug may cause digestive upset, headaches, or other side effects, but is generally well tolerated. It is taken as a pill once daily. Your doctor may suggest you use it for at least one to two years, maybe indefinitely.

Procedures

If your disease progresses despite the use of medications or other therapies and you develop severe liver scarring or cancer, you may be a candidate for a **liver transplant.** Recent advances in transplant surgery (*see box above*) have made liver transplants a viable option for many of those with advanced liver disease. Hepatitis C is now the primary reason for living transplants in the U.S. One-fourth of those with the disease may eventually need a transplant.

The transplant operation is intensive, requiring up to 12 hours to complete. It costs, on average, $250,000, which is often covered by insurance. The diseased liver is removed through an incision in the abdomen. The new organ is implanted the same way. Because of a shortage of donor livers, it is not uncommon to wait for several

The ABCs of Hepatitis

There are a number of different forms of hepatitis, each with its own viral plan.

Hepatitis A
The most common type, hepatitis A, may make you very sick for several weeks, but it doesn't often do lasting damage. There are no specific drugs or treatments, other than limiting your activities, eating small meals to keep up your strength, and abstaining from alcohol and all sexual contact while you're ill. Your doctor will review any medicines or supplements you are taking, because some may compromise your liver. Anyone in close contact with you will need a protective shot of an immune-boosting substance called immune globulin within 14 days to avoid catching what you have.

Hepatitis B
Spread through blood and sexual contact, hepatitis B may lead to a chronic, simmering liver infection. Long-term treatment with antiviral drugs can help halt progression of the disease.

Hepatitis C
Now the leading cause of chronic hepatitis in the United States, hepatitis C is considered a "stealth infection" because most people don't even know they have it. Many became infected by transfusions before 1990, before sophisticated blood screening techniques were widely used. Effective treatment is at hand.

Hepatitis D
Also called delta virus and found in the blood, hepatitis D piggybacks on the hepatitis B virus, causing a "super infection" that may progress rapidly. Antiviral interferon treatments may help.

Hepatitis E
Rare in the United States (but common in developing countries) and spread through tainted water, hepatitis E may cause an acute, flu-like illness. It does not usually cause lasting damage but may be especially dangerous if you are pregnant.

Hepatitis G
Discovered in 1995, hepatitis G is found in up to 2% of the population, but does not appear to cause liver disease.

---

months for a compatible organ. Doctors seek to match the new organ as closely as possible with your genetic makeup so that you will be less likely to reject it. Recovery from the operation takes about three months.

More than half of those who receive a donor liver are alive and well two years later. You will need to take **immune-suppressing drugs** such as cyclosporine indefinitely. Unfortunately, sometimes the hepatitis returns. Your doctor may suggest you take hepatitis medications such as interferon-alpha over the long term.

Natural Methods*

Certain herbs can help strengthen your liver's fight against hepatitis:
- **Milk thistle.** This herb, which contains a powerful antioxidant and liver protector called silymarin, also promotes the regeneration of new liver cells and improves liver function.
- **Dandelion root.** When taken as part of a liver-strengthening product called a lipotropic combination (which also includes milk thistle and the B vitamins choline and inositol hexaniacinate), this herb may help the liver rid itself of bile and toxins.
- **Chinese herbs.** In small European studies, a combination of the herbs schizandra, artemisia, and patrinia were shown to reduce levels of the hepatitis C virus. Further study is warranted.

Natural methods are not subject to the same testing and regulation as prescription medications. Please seek your doctor's advice and use caution.

FINDING Support

- Reliable information on hepatitis can be obtained from a number of government agencies, including the Centers for Disease Control and Prevention (1-888-4HE-PCDC or www.cdc.gov) and the National Institute of Diabetes & Digestive & Kidney Diseases (301-654-4415 or www.niddk.nih.gov).

- Interested in joining a support group for others living with hepatitis? The American Liver Foundation may be able to help. You can contact them at 1-800-GO-LIVER, check out their website, www.liverfoundation.org.

- The Hepatitis Foundation International offers physician referrals and phone support for hepatitis (1-800-891-0707 or www.hepfi.org).

High blood pressure

Some 50 million Americans have high blood pressure, but only about 30% of them know it. This is unfortunate, because this virtually symptomless—but potentially dangerous—condition is easy to treat with the right lifestyle choices and drugs.

LIKELY **First Steps**

- **Lifestyle changes** (low-sodium diet, stress reduction, weight loss, regular exercise) to lower your blood pressure naturally.

- If lifestyle measures fail, **medications**—or combinations of different drugs—to lower your blood pressure medically.

- For more complicated cases, **eliminating the cause**—whether it's a drug, illness, or other underlying problem.

QUESTIONS TO **Ask**

- Will the drug you just prescribed change the effectiveness of my other medications? Could it affect my sex life?

- Is it safe for me to exercise? My blood pressure levels went way up when I took a stress test.

- At what point do I need to see a heart specialist?

- How likely is it that I will be able to stop taking hypertension medication? What would I have to do?

What is happening

A doctor can explain why most diseases occur. Not so with high blood pressure, which is often a complex result of who you are (genetics), what you eat, and how you live. There are three main ways your body raises its blood pressure: 1. Your heart can change the rate and strength of its beats, forcing blood to move more vigorously through your system. 2. Your small arteries (arterioles) can constrict for various reasons—plaque on your vessels, for instance, or emotional stress—so higher pressure is needed to circulate your blood. 3. Your kidneys can retain more water in your body, creating more blood volume to pound through your vessels. The kidneys do this by releasing hormones that increase your body's supply of sodium (and a salty diet provides a ready source).

When blood pressure is routinely high, doctors diagnose it as hypertension. Most people with high blood pressure have primary (once called essential) hypertension. Even though its cause is unknown, it accounts for about 90% of cases. In only a few people (about 10%) can high blood pressure be linked to something specific, such as kidney disease or long-term use of certain drugs (NSAIDs, corticosteroids, oral contraceptives). This is secondary hypertension, and eliminating the underlying problem that causes it may be the only treatment you'll need.

Blood pressure fluctuates throughout the day, reflecting what you're doing. It drops during sleep, for instance, and spikes during exercise or in times of stress or pain. Most people know their "normal" blood pressure is supposed to be 120/80. The systolic number on the top (120) indicates the highest pressure exerted on your artery walls as the heart contracts to pump the blood out. The diastolic on the bottom (80) reflects the moment of lowest pressure, when it relaxes between contractions.

Over time, high blood pressure can inflict lasting damage. Your overworked heart muscle may become flabby and inefficient, causing heart failure. Vessels that supply blood to your eyes, brain, and various organs may become so stretched or strained that they leak or burst, causing stroke or internal bleeding.

Treatments

There are now many options for lowering your blood pressure, especially given recent drug advances. Treatment usually depends on how severe your condition is (*see table, page 172*). If your num-

Treatment options

Lifestyle changes

Diet	Follow DASH diet; reduce salt; get omega-3s.
Lower stress	Relax with yoga and/or tai chi.
Weight loss & exercise	Take off pounds and get moving.

Medications

Diuretics	Help body to excrete water and salt.
Beta-blockers	Ease heart's pumping action; widen vessels.
ACE inhibitors	Reduce an artery-constricting chemical.
Angiotensin II receptor blockers	Alternative to ACE inhibitors.
Calcium channel blockers	Decrease heart contractions; widen vessels.
Vasodilators	Expand blood vessels; improve circulation.
Alpha-blockers or central alpha-agonists	Interfere with nerve impulses that cause arteries to constrict.

(see page 354)

bers are only slightly elevated (130 to 139 mm Hg over 85 to 89 mm Hg), you may be able to avoid drugs altogether by making some sensible lifestyle changes. These might include altering how much you eat, exercise, and weigh, as well as how much alcohol you drink and how you deal with stress. As you work on lowering your blood pressure, check your levels often to be sure you're on course. Daily readings on a home monitor (*see page 354*) are good for more serious cases; biweekly checks on a do-it-yourself machine at a local pharmacy are fine for milder ones.

As a rule, many experts say if blood pressure in the range of 140 to 159 mm Hg systolic or 90 to 99 mm Hg diastolic hasn't responded to lifestyle changes after six months to a year, you'll need to start taking medication. A single drug is often very effective, although a second drug may be needed. If you're able to control your blood pressure very well for a few years, weaving lifestyle changes into your daily routine, your doctor might give you the green light to lower your dose or even stop taking the drugs.

Lifestyle Changes

The most powerful thing you can do to naturally lower mild hypertension is to **follow the DASH diet** (*see page 174*) and **slash your dietary sodium.** There's a 50% chance that you have the type of hypertension that is salt-sensitive. If that's the case, the more sodium you take in (through table salt and foods high in sodium), the higher your blood pressure will be. Anyone with hypertension can probably benefit from keeping sodium intake below 2,400 mg daily. **Eat lots of foods high in potassium.** A large part of the

TAKING Control

- **Choose nutrients with blood vessels in mind.** Omega-3 fatty acids found naturally in oily fish such as salmon will benefit hypertension by keeping your blood vessels flexible. Eat fish three times a week.

- **Stay alert for symptoms.** Although hypertension has a reputation as a mysterious "silent" condition, some people develop recognizable symptoms. If you have headaches and vision problems, see your doctor.

- **Watch for seasonal changes.** The weather affects blood pressure in some people. If you notice a significant increase during cold winter months, talk with your doctor about altering your treatment to compensate.

- **Keep an eye on your top number.** For years, doctors focused on the lower number—the diastolic. Now research indicates the top number—the systolic—is even more strongly linked to heart-related illness and death. If your top number begins to rise, ask your doctor what can be done.

- **Don't drink too much grapefruit juice** if you're taking a calcium channel blocker. It can boost the effects of this hypertension drug by inhibiting a small intestine enzyme that helps metabolize a number of medications. Not everyone has this problem and it doesn't happen with all grapefruit juice. It's most likely to occur when the medication is taken with the juice. Whole grapefruit may not have the same effect as the juice.

Promising
DEVELOPMENTS

■ **Sleep apnea** is the latest ailment to be fingered as a cause of hypertension. This is because some 6 million Americans with the sleep disorder have also been found to have high blood pressure. During sleep apnea, breathing stops or becomes very shallow, the throat muscles contract, there is a snort or gasp for air, and breathing starts again. This can happen dozens or even hundreds of times a night. The more severe one's apnea, the more likely a person is to develop hypertension. Sleep apnea can be treated (*see page 291*).

DASH diet success is thought to be its inclusion of many high-potassium foods (such as bananas). Potassium helps to lower blood pressure by relaxing the arteries.

In addition to diet, you need to get a handle on **reducing your stress.** Even mild tension or anger can raise blood pressure by triggering the release of hormones that constrict blood vessels. Stress sometimes accompanies depression and anxiety, conditions that can more than double your risk for hypertension. The best ways to de-stress are different for everyone: Find what works for you and stick with it. Studies have found that yoga or tai chi lower blood pressure almost as much as moderate-intensity exercise.

Whether you do tai chi or ride a bike, getting **regular exercise** is an essential part of any blood pressure reduction program. Vigorous exercise increases the feel-good hormones known as endorphins and lowers stress, anxiety, and depression. Getting your blood flowing helps keep your vessels flexible and less prone to narrowing, important in keeping blood pressure down. Exercise for at least 30 minutes, no fewer than three times a week. If you're concerned that exercise will raise your blood pressure more than a safe 20%, check it periodically with a monitor. Opt for aerobic exercises that

EVALUATING YOUR BLOOD PRESSURE

The blood pressure classifications below were developed by the Joint National Committee on Prevention, Detection, Evaluation, and Treatment of High Blood Pressure; they apply to adult men and women who aren't currently taking antihypertensive medications and who aren't acutely ill. To determine the category you fall into, use the more elevated number in the reading: For example, if you have 140 mm Hg systolic and 100 mm Hg diastolic you would be in the Stage 2 category.

Category	Systolic	Diastolic	Recommended Follow-up
Optimal	<120 mm Hg	≤80 mm Hg	Recheck in 2 years.
Normal	<120 mm Hg	<80 mm Hg	Recheck in 2 years.
High-normal	120–139 mm Hg	80–89 mm Hg	Recheck in 1 year.†
Hypertension			
Stage 1	140–159 mm Hg	90–99 mm Hg	Confirm within 2 months.†
Stage 2	≥160 mm Hg	≥100 mm Hg	Undergo complete medical evaluation and/or begin treatment within 1 month.
Isolated systolic hypertension	≥140 mm Hg	<90 mm Hg	Confirm within 2 months.†

† Applies only to initial blood pressure readings. Multiple readings at these levels may require more aggressive management.

About Low Blood Pressure

The lower the better when it comes to blood pressure, but only as long as you feel good. If your pressure drops too low—a condition called hypotension—your health can be compromised. Hypotension can result from overly aggressive treatment of high blood pressure or other factors. The most common form is postural hypotension, which occurs after you abruptly stand or sit up. Dizziness and fainting are common symptoms, the result of inadequate blood flow to the brain.

Treatment: If your doctor diagnoses postural hypotension, diet and lifestyle changes will probably be in order. Medications will be a last resort. Try to:

- Eat salty foods, especially in hot weather or when you're ill.
- Drink at least eight glasses of nonalcoholic beverages daily (sports drinks high in sodium and potassium are a good bet).
- Stretch your feet back and forth to stimulate circulation before rising from a prone or sitting position.
- Raise the head of your bed 5 to 20° (bricks are helpful).

get large muscles moving—brisk walking, swimming, bicycling—over strength training (weight lifting), which can temporarily but dramatically increase blood pressure.

Coupled with a reasonable diet, aerobic exercise will help you **lose extra pounds.** Being just slightly overweight doubles the risk that you'll have high blood pressure. (See page 355 to figure your Body Mass Index, an indicator of how you're faring weightwise.) Be aware that processed diet shakes and snacks often load up on salt to compensate for reduced fat and sugar.

Other smart moves include **getting plenty of sleep** (insufficient sleep can raise blood pressure) and **limiting alcohol and caffeine.** More than one or two alcoholic drinks or five cups of coffee a day can raise blood pressure, too.

If you have high blood pressure and diabetes, you may need to take more aggressive control of your hypertension. New guidelines suggest that blood pressure in such cases should be lower than 130/80.

Medications

You can't ever go wrong with good lifestyle choices, but sometimes medications (known as antihypertensives) are your best option. When you find the right drug—and take it regularly—you'll likely see your blood pressure return to normal, no matter how high it once was.

Drug side effects are a consideration, of course. They make some people feel worse than the hypertension itself, though if you're lucky, you won't notice any side effects at all. Everyone reacts differently, so be prepared for some trial and error. Eventually you'll

▶**Should I buy a home blood pressure monitor?**

It's an excellent idea for anyone with hypertension to check blood pressure at home using a monitor (see box, page 354). Results taken over several weeks will provide a much more accurate assessment of your real numbers than measurements taken in the doctor's office alone. (Lots of factors influence blood pressure, from time of day to diet and stress levels.) Keep a record, so you and your doctor can discuss whether your treatment plan is working.

To get an accurate reading: No caffeine, cigarettes, or alcohol for 30 minutes beforehand. Relax at least 3 to 5 minutes before starting your reading. Sit with your legs and ankles uncrossed. Wait 2 to 3 minutes before taking a new reading.

▶**Why does my blood pressure go up when I am in the mountains?**

Even a modest rise in altitude will slightly increase blood pressure—even if you don't have hypertension. This is a result of your body's natural attempt to deal with the lower amounts of oxygen available at higher elevations. During this process, complex changes occur throughout your body. You hyperventilate to get more oxygen, and your kidneys pump out hormones that constrict your blood vessels. Your blood pressure will probably acclimate naturally within 24 to 48 hours. If you're on medication and going above 6,000 feet, ask your doctor whether or not you need to alter your normal dosage.

Control Blood Pressure with the DASH Diet

Among the most compelling evidence for diet as a means of controlling blood pressure are two trials sponsored by the National Institutes of Health. These studies are known as the DASH diet.

Original DASH trial

The first study, done in 1997, was called "DASH," for Dietary Approaches to Stop Hypertension. It found that blood pressure levels could fall significantly with an eating plan low in total fat, saturated fat, and cholesterol and rich in fruits, vegetables, and low-fat dairy products. The diet was shown to prevent hypertension and, in some cases, reduce blood pressure as much as an antihypertensive drug. Results were seen within two weeks, and benefits remained eight weeks later, regardless of gender, ethnicity, or starting blood pressure.

DASH diet basics

The DASH diet calls for eating 8 to 10 servings of fruits and vegetables and 2 to 3 cups of low-fat dairy foods daily, more than most people are accustomed to. Here are the broad DASH guidelines you can follow in menu planning:

- Grains and grain products: 7 to 8 servings daily
- Fruits and vegetables: 4 to 5 servings of each daily
- Low-fat or nonfat dairy foods: 2 to 3 servings daily
- Meats, poultry, and fish: 2 or fewer 3-ounce servings daily
- Nuts, seeds, or legumes: 4 to 5 servings per week
- Fats: 2 to 3 servings daily; avoid saturated fat
- Sweets: 5 per week

DASH-sodium trial

A follow-up trial, held in 2000, examined whether reducing salt could enhance results. The sodium in table salt and other foods raises blood pressure by causing the body to retain water, increasing blood volume and blood pressure. Sodium also causes small blood vessels to constrict. This study showed that the DASH diet, combined with salt reduction, was superior to either strategy alone. All participants benefited from limiting their salt intake.

For details and recipes

For more information, contact the National Heart, Lung & Blood Institute's information line (1-800-575-WELL) or visit their website (www.nhlbi. nih.gov/health/public/heart/ hbp/dash).

▶**OVERINDULGING IN REAL LICORICE CANDY can raise your blood pressure by affecting your adrenal glands. "True" licorice is the culprit here. It's the costly type extracted from licorice plants and often found in European confections. If you have hypertension and must indulge in licorice, buy American-made licorice. It is typically flavored artificially or with natural oils, such as anise. The red variety contains no true licorice at all.**

zero in on the drug that's best for you and that has the fewest side effects. If side effects still are a problem, be sure to talk with your doctor. You might be surprised at all how many options you have if a beta-blocker is making you feel blue, or an ACE inhibitor is changing your sense of taste.

You probably won't need more than one or two antihypertensive drugs. Only a few people (typically those with diabetes or high systolic pressure) use three or more medications. A good doctor will be aware of how certain antihypertensives might harm—or even simultaneously benefit—any other ailments you may have. Until you find the right medication, be prepared to see your doctor every four to six weeks to discuss side effects and check your blood pressure levels.

If you need to start on an antihypertensive medication and are otherwise healthy, you'll probably be given a diuretic to eliminate excess fluid and sodium, or a beta-blocker, which eases the heart's workload by tempering the force and frequency of your regular heartbeats. Many studies have shown both of these drug groups to be safe and effective.

Diuretics prompt the kidneys to excrete excess salt and water. This reduces the volume of blood in your body and, therefore, the amount of fluid that needs to be forced through potentially narrowed arteries. Although they affect different sites in the kidneys, the three types of diuretics produce essentially the same reaction. Such drugs include thiazides (Diuril, Hygroton, Esidrix), loop diuretics (Bumex, Lasix, Edecrin), and potassium-sparing diuretics (Midamor, Aldactone, Dyrenium). Diuretics are particularly effective if you have fairly straightforward hypertension and are older or African-American.

The other top drug choice is **beta-blockers** (Inderal, Tenormin, or Corgard). When combined with other antihypertensives, beta-blockers are known for reducing heart-disease related deaths. In fact, these drugs are a good choice if you've already had a heart attack, are suffering from angina (chest pain), or have heart rhythm disturbances, tremors, hyperthyroidism, or migraine. They work because they mute the effects of adrenaline and slow your heart down, so it doesn't have to work so hard. Your doctor is unlikely to select a beta-blocker if you're prone to asthma (the drug can narrow bronchial airways), depression or have diabetes.

Over the past few years, research has homed in on another class of useful drugs, **angiotensin-converting enzyme (ACE) inhibitors** (such as Capoten, Vasotec, Prinivil). They lower blood pressure while they help control congestive heart failure and prevent stroke and heart attack in high-risk individuals. Because they reduce the risks and complications of diabetes, ACE inhibitors are an especially wise choice if you have that disease. This medication works by reducing the formation of angiotensin, a substance known to constrict blood vessels. Somewhat costly, ACE inhibitors are commonly taken along with certain other antihypertensives.

About 25% of those who take ACE inhibitors develop an annoying cough. If this side effect becomes overwhelming, a good alternative is **angiotensin II receptor blockers** (Cozaar, Avapro), which work in much the same way. They are associated with a high risk of birth defects, so tell your doctor if you're pregnant or trying to conceive.

Another option is **calcium channel blockers** (calcium antagonists), which include Norvasc, extended-release Cardizem CD, Dilacor-XR, Tiazac, and Procardia XL. They work by widening arteries and lightening the heart's workload. They're quick to reduce blood pressure and can ease angina (chest pain). You may find you like calcium channel blockers because they're so easy to take: just once a day. They're also pricey and not as effective as other drugs in preventing stroke and heart or kidney problems.

As a first drug, your doctor probably won't prescribe **vasodilators,** which lower blood pressure by widening blood vessels, or **alpha-blockers** or **central alpha-agonists,** which block nerve impulses that constrict small arteries. These medications are typically reserved for times when other antihypertensives have failed, or when a second drug is needed to round out a treatment regimen.

▶**HAVING TROUBLE COMMITTING to your drug regimen?** You're not alone: Millions of Americans stop taking antihypertensives because they view them as a nuisance. Compliance is crucial to your health, however. Here are a few tips to keep you faithful: Get a weekly drug-dosing box to help you keep track. An alarm clock can remind you when to take the drug. Strategize with your doctor to find a plan that works for your life. There may be a drug that doesn't cause side effects or that has to be taken just once daily.

FINDING Support

■ Feel like you have a multitude of unanswered questions after seeing your doctor? Log on to the NIH's National Heart, Lung and Blood Institute's website (www.nhlbi. nih.gov). Or try the National Library of Medicine's information site, which contains lots of links, from the latest research findings on high blood pressure to enrolling in a clinical trial (www.nlm. nih.gov/medlineplus/ highbloodpressure.html).

■ Want to chat with others about your high blood pressure? Contact the Dallas-based organization called Mended Hearts (1-888-HEART99 or www.mended hearts.org).

High cholesterol

Even if you're lean and healthy, high cholesterol could put you at risk for heart disease and stroke. Don't worry: There's plenty you can do to improve your outlook by lowering your cholesterol levels—safely and effectively.

LIKELY First Steps

- **Lifestyle changes,** with an emphasis on reducing the amounts of saturated fat and animal protein in your diet.

- **Medications**—most likely one of the statin drugs— if lifestyle measures are inadequate.

- **Natural remedies** can be effective for mildly elevated cholesterol levels.

QUESTIONS TO Ask

- Why didn't my strict diet plan make much of a dent in my cholesterol levels?

- Are there any tests to determine if my high cholesterol has damaged my health so far?

- Should I tell my children to get checked for high cholesterol?

- Could medicines I'm taking or other medical conditions I have be raising my cholesterol levels?

What is happening

The popular media portray cholesterol as a deadly villain, but you need a certain amount of it in your bloodstream to stay alive and well. This waxy, fatty compound is one of a group of lipids (blood-borne fats) essential to the manufacture of hormones, nerve fibers, and cell membranes. Only when you have too much of it does cholesterol become a problem. Your liver typically makes all the cholesterol you need. When you eat foods high in cholesterol or saturated fats, the liver responds by churning out even more. Over time, the excess is likely to build up in your arteries and harden into what's called atherosclerotic plaque. Untreated, this condition (atherosclerosis) can lead to angina, heart attack, or stroke.

Ideally, your total cholesterol level should be below 200 mg/dL (milligrams per deciliter). Two major subtypes of cholesterol must also be considered: low density lipoprotein (LDL), the so-called "bad" cholesterol, and high density lipoprotein (HDL), or "good" cholesterol. (Lipoproteins are tiny globules of fat and protein that help transport fats to cells throughout your body.) Each type of lipoprotein has a different impact on your health. The higher your LDL, for instance, the greater your risk of heart disease. On the other hand, high levels of HDL actually reduce your cardiovascular risk, because HDL carries cholesterol back to the liver, where it is metabolized and eventually excreted. (See the table on page 178 for a breakdown of cholesterol levels and what the numbers mean.) Doctors also pay attention to other blood lipids, especially triglycerides (*see box, page 179*).

Your risk for high cholesterol increases with age—and in men more than women (estrogen helps until menopause). Other risk factors include diabetes, an underactive thyroid, or a family history. Even though high cholesterol has no real symptoms, it is a major cause of coronary heart disease, the number-one killer of American adults (*see page 94*). On the bright side, if a blood test reveals high cholesterol, there are effective ways to get it under control.

Treatments

The first step is to try to lower cholesterol with lifestyle measures. Dietary changes, along with regular exercise, can often bring cholesterol levels down to an acceptable range. If these don't do the trick—which is common for people genetically predisposed to high cholesterol—your doctor can prescribe safe and effective medications. There are natural remedies you can try as well.

Treatment options

Lifestyle changes

Pay attention to diet	Avoid foods high in cholesterol, saturated fat.
Exercise & weight loss	Both protect against heart disease.
Enjoy a drink	Moderate alcohol use boosts HDL.

Medications

Statins	Highly effective, first-line treatment.
Nicotinic acid	Niacin, to lower LDL and raise HDL.
Bile-acid sequestrants	Work in GI tract to lower LDL.
Fibric acid derivatives	For high triglycerides, but will help LDL.

Natural methods

Relaxation techniques	De-stressing reduces blood lipid levels.
Herbs	Plant sterols, gugulipid, policosanol.
Vitamins	Inositol hexaniacinate (nonflushing niacin).

Lifestyle Changes

A few simple steps can cut cholesterol levels by 20% to 30%, or even more. First, **dietary changes.** Eat fewer high-fat, animal-derived foods, like red meat and whole-milk dairy products, which are high in cholesterol. Avoid processed foods that contain highly saturated vegetable oils (coconut oil, palm, and palm kernel oil). Even though these oils come from plant sources and don't contain cholesterol, they stimulate your liver to manufacture it. Always be wary of foods that flaunt "low cholesterol" or "no cholesterol" on their labels. They can still have saturated fat.

Trans fatty acids—also known as TFAs or trans fats—are bad news too. Found mainly in margarines and commercial baked goods, TFAs occur when hydrogen is added to make any liquid vegetable oil solid or semisolid. Like saturated fats, trans fats increase LDL and reduce HDL. Shun products with the phrase "contains partially hydrogenated vegetable oil." Use olive and canola oils instead. They're good sources of monounsaturated fat, which is considerably healthier than saturated fat. You should also follow the so-called Mediterranean Diet. Seek out foods that are low fat and high in fiber (fruits, vegetables, whole grains); get your protein from fish, legumes, and soy. Harvard scientists suggest that high-risk patients can benefit from the diet, but cardiologists disagree about whether or not it lowers the risk of fatal heart attack.

In addition to dietary changes, you should **lose extra pounds** if you are more than 20% overweight. Be sure to **exercise regularly:** Burning at least 250 calories a day (the equivalent of 45 minutes of brisk walking or 25 minutes of jogging) can raise your HDL and significantly protect you against heart disease. For best results, combine aerobic activity with resistance training and strength training. You

TAKING Control

- **Eat more omega-3s.** These fatty acids (found in olive and fish oils) are healthier than the more prevalent omega-6s (in corn, soybean, and cottonseed oils). To get a better balance, choose a salad dressing with olive oil. Cook with it, too. Look for mayonnaise made from canola oil.

- **Ask about low-dose aspirin therapy.** A daily low-dose aspirin may be a smart and inexpensive way to reduce your chance of heart attack. Don't initiate such a regimen without talking with your doctor.

Promising DEVELOPMENTS

- The biotechnology firm Avant Immunotherapeutics is working on a **cholesterol vaccine.** Administered twice a year, the vaccine has been shown in preliminary studies to increase HDL cholesterol by as much as 40% to 50%, while lowering LDL more than 20%. Further clinical trials are necessary, but the vaccine appears safe and may one day provide a useful alternative for those who don't respond well to statin drugs.

▶Is it really okay for me to eat an egg every day?
Some confusion has arisen from the American Heart Association's recent proclamation that eating an egg a day poses no great risk to people concerned about keeping their cholesterol levels down. The guideline still stands—with the important caveat that you need to consider everything else you eat that day. A single egg contains about 213 mg of dietary cholesterol; current guidelines suggest consuming no more than about 200 mg of cholesterol a day. If you have an egg, steer clear of meat, poultry, high-fat dairy products, and other sources of dietary cholesterol that day.

▶**ANGER MAY AFFECT YOUR CHOLESTEROL LEVELS,** according to a University of Maryland study of 103 healthy middle-aged women. Those prone to frequent angry outbursts had significantly poorer cholesterol profiles than their more even-tempered counterparts. Researchers speculate that poor anger control may be linked to the release of excess adrenaline and other hormones, which have been shown to affect blood lipid levels. On the positive side, the health risks associated with an angry temperament were offset in those women who exercised regularly and were otherwise physically fit.

might also consider **having a drink** every day (a glass of wine, a beer, or a cocktail). A number of studies have shown that moderate alcohol consumption may boost HDL. Men should have no more than two drinks a day. Women, no more than one. Exceeding that amount can increase your health risks. If you smoke, definitely **quit.**

Medications

A few months after making these lifestyle changes, have another blood test to see how you're doing. If your cholesterol is still too high, your doctor will probably prescribe medications to lower it.

The **statin drugs** are the safest, most effective, and most widely used cholesterol-lowering medications available. Formally known as HMG-CoA reductase inhibitors, statins interfere with the liver's ability to synthesize cholesterol. Popular statins include lovastatin (Mevacor), pravastatin (Pravachol), simvastatin (Zocor), fluvastatin (Lescol), and atorvastatin (Lipitor). Regular and careful monitoring by your doctor is essential. Although these drugs have a very low incidence of side effects, they can cause liver damage or serious muscle pain and weakness. Some evidence suggests that statins may help reduce your risk of osteoporosis and Alzheimer's disease.

Not everyone responds well to statin drugs. If you don't, your doctor may prescribe **nicotinic acid** (niacin), which lowers LDL and raises HDL. Extended-release forms of niacin (Niacor, Nicolar, Slo-Niacin, Niaspan) reduce the risk of bothersome side effects such as flushing and burning sensations in the skin. Combinations of nicotinic acid and lovastatin (Nicostatin, Advicor) are now available. Because you're getting smaller amounts of each component, the chances of side effects are considerably reduced.

Another possibility is the class of drugs known as **bile-acid sequestrants.** These drugs—including cholestyramine (Questran), colestipol (Colestid), and colesevelam (Cholestagel, Welchol)—bind

ASSESSING YOUR CHOLESTEROL NUMBERS

Total cholesterol	
Desirable	Less than 200 mg/dL
Borderline-high	200–239 mg/dL
High	240 mg/dL or higher
LDL cholesterol	
Optimal	Less than 100 mg/dL
Near or above optimal	100–129 mg/dL
Borderline-high	130–159 mg/dL
High	160–189 mg/dL
Very high	More than 190 mg/dL
HDL cholesterol	
High (protective)	More than 60 mg/dL
Normal	40–59 mg/dL
Low (CHD risk factor)	Less than 40 mg/dL

About Triglycerides

Cholesterol is only a part of the lipid story. Produced by the liver, triglycerides (also a lipid) are the most abundant fat in food (90% of dietary fat), and the body's main source of stored energy. They're measured in a blood test after a 12-hour fast.

According to new federal guidelines, a triglyceride reading of less than 150 mg/dL is considered normal (although some experts say it should be even lower). A reading of 150 to 199 mg/dL is considered borderline-high; 200 to 499 is high; 500 or more, very high. Triglycerides fluctuate quite a bit. Repeated testing may be needed to get an accurate picture. High levels are common in people with diabetes and are associated with obesity, a high-fat diet, excessive alcohol or carbohydrate consumption, hypothyroidism, kidney disorders, and use of certain medications.

If your triglycerides are high, the lifestyle measures recommended for high cholesterol apply. Medications usually start with a statin drug; a second drug may be added—possibly niacin or one of the fibrates, gemfibrozil (Lopid) or fenofibrate (Tricor). Although combination drug therapy helps successfully control both LDL and triglycerides, side effects—particularly severe muscle inflammation—can be troublesome.

with bile acids in your intestine, then are excreted in your stool. Because the liver manufactures bile acids from LDL cholesterol, these drugs stimulate it to make more, lowering your cholesterol in the process. **Fibric acid derivatives,** such as gemfibrozil (Lopid), fenofibrate (Tricor), and clofibrate (Atromid-S), are typically prescribed for people with unacceptably high triglyceride levels. These drugs may modestly reduce LDL and total cholesterol levels, but are generally not used alone to lower cholesterol.

Natural Methods*

Studies show stress can boost lipid levels. Therefore, find an activity or technique to help you **relax** and manage your stress better.

Several nutritional supplements may have cholesterol-lowering effects, but evidence on their efficacy varies. Among the most effective are **plant sterols** and **stanols** and the Indian herb **gugulipid,** which block absorption of cholesterol in the intestine. Another supplement, **inositol hexaniacinate,** is a safe form of niacin less likely to cause skin flushing and liver problems. **Policosanol,** a derivative of sugar cane wax, reduces the liver's ability to churn out cholesterol. Not very effective, studies show, are garlic and lecithin supplements, and antioxidants like vitamins C and E. They don't naturally reduce heart disease risk as has been theorized, but may actually interfere with statin drugs.

Natural methods are not subject to the same testing and regulation as prescription medications. Please seek your doctor's advice and use caution.

▶**HEART PATIENTS WHO STOPPED TAKING STATIN DRUGS** after being hospitalized for chest pain were more than three times more likely to suffer a heart attack or die than those who kept taking drugs, according to a study published in the journal *Circulation*.

▶**NATURAL SUBSTANCES CALLED** plant stanols and sterols, now incorporated into margarines (Benecol, Take Control) and other food products, have been shown to reduce total cholesterol by some 10% to 15%, if used regularly.

FINDING Support

■ The parent of the National Cholesterol Education Program (NCEP), the National Heart, Lung, and Blood Institute (1-800-575-WELL or www.nhlbi.nih.gov) offers health information, scientific resources, and information for patients interested in participating in clinical trials.

■ Contact the American Heart Association (1-800-242-8721 or www.americanheart.org) or the American College of Cardiology (1-800-253-4636 or www.acc.org) for more information about cholesterol and heart disease.

■ For daily nutrition tips and a guide to finding a registered dietitian in your local area, contact the American Dietetic Association (1-800-877-1600 or www.eatright.org).

Infertility

More than 6 million American couples struggle with infertility. Although you can't do much to turn back the biological clock, technological innovations are making it possible for many more people to ultimately bring a child into the world.

LIKELY First Steps

- Lifestyle measures, such as **tracking ovulation cycles** and **keeping your weight** within normal ranges.

- **Treatment of underlying medical causes** of infertility, such as fibroids, endometriosis, and menstrual problems.

- **Drugs** to boost ovulation.

- In more complicated cases, **artificial insemination** or **assisted reproductive technologies** with or without super-ovulation drugs.

QUESTIONS TO Ask

- What is the success rate of your fertility clinic? How does it compare with others?

- Are any of these hormones dangerous for me?

- I keep miscarrying. What are my options?

- How much will this therapy cost? Is any of the cost covered by medical insurance?

What is happening

Getting pregnant and carrying a baby to term may seem like the most natural thing in the world—until the requisite healthy machinery, exquisite timing, and luck aren't on your side. Consider what's involved. Well-shaped, active sperm must enter the uterus and swim up into the fallopian tube(s) at a time when one of the ovaries releases an egg. A single sperm has to wiggle its way into the egg, fertilizing it. The newly formed embryo must wend its way down to the uterus and snuggle firmly into the uterine wall.

If this scenario doesn't play itself out after 12 or more months of regular, unprotected sex, infertility is diagnosed. Having repeated miscarriages is also a form of infertility. The situation can leave you angry and heartbroken. In one in five cases no cause can be found, even after a full medical workup. Sometimes a problem with the male partner can be spotted and treated (*see box, page 182*). Often—in a third of cases—there's an issue with both partners. For women, age is always a factor. You're born with a finite number of eggs that start to run out in a fairly predictable way after age 30.

In most cases of infertility, doctors eventually identify and treat the problem. Nearly 30% of women with infertility, for instance, have blocked fallopian tubes, preventing the egg from traveling into the uterus. Pelvic inflammatory disease, a prior pregnancy in one of the tubes (called an ectopic pregnancy), endometriosis, or pelvic surgery can cause this kind of blockage. Another 20% of infertile women have an ovulation disorder, often infrequent ovulation because of hormonal imbalances, weight problems, heavy athletic training, or stress. Disorders of hormone-producing glands such as the thyroid and pituitary can also interfere with ovulation. In 20% of cases, fibroids or another disorder of the uterus disrupt embryo implantation or cause miscarriages.

Treatments

Whether you'll conceive and carry a baby to term depends on many things, from what's causing the problem to how severe it is. Proper timing of intercourse is crucial, of course. Hormone imbalance problems often respond to ovulation-promoting drugs. One in 10 women turn to high-tech options like in vitro fertilization (IVF). Surgery can repair damaged reproductive organs. Even if experts can't pinpoint a cause, it's extremely heartening to know that 60% of couples get pregnant within three years.

Treatment options

Lifestyle changes

Chart your cycle	Take your temperature to determine ovulation.
Improve your diet	Limit alcohol, caffeine; eat well; take vitamins.
Exercise	Consistently, but not too vigorously.

Medications

Clomiphene citrate	Induces ovulation.
Menotropins/follitropins	Stimulate follicles, egg development.
Gonadotropins	Improve implantation prospects.

Procedures

Artificial insemination	Sperm is inserted into uterus medically.
Assisted reproduction	Drugs incite ovaries to produce eggs.
In vitro fertilization	Developing embryo transferred to uterus.
Intrafallopian transfer	Fertilized egg(s) placed in fallopian tubes.

Lifestyle Changes

There are lots of simple things you can do to boost your odds of getting pregnant. You're most fertile in the five days before you ovulate, so **chart your menstrual cycle** by recording your basal body temperature each morning (right after awakening) for several months. Look for vaginal discharge that has become copious, clear, and slippery; this happens just before ovulation. Stay attuned to the slight pinching sensation in your abdomen that signals ovulation. **At-home ovulation tests** can also help identify the key time.

Many medications you might not suspect (asthma drugs, for example) can compromise fertility, not to mention potentially endanger your pregnancy once it occurs, so review what you take with your doctor. **Cut out alcohol.** Even one drink a day has been linked to compromised fertility. **Limit caffeine** as well. More than one cup of coffee daily may dump enough caffeine into your system to up your risk of miscarriage. (Fancy coffeehouse brews tend to be particularly high-octane.) Cigarettes are also linked to fertility problems—yet another reason to **stop smoking.** It seems smokers inhale a toxin that can trigger ovarian failure.

More than one in 10 cases of infertility are linked to too much or too little body weight. **Aim for a normal weight**, with a body mass index (BMI) of at least 20 if you're thin to start, and a BMI under 27 if you're heavier (*to figure out your BMI, see page 355*). **Exercise in moderation:** Working out too vigorously reduces levels of estrogen and progesterone. That may inhibit ovulation or make it impossible for an embryo to implant in the uterine wall. Aim for the equivalent of a two-mile daily stroll. **Eat a well-rounded diet** and take basic prenatal vitamins.

TAKING Control

- **Keep time on your side.** Over age 30? If infertility is an issue, don't wait a whole year before seeing a doctor. Go after six months if you're over 35. Always go if you aren't menstruating, have had three or more miscarriages, or have an infection of your reproductive organs.

- **Don't let $$ be the issue.** Before seeking treatment, check out your medical insurance coverage. Companies vary widely in how much testing or treatment they'll pay for—especially for a pre-existing condition. For a list of infertility-friendly employers and insurance carriers, log on to www.if.freehosting.net.

- **Express your feelings.** Infertility can undermine your sense of womanhood, self-worth, and identity. You may feel sorrowful, angry, or withdrawn. Relationships can fray from the pressure. Don't stuff these feelings away: Many other women are experiencing them too, and there are things you can do to ease your pain. Talk with your doctor about counseling or finding a support group.

- **Be wary of dietary supplements.*** Traditional treatments, from chasteberry to false unicorn root may not work. High doses of St. John's wort, echinacea, and ginkgo may damage eggs, sperm, and the fertilization process.

*Natural methods are not subject to the same testing and regulation as prescription medications. Please seek your doctor's advice and use caution.

▶ **Can fertility drugs cause ovarian cancer?**

Although the drugs stimulate the ovaries to produce more eggs, they don't increase the risk of ovarian cancer. At least that's the conclusion of a major 2000 study that looked at more than 12,000 women and was published in the American Journal of Epidemiology.

▶ **What can I do with embryos I don't use?**

You can have embryos (fertilized eggs) frozen for future use should you not get pregnant the first time, or if you want to try for another baby later on. If your ovaries are damaged or you have a genetic disease you don't want to pass on, consider donor egg IVF, in which eggs from another woman are fertilized by your partner's sperm in vitro, then transferred to your uterus.

▶ **Can I boost my fertility by reducing stress?**

This hotly debated topic is under study in clinical trials right now. If a link is made, you may be left with the unsettling idea that your fertility problems are partly your fault. Then again, programs that focus on the mind-body connection, using meditation, muscle relaxation, nutrition counseling, and emotional support, along with changing negative thinking patterns, have shown some small advantage. Bottom line: None of these techniques can hurt you, and they may improve your overall health.

Male Infertility

In 40% of cases, infertility is affected by a male factor—sparse or abnormal sperm or ejaculation problems. A basic exam and sperm analysis often reveals the problem. Less than 2% of infertile men are totally sterile, so odds are in your favor.

Low-tech approaches require some patience: Lifestyle changes to improve sperm work slowly. Eliminate or switch medications that could diminish your sperm count or quality. Eat right, lose excess weight, and pack in foods high in sperm-protectant antioxidants, such as vitamin C. Get good rest, reduce stress, and don't abuse drugs such as cocaine or marijuana, which can temporarily (but dramatically) reduce sperm count and quality. Tight clothing does not diminish fertility, as experts once thought. Protect the testes from overheating, avoiding extended hot baths and steam rooms. Because pressure from a bicycle seat can damage erection-sensitive blood vessels and nerves, avid bicyclists should take frequent rests and wear padded bike shorts. Counseling and medication can help you deal with feelings of guilt, low self-esteem, and anger, as well as intercourse problems such as impotence and premature ejaculation.

High-tech approaches include extracting sperm and preparing it for implantation. With a procedure called intracytoplasmic sperm injection (ICSI), a single sperm is inserted inside an egg in the laboratory, and the developing embryo is transferred to the woman's uterus. Surgery to correct a dilated vein around the testicle (a varicocele) can restore normal sperm flow.

Medications

Hormonal problems such as irregular—or absent—periods or long cycles are treated with **clomiphene citrate,** which induces ovulation. To increase their odds, some women take it to stimulate multiple eggs (and 10% to 20% of births resulting from fertility drugs are multiples). If you still don't ovulate, potent hormone stimulators can mimic natural steps leading to ovulation and encourage the development of egg-producing follicles on the ovaries. You may first be given continuous **gonadotropin-releasing hormone agonists** to turn off your natural hormones so that the artificial ones can take over.

Injected over several days, "super-ovulator" drugs are typically used in conjunction with various procedures. The **menotropins** act directly on the ovaries to stimulate follicle development. The **follitropins** (follicle-stimulating hormone, FSH), including Gonal-F, Follistim, and Bravelle, stimulate follicle and egg production. **Chorionic gonadotropins** mimic luteinizing hormone (LH) to release matured eggs, ripening prospects for implantation. **Progesterone,** taken after ovulation, primes the uterine lining. Many women ovulate after taking these drugs, but not all of them get pregnant, and the drugs are not risk-free. Be clear on benefits and risks. Other drugs can correct too much prolactin (a hormone that interferes with FSH and LH production) or a thyroid endocrine imbalance.

Procedures

With **artificial insemination (AI),** technology aids nature by injecting sperm directly into the uterus once or twice before ovulation, then during ovulation. The procedure is quick and relatively pain-free, and occasionally performed without drugs. With all other forms of **assisted reproductive technologies (ART),** egg-stimulating drugs are given to encourage multiple egg-containing follicles to develop. Ultrasound exams and blood tests identify when your follicles are large enough to contain mature eggs: Hormones made by the placenta—human chorionic gonadotropin (hCG)—are given to induce ovulation approximately 36 hours later.

For many procedures, surgeons guided by ultrasound retrieve eggs via a needle inserted through the vaginal wall. The egg(s) is fertilized with semen and incubated in a laboratory. Healthy embryos are then transferred into you. The developing embryos are transferred into your uterus through **in vitro fertilization (IVF)** (*see illustration below*). In **gamete intrafallopian transfer (GIFT)** sperm and eggs are placed directly into your fallopian tubes and fertilization occurs naturally. An IVF/GIFT hybrid and an option if GIFT fails is **zygote intrafallopian transfer (ZIFT);** here the laboratory-fertilized eggs are placed into your fallopian tubes.

Major **surgery** to repair damaged ovaries, uterus, or fallopian tubes is considered only if fertility prospects are good. If available, minimally invasive laparoscopic techniques are your best option.

IN VITRO FERTILIZATION (IVF)

With IVF, sperm from a man (**1**) and eggs harvested from a woman's ovaries (**2**) are combined in the lab to create embryos (**3**). When large enough, these embryos are transferred (**4**) to the woman's vagina using a catheter (**5**). Pregnancy occurs when an embryo implants in the uterus.

Promising DEVELOPMENTS

■ A small study found that the weak male hormone secreted by the adrenal gland, dehydroepiandrosterone **(DHEA),** improved pregnancy rates in women unresponsive to ovarian stimulation. When the follicles were mature, DHEA was administered first and continued while the women were given the normal FSH and hCG drugs.

■ A **blood test** may one day outsmart the biological clock—or at least figure out how quickly it's ticking—by predicting each woman's menopause. With this knowledge, a woman can get a better sense of how long she'll continue to have productive ovulation cycles. The exciting research comes from Dutch researchers who, while studying sisters, found that the onset of menopause is largely (87%) determined by genetics.

FINDING Support

■ The most useful association for infertility is RESOLVE: The National Infertility Association, a Massachusetts-based organization that provides extensive information on matters ranging from the success rates of various fertility clinics and clinical trials to getting emotional support. They also have an excellent list of questions to ask if you are considering surrogacy (1-888-623-0744 or www.resolve.org).

■ Find up-to-date information on clinical trials related to infertility, on the NIH website (www.clinicaltrials.gov).

Inflammatory bowel disease

Chronic abdominal problems can make you feel truly miserable, even debilitated. It doesn't have to be that way. Finding the right drug or therapy, and following some smart self-care strategies, can go a long way toward restoring a good quality of life.

LIKELY **First Steps**

- **Medications** to reduce inflammation and treat secondary problems.
- **Changes in eating habits** to relieve symptoms.
- **Regular screening tests** to check progress of the disease.

QUESTIONS TO **Ask**

- How do you know I have IBD and not irritable bowel syndrome?
- Will there ever come a time that I don't have to take medication?
- How likely am I to need surgery?

What is happening

Inflammatory bowel disease, often called IBD, has two main forms: ulcerative colitis and Crohn's disease. Both are chronic conditions, with flare-ups followed by periods of remission. If you have either ailment, you know the symptoms all too well: bloody diarrhea, abdominal cramps, and possibly constipation. With Crohn's disease, you may also have significant weight loss.

Ulcerative colitis is an inflammation that starts in the rectum but may progress to the rest of your large intestine, which is why getting it under control is important. This inflammation can lead to ulcers in the lining of the bowel, or colon, which may eventually become rigid and shrink. Crohn's disease may affect any part of your digestive tract, from your mouth to your anus. It most often occurs in only the last section of your small bowel, called the ileum. The affected area becomes swollen and brittle and forms deeper ulcers than ulcerative colitis. Eventually, Crohn's disease can cause abscesses, narrowings of the intestine called strictures, abnormal connections between organs called fistulas, and an overgrowth of surface fat tissue (*see illustration below*). Effective new treatments help prevent these complications.

No one knows for certain what causes IBD, but all signs point to a combination of genetic and environmental factors working

---

DISTINGUISHING THE TWO MAIN FORMS OF IBD

fat

thickened wall

excess fat

fissures

inflamed mucous lining

ulceration

Normal

Crohn's disease

Ulcerative colitis

A healthy intestine is a long muscular tube, with a mucous lining that absorbs nutrients from food. In Crohn's disease, inflammation causes swelling, fissures in the lining, scar tissue that narrows the opening, and an overgrowth of surface fat tissue. In ulcerative colitis, inflammation produces multiple erosions and ulcerations.

Treatment options

Medications

5-ASA agents	Reduce gastrointestinal inflammation.
Corticosteroids	Treat severe IBD inflammation.
Immunosuppressants	Slow down attacking immune cells.
Monoclonal antibodies	For Crohn's; combat inflammatory protein.

Lifestyle changes

Diet	Get fluids; avoid food irritants; watch weight.
Stop smoking & get exercise	To relieve Crohn's disease.
Work on stress	Practice stress-reduction techniques.

Procedures

Regular screening tests	Detect changes in IBD.
Surgery	If drugs don't control IBD.

Natural methods

Herbal supplements	Marshmallow, slippery elm, goldenseal.

together. IBD runs in families, and people with this disorder tend to have an overactive immune response to certain allergens, viruses, or bacteria, including the "friendly" bacteria that normally grow in the gut. IBD is not the same as irritable bowel syndrome (IBS), a less serious condition, which can also cause intestinal distress (*see Irritable Bowel Syndrome, page 192*).

Treatments

Most treatments for IBD are aimed at both controlling symptoms and halting the progress of the disease. People with IBD usually do very well when they're on the right medication and make some changes in their eating habits. As time goes on, some people may need to turn to surgical alternatives; with ulcerative colitis, surgery can provide a complete cure.

Medications

The medications your doctor prescribes will help reduce inflammation, control diarrhea or constipation, and treat infection and other secondary problems. If your disease is in the lower colon, your medication may be in the form of an enema or suppository. If it is higher in your digestive tract, pills or injections may be the best solution.

For moderate IBD (less than six stools per day) the first drug your doctor is likely to prescribe is a **5-ASA agent**, with an inflammation-controlling substance called mesalamine. These agents include sulfasalazine (Azulfidine), and the newer drugs Asacol, Dipentum, Colazal, and Pentasa (which is also available in enema form).

- Researchers at the University of Pennsylvania Medical Center have discovered that **thiazolidinediones,** which are drugs used by people with diabetes, can, in mice, decrease the symptoms of inflammatory bowel disease (especially those of ulcerative colitis) by an astounding 80%.

- Studies of **hepatocyte growth factor,** naturally produced in the liver and small intestine, have shown this substance can almost completely eliminate the symptoms of IBD in laboratory animals. Not only did it make all visible ulcers in the animals disappear, it got rid of half of the microscopic lesions. Researchers who presented the findings at a 1999 American College of Surgeons meeting hope to some day try the agents in humans.

- Most people aren't keen on having worms, but the opposite may be true if you have IBD. Researchers at the University of Iowa have had success treating IBD patients using intestinal worms called **helminthic parasites.** Patients swallow microscopic eggs in a glass of Gatorade. In studies to date, nearly all patients have gone into remission, with no side effects.

If you have **severe IBD** (more than six stools a day, mostly bloody) or 5-ASAs don't help, you might do well with **corticosteroids.** These are given as intravenous or oral medications, as an enema, or in a rectal aerosol foam, such as Cortifoam, which contains hydrocortisone.

For severe Crohn's disease, the next line of defense is powerful **immunosuppressant medications,** such as 6-mercaptopurine (Purinethol), azathioprine (Imuran), methotrexate (Folex), and cyclosporine (Neoral). These drugs are often prescribed in combination with corticosteroids. The newest FDA-approved medication for moderate to severe Crohn's disease is a **monoclonal antibody** (an immune cell that specifically targets a particular disease-causing agent) called infliximab (Remicade). This drug attacks tumor necrosis factor, an inflammatory protein associated with IBD, before it can reach your intestines. The largest study of a Crohn's disease medication ever done showed that after 54 weeks of infliximab therapy, patients were twice as likely to be in remission as those not using the drug. Many were able to discontinue corticosteroids.

To battle bacteria from blockages or fistulas in the small intestine, your doctor will prescribe **antibiotics** such as ampicillin or tetracycline. For diarrhea, you can get relief with over-the-counter medications such as **loperamide** (Imodium) or a prescription drug such as Lomotil, an **opiate.**

Lifestyle Changes

Although lifestyle changes won't make IBD disappear, they can significantly improve your quality of life by helping to minimize symptoms. Here are some good suggestions:

- **Drink plenty of water.** The diarrhea associated with IBD can dehydrate you, and you need to regularly replace lost fluid.

- **Avoid foods that may cause inflammation.** Everyone's system is different, but remain alert for bad reactions. Some well-known food irritants include saturated fats, milk products, alcohol, caffeine, sugar, dried fruit, high-sugar fruits (grapes, watermelon, pineapple), wheat, oats, barley, soy, eggs, peanuts, tomatoes, beets, chocolate, pepper, lamb, lime peel, nuts, parsley, poppy seeds, rhubarb, and spinach. Track what you eat. If any of these foods makes you feel bad, stop eating it.

- **Take omega-3 fatty acids.** There is some evidence that fish oil and flaxseed oil can minimize symptoms of IBD. Eat cold-water fish such as salmon three times a week. You can also use omega-3 supplements (follow the label directions for dosage).

- **Eat smaller, more frequent meals.** This will help keep gas to a minimum, especially if your diet has a high fiber content.

- **Try to maintain a normal weight.** If you're dropping too many pounds (which is likely with Crohn's disease), add high-calorie nutrition bars and shakes to your diet.

- **Stop smoking.** Research shows that smoking aggravates the progression of this disease. Symptoms of ulcerative colitis, on the other hand, actually seem to be improved by nicotine (*see box opposite*).

- **Do light exercise.** In a recent small study, people with mild or inactive forms of Crohn's disease who walked for 30 minutes, three times a week, experienced significant improvement in their quality of life. Consult a doctor before doing more vigorous exercise.
- **Reduce stress.** Evidence shows that stress aggravates inflammatory diseases. Try meditation or other stress-reduction techniques.

Procedures

After diagnosis, a gastroenterologist will monitor your intestinal health. The doctor may want to perform one of three **screening procedures** on a regular basis, probably annually. If you have ulcerative colitis, you may need a **sigmoidoscopy,** in which a thin, flexible, lighted viewing tube is passed into the rectum and through the lower third of the colon (*see page 359*). For either ulcerative colitis or Crohn's disease, a **colonoscopy** (*see page 360*) may be ordered. This procedure allows the doctor to examine the entire length of your colon with the aid of a flexible fiberoptic tube. If you have Crohn's disease, you may undergo regular barium swallows, in which you drink a chalky substance that lines the small intestine and allows your doctor to see abnormalities on an **x-ray.** Those with IBD are at a higher risk for colorectal cancer; a periodic colonoscopy is recommended.

If you have advanced IBD and drug therapy isn't helping, you may need **surgery.** In the case of ulcerative colitis, that may mean possibly removing your colon. This procedure, known as a **proctocolectomy,** will cure the disease. Afterward, you will need to collect your fecal matter in an external pouch connected to your intestine through your abdomen, called an **ostomy,** or in an internal pouch made of tissue from your intestines. Surgery for Crohn's disease usually involves removing the part of the intestine with a blockage or abscess. This won't cure the disease, but will allow fluid and food to proceed normally through your digestive tract.

Natural Methods*

Certain herbs may relieve IBD symptoms. To calm inflammation, try **marshmallow root.** For a tea, add 1 ounce of flowers to a quart of boiling water, steep, then strain out the petals. **Slippery elm** tea may help. Slowly add warm water to 1 heaping teaspoon of dried bark; strain before sipping. To combat unfriendly bacteria in the intestine, try **goldenseal.** For infections, take 15 drops of extract—sold at healthfood stores—every hour. To encourage normal immune function, take **echinacea.** In capsule form, you need to get at least 900 mg a day.

These herbs are generally safe, but don't take goldenseal if you're pregnant or echinacea if you have an autoimmune disease. Some evidence indicates that echinacea is more effective if you use it for three weeks, then abstain for one. Don't forget a daily **multivitamin/mineral.** With fluid leaving your body in copious amounts, you may become malnourished. A high-quality multivitamin supplement can help you combat this problem.

Nicotine Patch for Ulcerative Colitis

It's rare to hear anything good about nicotine, but if administered in the right way, it can be a godsend to ulcerative colitis patients. Although smoking can worsen Crohn's disease, it puts ulcerative colitis patients into remission. Obviously, smoking remains a bad idea for many reasons, but there are ways other than cigarettes to get nicotine into your system. A transdermal nicotine patch that smokers use to help them break their habit is one example. In a study published by the Mayo Clinic, 12 of 31 patients with mild to moderate ulcerative colitis showed improvement after four weeks on the patch. If you have ulcerative colitis, talk with your doctor about giving the nicotine patch a try.

FINDING Support

- For detailed information about IBD and its latest treatments, to find a doctor in your area, or to join a chat room, contact the Crohn's & Colitis Foundation of America in New York, NY (1-800-932-2423 or www.ccfa.org).

- For information on IBD in children, contact Reach Out For Youth, located in Melville, NY (631-293-3102 or www.reachoutforyouth.org).

Natural methods are not subject to the same testing and regulation as prescription medications. Please seek your doctor's advice and use caution.

Insomnia

Some 56% of American adults suffer from insomnia at least twice a week, yet only about half of them discuss the problem with their doctor. Too bad, because insomnia can almost always be put to rest with simple, fast-acting solutions.

LIKELY First Steps

- **Improve your sleep habits,** such as going to bed and getting up at the same time daily, and exercising regularly to promote sleepiness.

- **Meditation or other relaxation techniques** to reduce emotional stress.

- **Prescription or over-the-counter sedatives** for short-term relief of sleeplessness.

QUESTIONS TO Ask

- Do you think I might have sleep apnea or another sleep disorder?

- Could my insomnia be related to the depression I've been experiencing lately?

- Is there a way you can tell whether post-traumatic stress syndrome is what's keeping me awake at night?

- I seem to have more insomnia now that I'm going through menopause. Would HRT be good for me?

What is happening

Insomnia is a general term that refers to difficulty falling or staying asleep. It's not really a disorder, but a symptom with many causes. We all have occasional sleepless nights, and insomnia that sticks around for just a day or two isn't much of a problem, but if you have it for longer periods, you're likely to pay a high price. Research has shown that people who have frequent insomnia are four times more likely to suffer from depression than people who sleep soundly. You're also more likely to underperform at work and have difficult family relationships. More frightening, you could really hurt yourself (or your loved ones): The National Highway Traffic Safety Administration reports that insufficient sleep contributes to more than 100,000 car crashes annually.

It's hard to define insomnia because everyone requires different amounts of sleep. The bottom line, sleep experts say, is how you feel the next day. If you frequently wake up feeling dull and unrefreshed—either because it took you forever to fall asleep or you woke repeatedly at night or got up too early—there's a good chance that insomnia is taking its toll.

Most insomnia is triggered by temporary upsets—emotional stress, for example, or flare-ups of arthritis or other painful conditions. Once your life returns to normal, the quality of your sleep probably will, too, but sometimes it doesn't work that way. Some people get so frustrated when they can't sleep that they continue to feel anxious after the original problem is long gone. This can result in long-term, or chronic, insomnia—disturbed sleep at least three times a week for a month or more.

Treatments

Your doctor will most likely take a three-pronged approach to exploring the causes of your insomnia. The first step is to identify—and correct—any underlying physical or emotional problems that may be keeping you awake. After that, you'll probably be asked to make a few lifestyle changes to promote better sleep. Finally, you may be given over-the-counter or prescription drugs to break the "insomnia cycle" and help you get some much-needed rest.

Lifestyle Changes

Whether you've battled insomnia for years or are experiencing it for the first time, the best place to start is with what doctors

Treatment options

Lifestyle changes

Work on "sleep hygiene"	Maintain a regular sleep schedule; no naps.
Relax	Try yoga or meditation to reduce stress.
Limit caffeine & alcohol	No lattes after noon; no drinks before bed.
Exercise	Makes you tired and defuses stress.

Medications

Antihistamines	Act as mild sedatives.
Sleeping pills	Promote falling asleep and sleeping through.
Antidepressants	Can help depression-induced insomnia.

Natural methods

Herbal remedies	Try valerian, chamomile, or lemon balm.

Procedures

Sleep laboratory	Tests can determine underlying problems.

call "good sleep hygiene," habits that naturally promote better sleep. An hour before your usual bedtime, for example, **get into a relaxing routine.** Read or listen to soothing music. Avoid stressful activities, such as paying bills or completing work projects. Consider taking a hot bath. Your core body temperature will rise, then fall. That will help you fall asleep more readily— and stay asleep. Don't take a bath just before bed, however, because it will temporarily increase blood flow and make you more alert.

Maintain regular sleep habits. Go to bed and get up at the same times every day, even on weekends. And go easy on the naps. They're fine for catching up on occasional missed sleep, but napping regularly makes it harder to maintain a consistent sleep schedule.

A crucial part of sleep hygiene is to keep stress out of your bedroom. Limit what you do in bed to sleep or sex. Don't use the room as a second study. If you do, you'll start to associate going to bed with stress and anxiety. For the same reason, leave the bedroom when insomnia strikes. If you're going to be frustrated because you can't sleep, fret in the living room or kitchen. Go to bed only when you think you're really ready to fall asleep.

Two additional things: Shut out bright light and noise. Install heavy curtains or blinds if you need to. Earplugs will block external sounds, or you can mask noises by running a fan, setting the radio to the fuzz between stations, or using a white noise machine.

Your daytime habits are just as important for beating insomnia as what you do at night. **Don't drink caffeinated beverages** after about noon. **Limit your alcohol consumption** to one or two drinks in the evening. Alcohol can make it easier to fall asleep, but it causes more frequent nighttime awakenings.

TAKING Control

■ **Start a sleep diary.** A 10-day summary of your sleep habits can give you valuable clues about what's happening. Record when you go to bed, how long it takes you to fall asleep, how often you wake at night, how you feel the next day, and so on. Then pass this information along to your doctor.

■ **Avoid kava,** a popular sleep-inducing herb. Recent reports suggest that overuse could cause liver damage.

■ **Limit your ZZZZs at first.** Some experts advise starting with only four hours of sleep—say 3 AM to 7 AM. Once you're sleeping well during these hours, add another 15 to 30 minutes to either end or both—and keep adding time until you're getting the sleep you need.

■ **Eat tofu or other soy foods daily.** They're rich in estrogen-like compounds called phytoestrogens. Women who regularly eat them are less likely to experience menopausal hot flashes or other sleep-disrupting symptoms.

■ **Take care with sleeping pills.** The short-term use of sleeping pills—often up to a month—is very safe for most people. But there are some exceptions. Watch out if you drink: Combining the pills with alcohol intensifies the effects of each. If you're elderly or get up a lot at night, sleeping pills may increase your risk of falls or other accidents. The drugs may increase sleep-related breathing problems by depressing the vital "breathing center" in your brain.

Melatonin: Have the Benefits Been Exaggerated?

The hormone melatonin, produced by the pineal gland in the brain, has long been promoted in supplement form as a treatment for jet lag as well as insomnia. Until recently, scientists were pretty sure that the supplements worked. But new evidence suggests that while melatonin may have some benefits, it's hardly a panacea for interrupted sleep.

The "darkness hormone"
Melatonin has been dubbed the "darkness hormone" because levels in the body rise at night and fall during the day. It affects the sleep-wake cycle, and researchers have naturally assumed it might improve sleep and help reset the body's internal clock when travelers pass through multiple time zones.

In the last few years, however, melatonin has lost some of its scientific glow. Researchers now believe it has no effect on jet lag. Nor does it appear to improve overall sleep.

Internal clock regulator
Scientists have looked at melatonin's ability to affect the body's internal clock. They measured the activity patterns of baboons given melatonin and kept in a constantly dimmed room. Their findings showed that melatonin had no effect on the animals' usual cycles of behavior, which suggests that its ability to change the body's clock—and reduce the symptoms of jet lag—have been greatly exaggerated.

While melatonin does appear to help people fall asleep more quickly at night, it has little effect on the overall quality of their sleep. And it may cause a "sedative hangover."

Using melatonin
Even given these caveats, melatonin appears to be a safe supplement that may ease insomnia in some people. The optimal dose isn't known, so you may have to experiment a bit to find what works best for you. The only people who shouldn't take melatonin are children and pregnant women: It may interact with other hormones in the body.

▶ **I take a number of medications for different ailments, including high blood pressure. Could they be causing my insomnia?**
Some drugs have drowsiness as a side effect, but others promote sleep-disturbing alertness. Among the common offenders are blood pressure-lowering drugs, as well as allergy medications, nicotine patches, and some medications taken for depression.

Whether your insomnia is a recent problem or one you've fought for years, make sure that drugs aren't making things worse. Jot down all those you're currently taking, and show the list to your doctor or pharmacist. Changing one or more of your medications might be the solution you need.

Exercise is another key strategy for achieving better sleep. It tires you out and lowers levels of sleep-disrupting stress hormones. Just be sure to work out at least three hours before you turn in.

Another traditional remedy for insomnia is drinking a glass of **warm milk,** and there's good evidence that it works. Milk helps prevent hunger from disturbing your sleep; it also contains an amino acid called tryptophan, which is converted in the brain into a "relaxing" chemical known as serotonin. Once you're in bed, try **progressive muscle relaxation,** a technique that involves tensing, then releasing all the muscles in your body. Start at your feet and move toward your head.

Finally, try to **get a handle on the stressors in your life.** If you're in the throes of anxiety, it's harder to fall asleep and sleep soundly. Some of the best stress-beating activities include yoga, meditation, and listening to soothing audiotapes.

Medications

Good sleep habits are the best way to overcome insomnia in the long run. But when you need fast relief, your doctor may recommend over-the-counter or prescription drugs. These might include:

- **OTC antihistamines.** Two popular ones, diphenhydramine (Benadryl) and chlorpheniramine (Chlor-Trimeton) act as mild sedatives and are very effective for occasional sleepless nights.
- **Analgesics.** Aspirin, ibuprofen (Advil), naproxen (Aleve), or acetaminophen (Tylenol) often relieve sleep-disturbing pain.

- **Prescription sleeping pills.** Also called hypnotics, those commonly recommended for insomnia usually belong to a chemical family known as benzodiazepines. They're extremely effective and can be taken for months without losing their potency. They sometimes can be habit-forming, although not addicting. If you have trouble sleeping through the night, your doctor might recommend a long-acting benzodiazepine, such as flurazepam (Dalmane) or clonazepam (Klonopin). If your main problem is falling asleep, or if you tend to wake up very early in the morning, you might need a shorter-acting benzodiazepine, such as zolpidem tartrate (Ambien), triazolam (Halcion), alprazolam (Xanax), or zaleplon (Sonata). Any of these will help you fall asleep, but are unlikely to cause a "hangover" the next day.
- **Antidepressants.** These medicines are sometimes used to treat insomnia-caused depression. Some, such as amitriptyline (Elavil) and trazodone (Desyrel), cause drowsiness.

Natural Methods*

Certain herbs have been used for centuries to ease insomnia. **Valerian,** a natural herbal tranquilizer, works best when rotated with other sleep-inducing herbs. **Chamomile** is a sweet-tasting herb that depresses the central nervous system the way antianxiety drugs do. **Lemon balm** (also known as melissa) has a citrusy aroma; its leaves are the plant's medicinal part.

Procedures

Your doctor can probably recognize—and treat—many of the common causes of your insomnia. Some conditions, however, can only be detected if you spend one or more nights in a **sleep laboratory.** Don't let the name scare you. Sleep labs are like comfortable hotel rooms—except instead of a mini-bar by the bed, you'll see devices that measure everything from heart rate to brain waves and breathing patterns.

You'll arrive at the sleep lab about an hour before your usual bedtime. A technician will attach electrodes and other external monitoring devices to your body. Then it's lights out. The test will show how much (or how little) you sleep and whether you spend enough time in "deep" sleep. It will also pinpoint physical problems that interfere with normal sleep, such as sleep apnea (*see page 291*), limb movements, or a curious condition called "sleep state misperception," which means that you feel you're getting less sleep than you actually are. Treatment can be tailored to your specific problem.

FINDING Support

- For the latest information on insomnia and other sleep disorders, contact the National Sleep Foundation in Washington, D.C. (202-347-3471 or www.sleepfoundation.org).
- To find out about new research in the field of sleep medicine, log on to the website of the American Academy of Sleep Medicine at www.aasmnet.org.

Natural methods are not subject to the same testing and regulation as prescription medications. Please seek your doctor's advice and use caution.

Irritable bowel syndrome

It's been estimated that fully one-fifth of the American population suffers from this painful (and often inconvenient) digestive ailment. Even though there's no sure cure, IBS is definitely treatable—often with just diet and exercise.

LIKELY First Steps

- Identify possible **trigger foods** and cut back or eliminate them from your diet.

- If you suffer from constipation, boost **soluble fiber** and **exercise** more.

- Consider **medication** to treat specific symptoms.

- Practice some **relaxation techniques** to ease stress.

Is It IBS?

If you meet these criteria, you likely have IBS and will benefit from treatment:

- Abdominal pain or discomfort and a varying pattern of diarrhea and constipation (occurring 25% of the time) for 12 weeks out of the preceding 12 months. The pain or discomfort is relieved by a bowel movement or accompanied by a change in the frequency or consistency of the stool.

- The varying defecation pattern fits at least three of the following characteristics: altered bowel movement frequency; a change in stool form (hard or loose and watery); altered passage of stool (straining, urgency, or a feeling of incomplete evacuation); passage of white mucus; or bloating or the sensation of having a distended abdomen.

What is happening

The intestinal distress associated with irritable bowel syndrome (IBS) is responsible for more than 3 million doctor visits annually. Only the common cold results in more missed days of work. While no one is exactly sure what causes this mysterious, misery-making complaint, doctors now admit that it is definitely not "all in your head." They will also tell you it's not a life-threatening condition and confirm that it won't develop into a more serious illness like inflammatory bowel disease (*page 184*) or colon cancer (*page 86*).

The alternating bouts of diarrhea and constipation associated with IBS typically develop in the late teens or early 20s, primarily in women. Many people who have it are never diagnosed, however, because medical tests routinely show nothing out of the ordinary. That's why doctors have established a specific set of criteria to help identify the condition (*see box at left*). If you don't have a definite diagnosis of IBS, see if the criteria apply to you. Even if you have these key IBS symptoms, the underlying source of the problem remains elusive.

To better comprehend IBS, it helps to understand how it compares with normal digestion. When partially digested food leaves your stomach, it is usually moved through your intestines by the gentle, wavelike contraction and relaxation of muscles of the intestinal wall—a process known as peristalsis. When you have IBS, the muscles in your colon (part of your large intestine) go into spasm, contracting too quickly and forcefully (causing diarrhea) or too slowly and weakly (resulting in constipation).

There's plenty of speculation about why the colon misfires. Some suggest that hormonal problems play a role (women with IBS seem to have more symptoms on premenstrual days) or that a chemical imbalance in the brain may be present. Specific foods seem to trigger IBS flare-ups in some people, including the inability to digest lactose (*see "Taking Control," opposite*). Overuse of antibiotics could be another cause, as can a bacterial, viral, or parasitic infection. Another hypothesis is that people with IBS have extrasensitive pain sensors in their guts, overactive nerves that could cause the muscle spasms underlying this ailment. Stress appears to be another key factor. Even a healthy person experiencing the natural "fight or flight" response that occurs in a very stressful situation will have intestinal spasms and sometimes an involuntary emptying of the bowels. But, people susceptible to IBS experience this intestinal response to stress to an excessive degree.

Treatment options

Lifestyle changes

Dietary changes	Avoid trigger foods; eat smaller meals more often.
Exercise	To improve digestion and reduce stress.

Medications

Antidiarrheals	OTC and prescription to prevent spasms.
OTC laxatives	Don't use longer than two weeks.
Antispasmodics	To relax the muscles and relieve pain.
Antidepressants	Low-dose tricyclics help prevent spasms.
5-HT3 antagonist	Lotronex for severe diarrhea in women.

Procedures

Stress reduction	Try biofeedback or hypnosis to relax colon.

Natural methods

Peppermint oil	To relieve pain, bloating, and diarrhea.

Treatments

To be safe, your doctor will probably begin with tests to rule out more serious intestinal ailments, such as Crohn's disease, ulcerative colitis, diverticulitis, and colon cancer. Once these are out of the way, your IBS treatment plan will depend on your predominant symptoms—diarrhea, constipation, and/or abdominal pain and bloating. If you have a mild case (as two-thirds of patients do), your doctor will likely recommend that you start with self-care measures—including diet changes, stress reduction, and exercise. Drug therapy is usually reserved for those whose severe symptoms do not respond to lifestyle measures.

Lifestyle Changes

Many people feel much better simply by changing what they eat. Basically, you need to avoid foods that make your symptoms worse and stick with those that agree with you. Keeping a **food diary** will help you track the relationship between symptoms and diet. Write down what you eat and note which foods bring on what symptoms, so you'll be better able to pinpoint offenders. You may, for instance, have trouble with dairy, wheat, or corn products, or you might find acidic or spicy foods to be the problem. Artificial sweeteners, such as sorbitol and mannitol, as well as caffeine, alcohol, and even chocolate, can also cause spasms.

Eating too much at one time may trigger intestinal contractions, so you'll be advised to **eat smaller, more frequent meals.** You may also want to **experiment with getting more fiber.** Try gradually increasing the amount of soluble fiber in your diet over a period of weeks. This can be a big help if your primary IBS symptom is

QUESTIONS TO Ask

- Why aren't you testing me for colon cancer and other bowel diseases?
- Would I be a good candidate for a clinical trial? If so, what risks would I face?
- Do you think I'm anxious because of IBS or vice versa?
- Because there's no cure, will I feel this uncomfortable forever? What else can I do?

TAKING Control

- **Seek counseling.** If you're feeling down because IBS has taken such a toll on your life, you may want to consider professional advice from a psychotherapist or behavioral counselor.
- **Find out whether you're lactose intolerant.** For many people, symptoms of IBS can be hard to distinguish from those of lactose intolerance. But don't simply stop eating dairy. Try this quick test instead: Drink two glasses of nonfat milk on an empty stomach. If you experience symptoms (gas, bloating, diarrhea) within four hours, repeat the test with lactase-treated milk, such as Lactaid. If, after four hours, you are symptom-free, you may very well be lactose intolerant. Or ask your doctor about a reliable test to diagnose lactose intolerance.

Promising
DEVELOPMENTS

■ Besides Lotronex (*see box opposite*), more drugs specifically designed for IBS symptoms are on the way. **Cilansetron,** another 5-HT3 receptor antagonist now in clinical trials, may compete with Lotronex, helping to ease severe diarrhea.

▶**EAT MORE FISH. In a study published in the prestigious *New England Journal of Medicine,* more than half of those who had IBS reduced or eliminated symptoms when they took daily fish oil supplements along with their medication. Fish oil may help treat IBS because it contains omega-3 fatty acids, important fats known to reduce inflammation. Fish oil may also bolster levels of the brain chemical serotonin, normalizing the way your brain interprets bowel signals. Try to eat fatty, cold-water fish such as tuna or salmon at least twice a week.**

constipation or abdominal cramping. By absorbing water from the intestines, soluble fiber helps prevent the stool from becoming hard and painful to expel. Fiber also bulks up the stool, which in turn fills out the colon and reduces the chances of spasms. Foods high in soluble fiber include oatmeal, soy foods, barley, oat bran, and beans. You can try a bulking agent, such as psyllium seed (Metamucil, Citrucel), but be sure to take it with plenty of water and drink other fluids throughout the day to keep things moving.

When your main symptom is gas, try to **eliminate gas-forming foods** such as beans, peas, lentils, broccoli, cauliflower, onions, cucumbers, and leafy vegetables. As your symptoms improve, gradually start eating these foods again and see what happens.

Get more exercise, too. In studies of women with IBS, those who exercised reported fewer symptoms. Not only does exercise help stimulate digestion, it firms abdominal muscles, helping keep those out-of-control intestines in their place. Working out is also a great way to beat stress. Do some other form of aerobic exercise for at least 30 minutes, three times a week.

Medications

If your symptoms don't respond to lifestyle changes, your doctor may suggest one or more of the following medicines (be sure to discuss side effects and use the drug only as directed):

■ **Antidiarrheal agents,** such as OTC loperamide (Imodium A-D) and prescription diphenoxylate hydrochloride/atropine sulfate (Lomotil), help stop contractions that lead to diarrhea. While not for daily use, these work particularly well in preventing diarrhea at inconvenient and predictable times.

■ **Hyperosmotic laxatives,** such as magnesium hydroxide (Phillips' Milk of Magnesia) and lactulose (Chronulac, Duphalac), sold over-the-counter, may relieve constipation. As with antidiarrheal agents, don't make them a habit: Long-term use can worsen constipation. You may want to try a psyllium product first.

■ **Antispasmodics,** such as dicyclomine (Bentyl), hyoscyamine (Levsin), or atropine sulfate (Donnatal), are available by prescription. They help relax the intestinal muscles and are useful if you suffer from acute abdominal pain. Take the medication 30 to 60 minutes before a meal.

■ **Tricyclic antidepressants,** such as imipramine (Tofranil, Norfranil) and amitriptyline (Elavil), counteract the brain neurons responsible for telling your intestines to spasm. Prescribed at much lower doses for IBD than for depression, these drugs also stop pain receptors in your gut from relaying their signals to your brain.

■ **5-HT3 antagonists** are being developed specifically for treating IBS symptoms. The only one available to date is alosetron (Lotronex), which the FDA recently returned to the market on a limited basis after a two-year ban (*see box opposite*).

■ **Tegaserod maleate** (Zelnorm) has recently been approved for treatment of women whose primary IBS symptom is constipation.

Lotronex: Back by Popular Demand

In February 2000, the Food and Drug Administration approved alosetron (Lotronex) to treat women who had chronic diarrhea caused by irritable bowel syndrome. The manufacturer (GlaxoSmithKline P.L.C.) voluntarily removed the drug from the market less than 10 months later, because it was linked to cases of severe intestinal problems and several deaths.

After the withdrawal, thousands of women publicly protested—some in front of Congress—saying Lotronex was the only treatment that enabled them to lead normal lives for the first time in years. Their outcry helped persuade the FDA, and the manufacturer, to find a way to reinstate the drug.

Lotronex is again available, but with severe restrictions. Under new rules set by the FDA, doctors who want to prescribe Lotronex must enroll in a program run by the manufacturer that requires them to "self-attest" that they know how to diagnose and treat IBS, how to prescribe Lotronex, and how to recognize and treat complications. The doctors must also agree to explain the drug's risks and benefits to patients before prescribing it.

Women who want to use Lotronex must sign an agreement acknowledging its risks, which include a 1-in-1,000 chance of serious constipation problems and a 1-in-350 chance of developing ischemic colitis, an inflammation caused by interference with blood flow to the colon. Moreover, while Lotronex was originally prescribed for women with chronic diarrhea, it will now be recommended only for those who have very severe cases of diarrhea that have not responded to other drugs. To be extra safe, the daily dose has been cut in half—to just 1 mg.

Procedures

If stress clearly aggravates your IBS, relaxation techniques such as biofeedback and hypnosis may help. You can learn them from a trained professional, then do them at home. In a typical **biofeedback** session, you're hooked up to a machine that reads bodily functions such as heart rate, blood pressure, and muscle tension. As you try to relax, the machine provides constant feedback, letting you know exactly how relaxed you've become. Eventually you'll be able to generate the same results without the machine. During **hypnosis** for IBS, you enter a deeply relaxed state as the hypnotherapist talks you through a visualization that involves relaxing your intestinal muscles. In one study published in the *American Journal of Gastroenterology,* 250 IBS patients who underwent 12 hypnotherapy sessions over three months experienced fewer symptoms. After a few training sessions, you'll learn to place yourself in the hypnotic state, implant the positive suggestions you've been taught, and leave the hypnotic state at will.

Natural Methods*

Many people with IBS find relief by taking **peppermint oil** supplements, which can act as a natural muscle relaxant. In one recent study of 110 people with IBS, those who took one capsule 15 to 20 minutes before meals had less bloating, diarrhea, and pain within a month. Look for an "enteric-coated" supplement, which ensures that the peppermint oil is released in your intestine, where it's needed. Take one or two capsules (containing 0.2 ml of oil each) two or three times a day before eating. Don't take peppermint oil if you're pregnant (it relaxes the uterus) or if you have a hiatal hernia. Avoid peppermint tea, which may aggravate IBS symptoms.

FINDING Support

- The nonprofit Irritable Bowel Syndrome Association in New Haven, CT, sponsors support groups around the country and offers information on clinical trials and medical tests and treatments (416-932-3311 or www.ibsassociation.org).

- The Irritable Bowel Syndrome Self Help Group offers an online discussion list, tips, and information, such as how to take part in a clinical trial (www.ibsgroup.org).

- To find an acupuncturist near you, contact the National Certification Commission for Acupuncture and Oriental Medicine in Alexandria, VA (703-548-9004 or www.nccaom.org).

*Natural methods are not subject to the same testing and regulation as prescription medications. Please seek your doctor's advice and use caution.

Kidney stones

It seems amazing that something so tiny can cause so much suffering. But while a small minority of people are genetically destined to develop a kidney stone, some simple lifestyle changes may greatly reduce your odds of getting one.

LIKELY **First Steps**

- **Watchful waiting** to see if a kidney stone will pass on its own.
- **High volumes of water** to help flush the stone from the urinary tract.
- **Narcotic analgesics** and **anti-inflammatory medications** to control pain.
- **Antibiotics** if a urinary tract infection occurs.
- **Nonsurgical or surgical procedures,** if needed, to eliminate a stone.

QUESTIONS TO **Ask**

- If my pain is under control but the stone hasn't passed, must I still restrict my activities?
- Should I take a vitamin or mineral supplement? What about calcium?
- Could an undiagnosed condition be making me form kidney stones?

What is happening

Doctors don't entirely understand all the physiological changes that lead to formation of kidney stones (medically known as renal calculi), and aren't certain why some people are more susceptible than others to the most common types. Yet everyone agrees on one point: Kidney stones can hurt—a lot. In fact, it is commonly cited as the most painful reported condition. Even stones smaller than a pencil eraser can cause misery and a trip to the emergency room. It may not be much consolation, but you're not alone. About half a million Americans suffer at least one kidney stone each year, and men are four times more likely to have them. A kidney stone was even found in a 7,000-year-old Egyptian mummy.

Your kidneys are meant to efficiently flush microscopic particles of salts and minerals into the ureter—the long, narrow tube that leads to the bladder—and they're expelled when you urinate. Trouble looms when chemical imbalances and other processes cause these tiny particles to bind into crystals, which grow into a kidney stone. When the stone moves from the kidney into the delicate ureter, it produces anything from a nagging ache to excruciating pain, often accompanied by nausea and vomiting. This blockage may trigger a urinary tract infection. Sometimes stones get stuck in the kidney, causing an infection but not usually immediate pain.

Suspected causes of kidney stones include high levels of urinary calcium and oxalate (a chemical that enables stone formation); excessive absorption of calcium from the intestine; too much dietary sodium; chemical imbalances; diseases (such as gout, recurrent urinary tract infections, and hyperparathyroidism); and even some medications. Kidney stones are categorized by their chemical composition. It's likely made of calcium and oxalate, a combination responsible for 70% to 80% of all stones. About 7% are formed from uric acid, and a small fraction are either struvite stones (almost always caused by urinary tract infections) or cystine stones, which are due to a rare genetic disorder.

Treatments

If you think you're passing a kidney stone, call your doctor right away, or rush to an emergency room. You may be hospitalized if your pain is severe or you have signs of complications such as an obstruction or infection. However, about 85% of kidney stones are small enough (a quarter of an inch or less in diameter) to move through the ureter

Treatment options

Lifestyle changes

Lots of fluids	Help move and prevent stones.
Low-salt, low-protein diet	Keeps stones from forming.

Medications

Painkillers	Needed while a stone is passing.
Preventive drugs	Vary based on type of stone.

Procedures

Lithotripsy	Uses shock waves to shatter stones.
Ureteroscopy	For stones in the low or middle ureter.
PNL	Therapy for larger or cystine stones.
Chemolysis	Dissolves rarer types of stones.

and enter the bladder within about 72 hours after they're discovered by x-ray. Once the stone leaves the ureter, your pain leaves with it.

In the meantime, immediate pain relief will be at the top of your wish list. Anti-inflammatory medications and narcotics are very effective and work quickly. You'll also receive antibiotics if you've developed a urinary tract infection. Stones lodged in the kidney or ureter must be removed either surgically or nonsurgically.

Lifestyle Changes

If your doctor advises **watchful waiting** until the stone passes, you can lessen the wait by drinking fluids—three to four quarts a day. Walking can also help speed the stone along. Be sure to strain your urine (the doctor will provide a collection kit) so the stone can be sent for analysis. If you've had a kidney stone but take no precautions to prevent another, you have a 50% chance of repeating the ordeal within five years, but you can reduce your risk considerably with the following measures:

- **Drink lots of fluids**—mostly water. Your goal is to dilute your urine enough to prevent crystals from forming.
- **Lower your salt intake.** Too much salt can raise calcium levels in your urine. Aim to consume less than 2,400 mg of sodium a day.
- **Eat less meat.** Animal protein encourages the body to excrete calcium and uric acid. Get more of your protein from nonmeat sources like soy.
- **Get more potassium in your diet.** Foods rich in this mineral include orange juice, bananas, and other fruits and vegetables.

Although doctors typically recommend that patients reduce the oxalates in their diets (oxalate-rich foods range from spinach to cranberry juice), it's not clear if doing so really makes any difference. Doctors also routinely tell patients to cut back on calcium. Now, even the accuracy of that widely accepted piece of advice is under fire (*see box, page 199*).

TAKING Control

- **Treat a urinary tract infection promptly.** Struvite stones form only in infected urine. If you have an infection (*see Urinary Tract Infection, page 328, and Prostatitis, page 266*), call your doctor.

- **Rehydrate after sweating.** If you live in a warm climate or take part in strenuous physical activities, drink more than the recommended three to four quarts of water or non-caffeinated fluids a day— enough to keep your urine almost colorless. Carry a water bottle with you as a reminder.

- **Maintain a healthy weight.** Kidney stones seem to be more common among overweight people. If you need to lose some pounds, don't go on a crash diet: It can make you produce more uric acid, which promotes kidney stones. Lose weight gradually.

Promising DEVELOPMENTS

- In a study in Finland, men reduced their risk of kidney stones 40% for every bottle of **beer** they drank per day. According to researchers, this is not only because the alcohol and water in the drink dilute your urine, but possibly because certain substances in brewer's hops decrease the excretion of calcium. Of course, too many beers increases the risk of heart and liver disease, so experts advise that men limit their intake to two brews a day.

▶ **Why do I keep getting kidney stones?**

The reason someone is susceptible to kidney stones is not always clear, though a family history of this disorder makes you more prone to forming stones. Despite all sorts of diagnostic testing, doctors rarely find out why the stone appeared. What is known, is that if you pass one stone, you're more likely to have another. That makes it important for you to have blood and urine tests, and, if possible, have the stone itself analyzed. The results will arm you with what you need to know to help prevent a recurrence.

▶ **Should I avoid foods high in oxalates?**

That depends on what type of kidney stones you have. If your urine chronically contains high levels of oxalate, you may well benefit from a change in diet. If your stone was not composed of calcium and oxalate, reducing oxalate consumption won't make much difference. Unlike cutting back on calcium (needed for healthy bones), ingesting less oxalate won't do any harm because it doesn't have any nutritional value by itself. Foods high in oxalate include spinach, strawberries, nuts, rhubarb, beets, soy products, tea, cola drinks, apple juice, and cranberry juice.

Medications

If you have a kidney stone, your doctor will prescribe a **painkiller**, probably ketorolac (Toradol) or the narcotic meperidine (Demerol). You may also be given an **antispasmodic drug** so you can pass the stone more easily. If your urine chronically contains high levels of calcium, oxalate, or uric acid, your doctor might prescribe drugs to help prevent kidney stone formation. The decision will be based on the chemical makeup of your stone and whether your lab tests and blood work indicate you are at high risk for recurrence.

■ **For calcium-based stones:** Preventive medications include **thiazide diuretics,** commonly used to treat high blood pressure and eliminate fluid and sodium from the body. You will probably be given hydrochlorothiazide (Esidrix, Hydro-D), chlorothiazide (Diuril), or trichlormethiazide (Metahydrin, Naqua).

■ **For uric acid stones:** Commonly prescribed drugs include allopurinol (Zyloprim) and potassium citrate (Polycitra-K).

■ **For struvite stones:** Medications such as acetohydroxamic acid (Lithostat) and long-term antibiotics may help.

■ **For cystine stones:** Doctors will typically prescribe tiopronin (Thiola) and penicillamine (Cuprimine, Depen).

Procedures

Not long ago, the only option for removing a larger kidney stone was major surgery, lengthy recovery, and a big scar. Today, doctors can choose from several far gentler alternatives. **Extracorporeal shock wave lithotripsy (ESWL)** is the technique most frequently used to break up stones in the kidney or upper ureter (*see illustration*). Your doctor may place a small tube, called a stent, within the ureter to widen it and allow the stones to move more easily. You

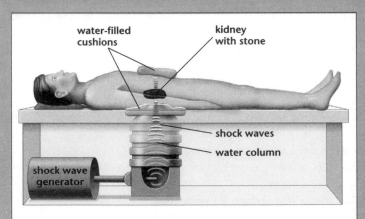

EXTRACORPOREAL SHOCK WAVE LITHOTRIPSY

water-filled cushions

kidney with stone

shock waves

water column

shock wave generator

During this procedure, water-filled cushions are positioned on either side of the sedated patient. The lithotriptor machine (*above*) then fires high-frequency shock waves (1,000 to 2,000 over 45 minutes or so) at the stone, literally shattering it into sandlike granules without harming the surrounding organs. The granules are then painlessly excreted in the urine.

The Calcium Question

Logic might dictate that if excess calcium in the urine is a prime cause of kidney stones, decreasing calcium intake should reduce your risk of developing a stone. Many urologists do instruct their patients to cut down on dairy products and other high-calcium foods.

This may not be good advice, however. In a clinical trial in Italy, 120 men with a history of calcium oxalate kidney stones (the most common type) were divided into two groups: One group ate a low-calcium diet with average amounts of animal protein and sodium. The other ate a normal-calcium diet with reduced meat and sodium.

After five years, nearly twice as many men on the low-calcium diet had formed new stones as those on the normal-calcium diet. There appeared to be two reasons why: The low-calcium group had higher levels of urinary oxalates (and thus stones) because there wasn't enough calcium in their intestine to bind (and render harmless) the oxalates. Those in this group didn't cut down on meat and sodium, which promote stone formation.

may go home just a few hours after an ESWL, although a day or two of hospitalization may be necessary as a precaution. Success rates range from 50% to 90%, depending on the stone's location and chemical composition. Multiple treatments may be needed. ESWL does not work for cystine stones or, usually, for larger stones (more than about an inch). After ESWL, expect to see blood in your urine and feel soreness in your side or abdomen for a few days. Complications are rare.

Stones caught in the middle or lower part of the ureter aren't good candidates for ESWL. Instead, your doctor may attempt a minimally invasive technique called **ureteroscopy,** in which a small fiberoptic scope (called a ureteroscope) is threaded into the urethra and through the bladder. Smaller stones are plucked out manually with small baskets or graspers. Larger ones may first be shattered with lasers, ultrasonic shock waves, or electric shocks delivered through the scope. The procedure is successful 90% of the time. Sometimes, ESWL is used prior to ureteroscopy to break up stones, making them easier to remove.

Larger stones wedged in the kidney or upper ureter and those that simply prove too stubborn for ESWL or ureteroscopy are candidates for **percutaneous nephrolithotomy (PNL).** This is the preferred therapy for cystine stones. For a PNL, the urologist cuts a tiny incision in your back, creates a tunnel into the kidney and, through an instrument called a nephroscope, locates and removes the stone. Ultrasound or a laser may be needed to break up very large stones. The success rate for PNL is a whopping 98% for stones in the kidney, 88% for those in the ureter. Serious complications are very rare.

The rarer types of kidney stones—uric acid, struvite, and cystine stones—may be chemically dissolved in a process called **chemolysis.** Special chemicals are delivered through a catheter inserted through the urethra in a series of treatments. Chemolysis may be used as a primary treatment or in combination with others but doesn't work for calcium stones. Fewer than 2% of people will require standard **open surgery (nephrolithotomy).** It's used only when all other attempts to blast or remove the stone have failed, or if there are special circumstances, such as obesity or an abnormal kidney structure.

FINDING Support

- For excellent overviews of kidney stone symptoms, treatments, and recommended lifestyle changes, contact the American Foundation for Urologic Disease in Baltimore, MD (1-800-242-2383 or www.afud.org) or the National Kidney Foundation in New York, NY (1-800-622-9010 or www.kidney.org).

- For in-depth information on kidney stones and other urologic conditions, go to the website of the American Urologic Association, at www.auanet.org, or take a look at the organization's *Journal of Urology,* www.jurology.com, which contains information written by leading researchers.

- If you have chronically high levels of oxalate in your urine, check with the Oxalosis and Hyperoxaluria Foundation (OHF) in St. Louis, MO (618-281-9450 or www.ohf.org).

Leukemia

While a diagnosis of leukemia is certainly frightening, many forms of this disease can be held in check for years with minimal treatment and appropriate follow-up. Some amazing new therapies are putting scientists closer than ever to a cure.

LIKELY First Steps

- Imaging techniques (**x-rays, ultrasound, bone scans**) may be done to check the chest, kidneys, liver, spleen, bones, or other areas.

- A **spinal tap** may be needed to see if leukemia has spread to the brain and nervous system.

- **For acute leukemia,** chemotherapy and a bone marrow transplant may be indicated.

- **For chronic leukemia,** a wait-and-watch approach may suffice. If the disease progresses, chemotherapy, interferon-alpha, or a bone marrow transplant may be indicated.

- Newer drugs like **Gleevec** may be an option for some.

QUESTIONS TO Ask

- What type of leukemia do I have? What's the treatment?

- What are the chances I will go into remission?

- What are my long-term chances for survival?

- Should I see a specialist? Where would you send a family member who was diagnosed with my illness?

- Am I eligible for a bone marrow transplant?

- What are the signs my leukemia is getting better or worse?

- What about alternative therapies?

What is happening

Leukemia is a cancer of the body's infection-fighting white blood cells. In most cancers, solid tumors form in specific organs. The malignant cells in leukemia appear in your bone marrow, where all blood cells are made, then spread throughout your body. No one is sure what causes leukemia, although pesticides, industrial chemicals, radiation, a virus called HTLV-1, and previous treatments for cancer have been linked to an increased risk for developing it. Some people may also have genetic susceptibility to certain forms of the disease.

The broad categories of leukemia are grouped according to the types of cells affected and how fast the disease progresses. Acute forms develop rapidly, chronic forms may remain stable for many years. There are four major types of leukemia: acute lymphocytic leukemia (ALL), chronic lymphocytic leukemia (CLL), acute myelogenous leukemia (AML), and chronic myelogenous leukemia (CML), as well as many subcategories. One of the rarer forms of the disease is hairy cell leukemia. In this chronic variation, the malignant cells look as though they have projecting hairs when they're examined under a microscope.

In all forms of leukemia, white blood cells proliferate or grow out of control. Your symptoms will depend on the type of leukemia you have. In acute leukemia (ALL or AML), you produce lots of white blood cells, but they are immature and can't perform their normal infection-fighting duties. That's why flu-like symptoms (respiratory or throat infections, fever, fatigue) often arise suddenly and repeatedly. By contrast, chronic leukemia (CML or CLL) often causes no symptoms at all: It's commonly discovered during a routine blood test. Over time, chronic leukemia sometimes develops into a more acute form.

As white blood cells run amok, they can crowd out platelets, red blood cells, and other cells made in your bone marrow. Platelets help your blood clot and keep you from bleeding. If your platelet counts are low, you may develop swollen and bleeding gums or nosebleeds, bruise easily, or have small purple splotches on your skin called petechiae. Red blood cells deliver oxygen to tissues throughout the body. If their levels drop, anemia results. You may then become pale, fatigued, short of breath, or suffer from headaches. You may also have headaches if white blood cells infiltrate the fluid around the brain, and bone pain if these cells congest your bone marrow. Huge numbers of white

Treatment options

Medications

Chemotherapy	Effective for acute and some chronic forms.
Anti-emetics	To help with nausea related to chemotherapy.
Antibiotics	To treat infections from reduced immunity.
Oral corticosteroids	Prevent chemo from attacking healthy cells.
Interferon-alpha	Often used to extend time in remission.
Gleevec	New drug that disables enzyme in cancer cells.

Procedures

Bone marrow transplant	New cancer-free stem cells grow in marrow.
Blood transfusions	Replace blood cells, platelets; fight fatigue.
Radiation	Kills leukemia cells; shrinks nodes, spleen.
Leukapheresis	Special filtering process for the blood.

blood cells may swell lymph nodes in your neck, armpits, or groin, as well as your spleen, liver, or, if you're a man, your testes. By monitoring such symptoms and body changes, you can provide information to help your doctor choose the best treatment for you.

Treatments

Innovative therapies are revolutionizing the treatment of leukemia, and exciting new approaches are in development. Once highly fatal, many forms of leukemia are now kept in check or even cured (*see table, page 202*). Treatment depends on the type of disease you have, its aggressiveness, your age, and other factors.

If you have acute leukemia, your doctor will begin prompt treatment with potent chemotherapy drugs. These can have strong side effects but can be very effective in bringing about remission, meaning that all evidence of the disease has disappeared, at least for a time. Other medicines such as interferon-alpha may be used to induce remissions or boost the effects of chemotherapy. Radiation, bone marrow transplant, surgery, and other procedures may be needed at some point.

If you have chronic leukemia, your doctor may suggest a wait-and-watch approach, holding off treatment but checking your blood regularly to see if your disease is changing in some way. Over time, some cases of chronic leukemia turn into more acute forms, requiring treatment. Doctors then use chemotherapy, bone marrow transplant, or other approaches designed to treat acute disease. Many older people with chronic leukemia, however, never need any treatment at all for their condition.

TAKING Control

■ **Work with your doctor to find a leukemia specialist**. An oncologist specializes in cancer care, a hematologist in diseases of the blood. A hematology-oncologist specializes in leukemia and other blood-related cancers. One of these specialists will likely work with you to coordinate your ongoing care.

■ **See your doctor for regular follow-up visits**. It's important that you report any new symptoms so your doctor can gauge treatment success and disease remissions.

■ **Try relaxation therapies**. Coping with leukemia can be emotionally exhausting. Relaxation therapies (guided imagery, meditation, biofeedback, massage) may improve your ability to deal with daily stresses.

■ **Start a healthy eating program** to bolster your strength and reserve. Leukemia treatment is hard on the body. A nutritionist can help you design an optimal diet.

■ **Avoid exposure to known toxins** such as benzene, which may increase your leukemia risk. Pesticides used in farming have also been linked to the disease.

▶**NEW TREATMENTS OFFER HOPE for the 2,500-plus children diagnosed with leukemia each year in the United States. In the 1960s, almost all children with leukemia died. In the 1980s, half survived. Today, chemotherapy drugs have boosted the cure rate for childhood leukemia to over 80%.**

▶ **I've been told I have multiple myeloma. What is it? How is it treated?**

Multiple myeloma is a leukemia that is due to the overgrowth of plasma cells in the bone marrow. These lymphocytes produce antibodies to protect you against infection. When multiple myeloma occurs, the plasma cells start to produce only a single type of antibody (immunoglobulin). That makes you more susceptible to infection. Symptoms include fatigue, weakness, and bone pain (due to bone damage). The good news is that promising research is under way to improve survival rates following traditional treatment regimens such as high-dose chemotherapy and bone marrow transplantation.

Medications

Cancer-fighting **chemotherapy drugs** are the mainstay treatment for all forms of leukemia. They are used for both acute leukemia and the acute phases of chronic leukemia. Most are given by injection, though some are available as pills. You may receive treatment during doctor visits or during a hospital stay. Many types of chemotherapy drugs may be used, including hydroxyurea (Hydrea), busulfan (Myleran), chlorambucil (Leukeran), cyclophosphamide (Cytoxan), and fludarabine (Fludara). Your drug or drug combination will depend on the type of leukemia you have. The aim of chemotherapy is to destroy proliferating leukemia cells so healthy cells can grow and perform their normal functions.

If you have acute leukemia, chemotherapy is given in phases. The first aims to quickly destroy cancer cells to bring a remission. Later treatments stabilize your condition and destroy hidden pockets of cancer, or "sanctuary sites," in the brain, testes, or other areas.

Chronic leukemia that is progressing is usually treated with monthly chemotherapy sessions, followed by a recovery period, then another treatment period, and so on.

When chemotherapy drugs attack cancer cells, they can damage normal cells, usually those with a fast growth rate, such as hair follicles, or those in the intestine and mouth. Chemo side effects often reflect damage to these systems and commonly include hair loss, nausea and vomiting, mouth sores, fatigue, and infections. To counteract this, your doctor may prescribe **anti-emetic drugs** to stop nausea and vomiting and improve your appetite, and sometimes **antibiotics** to prevent infections.

OUTLOOK FOR MAJOR TYPES OF LEUKEMIA

Type of Leukemia	Remission Success	Long-term Outlook
Acute lymphocytic leukemia (ALL), the most common form of leukemia in children.	The first round of chemotherapy brings about remission in more than 90% of patients.	Children tend to do better than adults. Half of children are free of disease 5 years after treatment.
Acute myelogenous leukemia (AML), the second most common adult form; almost half of child leukemias. Also called acute non-lymphocytic leukemia (ANLL).	Chemotherapy brings about a remission in up to 90% of younger people and 60% of older patients.	Up to 70% to 80% of patients achieve long-term remission with additional chemotherapy. Bone marrow transplant can lead to cure in more than 50% of patients.
Chronic lymphocytic leukemia (CLL), the most common type in adults, mainly over age 60.	Most cases require no specific therapy unless disease progresses and symptoms develop.	Many people live 10 to 20 years after diagnosis, although those with very advanced disease may live 2 years or less.
Chronic myelogenous leukemia (CML) affects mostly adults and is rare in children.	Interferon-alpha often induces remission for 2+ years. Early bone marrow transplant may offer cure in more than 50% of patients.	Median survival is 6 years. If disease worsens ("blast crisis"), chemotherapy may extend survival 8 to 12 months. Drug Gleevec shows promise, inducing remissions in 90%.

Your doctor may also recommend an **oral corticosteroid,** usually prednisone, prior or in addition to chemotherapy. Leukemia can cause your body to attack healthy cells, and these drugs suppress this reaction. Another drug that may be helpful is **interferon-alpha,** an immune booster that has been very successful in treating hairy cell leukemia and prolonging the period before CML worsens. Interferon therapy can be very taxing: It must be injected daily and those on it often feel as if they have a bad flu.

Gleevec is a promising alternative. Available as a capsule, and taken once a day, this new kind of cancer drug disables and destroys a defective enzyme in the cancer cell. Because it has little effect on healthy cells, Gleevec has fewer of the nasty side effects of chemotherapy drugs or interferon. In a study of 532 people with CML whose leukemia had worsened following six months of interferon therapy; doctors could find no evidence of disease in 41% of the patients who switched to Gleevec after 18 months. Doctors still don't know if the drug offers a reprieve or a complete cure, but results so far have been very promising. The downside is that it can cause muscle aches, nausea, a rash, and other side effects. Patients may have to take it for the rest of their lives.

Procedures

The best chance for a possible cure for many people with leukemia is **bone marrow transplant.** In the procedure, you receive healthy blood cells. If you have enough healthy cells, they may be collected from your own body, cleansed of leukemia cells, then returned to you, a procedure called autologous transplantation. Most cells come from a donor who is genetically compatible (allogeneic transplantation), often a sibling or donor located through a national registry. Before the transplant, you'll receive very high doses of chemotherapy and possibly total body radiation to kill leukemia cells in your bone marrow and suppress immune response so you don't reject the transplanted cells. Then about a pint of the cells harvested from the donor's hip is infused into one of your veins. These healthy cells take up residence in your newly sanitized bone marrow, where they carry out normal immune functions.

Other procedures may also be needed. If you are anemic and fatigued, **blood transfusions** will make you feel much better. **Radiation** may be tried for CLL with enlargement of the spleen or lymph nodes. If you have CLL or hairy cell leukemia, **surgery** may be necessary to remove a swollen spleen that's causing pain or other symptoms. If lots of leukemia cells are circulating in your blood, your doctor may recommend a procedure called **leukapheresis** before chemotherapy. This procedure takes blood from one arm, passes it through a filtering machine that removes white blood cells, and returns it to your body through the other arm. This will make you feel better and more able to cope with the effects of chemotherapy, which generally take effect several days later.

Promising DEVELOPMENTS

■ Advances in biotechnology are opening up potential new leukemia treatments. A promising but still experimental drug called **Genasense** made by Genta in New Jersey disables a protein that helps tumor cells thrive. Early studies indicate the drug prompted self-destruction of cancer cells already weakened by chemotherapy drugs, a type of natural cell death researchers call apoptosis. The drug is being tested against chronic lymphocytic leukemia (CLL), melanoma, and many other cancers. More studies are needed for FDA approval.

FINDING Support

■ For more information, contact The Leukemia & Lymphoma Society (1-800-955-4572 or www.leukemia-lymphoma.org). Nurses and social workers are available to answer your questions. The American Cancer Society also has useful educational overviews and information on locating an expert (1-800-ACS-2345 or www.cancer. org). To find a specialist, contact the American Board of Medical Specialties (847-491-9091 or www.abms.org).

■ Many people with leukemia enter clinical trials. Contact the National Cancer Institute (1-800-4-CANCER or www.clinicaltrials.gov).

■ Considering a bone marrow transplant? The Blood & Marrow Transplant Information Network has a directory of transplant centers (1-888-597-7674 or www.bmtnews.org).

■ For information on childhood leukemia, contact the Childhood Leukemia Foundation (www.clf4kids.com).

Lung cancer

This is the most common cancer in the United States in both men and women—and one of the most difficult to treat successfully. Each year, however, medical advances offer powerful new weapons to fight this disease more effectively.

LIKELY First Steps

- For early non-small cell cancer, **surgery** to remove the affected part of the lung.
- **Radiation and/or chemotherapy** for inoperable and more advanced tumors.
- In some cases, **clinical trials** to test new and hopefully more effective treatments.

QUESTIONS TO Ask

- Is surgery possible? How will it affect my breathing?
- What are the potential complications of the treatment you're proposing?
- Would I benefit from receiving my treatment at a major cancer center or even in another country?

What is happening

It's probably no surprise to learn that smoking causes about 90% of all primary lung cancers—meaning those that originate in the lungs. But this disease can also result from exposure to air pollution or industrial toxins such as asbestos or radon. Breathing in such poisons for years causes genetic mutations that make cells in the lungs multiply uncontrollably and form a tumor, also called a carcinoma. It can grow into nearby blood vessels and lymph nodes, then spread (metastasize) to the bones, brain, liver, and other sites in the body. Other types of cancer can also move into the lungs from elsewhere in the body. This is secondary lung cancer.

Lung tumors can grow undetected for years. Eventual symptoms may include coughing, shortness of breath, bloody sputum, chest pain, loss of appetite, and recurring pneumonia. The two main types of lung cancer are non-small cell and small cell. Accounting for about 75% of the cases, non-small cell cancers are divided into three categories. Squamous cell carcinoma (or epidermoid carcinoma) usually starts in a major airway and can grow slowly or quickly. Adenocarcinoma can occur anywhere in the lung and varies in size and speed of growth. Large cell carcinoma is typically sizeable when discovered. Small cell lung cancer (also called oat cell cancer) is very aggressive and has metastasized by the time it's diagnosed.

Once the type of lung cancer you have is identified, its stage is determined by the size of the tumor and whether it has spread to any

THE STAGES AND OUTLOOK FOR LUNG CANCER

Stage	Spread	Outlook
Non-small cell cancer		
I	Tumor is limited to the lung.	Five-year survival is 57% to 67%.
II	Cancer has spread to lymph nodes.	Five-year survival is 39% to 55%.
III	Cancer has spread to diaphragm, chest wall, or to lymph nodes in chest.	Five-year survival is 5% to 35%.
IV	Cancer has spread throughout the body.	Five-year survival is less than 5%.
Small cell lung cancer		
Limited	Cancer in one lung and nearby lymph nodes.	Two-year survival is about 20%.
Extensive	Cancer has spread to other parts of the body.	Two-year survival is less than 4%.

Treatment options

Procedures

Surgery	To remove part or all of lung.
Laser therapy	Intense light that destroys cancer cells.
Photodynamic therapy	Light-sensitive drugs kill small tumors.
Radiation therapy	In addition to or in place of surgery.

Medications

Chemotherapy	Before or after surgery and/or radiation.

Lifestyle changes

Stop smoking	Cuts risk of recurrence; improves health.
Get support	To help with emotional issues; depression.
Improve diet	Eat small protein- and calorie-packed meals.

lymph nodes or traveled to other parts of the body. There are four stages (I–IV) for non-small cell lung cancer, and two (limited and extensive) for small cell cancer. The earlier the stage for either type, the better your long-term outlook (*see table opposite*).

Treatments

With early stage non-small cell cancer, the goal is to remove the tumor and cure the cancer. While treatment can't cure cancer that has spread outside the lungs, it can control symptoms: This is called palliative care. With secondary lung cancer, you will be treated for the primary tumor and the lung tumor. The tools of lung cancer treatment are surgery, radiation therapy, chemotherapy, and clinical trials. Your doctor will recommend one or a combination.

Procedures

If you have early-stage non-small cell cancer and good lung function, your treatment is likely to begin with **surgery.** Some Stage I and II lung tumors can be completely removed with surgery alone. For other tumors, surgery may be just the first step, followed by radiation, chemotherapy, or investigative treatments in clinical trials. In a few cases, localized small cell cancers can be eliminated with one of several surgical procedures (*see illustration, page 206*).

Newer techniques help control symptoms. **Laser therapy** uses intense light to destroy cancer cells. If the tumor is small, you may be a candidate for **photodynamic therapy (PDT).** Your doctor will inject the light-sensitive drug porfimer sodium (Photofrin), which stays in the cancer cells. A laser activates it to kill the abnormal cells. Both procedures are used to eradicate tumors blocking an airway.

In addition to surgery, or in place of it, you may be given **radiation therapy,** which uses high-energy rays to kill cancer cells.

TAKING Control

- **Use a thoracic surgeon** (one who specializes in chest procedures) if you're scheduled for surgery. One study showed a much higher mortality rate when surgery is performed by general surgeons rather than by specialists.

- **Look for high volume.** If you're having lung surgery, choose a hospital where many lung cancer surgeries are performed. Researchers who analyzed lung cancer patients' records from 76 hospitals found that the more lung surgeries performed at a hospital, the longer patients survived.

- **Get relief from pain.** If your pain isn't well controlled, don't hesitate to talk with your doctor about more effective painkillers. Surveys show that 42% of people with cancer aren't adequately treated for pain, although 95% could get relief.

▶**Could I have a genetic tendency to develop lung cancer?**

Preliminary studies say it's possible. Researchers have found that people with mutations in the p53 gene have an increased risk for lung cancer if they smoke. This gene, a tumor-suppressor, is needed to repair DNA damage, or if there's too much damage, trigger cells to "commit suicide." When this process goes awry, cancer can occur. Variations in the p53 gene have been found most often in African- Americans, which may explain in part why this group has the highest lung cancer rates in the United States.

Promising
DEVELOPMENTS

■ A recent study offers new hope for people who have small cell lung cancer. Patients who took a combination of **CPT-11** (Camptosar or irinotecan) and **cisplatin** had a 55% improvement in one-year survival rates and were four times more likely to live two years than those who used the standard treatment of cisplatin and etoposide. This is the first trial to show a dramatic benefit for people with this type of cancer.

■ Doctors are very excited about **spiral computed tomography,** or spiral CT scan. In one study of 1,000 people at high risk for lung cancer, this new technique for detecting lung tumors earlier, found 23 early-stage tumors; standard chest x-rays picked up only four. All but one of the malignancies was removed successfully. Studies are under way to determine if this therapy should be used for widespread screening.

Radiation serves several purposes. Before surgery, it can shrink your tumor. After surgery, it may aid in killing any cancer left in lymph nodes. If you have early-stage non-small cell cancer but can't undergo surgery, radiation may even eliminate the tumor. For Stage III and IV small cell cancer and for cancer recurrence, radiation can shrink tumors and reduce symptoms such as pain, bleeding, and difficulty swallowing. When combined with chemotherapy, it lengthens survival in people with limited small cell lung cancer. Lung cancer that has spread to the brain may be treated with radiation (*see Brain Tumor, page 54*). Try to find a facility that uses a CT scan to guide the procedure. It shields the unaffected lung from unnecessary radiation.

If a tumor obstructs a tube leading to the lungs (a bronchus), your doctor may suggest **brachytherapy** in which radioactive seeds are inserted directly into the tumor site for a few minutes. Laser therapy and photodynamic therapy are also options, but rarely cure such a cancer. When cancer has spread, the best treatment may be **external-beam radiation,** which uses several beams of radiation from outside the body. A newer technique, called **3-D conformal radiation therapy,** provides a three-dimensional image of the tumor for the doctor to target. That makes it easier to avoid damaging normal tissue. Your doctor may order **continuous hyperfractionated accelerated radiotherapy (CHART)** for certain tumors, a regimen of two to three daily treatments that reduce the overall length of treatment. In one study, people with localized cancer who had CHART had a 24% lower death rate than those getting standard radiation.

Medications

With Stage I or II cancer, surgery to remove the growth may eliminate the need for **chemotherapy** (oral or intravenously administered

SURGICAL OPTIONS FOR LUNG CANCER

1) Wedge resection

tumor and tiny part of lobe removed

2) Segment resection

tumor and large part of lobe removed

3) Lobectomy

tumor and whole lobe removed

4) Pneumonectomy

entire lung removed

The extent of lung cancer surgery usually depends on the size of the tumor and how much it has spread. **1)** For very small tumors, a wedge resection procedure removes only a part of the lobe that contains the tumor. **2)** If the tumor is bigger, segment resection removes a larger part of a lobe. **3)** For a larger mass, a lobectomy removes one lobe of the lung (your right lung has three lobes and the left has two). **4)** A pneumonectomy, performed when a lobectomy cannot be done, removes one entire lung (you need only one lung to live).

Clinical Trials for Lung Cancer

Clinical trials are research studies on new drugs and procedures as well as new ways to use existing therapies. By taking part in a clinical trial you may benefit from cutting-edge research before treatments are widely available. For information on clinical trials, talk with your oncologist or visit the National Institutes of Health's website, www.clinicaltrials.gov.

Clinical trials for lung cancer include these categories:

- **Chemotherapy.** Some studies are examining if chemotherapy drugs now in use may work better combined with other drugs. Other studies investigate the most effective combinations of drugs and radiation. Still others look at the best ways to reduce chemo side effects.

- **Immunotherapy.** "Active immunotherapy" tests vaccines that force your immune system to treat substances in lung cancer cells as invaders, then kill them. "Passive immunotherapy" uses injections of manmade antibodies with toxins attached. The antibodies seek out lung cancer cells, which the hitchhiking toxins kill.

- **Gene therapy.** Researchers are studying ways to introduce extra DNA into lung cancer cells so your immune system can better recognize these abnormal cells and destroy them.

- **Biological therapies.** New drugs that interfere with the growth of lung tumors are being tested. One group, the angiogenesis inhibitors, prevents blood vessels from developing to nourish cancer cells. Another group (growth factor receptors) is intended to block hormone-like substances that signal cells to grow and divide. By blocking the receptors, they hinder the growth of cancer cells. Some of these drugs have already been approved to treat other types of cancer.

---

cancer-cell killing drugs) to ensure a good chance at survival. At later stages, however, chemotherapy can help by eradicating microscopic nests of cancer in other parts of the body. Chemotherapy is the standard method for temporarily controlling small cell lung cancer, which is notorious for spreading. It may also be used to reduce symptoms in the advanced stages of non-small cell lung cancer. Typically, cisplatin (Platinol) or carboplatin (Paraplatin), both platinum compounds, are combined with other drugs, including etoposide (VePesid) and paclitaxel (Taxol). Chemotherapy often causes temporary nausea, fatigue, and hair loss, and can make you more prone to infections. Drugs can minimize these side effects.

Many people experience pain from lung cancer treatments or from the spread of the disease. If this occurs, ask your doctor for **painkilling medications.** If you can't use or don't want standard treatment, consider joining a **clinical trial** (*see box above*).

Lifestyle Changes

One good way to have an active hand in your own treatment is to commit yourself to the following strategies:

- **Quit smoking.** It will make your treatment more effective, improve your overall health, and cut your risk of recurrence.
- **Get support.** When you have lung cancer, you'll encounter emotional and practical issues that you shouldn't try to deal with alone. Seek support from family, friends, a therapist, or a cancer support group.
- **Don't ignore depression.** Lung cancer and the rigors of treatment can add up to depression. Talk with your doctor about treating it.
- **Eat a nutrient-rich diet.** You may not have a big appetite, so eat lots of small meals packed with protein and calories.

FINDING Support

- For up-to-date information on lung cancer treatments, contact the National Cancer Institute (1-800-4-CANCER or www.nci.nih.gov).

- The Alliance for Lung Cancer Advocacy, Support, and Education in Vancouver, WA, offers a host of support services to people with lung cancer, including contact information for support groups around the country and phone buddies (a peer-to-peer support program). Call their hotline at 1-800-298-2436 or visit their website at www.alcase.org.

Lupus

As little as 50 years ago, only half the people diagnosed with lupus were alive four years later. Today, you can live with this chronic disease in relative comfort for many years, thanks to medical progress and numerous treatment options.

LIKELY **First Steps**

- With your physician, **development of a treatment regimen** for the disease.
- **Lifestyle choices** to keep the disease in remission as long as possible.
- **OTC and prescription medications** to relieve joint pain, fever, rashes, and other symptoms.
- **Steroids** to control inflammation and flares.
- If needed, **specialized procedures** for complications.

QUESTIONS TO **Ask**

- How can I avoid setting off lupus flares?
- Is there any medicine I can take instead of steroids?
- What are the chances I will need dialysis or a kidney transplant someday?
- Will I need to make big changes in my life because I have lupus?

What is happening

Doctors in medieval times named this disease lupus because its hallmark facial rash reminded them of a wolf bite ("lupus" is Latin for wolf). Not everyone with lupus develops this inflammation, however. Other symptoms might include achy swollen joints, fever, headache, extreme fatigue, and skin rashes aggravated by sunlight on other parts of your body. Lupus can also lead to more serious problems, such as anemia, inflammation of the lungs or heart, and serious neurological problems. About half of those with this kind of systemwide (systemic) disease develop kidney complications.

These symptoms may seem disconnected, but they all originate in your immune system, which creates antibodies to fight infection. When you have lupus, your immune system turns against you, creating antibodies that attack your vital organs. These antibodies react with your own tissues. They form protein clumps called immune complexes, which build up and cause inflammation, tissue damage, and pain where they lodge. The most common form of lupus, systemic lupus erythematosus (SLE), can affect nearly every organ or body system. While the course of SLE is unpredictable, you can count on periodic flare-ups (called flares by specialists) followed by periods of remission which might last for months. Another form, discoid lupus erythematosus (DLE), primarily makes the skin blotchy (see box, page 210).

The cause of lupus is unknown, but scientists think genetics sets the stage for sensitivities you develop later. Then, an unknown trigger—maybe an infection, antibiotics, ultraviolet light, or even hormones—unleashes your first lupus flare. You are more likely to get this disease if you are a woman between ages 15 and 45, and African-American, Asian, Hispanic, or Native American. On a brighter note, along with the rest of the million-plus Americans with lupus, you are likely to see a normal lifespan.

Treatments

The key to controlling lupus is to work with your doctor (usually a rheumatologist) to develop a plan to control symptoms. Your goals are to prevent flares, promptly treat those that occur, and prevent complications affecting your vital organs. In many cases, it's possible to keep a steady course with healthy lifestyle choices. When your disease does flare, a number of prescription and OTC medications are useful for quickly getting it under control and eas-

Treatment options

Lifestyle changes

Watch for flares	Early treatment minimizes damage.
Treat infections	Lupus makes you more susceptible.
Exercise	Builds strength and endurance.
Avoid sun & allergens	Either can trigger a flare.

Medications

Corticosteroids	Oral or IV for flares; topical for rashes.
NSAIDs	OTC/prescription for pain and inflammation.
Antimalarial drugs	Good for discoid lupus and skin problems.
Immunosuppressants	For severe flares or complications.

Procedures

Physical therapy	Strengthens weak, painful joints.
Plasmapheresis	Removes harmful antibodies from the blood.

ing milder symptoms. For serious complications, specialized therapies or even a kidney transplant may be required.

Lifestyle Changes

Bad habits certainly don't cause lupus, but good habits can help keep this disorder in check.

- **Be alert for the first signs of a flare.** Episodes are likely to follow a pattern. If you recognize a symptom—fatigue, joint pain, or feverishness—treat it promptly. This can minimize discomfort.
- **Get plenty of rest.** Sleep at least 10 hours a night, longer during a flare. When your body says it needs to rest, listen!
- **Treat infections ASAP.** Lupus and the drugs that control it make you more prone to strep throat, yeast infections, and viruses. At the first sign of any infection, contact your doctor.
- **Exercise within your limits.** It may seem counterintuitive, but exercise can make you feel less tired by building up your physical strength and endurance. Walking is energizing, but other good choices are swimming, water aerobics, and bicycling.
- **Keep stress to a minimum.** It worsens symptoms. Look into meditation, deep-breathing exercises, and other relaxation techniques.
- **Stay out of the sun.** Sunlight or ultraviolet (UV) light can bring on a flare. When you go outdoors, wear a sunscreen of SPF 15 or higher, and cover up with a hat and long sleeves.
- **Avoid allergens.** Hair dye, makeup, and drugs can cause lupus to flare.
- **Consult your doctor about pregnancy.** Having lupus can present special risks, both to an unborn baby and to you. Get the facts about minimizing these hazards before you try to conceive.

TAKING Control

- **Know your pain relievers.** Although acetaminophen (Tylenol) may help you with pain and is kind to your stomach, it doesn't reduce inflammation. You may need to test several different NSAID analgesics, such as aspirin, ibuprofen, and the prescription drug sulindac (Clinoril), to find which ones work best for you.

- **Get enlightened about light.** Ultraviolet-emitting lights (like those in tanning salons) may trigger flares. Standard fluorescent office lights won't: The National Electrical Manufacturers Association says eight hours' exposure yields the UV equivalent of just one minute under the July sun in Washington, D.C.

▶ Can prescription drugs cause lupus?

Lupus symptoms can develop as a side effect of certain medications, but this occurs in fewer than 10% of people who take such drugs long term. Possible culprits include arrhythmia medications procainamide (Procan, Procanbid) and quinidine (Quinaglute, Cin-Quin); blood-pressure drugs hydralazine (Apresoline, Unipres) and methyldopa (Aldoclor, Aldoril); the tranquilizer chlorpromazine (Thorazine); and the tuberculosis drug isoniazid (INH, Rifater). This form of lupus usually does no damage to the kidneys or nervous system. Symptoms typically fade within weeks or months of stopping the drug that caused them.

Promising
DEVELOPMENTS

- One of the newer treatments in the research pipeline, **LJP 394** targets damage factors more closely than ever before. This immune-regulating drug attaches to lupus-generated double-stranded DNA antibodies and ushers them out of the system. Researchers at Long Island's North Shore University Hospital found that LJP 394 reduced these antibodies by nearly 40% and was especially helpful for people with kidney complications.

- **Leflunomide (Arava),** an anti-inflammatory drug already used to treat rheumatoid arthritis (another autoimmune disease common in women), may have a new place in lupus treatment. In a study done at Cedars-Sinai Medical Center in Los Angeles, 10 of 14 participants taking leflunomide showed measurable improvement. Several were able to reduce their prednisone dose without causing a flare.

FINDING Support

- For the latest information on lupus and its treatments, and help finding a support group or a doctor in your area, contact the Lupus Foundation of America in Rockville, MD (1-800-558-0121 or www.lupus.org).

- If you'd like to talk with a specially trained registered nurse about your lupus care, contact the National Jewish Medical and Research Center for Immunology and Respiratory Medicine in Denver, CO (1-800-222-LUNG or www.njc.org).

Discoid Lupus

About 20% of people with lupus have discoid lupus erythematosus (DLE), also known as cutaneous lupus because it's confined to the skin. Its most distinctive symptom (small disk-shaped red patches on the cheeks, nose, scalp, ears, and elsewhere) usually responds well to topical steroids. If your rash is widespread, resistant, or in a tough-to-treat location such as the mouth, you may need oral steroids or immunosuppressant drugs.

Avoid making your DLE worse by treating sores promptly; they tend to spread and scar your skin if left alone. Avoid the sun, use sunscreen, and stay away from tanning salons. DLE doesn't usually affect your internal organs, and chances of it evolving into SLE are less than 1 in 10.

Medications

If you're having a flare, you'll need an **oral or intravenous corticosteroid** such as prednisone (Deltasone) or methylprednisolone (Medrol). These drugs reduce inflammation and slow your overactive immune system, bringing on a remission. High doses over long periods of time may have potentially serious side effects. However, your doctor will work to find the lowest possible dose. **Nonsteroidal anti-inflammatory drugs (NSAIDs)**—aspirin, ibuprofen (Motrin), naproxen (Aleve), and the prescription sulindac (Clinoril)—also reduce inflammation and relieve fevers. If these medicines upset your stomach, take them with meals, milk, an antacid, or a prostaglandin drug such as misoprostol (Cytotec). Or check out the newer **COX-2 inhibitors**—celecoxib (Celebrex) and rofecoxib (Vioxx)—which block stomach-inflaming substances.

If angry skin rashes are a problem, **topical cortisone** can be used short term. **Antimalarial drugs,** such as hydroxychloroquine (Plaquenil) or quinacrine (Atabrine), help relieve skin and joint symptoms and fever and are particularly effective for discoid lupus. However, they can damage your retinas, so have regular eye exams.

Immunosuppressant drugs, such as azathioprine (Imuran) and mycophenolate mofetil (CellCept), are used to treat severe flares in patients with kidney problems or other complications. These drugs are reserved for serious situations because the price for this firepower may be a reduced number of white blood cells, a susceptibility to infections, and other adverse reactions.

Procedures

If your joints are chronically weak and painful, **physical therapy** may help restore their range of motion and strength. If your blood tests show antiphospholipid antibody syndrome, in which antibodies react against a fat molecule found in cell membranes, a procedure called **plasmapheresis** (blood plasma exchange) can remove the harmful antibodies from your blood.

Lyme disease

If a tick becomes your blood brother, you could be infected with the *Borrelia* bacteria. But even if Lyme disease leaves its mark, a month-long course of potent antibiotics is likely to soon get you out of the woods.

What is happening

If you've got Lyme disease, you were recently host to an uninvited guest: an eight-legged tick, about the size of a poppy seed. It fell or climbed onto your skin and most likely hung on for 24 hours or more, feeding on your blood. While there, it infected you with spiral-shaped bacteria called *Borrelia burgdorferi,* which it probably picked up from a mouse or deer.

Although the ailment's common name comes from the Connecticut towns of Lyme and Old Lyme, site of a newsmaking outbreak in 1975, **Lyme disease** has been seen all over the United States and in many countries around the world. But that doesn't mean it is spread from person to person. You can get it only from a tick bite, and even in the areas where *Borrelia* is detected, just one or two of every 100 ticks carry the bacteria.

Symptoms change as the bacteria make themselves at home in your body's tissues. A few days to a month after you've been bitten, you may get a red rash or one resembling a bull's-eye, which burns rather than itches, or you may have no symptoms at all. With or without the rash, you might feel like you have the flu, with chills and fever, fatigue, and a headache.

If you don't have either of these early warning signs (20% to 50% of those with Lyme disease don't), your first symptom will probably be arthritis: aching, swelling joints, often with muscle pain early on or even months after you've been bitten. In rare cases untreated disease causes serious and prolonged complications, including meningitis, memory and concentration problems, heart arrhythmias, Bell's palsy (temporary facial paralysis), and pain in the lower spine. If you're diagnosed and treated soon after getting Lyme disease, it's very unlikely you'll have these problems.

In a small number of cases, symptoms persist even after treatment. This condition, known as **post-Lyme disease syndrome (PLDS),** is the subject of hot debate. Some experts believe Lyme disease requires much more aggressive treatment than is usually given. Others think people with lasting symptoms were misdiagnosed to begin with, and actually have some other health problem such as fibromyalgia. A third school of thought is that even if wiped out by treatment, *Borrelia* sometimes brings on an autoimmune disorder in which the body mistakes its own cells for the Lyme bacteria and attacks them. Scientists continue to pursue the answers to this puzzle.

LIKELY First Steps

- **Oral antibiotics** taken for 14 to 28 days.
- **OTC pain relievers** to reduce flulike symptoms and joint stiffness.
- For nerve problems and severe joint pain, **long-term treatment with oral or intravenous antibiotics**.
- If heart arrhythmia develops, temporary use of a cardiac **pacemaker**.

QUESTIONS TO Ask

- Should I take antibiotics every time I get bitten by a tiny tick, or wait to see if I develop symptoms of Lyme disease?
- When I'm taking the prescribed medications, will I continue to have symptoms?
- If I have joint problems, headaches, fatigue, or other lingering issues even after treatment, might I have another health problem besides Lyme disease?

TAKING **Control**

- **Take it easy until you feel better.** Nearly everyone with Lyme disease experiences fatigue. If you can, take a few days off work and rest.

- **Keep your doctor up to date on your symptoms.** You may need additional treatments if you have severe joint pain, dizziness, persistent head or neck ache, tingling sensations on your skin, muscular problems, heart arrhythmia, or depression.

- **Try Damminix to control ticks around your yard.** This pesticide-treated cotton comes in cardboard tubes (sold in hardware stores) that you put in underbrush. Mice take the cotton to line their nests, and the pesticide kills immature ticks that feed on the rodents.

The Vaccine that Vanished

A vaccine for Lyme disease called LYMErix was approved by the FDA in 1998, but taken off the market by its maker, GlaxoSmithKline, in early 2002. The vaccine had a number of drawbacks. It wasn't approved for people younger than age 15 or older than 70. For maximum effectiveness, anyone getting it needed three separate injections. Even then, it was only 68% to 80% effective in preventing Lyme disease. In some, it caused nausea and vomiting, or even the Lyme disease-like symptoms it was supposed to prevent. All this added up to a weak demand for the drug.

Treatment options

Medications

Antibiotics	Oral or IV against bacteria and complications.
OTC pain relievers	For flulike symptoms and joint pain.
Anti-inflammatories	For persistent arthritic pain.

Procedures

Fluid drainage	To ease swollen joints.
Joint replacement	For severe arthritic complications.
Pacemaker	Used short-term for arrhythmia.

Natural methods

Tai chi	To help Lyme-related joint problems.

Treatments

A short round of oral antibiotics is usually enough to treat Lyme disease. Symptoms that persist may require additional medications. If you develop arthritic joints, an extended regimen of oral antibiotics is usually required. A few people who develop serious joint or heart problems may need surgery.

Medications

If you have clear symptoms of Lyme disease, your doctor will prescribe **oral antibiotics** for two to four weeks. Among those effective for *Borrelia* are doxycycline (Doryx), amoxicillin, cefuroxime (Ceftin), and erythromycin. These can sometimes have side effects such as cramps, nausea, vomiting, and diarrhea. Let your doctor know about any reactions, and keep taking the drugs unless you're told to stop. In the meantime, reach for **OTC pain relievers** (acetaminophen or aspirin) to relieve flu-like symptoms, headache, and joint pain.

Some doctors prescribe preventive antibiotics for people with tick bites who do *not* have symptoms of Lyme disease. Many experts don't condone this practice, however, because antibiotic overuse can reduce the drugs' effectiveness. On the other hand, one study showed that a single dose of doxycycline taken within 72 hours of a tick bite was very effective in preventing Lyme disease. Ask your doctor.

If you've developed Lyme-related arthritis, your doctor may prescribe oral doxycycline for two months, or the **intravenous (IV) antibiotic** ceftriaxone for a month (this can be taken at home or as an outpatient). Although the oral medication has fewer side effects and costs less than IV antibiotics, some who take it still develop neurological Lyme symptoms, which must be treated with IV drugs. If your arthritis persists even after IV antibiotics, your doctor may suggest a nonsteroidal anti-inflammatory medication, either OTC ibuprofen or a prescription **COX-2 inhibitor** such as celecoxib (Celebrex).

Tips to Stop Ticks in Their Tracks

It's possible to get Lyme disease more than once, especially if you frequent areas where *Borrelia*-bearing ticks are prevalent. Here are some key precautions:

- **Look to your lawn.** Mow regularly, and treat it with an insecticide in the late spring or early fall. Try Pyrethrins (called permethrin in its synthetic form), which can eliminate 90% of tick infestations.
- **Dress for success.** Wear long pants tucked into high socks when you're in grassy or wooded areas. Light-colored pants and socks make it easier to spot the ticks. To kill any ticks hiding in folds or seams, put your clothing in a dryer on high heat for 30 minutes.
- **Use a strong repellent.** Look for a product that contains the insecticide DEET (N,N-diethyl-meta-toluamide) in a concentration up to 35%. Spray it on your pants, shoes, socks, and exposed skin. But never use DEET-containing products on very young children.
- **Do a thorough tick inspection.** If you're in a tick-infested area, take a shower and wash your hair as soon as you go inside. Then look over your skin carefully and ask someone to check the areas you can't see. Most ticks that carry Lyme bacteria are tiny and look like moles or freckles.
- **Remove it the right way.** Using curved, sharp-tipped tweezers, grasp the tick and pull up steadily, without twisting. Once the tick is extracted, don't touch it: Drop it into a jar of alcohol. Wash the site and dab some antibiotic ointment on it. If you want to know whether that tick carries *Borrelia* bacteria, take it to your doctor.

In the rare case that you develop neurological symptoms, you're likely to be put on IV antibiotics for 21 to 30 days. The first choice is usually ceftriaxone, but good alternatives are cefotaxime or penicillin G. Intravenous antibiotics are also used for cardiac arrhythmia.

If symptoms persist despite treatment and your doctor believes the Lyme bacteria are still hiding out in your body, you may be prescribed 30 days of IV antibiotics, followed by 30 days of oral doxycyline. But if your doctor thinks that you actually have a different ailment (such as chronic fatigue, fibromyalgia, or major depression), or that you have an autoimmune response to Lyme, other medications will be chosen to treat your symptoms.

Procedures

In those rare instances when Lyme disease creates neurological problems, cardiac arrhythmia, or severe joint pain and fatigue, surgical and nonsurgical procedures can help. If your joints are affected, **draining the joint fluid** can make you more comfortable. If a joint has been hampered by severe and persistent arthritis, your best bet to regain mobility may be **surgical replacement of that joint** (*see page 38*). For Lyme-associated heart arrhythmia, a cardiologist may implant a **pacemaker** for one or two weeks (*see page 93*).

Natural Methods*

If you have joint pain from Lyme disease, try **tai chi.** This ancient Chinese discipline incorporates meditation and deep breathing into slow-moving exercises to strengthen the muscles surrounding arthritic joints. It also improves flexibility.

Natural methods are not subject to the same testing and regulation as prescription medications. Please seek your doctor's advice and use caution.

▶ **Are there any natural supplements that will help treat Lyme disease?**
You may have heard that vitamin-B complex, magnesium, and omega-3 and omega-6 fatty acids work against Lyme disease. But when these and other supplements have been evaluated by researchers, none has been found effective for this ailment.

FINDING Support

- You can obtain extensive, up-to-date information on Lyme disease through the Lyme Disease Network (www.lymenet.org).

- For Lyme-related information of all kinds, contact the Lyme Disease Foundation in Hartford, CT (860-525-2000). Their easy-to-navigate, well-designed website is www.lyme.org.

Lymphoma

Advances in therapy have led to numerous treatment approaches for cancer of the lymphatic system. Team up with your doctors, and you have a very good chance of a long (possibly even life-long) victory in your fight against lymphoma cells.

LIKELY **First Steps**

- **Discussion of a treatment plan** with an oncologist.
- **Initiation of therapy** (radiation, chemo, and/or bone marrow transplant), depending on the particulars of your case.

QUESTIONS TO **Ask**

- What kinds of treatments are recommended for the type of lymphoma I have?

- Should I see a doctor who specializes in lymphoma or travel to a distant hospital?

- Could radiation or chemo-therapy cause other diseases?

- What clinical trials are currently underway for the type of lymphoma I have? Where are those studies being done? Should I try to enroll?

- How much time will I be spending in the hospital or clinic for treatments? How often will I have to go?

- Should I make special home-care arrangements?

- After I have completed my treatment, what kinds of symptoms should I report to you?

What is happening

Your lymphatic system is an elaborate network of vessels and white blood cells designed to defend your body against bacteria, viruses, and other disease-causing agents. Lymph nodes (or glands) strategically located throughout your body serve as boot camps for these cells, called lymphocytes. They include B-cells (because they develop in bone marrow) and T-cells (which develop in the thymus gland). Once these ace fighters leave the nodes, they patrol the entire body. Some circulate in the blood. Others gather in specific organs.

Sometimes the defenders themselves become malignant, leading to cancer of the lymphatic system. This cancer is called leukemia if it involves the blood or bone marrow (*see Leukemia, page 200*); lymphoma if it centers on lymph nodes or organs. There are two main types of lymphoma. Non-Hodgkin's lymphoma, in which cancerous B-cells or T-cells appear in your lymphatic system and proliferate, is usually more serious. About 85% of people with lymphoma have non-Hodgkin's. The other major form, Hodgkin's lymphoma (usually called Hodgkin's disease), features a distinctive type of cancer cell that appears in the lymphatic system (*see box, page 216*).

The lymphatic system affects many parts of your body, so a lot can go wrong if a malignancy develops. Lymph nodes may be tender, organs affected, and the spleen (a key site of lymphatic activity) may swell as cancer cells crowd in. Before treatment begins, you'll be referred to a cancer specialist (an oncologist) for "staging" to determine how advanced the disease is. Stages range from the mildest at Stage I (tumors are limited to a single node region) through the most advanced at Stage IV (disease has spread to other areas).

Treatments

At one time, lymphomas were fatal. But this cancer is now better understood, and sophisticated chemotherapy regimens cure many people. The treatment is largely influenced by the grade (aggressiveness) of the lymphoma. For non-Hodgkin's lymphoma, chemotherapy, radiation, and bone marrow transplants are used singly or in combination. Ask about potential side effects and outcomes for your doctor's recommended approach. Talk it over with your family as well as veterans of lymphoma, if possible. Although a specialist's recommendations carry a lot of weight, remember that you can choose whether or not to begin or continue a specific type of treatment.

Treatment options

Procedures

Radiation	Used alone or with other therapies.
Surgery	For lymphomas isolated to a single organ.
Bone marrow transplant	For more advanced lymphoma.
Clinical trials	Test new treatments.

Medications

Chemotherapy	Most common approach; kills cancer cells.

Lifestyle changes

Rest	Helps promote recovery.
Moderate exercise	Battles fatigue.
Support group	Provides practical and emotional advice.

Procedures

If your non-Hodgkin's lymphoma is low grade (nonaggressive) in Stage I or II, your doctor is likely to recommend **radiation therapy** alone. For other stages or if the lymphoma causes symptoms, radiation may be combined with chemo or other therapies. Radiation directs high-energy x-rays at tumors. There's an added risk of temporary or permanent infertility from radiation damage to sexual organs for both sexes. Consider talking with a fertility expert about **freezing sperm** or **banking eggs** before undergoing radiation.

If the lymphoma is isolated in a specific organ, **surgery** alone may cure it. When other procedures are ineffective, however, a **bone marrow transplant** may be the best route, using cells from a donor or your own. Prior to bone marrow transplant, aggressive chemo or external radiation rids the body of lymphoma cells, but the treatment also destroys healthy bone marrow cells. If you don't respond well to established treatments, ask your doctor about joining a **clinical trial** that's testing new therapies for cases like yours. You may benefit from innovations before they are widely available.

Medications

For aggressive lymphomas, your oncologist may recommend **chemotherapy,** often the treatment of choice for relapses. (Less aggressive, low-grade lymphomas are generally treated with chemo only when symptoms develop.) Given intravenously or orally, these drugs are often used in combinations, such as CVP, or cyclophosphamide (Cytoxan), vincristine (Oncovin), and prednisone.

Chemotherapy targets all fast-growing cells—not just the cancerous ones—so the side effects of these powerful drugs will affect your blood, hair, and digestive tract. In addition, chemo increases your risk for infection, and some of the chemicals may up your chances of heart failure or infertility.

TAKING Control

- **Read up.** Lymphoma is a complex disease, and there are many types. Therefore, you will need specialized books, articles, and online sources to help you understand your doctor's advice and make informed decisions about your treatment.

- **Contact siblings.** For environmental or genetic reasons, the risk of some lymphomas is higher among family members. Your brothers and sisters should know the details of your lymphoma so their doctors can be alert for any signs of onset in them.

- **Schedule frequent mammograms and other cancer screenings.** Cancers caused by lymphoma treatment aren't uncommon, so get regular screenings for diseases like colon cancer, leukemia, breast cancer, and thyroid function. Researchers at Boston's Dana Farber Cancer Institute found an increased risk of breast cancer in their eight-year study of 90 women who received radiation treatments for Hodgkin's.

- **Avoid alternative "cancer cures"** like Laetrile and Essiac. Some alternative remedies may improve your health in other ways, but there is no proof that any of these therapies is effective in treating cancer. The product promoted as Laetrile (amygdalin), found in apricot and cherry pits, does not have any measurable impact on lymphoma. Essiac contains burdock root, turkey rhubarb, slippery elm bark, and sheep sorrel. There are no studies to support claims that it has healing power, and even most alternative doctors are skeptical of it.

Promising DEVELOPMENTS

- Scientists are currently figuring out ways to use **monoclonal antibodies** (MAbs), such as rituximab (Rituxan), to single out lymphoma cells and destroy them. Other kinds of MAbs might be developed that would collect at tumor sites, triggering an immune response.

- Doctors are also testing **nucleoside analogues**, antiviral agents that have been effective against some low-grade lymphomas. Interferon-alpha is one kind of antiviral drug that seems to be successful in fighting some forms of non-Hodgkin's lymphoma.

- Lymphoma **vaccines** have shown promising results. Using specific lymphoma cells, a vaccine is created to fight the disease. The immune system destroys this antigen as it goes after look-alike lymphoma cells.

FINDING Support

- For more information, contact the Lymphoma Research Foundation in Los Angeles, CA (1-800-500-9976 or www.lymphoma.org). The website has message boards where people with lymphoma discuss therapies and share information about new breakthroughs.

- To find clinical trials worldwide, you can log on to www.clinicaltrials.gov, maintained by the National Institutes of Health. The website provides the location of the trial sites and descriptions of the types of lymphoma that are being treated.

Hodgkin's Disease

About 15% of people with lymphoma have Hodgkin's disease. It occurs most often from the late teens to early 20s, and then over age 60. It also sometimes appears in children. Doctors don't know its cause, although some suspect a virus, such as Epstein-Barr. Hereditary factors may also play a role. There are four subtypes of classic Hodgkin's disease (HD): The rarest is **lymphocyte predominance,** which grows slowly; the most common, responsible for 65% to 80% of HD cases, is **nodular sclerosis,** which has moderate growth. **Mixed cellularity** makes up 3% to 15%, and **lymphocyte depletion** accounts for less than 1%.

Reed-Sternberg cells, the cancer cells responsible for this disease, are easy to spot under the microscope, so doctors can make a quick diagnosis and zero in on specific therapies. For Stage I and II Hodgkin's disease, treatment is often radiation alone. For later-stage Hodgkin's, or situations in which the lymphoma has spread in detectable ways, it may be chemotherapy, followed by measured doses and special kinds of radiation. Many people with advanced Hodgkin's (Stage IV) can be cured with chemotherapy. The best news is that in 9 out of 10 people with early-stage Hodgkin's, treatment brings about cure.

Lifestyle Changes

Lymphoma and its treatments can deplete you physically and emotionally. The following can help you maintain your equilibrium:

- **Get as much rest as possible.** People being treated for lymphoma generally feel fatigued, yet don't sleep well due to night sweats, fever, coughing, or nausea. Plan on resting whenever you can.
- **Exercise in moderation.** Try walking, cycling, or swimming, as long as your doctor approves. One study showed that aerobic exercise significantly lessened fatigue.
- **Join a support group.** It can be helpful to talk with people having similar experiences. Your doctor can guide you to such a group, or you can correspond through online message boards and forums.

Natural Methods*

Good nutrition is always advisable, especially when your immune system is in trouble. Ask your doctor about taking a **daily multivitamin,** particularly if you are suffering from loss of appetite.

Outlook

There are many new developments in lymphoma research, and therapies are constantly being scrutinized to improve outcomes and lessen side effects.

Natural methods are not subject to the same testing and regulation as prescription medications. Please seek your doctor's advice and use caution.

Macular degeneration

Age-related macular degeneration (AMD) is the leading cause of severe vision loss among older Americans. Although the disease is not yet curable, promising new therapies in the research pipeline may be available soon.

What is happening

Roughly the size of an eraser on a pencil, the macula occupies the center of the retina in your eye. Despite its small size, it is responsible for the sharp, high-definition, central vision that allows you to read, drive, recognize faces, and distinguish fine details. When you have macular degeneration, the macula in one or both eyes has irreversibly deteriorated over time. Your vision may become blurred. A blind spot may develop in the center of your visual field, and many fine-detail activities, such as reading and writing, may become difficult or impossible to do with accustomed ease. Your peripheral vision remains intact.

No one knows what causes age-related macular degeneration (AMD), but by some estimates, about one-quarter of people over age 65 and fully one-third of those over age 80 show evidence of this condition. Nearly 90% of those with AMD have the dry (or nonexudative or atrophic) form, in which the light-sensitive cells in the macula slowly decay and yellow spots of fatty deposits called drusen appear on the macula (*see illustration below*). Dry AMD is the less severe of the two forms, progressing slowly and sometimes stabilizing for a time. You might not even notice symptoms of

LIKELY First Steps

- **Monitoring your vision** for signs of change.

- For some people, daily supplements of **high-dose antioxidants and zinc.**

- **Laser surgery or photodynamic therapy** to stop certain cases of wet AMD.

QUESTIONS TO Ask

- How often should I have the status of my AMD re-evaluated?

- What are some signs that my AMD might be worsening?

- Am I a candidate for laser surgery or photodynamic therapy?

DRY FORM OF AMD

cornea
rods and cones
retina
blood vessels
lens
drusen
Close-up of macula with AMD
macula   optic nerve

In dry macular degeneration, cells in the center of your eye's retina slowly deteriorate. Tiny yellowish fatty deposits called drusen appear and may grow over time. Vision loss is gradual, and self-care measures can help keep it in check.

- ■ **Keep up with the news about AMD.** Researchers are currently testing and developing new treatments that may turn out to be just what you need. Ask your doctor about clinical trials of therapies that might help your particular case.

- ■ **Don't be afraid to use your eyes.** Your normal activities won't make your AMD get worse. So go ahead and read, watch television, and use a computer as much as you want.

▶ **Are there measures I can take to compensate for my poor vision?**

Ask your eye doctor for a referral to a low-vision specialist or low-vision center, where you can get training in the use of low-vision aids, devices designed to help you maximize your vision and help with reading and writing (see box, page 220). Brighten your home with more illumination, and remove or secure clutter that could cause a fall. To get around outside, use miniature telescopes focused for distance vision, either mounted in your glasses or hand-held. Use protective filters and sun lenses to improve contrast and reduce glare.

Treatment options

Lifestyle changes

Vision watch	Regular checkups and home monitoring.
Healthy diet	Low in fat, high in fruits and veggies.
Avoid smoke & UV rays	Can make AMD worse.

Natural methods

Antioxidant & zinc supplements	Shown to be very helpful for people with intermediate dry AMD.

Procedures

Laser photocoagulation	Seals leaking blood vessels of wet AMD.

Medications

Photodynamic therapy	Drug/laser treatment for wet AMD.

vision loss, especially if it is restricted to one eye and your "good" eye compensates.

In the less common form, called wet (or exudative or neovascular) AMD, fine blood vessels grow beneath the retina, leaking and damaging the macula. Wet AMD progresses more quickly than dry AMD and causes more severe vision loss, sometimes within days or weeks. Left untreated, wet AMD can lead to legal blindness (defined as vision of 20/200 or worse) although not to total blindness. About 15% of people with dry AMD develop wet AMD.

Although they rarely do, young people can develop macular degeneration due to a genetic disorder or as a drug side effect. Most often, though, the condition is related to the aging process. Your odds of getting AMD are higher if you have a family history of it, or if you're female, white, and have light-colored eyes. Other risk factors include exposure to smoke and direct sunlight and conditions such as high blood pressure, high cholesterol, or obesity.

Treatments

The cause of AMD is still unknown. There is no cure for it at present and no sure way to reverse the vision loss that may result. There are no proven remedies for dry AMD, and there are treatments for only certain cases of wet AMD. Still, there is plenty of cause for optimism. AMD is currently a hot area for research, especially as the population ages and the disease becomes more prevalent. There is also growing evidence that diet and nutritional supplements can make a real difference. Further, macular degeneration does not cause total blindness. In fact, dry AMD causes no serious vision loss in most people. Even if you have the wet form, with its more severe ramifications, you'll still be able to see well enough to perform most activities of daily living.

Because having dry AMD puts you at risk for developing wet AMD, you'll need regular vision tests (*see page 367*). If wet AMD is caught early, the chances are better that it can be halted with laser surgery or a treatment called photodynamic therapy.

Lifestyle Changes

Even though effective treatments for AMD are scarce, there is much you can do on the lifestyle front to preserve the vision you have:

- **Monitor your eyes.** Your best defense against vision loss is to act promptly. See your eye doctor regularly, and monitor your eyes at home with an Amsler chart, a piece of paper with a grid of black lines (ask your doctor for one). Cover one eye at a time so you can test each eye individually. If straight lines look wavy or there is a gap in the lines, call your eye doctor at once.
- **Eat your fruits and vegetables.** The old saw that carrots are good for the eyes is true. Studies have shown that a balanced diet rich in fruits and vegetables—especially those containing carotenoids such as beta-carotene and lutein—can help preserve eye health. This means eating foods of green, red, orange, or yellow hue (tomatoes, corn, squash, kiwis, oranges), as well as green leafy vegetables.
- **Cut down on fat.** A high total fat intake is associated with increased risk of AMD. This is especially true of animal fats but also includes the omega-6 fatty acids (found in vegetable oils). There's one exception: The omega-3 fatty acids in salmon, mackerel, tuna, and other fish may help preserve your vision.
- **Keep up your health.** High blood pressure is associated with AMD. Diabetes can also affect eye health. If you have it, continue your efforts to keep your blood sugar levels under tight control.
- **Don't smoke.** People who smoke are at a greater risk for AMD, and more likely to respond poorly to laser surgery.
- **Avoid bright sunlight.** When you go outdoors, wear sunglasses that absorb all UVA and UVB radiation, and shade your eyes with a wide-brimmed hat.

Natural Methods*

In some people, nutritional supplements can help prevent AMD from progressing. The Age-Related Eye Disease Study (AREDS), a 10-year trial sponsored by the National Eye Institute, found that people with intermediate-stage dry AMD who took high-dose antioxidants and zinc supplements every day reduced their risk of advanced AMD by about 25%. The benefit was greater when both antioxidants and zinc were taken.

To get this result, you'll need daily doses higher than you can get from diet alone or from ordinary multivitamins: 80 mg of **zinc picolinate**, along with the antioxidants **vitamin C** (500 mg), **vitamin E** (400 IU), and **beta-carotene** (15 mg). You should also

Natural methods are not subject to the same testing and regulation as prescription medications. Please seek your doctor's advice and use caution.

Promising
DEVELOPMENTS

- **Steroids** may inhibit abnormal blood vessel growth in the eyes and halt progression of wet AMD, according to preliminary studies. Anecortave acetate, a modified steroid developed by Alcon Laboratories, is one candidate; another is triamcinolone (Kenalog).

- **Anti-angiogenic drugs** prevent new blood vessels from forming. They show evidence of being able to inhibit the growth of new vessels in the eyes. This would certainly help prevent wet AMD.

- Several experimental surgical procedures are very promising. One is **macular translocation**, in which the macula is moved from the diseased area of the retina to a healthier part. To restore lost vision, scientists are experimenting with **transplantation of healthy cells** into diseased retinas, and **implantation of a silicon chip** that serves as a "bionic eye."

- Experimental new medicines have had startling results in stopping vision loss, and in some cases, actually restoring the vision of people with wet AMD. One of the drugs used is **rhuFab**, made by Genentech. Most people who had injections of this medication, soon after they noticed AMD symptoms, stopped losing their sight. From one-quarter to one-third experienced significant improvement in their vision.

Easier Reading and Writing

There are a number of simple things you can do to make newspaper reading and check writing easier on your failing eyes:

- Use adjustable lamps for close work.
- Position a book or newspaper on a reading stand, and when possible, get large-print publications.
- Make type look bigger with a magnifier lamp. Consider a mobile electronic magnifier, such as the Jordy, worn like a pair of glasses. Another option is a closed-circuit television system designed to magnify and enhance type.
- Use bold-lined paper to help with writing and stencils to guide check writing and envelope addressing.
- If you're a computer user, try special screen display software or a system that converts computer text into sound.

FINDING Support

- Want the latest news on macular degeneration? The National Eye Institute in Bethesda, MD, is the lead federal agency for vision research (301-496-5248 or www.nei.nih.gov).
- The Macular Degeneration Foundation in Henderson, NV, offers information and support for those with AMD (www.eyesight.org).
- For referrals to vision rehabilitation services, contact Lighthouse International in New York, NY (1-800-829-0500 or www.lighthouse.org).

take **copper** (2 mg) to counteract the tendency of large doses of zinc to interfere with copper absorption. Bausch & Lomb offers a whole package of vitamins and minerals as **Ocuvite PreserVision,** the supplement used in the AREDS trial. If you are interested in this nutrient mix, talk with your doctor: Not everyone can benefit from it. It doesn't prevent AMD, and it doesn't keep early stages of the disease from progressing.

Supplements for **lutein** and **zeaxanthin**—both carotenoids like beta-carotene—are widely used by people with AMD, but their ability to prevent or slow down this ailment are still unproven. Taking beta-carotene in high doses (without other carotenoids) may actually increase a smoker's risk of developing lung cancer.

Procedures

If you have wet AMD, your doctor may use laser surgery to seal the leaking blood vessels under your macula. This outpatient procedure, known as **laser photocoagulation,** takes about half an hour and requires only local anesthesia. However, it is recommended for only a small percentage of people with wet AMD. Leaking vessels the doctor can't see are called occult (hidden). Laser photocoagulation is not an option for people who have them, nor is it advised if the leakage has reached the central part of the macula (called the fovea), an area the laser would damage.

The procedure works best on newly formed, well-demarcated vessels clustered in a specific area. To locate the vessels, your doctor will use a procedure called **fluorescein angiography,** in which a dye called fluorescein is injected into your arm and circulates through your eyes. If you have this treatment, the laser will cause some vision loss, but less than if you were completely untreated. Such surgery can halt the progress of wet AMD, but can't restore lost vision, and there is at least a 50% chance that the disease will recur. If this happens, it can be treated with more laser surgery.

In **photodynamic therapy,** a drug is injected, then activated by a laser to seal the leaking vessels. This process has an advantage over standard laser surgery: The laser in photodynamic therapy uses much less heat, and so is less likely to damage healthy eye tissue. Like laser surgery, however, photodynamic therapy does not restore vision or cure wet AMD. It may need to be repeated. It is approved only for patients whose new blood vessel growth is deemed "predominantly classic," or plainly apparent, which is true of 40% to 60% of patients. Studies are under way to see if it can help people whose blood vessel growth is hidden.

Medications

The first-ever drug therapy for wet AMD was recently approved by the FDA. Here's how it works: A medication called **verteporfin (Visudyne)** is injected into your arm and absorbed by the abnormal blood vessels in your eye. Then photodynamic therapy (*see above*) is performed. In clinical trials using Visudyne, 67% of people found their vision loss halted after this therapy.

Memory loss

If those "senior moments" are occuring more often, don't get too upset: It's probably just natural age-related memory loss. Treatment can be as easy as exercise classes, nutritional supplements, or a simple change in your diet.

What is happening

Most age-related memory loss is normal. Still, it's hard not to be a bit concerned when you suddenly have trouble remembering your best friend's first name or have misplaced your house keys for the umpteenth time. So what is really going on upstairs? Why isn't your brain as sharp as it used to be? One theory is that there's a slowdown in the production of neurotransmitters— the chemicals that relay signals between the approximately 100 billion nerve cells (neurons) in your brain. Another suggests that as you age, blood flow to your brain is reduced—up to 20% by the time you're 70. More mundane causes are probably responsible for why you have no remembrance of things past. Inadequate nutrition, lack of sleep or exercise, hormone imbalances, your medication mix, blood pressure problems, and stress can all contribute to reduced recall. Depression is also a mind-muddler.

While forgetting where you left your keys is nothing to worry about, not knowing what your keys are used for should be a cause for concern. Persistent inability to recall familiar facts, failure to navigate known surroundings, or repeating the same question and forgetting the answer could all signal the onset of what's called mild cognitive impairment (MCI). Individuals with MCI (which doesn't seem to affect perception, abstract reasoning, or language) are 10 times more likely to develop Alzheimer's disease than the general population. The good news is that if you're concerned about your memory, it's unlikely that you're in the first stages of Alzheimer's (*see page 28*).

Another bit of good news is that scientists now believe that your brain cells are simply shrinking, not dying off, as previously thought. Recent research shows that even if you're older, you may be generating some healthy new cells in your hippocampus, the seahorse-shaped part of your brain that houses your memories.

Treatments

If your memory problems are the natural result of aging, there's plenty you can do to keep yourself on the ball well into your 70s and 80s. In fact, evidence strongly suggests that making some basic lifestyle changes can go a long way toward preserving, and even boosting, your mental capacity. Studies show that the old "use it or lose it" adage really holds true. Your doctor probably won't

LIKELY First Steps

- **Rule out underlying ailments.** Have your thyroid levels checked.

- **Adopt lifestyle changes**—improve diet, get more exercise, and challenge your brain.

- **Drugs** may be necessary for mild cognitive impairment (MCI) or hormonal problems.

QUESTIONS TO Ask

- Can you tell if my memory problem is early Alzheimer's?

- Could my memory loss be related to depression?

▶ **EAT MORE BLUEBERRIES (MAYBE).** A study conducted at Tufts University found that blueberries reversed mental decline in elderly rats. The animals were better able to remember the correct path through a maze after having their diets supplemented with blueberry extract for two months. Although there are plenty of good reasons to eat blueberries whenever you can, keep in mind that what smartens up lab rats may not have the same effect in humans.

TAKING Control

■ **Systematize your life.** Getting organized can do wonders for your memory. Hang up a key rack, keep a journal or appointment log, and scrupulously maintain to-do lists.

■ **Keep your brain agile.** This means regularly challenging yourself. Take up a foreign language. Play word games. Do complicated jigsaw puzzles, or learn to play the tuba. It doesn't so much matter what you do as long as you set out to actively participate in some mentally invigorating activities.

■ **Learn a few tricks** to stimulate recall. Try saying what you're doing out loud while you're doing it ("I'm unplugging the electric curlers!"). Or come up with good associations (think of a whirling eddy when you're introduced to someone named "Eddie"). MRI scans have shown that elderly people who are taught to use memory-enhancing tricks recruit more parts of their brains during word memorization tests.

■ **Decrease your use of non-prescription medications.** Overuse of OTC drugs may be the single biggest cause of memory loss or confusion in older adults.

■ **Try meditation.** This age-old technique has been found to heighten ability to focus and concentrate, and improve creativity and problem-solving.

■ **Break with routine.** You can stimulate new neurons by simply brushing your teeth with your nondominant hand or using a map to find a location instead of asking directions.

Treatment options

Lifestyle changes

Healthy diet	Low-fat; high in B vitamins and antioxidants.
Exercise	Gets blood to brain; increases brain activity.
Brain stimulation	Preserves nerve cells.

Medications

HRT	If brain fog is attributed to menopause.
Galantamine	Stimulates neurotransmitter acetylcholine.
NSAIDs	May work to prevent brain inflammation.

Natural methods

Supplements	Stimulate various brain functions.

need to prescribe drugs unless you have memory problems related to hormone deficiencies or MCI.

Lifestyle Changes

One good way to boost your brain power is to eat a **well-balanced, low-fat diet** (with only 20% of your daily calories from fat). An analysis of 19 studies on the effect of diet on memory loss found that a high calorie consumption added to a high fat intake was a risk factor for cognitive decline. In addition to diet, **exercise** can do wonders for your mental agility. Because your brain requires more oxygen than any other organ (it uses 25% of the oxygen taken in by the lungs), brain cells need a continuous supply of oxygen-laden blood. Regular, vigorous aerobic exercise (a brisk 30-minute walk, for example, at least three times per week) not only gets blood heading to your brain: It also increases levels of trophic factors, naturally occurring proteins, necessary for healthy brain functioning. If you really want to stay on the ball, you must also **exercise the brain itself.** (See "Taking Control," at left, for some key ways to do this.)

Medications

There are no "official" drug remedies for mild age-related memory lapses, but some physicians prescribe useful drugs that were originally approved for other diseases. This "off-label" use means that it's fine for your doctor to prescribe a particular drug for memory, but that the manufacturing company isn't allowed to advertise it for this purpose. Your doctor may also prescribe drugs if your brain fog is due to an underlying condition, such as an underactive thyroid. Keep in mind that the side effects of certain drugs may prove more problematic than your memory loss.

■ **Galantamine.** Known to raise levels of the neurotransmitter acetylcholine, galantamine has for years been available over the counter and used by many people as a "smart drug." In 2001, the FDA approved prescription-strength galantamine (Reminyl) for treating mild to moderate Alzheimer's disease. Some doctors now prescribe it "off label" for age-related memory loss. Like other powerful Alzheimer's drugs, galantamine can cause nausea, vomiting, and diarrhea, and should be used only under a doctor's supervision. If you have been diagnosed with MCI and are at risk for developing Alzheimer's, you may also want to consider other drugs to forestall its progression (*see Alzheimer's Disease, page 28*).

- **NSAIDs.** Some studies show that patients taking nonsteroidal anti-inflammatory drugs (NSAIDs) such as Celebrex (usually prescribed for arthritis) are at reduced risk for memory loss and dementia. (It is also conjectured that because Alzheimer's may represent a brain inflammation, NSAIDs may keep it in check.)

Natural Methods*

To supplement your diet, your doctor may recommend that you take a daily **multivitamin/mineral supplement** as well as an antioxidant complex. A study published in the *Journal of the American Medical Association* showed that individuals using daily antioxidants (especially vitamins C and E) had some protection from developing Alzheimer's. Because many people over age 50 are deficient in vitamin B_{12}, which is essential for healthy brain functioning, taking extra B_{12} may be a good idea. The herb **ginkgo biloba** may improve cerebral blood flow and act as an antioxidant and anti-inflammatory. Most trials have used 120 to 160 mg of ginkgo biloba extract a day, divided into three doses.

Huperzine A, a Chinese medicinal herb, has been reported to help people who produce insufficient amounts of the neurotransmitter acetylcholine. Take it in doses of 50 mcg twice a day. In addition, **phosphatidylserine (PS)** supplements may increase levels of neurotransmitters, if you've been diagnosed with mild cognitive impairment (it doesn't appear to work for those who simply want to improve already good memory). In one 12-week study of 149 adults ages 50 to 75, those who took 300 mg of PS a day were better able to learn and recall names, faces, and numbers than those taking a placebo.

The Brain Chain

When you think of your dog, you may not be drawing up the memory from a discrete, tidy part of your brain. Researchers from the University of Arkansas for Medical Sciences suggest an elaborate choreography of electrical rhythms may pull up the memory of Fido from diverse brain sites responsible for recalling how your dog smells, looks, and sounds.

The researchers say that the thalamus portion of the brain acts as a sort of switchboard operator for the electrical rhythms that, ideally, cause the different brain regions to work together. It might be a disruption in these rhythms that makes you unable to access the name of something or someone, they suggest.

Patients with memory loss may not be "losing" information so much as experiencing glitches in the elaborate circuitry of neurotransmitters that connect the different regions of the brain. That would explain, the researchers say, why you are able to remember names with ease at certain times, but at other times be at a complete—and embarrassing—loss.

FINDING Support

- For the latest research on memory loss, check out these websites: www.memorylossonline.com and www.earlymemoryloss.com.

Natural methods are not subject to the same testing and regulation as prescription medications. Please seek your doctor's advice and use caution.

Menopause

Menopause is your body's adjustment to a downshift in hormones. Because of recent concerns about hormone replacement therapy (HRT), now may be the time to consider natural options such as soy foods, herbs, and exercise.

LIKELY **First Steps**

- **Talk with your doctor** to determine whether low-dose, short-term HRT or other symptom-related medications are right for you.

- **Make dietary changes** (low-fat, high-fiber diet, rich in calcium and soy foods) to maintain a healthy weight, protect bones, and control symptoms.

- **Get regular exercise,** with a focus on weight-bearing activities for stronger bones.

QUESTIONS TO **Ask**

- Could low-dose, short-term HRT be good for me?

- Will using HRT after years of birth control increase my risk for breast cancer?

- Is my failing memory a symptom of menopause?

- Can I still get pregnant now that I'm going through menopause?

What is happening

Strictly speaking, a woman is in menopause when her ovaries stop producing estrogen and progesterone, and she hasn't had a menstrual period for a full year. This signifies the end of a natural ability to bear children. The average age most women experience menopause is 51 (although it can occur as early as your late 30s or as late as your 60s). The loss of hormones is usually gradual, often beginning a decade earlier. This time frame is now commonly known as perimenopause.

As estrogen levels decline, many women begin to experience some decidedly unpleasant symptoms: an intense heat, flushing, and sweating known as hot flashes (felt by 75% of women), night sweats, insomnia, vaginal dryness, less interest in sex, mental fuzziness, and/or mood changes. These symptoms may be subtle and short-lived, ending after just a few months, or you may experience several years of sudden sweats, sleep loss, and surliness. Once your body adjusts to the hormone reduction, though, symptoms diminish.

Decreased hormone levels can have long-term effects. After your final period, estrogen declines rapidly, as does your body's ability to absorb bone-building calcium. This leaves you more vulnerable to a thinning of the bones known as osteoporosis (*see page 242*). Almost half of women over age 50 are at risk for this condition. Left untreated, it can result in an annual 3% loss of bone during the first five postmenopausal years (after that, bone loss continues at a rate of 1% to 2% a year). Reduced estrogen also raises levels of blood cholesterol, which may explain increased risk for cardiovascular disease and heart attack in postmenopausal women.

Treatments

There's no doubt that the drop in female hormones during menopause profoundly affects your body, but don't make the mistake of thinking of menopause as a "disease." Menopause may actually bring about a feeling of freedom—namely, freedom from menstruation and concerns about contraception. Still, for many women, menopause can be decidedly uncomfortable, and it can carry with it the potential for future health problems.

Until recently, the most widely prescribed treatment for women experiencing unbearable hot flashes, irritability, insomnia, and other menopausal symptoms was hormone replacement. Doctors believed that resupplying a woman's body with estrogen not only offered

Treatment options

Medications

| Hormone replacement | HRT (low-dose, short-term) for severe symptoms; ERT if you've had a hysterectomy. |
| Bisphosphonates/SERMs | Alternatives to HRT for bone protection. |

Lifestyle changes

Better diet	Helps symptoms, strengthens bones; try soy.
Exercise	Protects bones; Kegels tone pelvic muscles.
Support group	To improve self-esteem; combat depression.

Natural methods

| Supplements | Vitamins and herbs to lessen symptoms. |
| Acupuncture | Relieves symptoms in some women. |

short-term symptom relief, but provided lasting protection against osteoporosis and heart disease. New research proves that long-term use of hormones may not be safe. Many women are opting for natural treatment approaches.*

Whichever treatment you choose, your personal health profile must be a key factor in your decision. If you have a history of breast cancer or heart trouble, for instance, your treatment may be different from another woman's. What works for your best friend, your neighbor—or even your sister—may not be right (or even safe) for you. Look to your doctor for help in reviewing the pros and cons of the treatments you're considering.

Medications

For more than 50 years, the first-line drug treatment for menopausal symptoms has been supplemental hormones. Estrogen alone ("unopposed estrogen"), known as **estrogen replacement therapy (ERT)**, was the earliest option. Later, estrogen in combination with progestin (a form of progesterone), known as **hormone replacement therapy (HRT),** became the choice for most women. Today the benefits of both have been studied and re-evaluated. Because unopposed estrogen can increase the risk of cancer of the uterus, it is now recommended for treating symptoms only in women whose uterus has been removed (hysterectomy). Its long-term risks are still being examined: One study showed that estrogen alone increased a woman's chance of developing cancer of the ovaries.

HRT, which was used by more than 12 million menopausal women at its peak, has also suffered a setback. In July 2002, the Women's Health Initiative, a planned 8½-year study investigating the long-term effects of the popular HRT drug Prempro on more than 16,000 postmenopausal women, was stopped abruptly after only five years. As expected, researchers found a slightly increased

TAKING Control

■ **Dress for success.** Pull on layers of breathable cotton garments—a tank top, T-shirt, or cardigan—that can be easily removed when a hot flash hits. You also might want to sleep on cotton sheets, which wick away moisture better than polyester ones.

■ **Breathe from your belly.** Deep-breathing exercises, such as inhaling slowly through your nose and down to your belly, have been shown to reduce hot flashes by 50%.

■ **Use drops for dry eyes.** Women on ERT may be at greater risk for dry eye syndrome, according to a study of 25,000 postmenopausal women. The longer the therapy continued, the greater the risk.

■ **Stay sexually active.** Regular intercourse increases the tone and lubrication of vaginal tissues. If necessary, use a vaginal cream containing a nonestrogenic water-soluble lubricant to relieve dryness. Popular choices include Astroglide, Replens, or K-Y Jelly. Progestin-free estrogen products that are minimally absorbed by the body include a tablet that dissolves in the vagina (Vagifem), a ring that slowly releases estrogen over three months (Estring), and a vaginal cream (Estrace).

■ **Keep up with regular physicals.** After menopause, continue with yearly Pap tests and pelvic exams, along with such appropriate screenings as mammograms and lipid profiles to check cholesterol levels, and continue to do a monthly breast self-exam (*see page 356*).

▶**I have heart disease and was considering HRT. Is the HERS Study something I should heed?**

Even before the Women's Health Initiative was canceled in 2002 (see page 225), results from the Heart and Estrogen/Progestin Replacement Study (HERS) shook experts' confidence in the role of HRT as a heart protector. The five-year HERS study, which concluded in 1998, found that women who already had heart disease were 50% more likely to have a heart attack during their first two years on HRT than those who didn't take hormones. But during the study's fourth and fifth years, those on HRT had fewer heart attacks and deaths from heart disease. The original trial was extended for an additional 2.7 years (called HERS II). Its results support the conclusions of the original trial: HRT neither worsens nor improves a heart condition.

Promising
DEVELOPMENTS

■ While ongoing studies attempt to sort out the benefits and drawbacks of HRT, researchers are testing other drugs to determine their ability to manage menopausal symptoms. Future treatments may include **tibolone** (Livial), a progestinlike synthetic hormone to protect against bone loss; combinations of **estrogen and testosterone** (Estratest), to increase bone mass, improve sexual drive, and sharpen alertness; and **gabapentin** (Neurontin), a neurological drug that may alleviate hot flashes.

rate of breast cancer and blood clots in the group taking the estrogen/progestin combination. They also discovered a very disturbing increase in incidence of heart attack and stroke—precisely the ailments they had believed HRT would protect against.

While these results have caused many women to re-evaluate HRT, doctors point out that your personal risk for developing these problems is less than one-tenth of 1% per year. In spite of the data from the study, HRT may eventually be recommended to women who have especially severe menopausal symptoms and no history of breast cancer or heart disease. Rather than using HRT for years, your doctor may prescribe a low-dose short course for the period your symptoms are at their worst. You'll gradually taper off the hormones to avoid bringing on the symptoms all over again.

If osteoporosis is your primary concern, you might try a **bisphosphonate,** such as alendronate (Fosamax) or risedronate (Actonel). These reduce fracture risk by 40% to 50%, contain no hormones, and some need be taken only once a week. A newer choice for preventing osteoporosis is the so-called "designer estrogen" drug raloxifene (Evista), a selective-estrogen receptor modulator (or SERM) that mimics the effects of estrogen to keep bones strong. A statin drug such as lovastatin (Mevacor) might help for heart disease prevention (*see High Cholesterol, page 176*), and for hot flashes, ask your doctor about using an **antidepressant** or **a blood pressure medication.** Discuss side effects before you start. They might be worse than your present symptoms.

Lifestyle Changes

Whether or not you're on medications for your symptoms, changes in your daily habits will help keep you physically and mentally agile. Because unwanted weight gain tends to go hand in hand with menopause, adopt a **low-fat, high-fiber diet** that includes lots of whole grains and fresh fruits and vegetables. To keep hot flashes in check, cut way back on alcohol, caffeine, chocolate, and spicy foods. If your diet's shy on bone-building **calcium** (aim for 1,200 to 1,500 mg daily), include more reduced-fat dairy products, fortified orange juice, and canned salmon (with the bones). You might also want to eat more tofu and other **soy products,** which are rich in isoflavones, estrogen-like compounds found in plants. Research shows that isoflavones may help relieve hot flashes and night sweats, and may protect against osteoporosis and breast cancer. Soy isoflavone supplements have never been found to have the same effects as dietary soy, and some research suggests that very large doses of the supplements may cause a hormone imbalance that increases the risk of certain estrogen-sensitive cancers.

Another way to keep your bones in good shape is to engage in about 30 minutes of **weight-bearing exercise**—any activity that's carried out on your feet, such as walking, running, jumping rope, or playing tennis. Try to exercise at least three times a week. If urinary incontinence is a problem, **Kegel exercises,** which strengthen and tone the pelvic-floor muscles, can help (*see page 325 for information*

Herbal Remedies for Menopausal Symptoms

If you favor a natural approach to the natural changes in your body, consider these popular herbal remedies for menopausal symptoms.*

- **Black cohosh.** This buttercup relative has long been used for hot flashes and vaginal dryness. Its properties resemble estrogen, and studies are needed to confirm its long-term safety and effectiveness. Until then, experts suggest using it no more than six months at a time. One such product is Remifemin Menopause, available in drugstores.
- **Siberian ginseng.** Used for centuries in China, this all-purpose herb helps relieve stress, boost mood, enhance immunity, and increase mental alertness. It may also alter hormone levels and reduce menopausal symptoms.
- **Dong quai.** Often referred to as the "female ginseng," this herb seems to have a balancing effect on the female hormone system. It's best taken in combination with herbs such as black cohosh and Siberian ginseng. Studies are inconclusive as to whether it works on its own.
- **Red clover.** Available in a menopause-targeted formula called Promensil, red clover contains powerful phytoestrogens called isoflavones. In a study at Tufts University, menopausal patients reported that Promensil cut hot flashes by half. Two other studies, however, revealed no benefits.
- **Menopausal formulas.** A number of "women's formulas" for menopause feature various herbs, including black cohosh and dong quai. The amount of each herb may be so low that it pays to take them separately. Remember that such a combination product is an alternative to, not an addition to, using black cohosh or other "female" herbs.

on how to do them). Don't buy into the myth that menopause makes you less of a woman: Many women report feeling sexier than ever once they're in menopause—and remaining sexually active helps preserve the elasticity of your vaginal walls.

If you are feeling anxious or worrying about your self-esteem or sexuality, consider seeing a counselor or psychotherapist or joining a **women's support group.**

Natural Methods*

In addition to getting plenty of calcium in your diet, it's also important to get enough **vitamin E, vitamin D,** and **magnesium.** These can be taken in supplement form to boost the amount you get from foods. Vitamin E stimulates the body's estrogen production and as one of the antioxidant vitamins (along with the carotenes and vitamin C), acts to prevent LDL ("bad") cholesterol from causing plaque in your artery walls. Magnesium and vitamin D help prevent osteoporosis and are often combined with calcium in a "bone-building" supplement. There are a number of other **herbal supplements,** such as black cohosh and red clover, which you also might want to consider (*see box above*) to help keep menopausal symptoms in check. In addition, some women have found success with **acupuncture,** an ancient Chinese technique in which thin needles are inserted at key points on the body to relieve headaches, sleep disturbances, and other menopausal symptoms.

Natural methods are not subject to the same testing and regulation as prescription medications. Please seek your doctor's advice and use caution.

FINDING Support

- Need a physician to guide you in treatment of menopausal symptoms? Contact the American College of Obstetricians and Gynecologists in Washington, D.C. (202-863-2518 or www.acog.org).

- The North American Menopause Society in Cleveland, OH, offers both online and printed materials about menopause, perimenopause, and health-enhancing therapies (1-800-774-5342 or www.menopause.org).

- For more information on dealing with menopause, including information on hormone replacement therapy, visit the website of the National Institute on Aging at www.nia.nih.gov.

Migraine

An estimated 28 million Americans suffer from migraine headaches, but only about half of them seek the medical treatment that could bring relief. There's no reason to suffer in silence. Powerful new medicines offer hope for breaking the cycle of pain.

LIKELY First Steps

- See your doctor to identify the **best prescription medications** for your symptoms.
- **Lie down** and rest in a dark, quiet room **with an ice pack** for immediate relief.
- Identify possible migraine **triggers,** such as food, drink, sleep patterns, and stress.

QUESTIONS TO Ask

- How can I tell if certain foods are triggering my migraine attacks?
- Am I a candidate for a medication to prevent migraines?
- Does the medication I'm on have a rebound effect if used too often?
- Can I become addicted to my migraine painkillers?
- Is there a danger that beta-blockers or calcium channel blockers will cause my blood pressure to drop too low?

What is happening

During a migraine, blood vessels deliver too little blood to the brain, irritating the nerves around them. The word itself comes from the Greek, meaning half a skull, which describes a distinguishing characteristic of migraine headaches: They often involve a stabbing pain on one side of the head. For centuries, migraines were seen as a psychological problem or, worse, a sign of weakness in those who had them. People with migraines were, in effect, often blamed for their own pain. Nothing could be further from the truth. They are now recognized as a chronic disease, not just painful headaches. The excruciating, often debilitating pain is a symptom, not the underlying problem. This is a key distinction.

Although the exact cause of migraines is uncertain, there's a strong genetic link. If one of your parents has migraines, you have about a 50% chance of having them too. Many researchers say that people prone to migraines inherit an acutely sensitive nervous system. Changes in your body (diet, sleep, hormones, or stress) or in your environment (weather or lighting) can "trigger" a migraine attack. Low levels of the brain chemical serotonin are also believed to play a role.

Most migraines have four stages. During the **prodrome** (the period before an attack), you may be sensitive to light, smell, or sound. About 20% of people with a migraine experience an **aura**—bright, flashing lights or partial loss of vision. During the **attack,** a throbbing or pulsating pain often starts on one side of the head and gradually worsens; sometimes it spreads to the other side. You may also have vomiting, blurred vision, neck and shoulder pain, tingling, or difficulty concentrating. An untreated attack can last from a couple of hours to several days. Afterward, in the **postdrome,** you may feel drained, irritable, and foggy, or refreshed and even euphoric.

About 13% of Americans suffer from migraines. Women are three times more likely than men to have them, and an estimated 80% of people with migraines have a family history of the condition. The National Institute of Neurological Disorders and Stroke estimates that 157 million workdays are lost each year due to migraines.

Treatments

There is no permanent cure for a predisposition to migraines. But treatments can prevent attacks and relieve symptoms, thereby restoring quality to your life. The key is understanding that a migraine isn't just a headache you have to ride out. It's a complex medical condition. You

Treatment options

Medications

Triptans	First-line drugs; constrict blood vessels.
Ergot derivatives	Second-line; often used with antinausea drug.
Local anesthetic	Lidocaine in nasal spray brings quick relief.
Opiates	If no other drugs work for pain.
OTC pain relievers	From aspirin to special migraine products.
Preventive medications	Wide choice to stop a migraine before it starts.

Lifestyle changes

Diet	Determine if foods are migraine triggers.
Sleep	Keep to a regular schedule.
Relax	Stress can trigger migraines.

Natural methods

Herbs & vitamins	Feverfew and vitamin B_2.
Alternative therapies	Biofeedback, chiropractic, acupuncture.

need to consult your doctor about the appropriate medication for you. There are many choices, and they can bring fast relief. One survey showed that those who took prescription medications were twice as likely to experience complete headache relief within two hours as those who used over-the-counter products. In addition, lifestyle factors such as food, stress, exercise, and sleep can make a big difference, and there are a number of natural methods that have helped many find relief.

Medications

Prescription drugs are the first-line treatment for migraine attacks, and the particular medication you end up taking will depend on your symptoms as well as your response to different medicines. The most effective are probably the **triptans,** a group of drugs that enhance levels of the brain chemical serotonin and constrict blood vessels. Sumatriptan (Imitrex), the key drug in this category, can be self-injected for fast relief, taken orally, or inhaled as a nasal spray. In clinical trials, up to 80% of those who had sumatriptan injections reported milder headaches or complete relief within an hour. When taken orally, two other triptans—rizatriptan (Maxalt) and zolmitriptan (Zomig ZMT)—work faster than sumatriptan.

Other triptans include almotriptan (Axert), eletriptan (Relpax), and frovatriptan (Frova), as well as the longer-lasting naratriptan (Naramig, Amerge). Some people who take triptan experience flushing, jaw tightness, neck pain, and other side effects. Because these drugs constrict blood vessels, people with heart disease should not use them without a doctor's approval.

TAKING Control

- **Have a cup of coffee**—strong and black—at the first sign of an attack. Too much caffeine can trigger a migraine attack, but a little bit can relieve oncoming pain. This is especially helpful for people who only rarely have caffeine.

- **Avoid the rebound.** Overusing headache medications—even common OTC products—can lead to a vicious cycle of rebound headaches. Your body becomes so dependent on the medication that you get a new headache as soon as the drug wears off. Anyone who uses migraine medication more than two or three times a week is at risk for this effect. Once you're locked into the cycle, the best way to break out is to go off all medication, possibly in the hospital.

- **Eat more fish.** Varieties high in omega-3 fatty acids (salmon, tuna, sardines) may help prevent migraines from recurring. Omega-3s seem to alter blood chemicals, reducing the risk of blood vessel spasms associated with this type of headache.

- **Watch out for additives.** The artificial sweetener aspartame, found in many diet sodas, may trigger migraines in some people. Saccharin does not. The food coloring FD & C yellow #5, found in candy, beverages, some cereals, and ice cream, has also been known to trigger migraines in certain individuals.

The next group is the **ergot derivatives.** Ergotamine (Ergomar, Wigraine, Ercaf) has been around longer than the triptans and also works by constricting blood vessels. But it can cause nausea and vomiting, so your doctor may prescribe an antinausea drug to go with it. Dihydroergotamine (D.H.E. 45), a nasal spray, has milder side effects and is less likely to upset your stomach. Methysergide (Sansert) is very effective, but used only if other choices don't work. Its side effects range from nausea, vomiting, abdominal pain, diarrhea, and depression to a rare but potentially fatal lung fibrosis (excessive scar tissue). Lidocaine, a **local anesthetic** available as a nasal spray, can provide relief for many sufferers within 15 minutes. If pain relief continues to elude you, the next step is a powerful **opiate,** such as morphine, codeine, meperidine (Demerol), or hydrocodone (Vicodin).

Less effective than prescription drugs but useful only for mild cases, **OTC pain relievers** include acetaminophen (Tylenol, Excedrin) and nonsteroidal anti-inflammatory drugs (NSAIDS) such as aspirin, naproxen (Aleve), and ibuprofen (Motrin, Advil). Some OTC migraine formulations combine caffeine with acetaminophen and aspirin.

Preventive medications may stave off migraines. Options include a daily aspirin; prescription beta-blockers, such as propranolol (Inderal), which provides long-term relief for about half of those with frequent migraines; calcium channel blockers, such as verapamil; tricyclic antidepressants, such as amitriptyline (Elavil, Endep), nortryptiline, and protriptyline (Vivactil); and selective serotonin reuptake inhibitors (SSRIs), such as fluoxetine (Prozac), sertraline (Zoloft), and paroxetine (Paxil). Divalproex sodium (Depakote)—a drug used to prevent epileptic seizures and control bipolar disease—is approved by the FDA to reduce the severity and frequency of severe "common" migraines, the kind without auras.

Lifestyle Changes

Medications aren't your only defense. When a migraine strikes, **lie down** in a dark room. Place an **ice pack** or **gel pack** (Migraine Ice or TheraPatch Headache Cool Gel) wherever the pain is. A **headband**— either elastic or gel-filled (and cooled)—can also offer relief. Other lifestyle measures can minimize your attacks, too. The key is to identify and eliminate your triggers. Here's how:

- **Watch your diet.** Many foods have been linked to migraines. Among the likely suspects are foods with nitrates (bacon, corned beef, ham, hot dogs, lunch meats, and sausage); the chemical MSG (monosodium glutamate); aged cheeses (Cheddar, Swiss, Stilton, Brie); chocolate; nuts; peanut butter; sour cream; caffeinated beverages; aspartame (artificial sweetener); and alcohol.
- **Eat regularly.** Skipping meals is a common migraine trigger.
- **Get a good night's sleep.** Too much or too little sleep can cause a migraine. Your best bet is to establish a consistent sleep pattern of seven to nine hours nightly. Keep in mind that changes to this pattern, including jet lag, can trigger a migraine.
- **Exercise smart.** Always warm up properly and ease into your workout. Aerobic exercise can sometimes make migraines worse.

Cluster Headaches

This rare form of headache strikes about 1% of the population. The overwhelming majority of sufferers—an estimated 85%—are men. Its key symptom is distinctive: intense pain around one eye, lasting from 15 minutes to two hours. These headaches tend to come in clusters, occurring repeatedly (often at the same time of night) for weeks or months. A common pattern is for the headache to attack a few hours after you fall asleep.

The cause of cluster headaches remains a mystery. Cigarettes and alcohol are often triggers, so heavy smokers and drinkers are at the greatest risk. Lying down may help relieve migraine pain, but it can have the opposite effect on a cluster headache. Since the attacks are short and intense, it's difficult for any drug to work quickly enough to help. Breathing pure oxygen through a mask from an oxygen tank for about 10 minutes at the start of an attack provides the most effective relief for some people. Because the headaches come in clusters, your best bet for preventive medication may be naratriptan (Naramig, Amerge), which gives you long-term coverage.

■ **Relax.** Stress can be a trigger, so take time each day to sit quietly and relax your muscles. Learn to let go of things you can't control.

Natural Methods*

One of the oldest non-drug approaches is **feverfew,** long recommended by herbalists to prevent migraines. Fresh leaves of this herb are very bitter, so you might want to try standardized capsules or a tea. Don't use feverfew if you're pregnant or taking aspirin. **Vitamin B₂ (riboflavin)** may help by boosting your brain's energy reserves. Good food sources include mushrooms, poultry, and quinoa. It can also be taken in supplement form.

Several alternative therapies for migraine relief may be worth checking out. **Biofeedback** hooks you up to a small machine that allows you to monitor your ability to regulate muscle tension, skin temperature, and other things. The relaxation techniques you learn can then be applied without the machine. Some people learn to raise their hand temperature, which draws blood away from the constricted vessels in the head that cause migraine pain. Those using biofeedback techniques report reduced frequency, severity, and duration of attacks.

A session with a **chiropractor,** who uses massage, spinal manipulation, and adjustments to joints and soft tissues, can provide relief for certain people. Proponents of **acupuncture** say this ancient Chinese technique can help relieve migraine pain by balancing serotonin levels and relaxing tense muscles.

Natural methods are not subject to the same testing and regulation as prescription medications. Please seek your doctor's advice and use caution.

Promising DEVELOPMENTS

■ A daily cup of **yogurt** may help prevent migraine headaches, according to Italian researchers. They estimated that 18% of chronic migraine sufferers are infected with the bacteria *Helicobacter pylori,* which has been linked to ulcers, heart disease, and other health problems. The researchers split 130 people who had migraines and *H. pylori* into two groups. They gave half of them antibiotics and gave the other half antibiotics plus the friendly bacteria *Lactobacillus,* found in certain yogurt brands. After a year, 80% of those who took *Lactobacillus* and the antibiotic reported their migraines had ceased. Only 50% of those on the antibiotic alone were better. Such results are encouraging, although not definitive.

FINDING Support

Three of the best sources of headache information on the Internet include:

■ The National Headache Foundation (www.headaches.org), which offers treatment information, the latest news, and current clinical trials.

■ The Migraine Awareness Group (www.migraines.org), which offers an online discussion forum and a message board.

■ The American Council for Headache Education (ACHE) (www.achenet.org), which features an "Ask the Expert" discussion forum with participating physicians, along with an open forum, background information and resources, and a physician listing.

Multiple sclerosis

Hearing that you have multiple sclerosis can be frightening and bewildering, but this nerve disorder often progresses very slowly—or not at all. Now even the more aggressive forms of MS can be treated to delay the disease's progress.

LIKELY **First Steps**

- **Medications** to bring an acute attack under control and delay the onset of another attack.

- Once an attack is under control, **lifestyle changes** to prepare you, mentally and physically, for the challenge of living with MS.

QUESTIONS TO **Ask**

- Does my condition merit seeing an MS specialist?

- How long will I be able to continue with my usual activities?

- Do you know of any clinical trials that might be appropriate for me?

- How do I know if a particular product or program is bogus?

- Are there support groups that my family can join?

- Do any of the special MS diets work?

What is happening

Your central nervous system—including your brain and spinal cord—is a jumble of wires, or nerves, that transmit messages all over your body. To prevent short circuits, nerves are covered with an insulation called a myelin sheath. Researchers have long believed that multiple sclerosis (MS) occurs when the immune system attacks myelin, which it may mistake for a virus, and damages nerves. Recent findings suggest the myelin may die before the immune system attacks. Your symptoms will depend on where the damage occurs. Problems range from vision abnormalities and fatigue to poor coordination and tingling sensations.

The course of MS is unpredictable, but an acute flare-up is usually followed by a remission that can last for months or years before another episode occurs. After an acute attack, your nerves begin to heal, forming scars, or plaques, over areas of myelin damage. (This process gives MS its name: Sclerosis is from the Greek *skleros*, which means hard, and multiple sclerosis connotes hard, patchy scarring along the nerves.) If this acute damage is too great, weakness, fatigue, sensory loss, visual changes, dizziness, tremors, speech difficulties, trouble swallowing, urinary and bowel problems, mood swings, and other residual symptoms may persist. If MS continues unchecked, your muscles become increasingly difficult to control. You may lose the ability to walk.

Some 250,000–300,000 Americans have MS, which affects twice as many women as men. About 20% of cases are called **benign MS:** A single attack is never repeated, but most people (up to 75%) have **relapsing-remitting MS:** You may be symptom-free between attacks, and months (even years) can go by before another flare-up, or relapse. Then there are the more serious forms of the disease: **secondary progressive,** in which years of relapsing-remitting MS changes to continuous deterioration; **primary progressive,** in which deterioration is slow but constant, with no remission; and (very rarely) **progressive-relapsing,** in which continuous deterioration is interspersed with sudden episodes of new symptoms or worsened old ones.

Treatments

The goal of MS treatment is to stave off acute attacks (when nerve damage is likely to occur) as long as possible and then manage symptoms effectively. Your success will likely depend on the type of MS you have. Effective treatments for MS have existed only since the 1960s. Since then, doctors have continued to develop treatments for making life with MS easier to manage.

Treatment options

Medications

Interferon	Limits nerve damage; may slow progression.
Glatiramer acetate	Protects myelin sheath to limit nerve damage.
Corticosteroids	Reduce inflammation; control immune system.
Mitoxantrone	Slows secondary progressive MS symptoms.
Other drugs for symptoms	For spasms, urinary problems, depression.

Lifestyle changes

Exercise & diet	Keep muscles strong; good nutrition helps.
Keep cool	Overheating can make symptoms worse.

Natural methods

Supplements	Antioxidants, magnesium, essential fatty acids.
Acupuncture	Helps reduce symptoms.

Procedures

Plasma exchange	Blood processing to reduce myelin damage.
Therapy	Physical, occupational, and psychological.

Medications

Pharmaceutical options for treating MS are available only through prescription, so you'll have to keep in close contact with your doctor, detailing what's working and what isn't. If a drug doesn't work, don't despair. There's usually something else to try.

For treating the disease itself, evidence suggests that **interferon** medications, if used early enough, can limit irreversible nerve damage and may slow the disease's progression. If you've had an initial attack, and are not on interferon, ask your doctor if it makes sense to start. Drugs often prescribed include interferon beta-1a (Avonex, Rebif) and beta-1b (Betaseron). Studies have found that all three reduce flare-ups for relapsing-remitting MS by 30%, and make attacks less severe if they do occur. Interferon works by suppressing inflammatory mechanisms in the immune system and blocking molecules that target myelin for attack. These drugs also have potentially beneficial antiviral properties: Many experts believe a virus may be one cause of MS.

Another helpful drug is **glatiramer acetate** (Copaxone), a synthetic molecule similar to a protein found in myelin. It works by tricking your immune system into attacking the drug instead of the myelin sheath. It's most beneficial if started early in the disease, and its effectiveness increases the longer you take it.

For severe flare-ups, your doctor may prescribe **corticosteroids**, such as oral prednisone or intravenous methylprednisolone (Medrol). They reduce inflammation in the central nervous system

■ **Consider taking part in a clinical trial** (there are usually a dozen or so for MS at any one time). New and potentially better medications depend on clinical trials to get FDA approval before they can be marketed. Go to www.clinicaltrials.gov to find studies that might be appropriate for you.

■ **Don't ignore pain.** Pain is the "hidden symptom" of MS and may not be adequately treated. Because pain can really affect the quality of your life, be sure your doctor knows you're experiencing it and it is treated accordingly.

■ **Get a flu shot.** Flu-related fever means overheating, which worsens MS symptoms.

■ **De-stress.** Too much stress is usually harmful to people with MS. One study found a connection between increased levels of stress (both everyday hassles and major life events) and new nerve damage in the brain.

▶ THE CLOSER YOU GET TO THE EQUATOR, the rarer multiple sclerosis becomes. Most cases are found in people living in temperate climates.

► **Will MS affect my ability to have children?**
Rest assured that it won't. Studies have repeatedly shown that women with multiple sclerosis can safely become pregnant and deliver children. Relapses become less common late in pregnancy, although they may increase in frequency during the first three months following childbirth.

► **I've just been diagnosed with MS. Should I quit my job? I'm worried that I won't be able to keep up.**
It's normal to want to stop working when you're going through a crisis, but experts say it's vital that you stay employed through this time. Too often, people quit, then regret it later once they realize the decision was premature. It's far easier to keep a job than to find a new one when you're not feeling well. Talk with your employer about part-time status, or start telecommuting.

► **What is the Swank Diet?**
Devised by Dr. Roy Swank of Oregon Health Sciences University, this plan is very low in saturated fat and recommends specific amounts of polyunsaturated oils (like canola and safflower). Many patients say following the Swank Diet has slowed the course of their MS and reduced the number of attacks they have. There is no scientific evidence that this diet has specific benefits for treating this disease beyond what a healthy, balanced diet would provide.

and inhibit your immune system from attacking myelin. Steroids don't change the progression of the disease. They are not prescribed for milder flare-ups because they lose effectiveness if overused.

For the more serious forms of MS, your options are more limited. A drug called **mitoxantrone** (Novantrone) is the first to be approved for treating secondary progressive MS. It's shown some effectiveness at slowing relapses and progression of the disease. Side effects, including heart complications, can be serious.

For relieving MS symptoms, a wide array of drugs can be extremely helpful, especially in milder cases. **Antispasmodics** ease muscle spasms that can accompany MS. These include botulinum toxin injections (Botox), tizanidine (Zanaflex), and diazepam (Valium). Tremors can be controlled with drugs like clonazepam (Klonopin) and primidone (Mysoline). Some people with MS develop urinary complications. For urge incontinence, in which the need to urinate comes on suddenly (*see Urinary Incontinence, page 325*), **anticholinergic drugs,** such as oxybutynin (Ditropan), are useful. If urinating is a problem, drugs like maprotiline (Ludiomil) are a good choice. There are also medications to relieve sexual dysfunction: sildenafil (Viagra) for men, low-dose corticosteroids for women.

Depression is common if you suffer from MS. It's due to the effects of the disease on the brain as well as to the impact of living with a degenerative condition. **Tricyclic antidepressants** work well and may confer other benefits. It's important to talk with your doctor about the emotional side of this disease. Too many people try to conduct their lives in a "business as usual" fashion when they could be getting effective professional help.

Lifestyle Changes

One of the greatest challenges of MS is dealing with its impact on daily life. The following lifestyle measures may not slow the disease itself, but they will help you deal with it much more successfully.

- **Start a regular exercise regimen.** Your muscles can weaken when you have MS, so it's essential to stay in the best shape you can. Exercise helps maintain strength, coordination, and balance, and can reduce spasticity. Try riding a stationary bike, walking, swimming, or doing tai chi or yoga. Just don't get too warm: Many people with MS find that being overheated worsens their symptoms.
- **Eat a well-balanced diet.** Proper nutrition helps boost your immune system and prevent colds and flu, which can worsen MS. Get lots of fiber from fruits, vegetables, and whole grains to prevent constipation, a common problem with MS. Drink at least two quarts of water a day. Keeping well hydrated not only beats constipation, but also will prevent the urinary tract infections that occasionally occur among some people with this disease.
- **Keep cool.** Make sure your air conditioners are working well in summer. Avoid hot tubs, and choose swimming pools that aren't kept too warm.

Natural Methods*

Nearly 60% of people with MS try some form of nontraditional therapy. Sometimes these approaches can be very helpful, but be sure to talk with your doctor so you'll know what to avoid. Some popular dietary supplements, including echinacea, garlic, and ginseng, can worsen MS symptoms by overstimulating the immune system. The following therapies have shown some promise:

- **Antioxidants.** Because the nerve damage of MS is partly due to oxidation, antioxidants may make sense. In addition to plenty of fruits and vegetables, try vitamin A, C, and E supplements, as well as coenzyme Q_{10}, grape seed extract, and N-acetylcysteine (NAC).
- **Acupuncture.** Many report this ancient Chinese therapy helps lessen symptoms. Find a licensed practitioner experienced with MS.
- **Magnesium.** This mineral may help reduce uncomfortable muscle spasms that often accompany MS.
- **Essential fatty acids.** Flaxseed oil and evening primrose oil, both fatty acids, may help protect the myelin sheath.

Procedures

Usually recommended only for people whose sudden, severe attacks aren't helped by steroids, **plasmapheresis,** or plasma exchange, involves removing blood, spinning out the blood cells from the plasma, and replacing the plasma with a synthetic fluid. The new mix is pumped back into the body. Doctors think the technique may remove destructive factors in your blood, turning off the process that's destroying your myelin.

Physical and occupational therapy can help you navigate physical limitations. **Psychological counseling** helps you deal with the mental distresses of a chronic condition. Family counseling is often a good idea, because your loved ones also need coping skills.

Outlook

There's a lot of exciting research focusing on new treatments and potential cures for multiple sclerosis. Given the slow progression of the disease, you may well benefit from innovative treatments over the next few years.

▶ **SOME PEOPLE SWEAR BY BEE VENOM and regularly arrange to be stung by bees to ease MS symptoms. This therapy should be undertaken only under the care of a doctor experienced with its use. Those with bee-sting allergies should avoid it.**

FINDING Support

- Make sure you stay abreast of the latest treatments for MS. One of the best sources for information is the National Multiple Sclerosis Society in New York, NY (1-800-FIGHT MS or www.nationalmssociety.org).

- The Multiple Sclerosis Foundation in Fort Lauderdale, FL (888-MSFOCUS or www.msfacts.org) and the Multiple Sclerosis Association of America in Cherry Hill, NJ (1-800-532-7667 or www.msaa.com) are good resources. The latter is a great place to find a support group.

Natural methods are not subject to the same testing and regulation as prescription medications. Please seek your doctor's advice and use caution.

Obesity

After smoking, obesity is the most preventable cause of death in the United States today. It's heartening to realize that losing as little as 5% to 10% of your total body weight can make you much healthier. The secret weapon is commitment.

LIKELY First Steps

- **Diet and exercise** to help you shed pounds gradually—and keep them off.
- **Counseling and support groups** to clarify emotional issues and keep you motivated to continue.
- **Medications** in conjunction with diet and exercise.
- **Surgery** to reduce stomach capacity in the severely obese.

QUESTIONS TO Ask

- Could I be overweight due to a metabolic disorder? Can you test my thyroid levels?
- With so much extra weight, is it safe for me to exercise?
- Am I a candidate for a weight-loss drug?
- If I get my stomach stapled, will it affect other medical problems I have?

What is happening

If you're carrying extra pounds, you've got lots of company. Two-thirds of American adults are overweight. One-third of them suffer from obesity, defined as being 20% or more over your ideal body weight, with an abnormally high proportion of body fat. (More than 100 pounds overweight is considered morbidly obese.) Even more alarming, these numbers are growing markedly every year. Many doctors now call the nation's weight gain a public health emergency. That's because extra weight in adulthood dramatically increases your risk for high blood pressure, diabetes, cardiovascular disease, arthritis, and several kinds of cancer. The more pounds you gain, the higher your risk.

So what's making so many Americans so fat? The major culprit is lifestyle. Most of us spend hours sitting—at computers, in front of TVs, in our cars. Fast food and vending machines can't be avoided. We've grown accustomed to "supersized" everything, from candy bars to restaurant meals. Genetics certainly plays a part: If your parents and grandparents were heavy people, you may well have inherited their body type. You could also have an underfunctioning thyroid or neurological problems. Maybe you're gaining weight because you're taking certain medications. Ask your doctor about these possibilities. Another conflicting factor: Some 30% to 40% of obese patients who seek help with weight are suffering from depression or another psychological disturbance.

Does all this add up to "situation hopeless"? Not at all. Even if you've tried to lose weight and never succeeded, don't despair: The National Weight Control Registry, a database of people who are maintaining their weight loss, shows that the majority of people who successfully lose a minimum of 30 pounds—and keep the weight off for at least a year—have done so after repeated failures at dieting.

Treatments

Weight loss choices depend on your medical profile and how many pounds you need to lose to lower your risk of disease. To see how you measure up, consult the chart on page 355 and figure out your Body Mass Index: Experts use this standard method to evaluate body weight according to height. If you have a BMI of 25 to 29, you're "moderately overweight." If it's between 30 and 40, you're considered "severely overweight" or obese.

Treatment options

Lifestyle changes

Track eating habits	A food diary reveals unhealthy patterns.
Maintain a healthy weight loss diet	Talk with your doctor or a dietitian to find the right program for you.
Join a support group	It increases success and provides motivation.
Exercise	Essential for faster weight loss and toning.

Medications

Weight loss drugs	Xenical or Meridia for long-term treatment.

Natural methods

Supplements	Get mixed reviews.

Procedures

Bariatric surgery	Only for the seriously obese.
Liposuction	For body contouring, not weight loss.

If you're in the moderately overweight category, you should be able to lose sufficient weight with diet and exercise. However, if you're severely overweight, lifestyle methods alone may not correct your problems. Medications and physical therapy may be required, possibly even surgery (although surgery is usually reserved for people who are at least 100 pounds overweight and at high risk for early death).

In working out any realistic treatment plan with your doctor, consider whether you're under lots of stress or often feel out of control when you're around food. If so, ask your doctor about counseling or psychotherapy, which can help control binge eating.

Lifestyle Changes

Whether you are overweight or obese, the principle of weight loss is maddeningly simple: Burn more calories than you take in and you'll lose weight. But if it were that easy, there wouldn't be so many best-selling diet books or quick-fix over-the-counter weight loss products. As you're undoubtedly aware, beating obesity requires an ongoing commitment to change.

To start, many experts recommend that you keep a **food diary** to record not only what you eat, but your hunger levels and emotions when you eat. After a couple of weeks you'll have a good idea of your eating habits. You can then talk with your doctor (or a dietitian) about a specific **low-calorie eating plan** and how you might modify your diet. You might also want to discuss finding a **support system** beyond family and friends. Weight-loss support groups offered by university or hospital clinics typically meet weekly for 16 to 26 weeks and have led to average reductions of 8% to 10% of initial weight. Many people find such groups—and

TAKING Control

When you change your diet, you need to develop new habits. Here are some that have been found to work well for gradual weight loss:

- **Don't skip meals.** Your body goes into deprivation mode, and this leads you to eat more at the next opportunity. Eat often enough to keep your energy level steady— maybe as often as every three to four hours.

- **Drink lots of water.** Eight glasses daily is good for your overall health and helps stave off hunger. One good tip: Drink a glass right before eating.

- **Watch serving size.** That means measuring your morning cereal until your eye knows how a portion looks in a bowl. A serving of chicken or lean meat should be no bigger than a pack of cards. Use smaller plates and bowls to help you adjust.

- **Follow the 20-minute rule.** If you're tempted to go for second helpings, wait. It takes 15 to 20 minutes for your stomach to signal your brain that it's full.

- **Think volume.** Research has shown that a bowl of low-fat, low-calorie soup or plain popcorn helps assuage hunger. Make your own healthy soup with low-fat broth and onions, carrots, greens, or other vegetables; eat it before lunch or dinner.

- **Reward yourself regularly.** If you stick to your eating plan, buy a book, some flowers, a new CD, or take time off from work. We often "reward" ourselves with food; it's good to remember there are noncaloric treats as well.

The Allure of Fad Diets

Who doesn't want to lose weight fast? Who doesn't want to believe Dr. Atkins and others who promise you can eat steaks, bacon, and butter every day and still shed pounds?

Every generation has its fads (remember the Scarsdale Diet?), and some come back again and again. Consider the "Hollywood Diet," born in the '30s: It has you eat half a grapefruit with every (low-calorie) meal, because grapefruit supposedly contains a unique fat-burning enzyme. It doesn't.

The reason such diets work—at least over the short term—is that they limit calories. However, from a health standpoint, they often fail to provide enough key nutrients. Nobody can stay on one forever, so the weight inevitably comes back.

Not surprisingly, physical problems can result. High protein/very low carbohydrate regimens can lead to higher LDL (the "bad" cholesterol), high blood pressure, even osteoporosis.

Moreover, diets of this sort do psychological damage. When you lose weight on so-and-so's miracle diet, you credit the diet. Yet when you go off it, you inevitably blame yourself—forgetting that it's human nature to revolt against rigid rules.

Bottom line: Most people who lose weight and keep it off find greater pleasure and greater success when they eat a wide variety of nutritionally sound foods.

commercial programs like Weight Watchers—extremely helpful. They provide social support along with sound advice on diet and nutrition. Some have online services.

Weight loss plans that work for most people encourage eating a **wide variety of foods**—in smaller amounts. The focus is on lowering your fat intake (especially saturated fat) and eating more whole grains, legumes, fruits, and vegetables. Many of these foods are high in fiber, which makes you feel satisfied sooner. Make it your goal to get the greatest "bang for the buck" with every calorie.

If you're in the moderately overweight category, your goal will probably be to lose one to two pounds a week. This can usually be accomplished by creating a daily "deficit" of 500 calories through eating less and exercising more. Most overweight women will lose about a pound a week by consuming 1,200 to 1,500 calories daily; men, by eating 1,500 to 1,800 calories. Getting fewer calories is usually not recommended, because it's difficult to get a good nutritional balance. However, a study reported in the *American Journal of Clinical Nutrition* showed that very-low-calorie programs that rely on fortified liquid meal replacements, low-calorie entrees, and energy bars have helped people lose as much as 45 to 50 pounds—and keep them off for five years. According to this same study, those who exercised were more likely to keep weight off than those who didn't.

Why does **exercise** work so well? Because it burns calories while you're doing it, and because regular exercise increases the rate at which you burn calories even when you're just sitting around. Exercise is also a great mood elevator, and seeing quick results helps people stick to their eating plans.

Before you begin any sort of exercise program, your doctor may recommend a **stress test** (*see page 366*) to record your heart's performance while you work out. Once you get the medical go-ahead, begin to increase your daily activity. If you're not used to exercise, this could mean starting with five-minute walks, plus some strengthening exercises. Your goal is to work up to 30 minutes of aerobic exercise daily (brisk walking, jogging, swimming, biking); 30 minutes of strengthening exercises two to three times a week; and regular stretching to gain flexibility.

Medications

Maybe you've tried and tried to lose weight and kept putting it back on. If so, ask your doctor whether a medication can help you succeed. There are several drugs available for short-term use. Since keeping the weight off is the point of weight loss, many doctors focus on the following two prescription drugs, which are FDA-approved for long-term treatment:

- **Orlistat (Xenical).** Taken before, during, or after a meal, orlistat prevents the digestion of about 30% of the fat you eat. In clinical trials, it worked better than a placebo to help overweight people lose pounds—and keep them off—when combined with a healthy diet. The downside? Important fat-soluble nutrients can be lost. Not all of them can be replaced by supplements. Some

Diet Busters: Don't Let Them Get You Off Track

There are a million ways to get into trouble when you're trying hard to stick to a diet. Avoid the following:

- **Soft drinks and alcohol.** Soft drinks are loaded with sugar. Even healthy-sounding fruit drinks may have as many as 200 calories a bottle. You can choose diet soda, but many successful dieters do better when they let go of sweet-tasting drinks altogether. Alcohol is another calorie-expensive habit, and because it reduces inhibition, you may eat more than you intended. Choose sparkling water instead.

- **"Fat-free" packaged goods.** They're often made with refined grains and loaded with sugars, so they're not low in calories. Studies show that people tend to eat more of these "diet foods" anyway, which defeats their apparent purpose. Even those with "low-fat" or "cholesterol-free" on the label may contain bad-for-your-heart hydrogenated oils.

- **Eating while watching TV.** Experts say mealtime in front of the TV isn't good for the waistline. You don't really savor your food—a necessary ingredient in healthy eating—because you're too busy watching those food-touting commercials. Save TV for other times.

- **Self-punishing thoughts.** It's important to remember that you will occasionally slip off your eating plan. Every successful dieter has. Tell yourself you're not a bad person doomed to failure. Then forgive yourself and get back on track.

---

patients report gas and frequent bathroom trips. Certain people develop high blood pressure while on the drug.

- **Sibutramine (Meridia).** This drug affects brain neurotransmitters that influence appetite and satiety (fullness) mechanisms. In clinical trials, those who took the drug and got advice on diet lost significantly more weight over one year than those who got diet advice alone. Side effects include dry mouth, insomnia, heart arrhythmia, and elevated blood pressure. Studies suggest that taking Meridia in 12-week on/off cycles minimizes side effects without affecting its ability to suppress appetite.

If taking either drug, you should be monitored closely by your doctor. Some people shouldn't take diet drugs at all—including pregnant women and those who have a history of drug or alcohol abuse, or who have an eating disorder, severe depression, migraine headaches, or an unstable medical condition. The bottom line on drugs: There is no magic bullet, and diet and exercise still count.

Natural Methods*

Most experts (including those at the National Institutes of Health) don't recommend herbal supplements as part of a weight loss program, yet people continue to buy them. Do any of them work? Maybe. Studies show mixed results (and some dangers) with certain herbs. A recent review of weight loss supplements by an independent laboratory found that many brands do not contain the amount of active ingredients the labels proclaim. Despite these drawbacks, a number of supplements can prove a beneficial addition to a weight-loss program:

Natural methods are not subject to the same testing and regulation as prescription medications. Please seek your doctor's advice and use caution.

▶ **Is it true that I can write off the cost of my weight-loss program on my taxes?**
In April 2002, the Internal Revenue Service decided to recognize obesity as a disease, instead of a precursor to other diseases. This means you can claim weight-loss program expenses as a medical deduction. In prior years, you could deduct weight-loss expenses for diabetes or heart disease, say, but not for obesity itself. The ruling may lead insurance companies and Medicare to offer coverage specifically for obesity treatment. And because the ruling covers tax returns as far back as 1998, you may recoup some past expenses. To qualify, you must participate in a weight-loss program under a physician's guidance (the cost of diet foods is not included).

Promising DEVELOPMENTS

Drug research may eventually provide some surprising solutions in the battle against obesity.

- **Metformin (Glucophage),** a diabetes drug, improves insulin sensitivity in people with diabetes, and has a "side effect" of preventing weight gain. Studies are ongoing to see if it will help people who don't have diabetes lose some weight.

- A study at McGill University has found that mice with low levels of **protein tyrosine phosphase (PTB1B),** a signaling protein in the brain's hypothalamus, gain less weight. Drug companies are already busy trying to identify drugs that could turn off PTB1B in people.

- **Green tea** is good for you because of its antioxidants. One Swiss study showed that three daily doses of green tea extract helped burn more calories than similar doses of caffeine.

- **Psyllium,** the soluble fiber from the husk of psyllium seeds, absorbs water in the stomach and may create a feeling of fullness.

- **Chromium picolinate** supplements can help those with diabetes who have mild glucose intolerance and may help lower cholesterol, but most studies don't support claims that chromium increases weight loss or changes body composition. Still, some dieters report that the supplement reduces sugar cravings.

Procedures

Advances in stomach-shrinking (bariatric) surgery offer some hope for the severely obese. You could be a candidate for an operation that blocks off part of your stomach if you are more than 100 pounds overweight, have a BMI of 35 to 40, and perhaps a related medical condition such as diabetes or high blood pressure. Dramatic weight-loss results occur because, after surgery, you feel full even if you eat only a small amount of food.

There are a number of variations on bariatric surgery. The most popular method is **Roux-en-Y gastric bypass surgery (RNY).** In this procedure, the surgeon creates a small pouch (which holds a

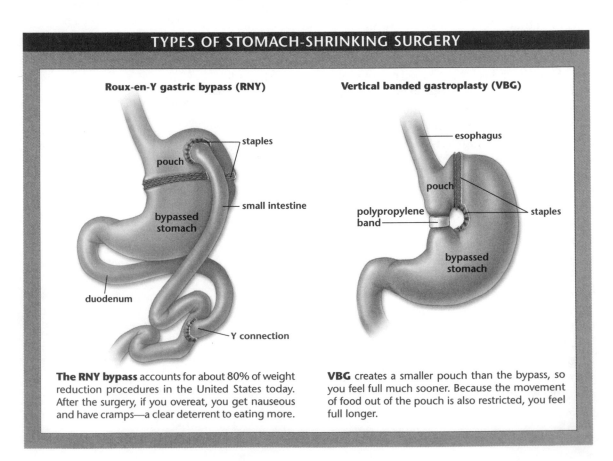

TYPES OF STOMACH-SHRINKING SURGERY

Roux-en-Y gastric bypass (RNY)

staples
pouch
small intestine
bypassed stomach
duodenum
Y connection

Vertical banded gastroplasty (VBG)

esophagus
pouch
polypropylene band
staples
bypassed stomach

The RNY bypass accounts for about 80% of weight reduction procedures in the United States today. After the surgery, if you overeat, you get nauseous and have cramps—a clear deterrent to eating more.

VBG creates a smaller pouch than the bypass, so you feel full much sooner. Because the movement of food out of the pouch is also restricted, you feel full longer.

Liposuction: It's Not a Magic Bullet

Every year millions of women (and men) fail to win their battle against "love handles" and excess fat in the hips, thighs, buttocks, and other problem areas. Frustrated, they turn to liposuction, a type of cosmetic surgery that literally vacuums fat out of the body.

Think carefully before committing yourself to surgery. Liposuction doesn't let you eat anything you want afterward. Nor does it mean you'll be in a bikini the next day (it can take six weeks or longer for the swelling to go down). While the procedure may improve the look of your cottage-cheese thighs, it won't transform you from a size 16 to a size 6. Moreover, liposuction is not without risks.

The American Society for Aesthetic Plastic Surgery (check out www.surgery.org) offers the following guidelines for those considering liposuction:

- **Be sure** your expectations are realistic. Liposuction is meant for body contouring and recommended only for people who want to remove small amounts of fatty deposits. As a general rule, this means only those within 30% of their ideal body weight.
- **Select** a surgeon certified by the American Board of Plastic Surgery. Ask for written verification of the doctor's privileges to perform liposuction in an accredited acute care hospital. If the doctor does the surgery in an office, ask for proof of the facility's accreditation.
- **Give** an accurate medical history and be sure to report all medications you take, even herbal supplements.
- **Discuss** the procedure thoroughly with your doctor. Make sure you understand the differences between the various types of liposuction. Ask questions. If your doctor can't answer them or dismisses them as unimportant, find another doctor.
- **Understand** which type of anesthesia is recommended. If it includes deep sedation, be sure certified staff who have appropriate training will administer it.
- **Talk about** pre- and postoperative care and any risks.

maximum of about four tablespoons of food at a time) by stapling the upper end of your stomach and completely blocking off the lower part. A section of the small intestine is attached to the new stomach pouch to create the bypass (*see illustration opposite*). In another method, called **vertical banded gastroplasty (VBG)**, both staples and a polypropylene band are used to create an even smaller pouch, which holds only about one tablespoon of food at a time.

Although there seem to be fewer complications and better weight loss with RNY, some surgeons prefer VBG because any necessary band adjustments can be made more easily. Exciting advances in laparoscopy (use of a tiny video camera to guide the surgeon) are making stomach-shrinking surgery less taxing on the patient. The surgery carries risks, of course—including infection, bleeding, hernia, ulcers, and vitamin deficiencies—but fatal complications are rare. Compared with the risks of extreme obesity, they may seem slight indeed.

If you're moderately overweight, bariatric surgery isn't for you. However, many overweight women and men are turning to a type of cosmetic surgery called **liposuction** (also known as lipoplasty or suction-assisted lipectomy) to get rid of unsightly fat ripples (*see box above*). In recent years, some 75,000 people have had liposuction at a cost ranging from $14,000 to $35,000. Not a substitute for conventional weight loss, liposuction is most successful at improving body image. Even if you have it, you'll still be encouraged to eat right and exercise to maintain your new look.

FINDING Support

- The American Dietetic Association's website features nutrition fact sheets, daily tips, and information on vegetarian eating and using dietary supplements (www.eatright.org).

- The American Obesity Association can keep you informed of solid scientific studies, consumer alerts, and advocacy efforts (www.obesity.org).

- The website run by the American Heart Association has lots of specific tips on exercise, diet, and a healthy lifestyle (www.americanheart.org).

Osteoporosis

Called the "silent disease" because it steals strength from your skeleton, osteoporosis has few warning signs—until suddenly you break a bone. Now, thanks to new targeted medications, you can slow bone erosion and even reverse your losses.

LIKELY **First Steps**

- Adequate intake of **calcium** and **vitamin D** to build bone.
- **Medication** prescribed to strengthen bones and reduce your risk of fractures.
- **Weight-bearing exercise** to increase bone density.
- **Alterations in home and office** to prevent falls.

QUESTIONS TO **Ask**

- How severe is my condition?
- Taking into account my general health and family history, is hormone replacement therapy the right choice for me?
- Are there specific physical activities I should avoid?
- Can I avoid getting the hunched back my grandmother had?

BONE LOSS

Degenerating hipbone

With osteoporosis, your bones (especially the hip, wrist, and spine) lose vital calcium and become brittle, porous, and prone to sudden fracture.

What is happening

Some 10 million Americans—8 million women and 2 million men—have osteoporosis. Another 18 million are at risk for it. Put simply, osteoporosis is an extension of the natural aging process. When you're young, your bones get longer and denser until you reach your full height. Even as you grow, your bone tissue is constantly being broken down and rebuilt. Then, in your early 30s if you're a woman, and at about age 40 if you're a man, your skeleton begins to slowly lose bone faster than your body can replace it.

From this point on, the skeleton very gradually thins as you age. But if you have osteoporosis, it's a different story. By the time you're diagnosed, your bones will already have lost significant density, making them fragile and easy to break—often spontaneously or after a very minor accident. You'll have a special risk for fracturing wrists or suffering painful compression fractures of the spine, causing your upper back to curve forward. The greatest danger, however, is hip fractures, which can cause permanent disability. Even worse, studies show that 20% of people over age 50 who break a hip die of complications within a year.

Bone loss is mainly a depletion of the mineral calcium. It affects more women than men because the hormone estrogen plays a crucial role in the female body's ability to use dietary calcium to build new bone. When you approach or are in menopause, the reduction in your body's estrogen production deprives your bones of the calcium they need. Some 20% to 30% of bone loss in women occurs in the first five years after menopause. Osteopenia often develops during this critical time. Without treatment, this bone-thinning condition can lead to osteoporosis.

Bone loss can also occur in younger women whose estrogen levels fall after hysterectomy or in athletes whose ability to produce estrogen may be hindered by low body fat. Hormonal changes can also contribute to osteoporosis in men (*see page 245*), as can long-term use of medications such as anticonvulsants and corticosteroids.

Treatments

To begin, treatment for your osteoporosis will focus on medications to slow bone loss and reduce your risk of fractures, as well as lifestyle changes to improve your general health and feelings of well-being. If you've got osteopenia, your doctor may recommend the same approach to keep your bone loss in check. For severe cases and fractures, surgery may be an option.

Treatment options

Medications

Calcium & vitamin D	Supplements to build and strengthen bones.
Bisphosphonates	Fosamax, Boniva, Actonel, first-line treatments.
Hormone replacement	Short-term at menopause can be beneficial.
SERMs	Promising drugs Evista, Nolvadex, Livial.
Calcitonin	Hormone given as injection or nasal spray.

Lifestyle changes

Dairy products	Rich sources of calcium.
Weight-bearing exercise	Strength-building helps calcium work.
Safety measures	Practical precautions prevent injury.

Procedures

Joint replacement	For severe injuries, especially fractured hips.
Kyphoplasty	Restorative therapy for collapsed vertebrae.

Medications

You already know that **calcium** helps your body make bones, but how much do you need? Adults up to age 50 require 1,000 mg of calcium daily. Postmenopausal women (and men over age 65) should get 1,200 to 1,500 mg a day. If dietary sources aren't enough, add supplements. The two with the highest levels of calcium are calcium carbonate (take it with food) and calcium citrate (which can be taken without food). For best absorption, don't take more than 500 to 600 mg at a time. Calcium needs a partner in its bone-protection work: **vitamin D.** Most adults need 400 IU of vitamin D daily. If you have osteoporosis, you may require 600 to 800 IU daily. Your doctor may suggest a prescription form of the vitamin called calcitriol (Rocaltrol).

You'll also need medication to slow bone loss and increase bone mass. What's best for you depends on the cause of your osteoporosis, the part of your skeleton most affected, and your overall health history. The first choice for many patients are drugs called **bisphosphonates:** alendronate (Fosamax), risedronate (Actonel), and ibendronate (Boniva). These drugs have been approved by the FDA (for men and women) to prevent and treat osteoporosis related to hormones or induced by corticosteroids. All three drugs have been shown to lower the incidence of fractures, including those of the hip. Each morning, you take the medication on an empty stomach with plain water, and stay upright without eating or drinking for at least 30 minutes in order to prevent irritation of the esophagus. Some people prefer the once-a-week forms.

TAKING Control

- **If a physical activity feels too strenuous or unsafe, stop immediately.** Tuning into the signals your body is sending may help prevent serious injury. If the activity is something you still wish to pursue, talk it over with your doctor.

- **Take tea and see.** A study in Taiwan found that long-time tea drinkers had the highest overall bone density. Researchers determined that drinking two cups of black, green, or oolong tea a day for at least six years protected the bones. This could be because tea contains flavonoids, estrogenlike substances that may keep bones strong.

- **Bone up on nondairy sources of calcium.** Even if you drink plenty of milk, make sure your diet includes such calcium-rich foods as canned salmon and sardines (eaten with the bones), dark-green leafy vegetables, and white beans. A variety of processed foods, including juices and cereals, are now fortified with calcium.

▶**Is it possible to get too much calcium?**
Yes. Most adults can safely consume up to 2,000 mg of calcium a day, but larger amounts can lead to a variety of problems, including nausea, vomiting, and kidney stones. In two studies, men who consumed very high levels of calcium appeared to have an increased risk of developing prostate cancer. Excessive doses of vitamin D can cause similar problems.

Promising
DEVELOPMENTS

■ Doctors are studying the benefits of taking extra **parathyroid hormone (PTH),** a substance all people naturally secrete and that appears to stimulate growth of new bone tissue. In studies, PTH injections dramatically reduced the risk of all fractures in postmenopausal women, especially those of the spine. Benefits may continue even after PTH treatment is completed. The FDA has approved daily injections of teriparatide (Forsteo), a form of parathyroid hormone, for treatment of osteoporosis. Researchers are also looking at combining injections with other osteoporosis treatments to offer patients the best possible therapy.

If you are a postmenopausal woman, your doctor may recommend **hormone replacement therapy (HRT).** Because HRT replaces lost estrogen, it prevents rapid bone loss and increases bone density in the hip and spine. Long-term treatment with HRT is controversial, however, because it carries increased risk for gallstones, blood clots, breast cancer, and other problems. For estrogen's protective benefits without its side effects, ask about a new class of drugs called **selective estrogen receptor modulators (SERMs),** such as raloxifene (Evista). SERMs prevent bone loss throughout the entire body, but carry an increased risk of blood clots. They are not right for everyone.

If you can't take other medications, your doctor may recommend **calcitonin.** This naturally occurring hormone inhibits the breakdown of bone and reduces the risk of a fractured vertebra. (It's not yet known if it protects other bones, too.) This drug also relieves pain in people who already have spinal fractures. Calcitonin is given as an injection (Calcimar) or used as a nasal spray (Miacalcin).

Lifestyle Changes

As with other medical conditions, lifestyle changes can make a big difference when you have osteoporosis. Keep the following bone-building and safety tips in mind:

■ **Have milk** or other low-fat dairy products, on a regular basis. These foods are richest in the calcium you need for strong bones.

■ **Do some strength-building.** For your bones to make the best use of calcium, you need to do weight-bearing exercise (which may also increase bone density). Try brisk walking, jogging, dancing, lifting weights, or climbing stairs. Be sure to ask your doctor for guidelines on what, and how much, exercise is safe for you.

Spare Your Bones: Do Things Right

To prevent osteoporosis-related injuries:

● **Always sit up straight.** Pick a chair that supports the curve of your lower back (or use a rolled-up towel or lumbar roll). Sit with spine lengthened, shoulders wide.

● **Prepare for a sneeze (or cough).** A sudden sneeze can jerk your weakened torso forward, injuring your spine. If you feel one coming on, bend your knees. Keep your back straight, and put one hand on your thigh for support (*see illustration*). Or brace

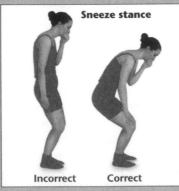

Sneeze stance

Incorrect   Correct

your lower back with your hand to stay upright.

● **Do chores correctly.** Take care as you vacuum, mop floors, or rake the yard. Bend from your knees and hips, not

your waist. Don't twist; push rather than pull.

● **Bend from your hips.** When you lean down to load the dishwasher or make the bed, don't sag from your waist. Bend at your knees and hips, keeping your lower back straight.

● **Open with care.** Trying to lift a "stuck" or especially heavy window is a common cause of compression fractures. That's because it puts a great deal of pressure on your spine. Instead of opening the window by yourself, ask someone to help.

Osteoporosis in Men

While it's true that men start out with greater bone density and lose calcium more slowly than women, hormonal changes may also contribute to men's development of osteoporosis. A decline in testosterone, which occurs naturally after age 60, reduces ability to use dietary calcium to build new bone. (Men also produce a small amount of estrogen, and fluctuations in this hormone may play a role.) Prostate cancer treatment can also cause abnormally low testosterone.

Treatment: Men who develop osteoporosis and have low testosterone may be treated with alendronate and/or androgen replacement therapy. It's often applied as a skin patch. If long-term steroid use is the culprit, Fosamax, Actonel, or Boniva are good options.

- **Limit beverages that leach calcium from your bones.** Restrict alcoholic drinks to one a day if you're a woman or two if you're a man. Hold the line at two cups of caffeinated coffee a day.
- **If you smoke, quit.** Tobacco interferes with normal bone metabolism, contributing to osteoporosis.
- **Secure rugs firmly to the floor.** Tack area rugs down, or use a slip-proof backing, to lessen chances of falls.
- **Install handrails** in the bathtub, shower stall, or wherever you feel you might need assistance in changing position.
- **Check the lighting.** Be sure your rooms are well lit during waking hours and that you can find light switches easily in the dark.
- **Don't run for a train or bus.** Rushing increases your risk of tripping and falling. Always allow enough time to get there safely.

Procedures

Your doctor will check your progress with bone density tests called dual energy x-ray absorptiometry, or DEXA (*see page 355*). If you have a severe break or problems such as osteoarthritis, **joint replacement** is an option. This surgery, which replaces part of a hip or knee with manmade materials (*see page 38*), can greatly improve your ability to participate in daily activities. If you have a collapsed spinal vertebra, a new therapy called **kyphoplasty** may relieve pain and prevent kyphosis (dowager's hump). In this procedure, a tiny balloon expands the collapsed vertebra. Bone-like material is then injected to restore the spine to its normal structure.

▶**IF YOU TAKE FOSAMAX,** be careful about using NSAIDs like aspirin or ibuprofen (Advil). A new study has found that the combination of the two drugs magnifies potential irritation of your stomach lining and increases chances for developing a stomach ulcer.

FINDING Support

- For an excellent overview of osteoporosis and its treatment, as well as discussions of more specific concerns such as fashion tips for people with spinal compression fractures, contact the National Osteoporosis Foundation in Washington, D.C. (1-800-223-9994 or www.nof.org). You'll also find information on how to join or start a support group in your area.

- Interested in joining a clinical study of new medications? A trial that explores new forms of existing medications? Or one that looks at how lifestyle changes influence osteoporosis? Many researchers are seeking participants. You can find out what's available and where the study sites are by logging on to www.clinicaltrials.gov and entering the word "osteoporosis."

- To help the girls in your family start caring for their bones at an early age, check out www.cdc.gov/powerfulbones. Designed for young people by the Centers for Disease Control, this website includes a discussion of the importance of prevention, fun recipes for calcium-filled treats, ideas for weight-bearing activities, and more.

Parkinson's disease

Symptoms are so subtle and develop so slowly that it usually takes 5 to 10 years before you know there's a problem. Even then, this disease can almost always be managed, often for decades, with specialized medications and good self-care.

LIKELY **First Steps**

- **Medications** to preserve or replace the natural nerve chemical dopamine in the brain.
- **Regular exercise** to improve coordination and strength.
- **Nutritious diet** to prevent constipation and increase antioxidant levels.
- **Surgery** to reduce symptoms, if drugs don't work, or side effects are unbearable.

QUESTIONS TO **Ask**

- Is there any way to slow the progression of my symptoms?
- Will this disease shorten my life span?
- Do I need physical therapy or a special diet?
- Would surgery help reduce my symptoms?

What is happening

More than a million Americans may have Parkinson's disease. About 50,000 new cases are discovered every year. If you've recently been diagnosed, you are probably already displaying some symptoms: maybe a slight trembling (tremor) in your hands, legs, or face, or muscle stiffness, coordination problems, or a slowness of movement (bradykinesia). These and other Parkinson's symptoms indicate that nerve cells (neurons) in a relatively tiny part of your brain called the substantia nigra have started to die off. This causes a drop in dopamine, a nerve chemical that carries the signals that allow your muscles to move quickly and smoothly.

Parkinson's disease usually occurs between the ages of 55 and 70, and men get it slightly more often than women. Up to 10% of those afflicted, however, are under age 40. They have what's called "young-onset" Parkinson's. But whether your symptoms start when you're young or old, the cause of Parkinson's remains a mystery. One theory is that naturally occurring oxygen molecules called free radicals damage nerve cells in the brain. Research has shown that some Parkinson's patients have a 30% to 40% decrease in complex I, an enzyme that normally controls this free radical onslaught. Genetic factors are occasionally involved as well. If you have a close relative with Parkinson's disease, your chances of getting it are three times greater than those of someone without a family link. It's also possible that exposure to herbicides and pesticides plays a role, but this has not been proven.

Whether you've had Parkinson's for years or have just learned your diagnosis, the outlook is good. Among the degenerative diseases of the nervous system, Parkinson's is one of the most treatable. Symptoms worsen over time as dopamine steadily decreases, but many individuals continue to live full, active lives.

Treatments

There isn't a definitive test for Parkinson's disease, but neurologists have little trouble recognizing it once symptoms progress beyond the earliest stages. Early symptoms are often so mild that people don't bother to call their doctors. That's unfortunate, because early treatment can make a difference in how you function.

The goals of Parkinson's treatment are to relieve your symptoms and effectively balance the challenges of the disease with medication side effects that can be troubling. Treatment is

Treatment options

Medications

Levodopa	First-line therapy; often with carbidopa.
COMT inhibitors	Tasmar, Comtan prolong effects of levodopa.
Dopamine agonists	May be prescribed before levodopa.
Anticholinergics	Artane et al. reduce tremors in early stages.
Antivirals	Symadine, Symmetrel for rigidity, slowness.

Lifestyle changes

Exercise	Essential for balance, mobility, strength.
Diet	Low-protein, high-antioxidant best.
Hobbies & support groups	To keep the mind agile; prevent depression.

Procedures

Pallidotomy	Treats involuntary movements.
Thalamotomy	For tremor; destroys thalamus tissues.
Deep brain stimulation	To control symptoms via electrode implants.

extremely individualized. As the disease progresses, you'll need to work closely with a neurologist to customize your program. Parkinson's can't be prevented or cured, but there have been exciting breakthroughs. A number of new drugs (and combinations of old ones) can control or even eliminate symptoms for a time. And as the disease progresses, a mix of lifestyle adjustments and drug and surgical options can help keep symptoms from taking over your life.

Medications

The main treatment for Parkinson's is a drug called **levodopa (L-dopa),** which the brain converts to muscle-controlling dopamine. It's most effective against rigidity and slowness. Most levodopa preparations (such as Sinemet and Atamet) include the drug **carbidopa.** It helps levodopa work more efficiently and helps reduce nausea or other side effects. The drawback to levodopa is that the "honeymoon" usually lasts only five years on average. After that, the drug may gradually stop working.

A relatively new class of drugs, the **catechol-O-methyltransferase (COMT) inhibitors,** are taken along with levodopa to block a liver enzyme that breaks down levodopa before it reaches your brain. These drugs, which include tolcapone (Tasmar) and entacapone (Comtan), prolong the effects of levodopa and allow you to manage on smaller doses.

Because levodopa works for only a short time, your doctor may not want to start you on it right away. So as an initial treatment,

TAKING Control

- **Eat more fava beans.** If you're at the earliest stages of Parkinson's disease and aren't yet taking medications, your doctor might advise you to eat these legumes. They contain a hefty amount of levodopa, the same therapeutic compound that's used in some medications. If you're already taking drugs, however, don't add favas to your diet without checking with your doctor. You could wind up getting too much of the active ingredient.

- **Work on "muscle freezing."** If, like many Parkinson's sufferers, you literally freeze in place and find it hard to take a step, you can usually break free by rocking from side to side or by pretending you're stepping over a small object. You can also divide each movement into several steps. For example, if you're going to walk through a door, approach the door, pause, open the door, pause, then walk through. Some people also have success improving their gait by walking to the ticking of a metronome.

- **Wear clothes that are easy to get on and off.** As the disease progresses, you may have trouble even with simple activities like dressing. Make it easy on yourself by buying pants and skirts with elastic waistbands and simple slip-on tops. Avoid hard-to-fasten buttons or snaps.

- **Take small bites when eating.** It puts less strain on your chewing and swallowing muscles, which may become less responsive over time.

The Search for Clues in the "Fox Cluster"

Parkinson's disease overwhelmingly affects older adults. Yet actor Michael J. Fox was only 30 when he was diagnosed in 1991. Scientists want to know why—especially because Fox was one of four people working on the TV sitcom "Leo & Me" who later got the disease.

Experts are intrigued by the "Fox Cluster," which suggests that environmental factors or virus might be responsible. Clusters of Parkinson's disease are not new, but health experts rarely have enough time or money to investigate them. Fox's celebrity status guaranteed that this particular cluster would get a second look.

So far, no one's figured out what causes Parkinson's disease. Genetic factors have been linked to the disease. So has exposure to pesticides and herbicides. The Fox Cluster may provide additional clues by allowing experts to investigate a small group of people who appear to have had an abnormally high risk of getting the disease. The goal will be to determine what, if anything, they had in common.

The viral theory

The theory that a virus was the culprit makes sense: An infectious agent could readily pass from person to person in the insulated confines of a production studio. The viral theory is further bolstered by the fact that Parkinson's disease is slightly more common among teachers, doctors, and nurses, who are regularly exposed to infections. Loggers and miners, who often share tight quarters at work camps, also have a slightly higher risk for it.

The environmental theory

The other suspect in the Fox Cluster is environmental toxins. Any group of people that shares a work space—especially one with limited air circulation—would be exposed to similar levels of chemicals or other substances. If one or more of these substances caused Parkinson's, it would make sense to see a "spike" of disease among the coworkers.

Or was it chance?

It's possible that the Fox Cluster arose purely coincidentally. But the odds of four people getting the disease, out of a crew of 125 has been estimated at less than 1 in 20,000. Researchers studying the case hope it will eventually provide much-needed clues about the origin of this mysterious disease.

▶ Is it true that coffee and cigarettes protect against Parkinson's?

They might, research suggests. A study in the journal Neurology *compared 196 people with Parkinson's disease to an equal number of healthy people. It found that coffee drinkers were significantly less likely to be in the Parkinson's group, and the more they drank, the lower their risk. It's possible that something in coffee (caffeine, perhaps) protects cells or improves the action of dopamine. The nicotine in cigarettes may have similar protective effects, with far fewer smokers affected by Parkinson's. Since cigarette smoking is so unhealthy, patches and other nicotine delivery forms are being studied.*

some doctors are trying another class of drugs—the **dopamine agonists.** These include bromocriptine (Parlodel), pergolide (Permax), and pramipexole (Mirapex). These drugs mimic the effects of dopamine to reduce Parkinson's symptoms by activating certain chemical receptor sites in the brain.

Your doctor can also choose among a variety of other drugs to control specific Parkinson's symptoms. For muscle tremors in the early stages, for example, you might need to take an **anticholinergic drug,** such as trihexyphenidyl (Artane). To reduce tremor, muscle rigidity, and slowness, an **antiviral drug** called amantadine (Symadine, Symmetrel), often prescribed for treating bouts of the flu, may be recommended.

Lifestyle Changes

Because Parkinson's affects muscle movement, it's important to stay as strong and fit as you can. **Regular exercise** is essential. It improves your mobility, balance, and range of motion and keeps up your strength. Any physical activity, such as stretching, walking, swimming, or even weight-lifting, will help you move better and could enhance your endurance. If you're new to exercise or could simply use some extra motivation, begin by working with a physical therapist who can design an exercise plan that will be effective for you.

To prevent falls, safety-proof your home. Install handrails along stairways, and grab rails in the shower and next to the toilet. Keep electrical or phone cords out of the way. Once the disease progresses, carry a small cellular phone with you in case you fall and can't get up.

Diet is another self-care cornerstone. If you're taking L-dopa medications, limit protein to about 12% of total daily calories. More than this makes it harder for the levodopa to reach your brain. Eat plenty of fiber-rich foods, such as vegetables, fruits, and legumes. Fiber prevents constipation, a common symptom of Parkinson's. Plant foods are also rich in vitamin C and other antioxidant nutrients, which may help curtail nerve-cell damage caused by free radicals. Consider working with a nutritionist.

Don't forget that a good mental attitude can be just as important as keeping yourself physically healthy. One good way to avoid dwelling on your condition is to **take up a hobby.** Tasks that involve both the mind and the hands, such as sewing, carpentry, or even playing cards, may slow the progression of the disease. Joining a Parkinson's **support group** can also be beneficial for you as well as family members and caregivers.

Procedures

Surgery for Parkinson's disease fell out of favor when scientists developed levodopa and other medications. But a number of procedures have been revived as advances in magnetic imaging provide new understanding of how motor information is processed. You may be a candidate for one of the surgeries below if drugs become ineffective or side effects unbearable.

- **Pallidotomy.** This procedure uses electrical current to destroy cells in the globus pallidus, the part of the brain responsible for some Parkinson's symptoms. The procedure is sometimes used to reduce involuntary movements such as twitching, nodding, or jerking (called dyskinesias), which may be due to taking large doses of levodopa for a long time.

- **Thalamotomy.** The surgery that actor Michael J. Fox (*see box opposite*) underwent in 1997, thalamotomy uses the same technique as pallidotomy, but it reduces tremors by destroying a small amount of tissue in the thalamus, the brain's message relay center. It has successfully eliminated tremors in 80% to 90% of patients.

- **Deep brain stimulation (DBS).** Used in Europe for many years and in the United States only since 1997, this procedure involves inserting an electrode in the brain's thalamus. Connected to a pacemaker-like device that's implanted in your chest and that you control, the electrode delivers electrical signals to the brain to interrupt tremor-causing nerve signals. In 2002, the FDA approved Medtronic's Activa Parkinson's Control Therapy, a more advanced form of the surgery in which electrodes are implanted in both sides of the brain. The new procedure is expected to improve not only tremors, but other symptoms as well. The advantage of DBS over pallidotomy and thalamotomy is that it is reversible.

Promising DEVELOPMENTS

- Implanting cells into the brain's substantia nigra to replace dopamine-producing cells may hold the greatest promise for Parkinson's treatment. While many novel methods are being investigated, including the implantation of fetal brain cells, recent research suggests that **implanting cells from your own brain** may produce dramatic symptom improvement.

- The dietary supplement **coenzyme Q_{10}** slowed the progression of Parkinson's disease in a small but widely publicized study published in the *Archives of Neurology* in 2002. Produced naturally in the body, this compound is thought to be at unusually low levels in people with Parkinson's. Available over the counter, CoQ_{10} is believed to help cells' energy-supplying structures to function better. In the 16-month study of 80 Parkinson's patients, the 23 on the highest daily CoQ_{10} dose experienced 44% less decline in mental function, movement, and ability to carry out daily tasks.

FINDING Support

- For the latest developments in Parkinson's disease treatments, contact the American Parkinson Disease Association (1-800-223-2732 or www.apdaparkinson.com).

- Another helpful group is the National Parkinson Foundation (1-800-327-4545 or www.parkinson.org).

Peripheral vascular disease

If you feel pain in your legs after walking only a block or two, it may be peripheral vascular disease, an ailment that affects 10 percent of Americans over age 85. Surprisingly, more exercise is part of the treatment—and it can bring real relief.

LIKELY First Steps

- **Daily exercise** to build endurance and blood flow.
- **Lifestyle changes**—stop smoking, lose weight, and follow a heart-healthy diet.
- **Aspirin or prescription medications** for circulation.

QUESTIONS TO Ask

- Should I purchase a treadmill to exercise at home?
- What if my legs hurt even when I'm not walking?
- How likely am I to develop a more serious problem?

BYPASS SURGERY

In this procedure, a healthy vein is removed from your leg or arm (or an artificial blood vessel is used). Doctors graft it into place, rerouting the blood flow around the blockage.

What is happening

Peripheral vascular disease (PVD) occurs when arteries in the "periphery" of your body—typically your legs—narrow or become blocked by the buildup of a fatty substance called plaque. The blockage usually develops over many years and is due to atherosclerosis (also known as hardening of the arteries), the same problem that gives rise to coronary heart disease, heart attack, and stroke. The risk factors for all these illnesses are similar: smoking, high blood pressure, high cholesterol, diabetes, and a sedentary lifestyle.

When your leg arteries are blocked, not enough oxygen-rich blood can get through the vessels to replenish your muscles. The resulting pain when you walk, which is relieved when you stop, is termed intermittent claudication. An MRI will probably show blockages within your arteries. As blockages worsen, you may feel pain after walking a short distance or even at rest. Your feet may develop sores, and tissue may die off. This dangerous condition is called gangrene.

Treatments

The good news is that virtually no one dies from peripheral vascular disease. The bad news is that the condition will deteriorate unless you make significant lifestyle changes. The aim of therapy is to relieve pain and, over the long term, prevent your condition from becoming worse. Regular exercise, a healthy diet, and weight maintenance can go a long way toward helping you achieve these goals. These strategies will also lessen your likelihood of having a heart attack or stroke. Medications and surgery can also help.

Lifestyle Changes

In milder cases of PVD, an **exercise program** can dramatically relieve leg pain and be as effective as medications or surgery for increasing the distance you can walk without pain. When you exercise regularly, the body naturally uses smaller blood vessels. With PVD, this added circulation will help compensate for a blocked artery. You'll need to push yourself a bit by walking every day. Pick a realistic distance, say a quarter mile. Then walk until you feel pain. Stop and rest, checking how far you've come and how long it took. When the pain passes, start walking again. Keep up this cycle for the full distance. In a few weeks, your "points of pain" will improve, and you can start increasing your daily distance and your speed.

Treatment options

Lifestyle changes

Exercise	Can be as effective as drugs or surgery.
Stop smoking	Key change to help your circulation.
Healthy diet	Fruits, vegetables, and no saturated fats.
Treat related conditions	Usually diabetes, cholesterol, hypertension.

Medications

Circulation-improving	Aspirin, Plavix, Ticlid, Pletal.

Procedures

Angioplasty	Compresses plaque to clear vessel.
Bypass surgery	Reroutes blood around clogged artery.

The conditions causing blocked arteries in your legs also affect arteries in your heart. Heart-healthy lifestyle changes will help both (*see Coronary Heart Disease, page 94*). The single most important action you can take is to **stop smoking:** Smoking decreases the elasticity of your blood vessels and increases your risk for blood clots. You should also eat a **healthy diet.** Get plenty of fruits and vegetables, avoid saturated fats, and keep your weight down. Treat **related conditions,** including high cholesterol (*page 176*), diabetes (*pages 104–109*), or high blood pressure (*page 170*).

Medications

Your doctor may prescribe various drugs to improve blood circulation, ease pain, and prevent heart attack and stroke, and suggest a daily **aspirin** (either a baby or adult tablet) to keep blood from becoming too sticky. Prescription drugs, such as **clopidogrel** (Plavix) or **ticlopidine** (Ticlid) may also be prescribed. **Cilostazol** (Pletal) may allow you to walk further without pain and be more effective than pentoxifylline (Trental), the first drug to be approved for claudication. Many other medicines are in the pipeline.

Procedures

If pain persists, your doctor may try a procedure called **angioplasty** (*see page 97*). A thin tube called a catheter is threaded into the problem artery. The doctor then inflates a balloon to compress the blockage and reopen the clogged vessel. A metal device called a stent may be used to help keep the artery propped open, but in about half of those who have angioplasty, the artery closes again after several months. Doctors are investigating related techniques, such as atherectomy, in which a small tool shaves away plaque buildup, but similar problems can occur. If the disease becomes severe, **bypass surgery** is an effective option (*see illustration opposite*). More than 75% of patients who undergo it are fine five years later.

TAKING Control

- **Find a podiatrist,** a foot-care specialist, to help prevent PVD-related infections. Inspect your feet daily for cracks, sores, or calluses. If infection develops, a prescription antibiotic ointment called becaplermin (Regranex) may help. Take note: Left untreated, an infection can lead to gangrene. This serious complication may require amputation.

- **Consider natural therapies.** In some European countries, the herb ginkgo biloba (120 mg daily) is medically approved for "circulatory disorders" like claudication. Vitamin E (400 IU a day) and the amino acid arginine (1,000 mg twice a day) may also promote blood vessel health. Let your doctor know of any remedies you are taking; some can interfere with medications or surgery.

- **If pain keeps you up at night,** elevate the head of your bed four to six inches to increase blood flow to the legs.

- **If pain is sudden and severe** or the leg becomes cold or blue, seek help immediately. You could have a blood clot and need an injection of a clot-dissolving drug.

FINDING Support

- For additional information, contact the American Heart Association (1-800-242-8721 or www.americanheart.org). Local chapters are available in many cities.

- The American Medical Association physician locator can help you find a vascular surgeon, or other specialist (www.ama-assn.org/aps/amahg.htm).

Pneumonia

The diagnosis of pneumonia can be alarming—and this disease can be serious. Given the advances of modern medicine, however, most cases now clear up rapidly when treated with the right combination of drugs and a dose of common sense.

LIKELY **First Steps**

- **Antibiotics** if your pneumonia is caused by bacteria.
- **Bed rest** and plenty of fluids to allow your body to begin to heal.
- **Expectorants** for your cough to bring up sputum and help clear your lungs.

QUESTIONS TO **Ask**

- What should I do to prevent passing pneumonia to other members of my family?
- When can I return to my daily activities?
- Am I likely to develop any lingering after-effects, asthma, or other chronic health problems?

What is happening

Pneumonia is not one illness, but many. This lung infection is caused by inhaling some sort of nasty organism when your immune defense system is down, usually due to a cold, the flu, or a chronic disease. The perpetrator may be any of hundreds of strains of viruses, bacteria, or other microorganisms. These germs get into your alveoli, the small air sacs deep in your lungs. They inflame the lungs and fill the alveoli fill with mucus.

Symptoms of pneumonia vary widely. If bacteria is the cause of the infection, you'll probably have a sudden onset of illness, with fever, shaking, chills, chest pain, and a productive, or "wet" cough that expels sputum from your lungs. Viruses and organisms called mycoplasma usually cause milder symptoms, including headache, low-grade fever, hacking ("dry") cough, and general malaise. (It is mycoplasma, for instance, that produces walking "pneumonia," which is usually not severe enough to confine you to bed or send you to the hospital.) When pneumonia strikes an elderly person, the signs can be very different—often just rapid breathing and sometimes confusion.

If you contract pneumonia when you're not in the hospital—a condition formally called community-acquired pneumonia—you probably won't be as sick as a hospital-acquired case. Infants, young children, and adults over age 75 are much more likely to get pneumonia than the general population, as are people with compromised immune systems. It is reassuring to note that when pneumonia fatalities do occur, they are usually the final complication of some other serious condition.

Treatments

Because pneumonia has so many different causes, there are various ways to treat it. Fortunately, up to 75% of cases can be dealt with at home. Unless your doctor wants you hospitalized, your best plan is to rest in bed and take your medication. You'll likely feel better within a few days. For several days or weeks after that, you may still cough and feel more tired than usual, but in time, your lungs will be as good as new. Certain patients, especially heavy smokers or the chronically ill, may take months to recover fully, however. Four to six weeks after treatment, see your doctor for a follow-up visit to make sure the entire episode is history.

If you are at home, be on the alert for any of the following: A fever that reaches 104°F, difficulty breathing, a rapid pulse rate

Treatment options

Medications

Antibiotics	For bacterial or mycoplasmal pneumonia.
Antivirals/antifungals	Depending on type of infection.
Cough medicine	Suppressants or expectorants, as necessary.
Analgesics	Good for fever and pain related to coughing.
Flu/pneumonia vaccines	Protect against germs that cause pneumonia.

Lifestyle changes

Bed rest	Until fever passes.
Fluids	Prevent dehydration; loosen mucus.
Steam inhalation	Helps you loosen and expel infected sputum.
Heating pad	Relieves chest pain.

Procedures

Supplemental oxygen	Makes breathing easier; rarely needed.

(125 beats a minute or faster), a drop in blood pressure that makes you feel dizzy, or bluish skin. These are signs of a severe infection. If you have any of them, go to an emergency room right away.

Medications

If your pneumonia is bacterial or mycoplasmal, your doctor will prescribe **antibiotics.** Those commonly used include a group called macrolides, such as erythromycin and azithromycin (Zithromax). Another possibility is fluoroquinolone antibiotics, such as levofloxacin (Levaquin), or the tetracyclines, such as doxycycline or the combination of amoxicillin-clavulanate (Augmentin). Most mild viral pneumonias clear up by themselves; for severe cases, you may need an **antiviral drug,** such as acyclovir or ribavirin. Fungal pneumonia is treated in the hospital with intravenous **antifungal drugs,** such as amphotericin B.

For pain, ask your doctor about taking **analgesics** such as aspirin or acetaminophen (Tylenol). There are also a number of **cough medicines:** Expectorants with guaifenesin (found in Robitussin and Glycotuss) help loosen mucus while allowing your cough to bring up infected material. Cough suppressants turn off your cough reflex and may slow recovery, because your lungs need to expel the infected material. For a dry, persistent, and nonproductive cough, your doctor may recommend a suppressant (Robitussin Maximum Strength, Halls), so that you can get some sleep.

If you are age 65 or older, get the **pneumonia vaccine,** which is effective against 88% of strains of *Streptococcus pneumoniae,* the most common pneumonia-causing bacteria. You should also get the vaccine if you are in a high-risk group—if you have heart, lung, or

TAKING Control

- **Avoid polluted air.** Exposure to high levels of automobile exhaust or industrial smoke increases the risk of developing pneumonia and other cardiopulmonary diseases.

- **Eat your veggies.** Orange, yellow, and dark-green vegetables (and fruits), such as oranges, carrots, and broccoli are rich in antioxidants that boost your immune system.

- **Don't take antibiotics** at the first sign of a cold in an effort to prevent future bouts of pneumonia. Antibiotics cannot fight a viral cold. Take all of any antibiotic your doctor does prescribe for you. This will ensure complete recovery and prevent development of antibiotic-resistant bacteria.

▶ **When I got pneumonia last year, the doctor hospitalized me even though I didn't feel very sick. Was this necessary?**

Some types of pneumonia can become severe within hours, so your doctor may want to keep you under hospital supervision in the early stage. This is especially true if you're an older person, a smoker, or have a compromised immune system. Your doctor may also decide that you need intravenous drugs. Studies reveal too much unnecessary hospitalization for pneumonia. According to one study, 30% of pneumonia patients now routinely hospitalized could be treated safely at home and another 20% could be sent home after a brief in-patient observation. So always ask your doctor why hospitalization is required.

How to Clear Your Lungs

Clearing your breathing passages makes it easier to get rid of infected sputum. Here are some suggestions:

- **Inhale steam.** Loosen mucus by breathing in steam from a pot of hot water for 10 minutes morning and evening. Add a drop of eucalyptus oil to the water.
- **Use a humidifier.** Moistening the air will help thin sputum. Clean the device with bleach every week to keep it free of fungus.
- **Take hot showers.** Let the water stream over your face and breathe in the steam.
- **Try postural drainage.** Lie with your head below your torso, so gravity pulls fluids toward your throat.
- **Ask about an incentive spirometer.** This device has a breathing tube and gauge to measure air entering and leaving your lungs. Exhale, then inhale as strongly as possible to raise the gauge. This exercises your lungs while it measures how well you're recovering.
- **Try deep or rhythmic breathing.** Tap lightly on your chest to loosen mucus, or have someone else tap on your back. Inhale deeply and rhythmically three or four times. Cough deeply to try to produce sputum. To reduce any pain during coughing, hold a pillow tightly against your chest or lie on the side that hurts. Repeat the entire procedure every four hours.

Promising
DEVELOPMENTS

- The FDA recently approved a **new antibiotic, telithromycin (Ketek)**, for treatment of community-acquired pneumonia in certain patients. A new type of antibiotic called a ketolide, Ketek is intended to combat bugs resistant to older antibiotics.

FINDING Support

- Being bedridden with pneumonia can leave you feeling isolated. For more information and services, contact the American Lung Association in New York, NY (1-800-LUNG-USA or www.lungusa.org).

kidney disease, for example, or are HIV-positive. In the past, the vaccine was given just once in a lifetime, but your doctor may opt to give you a booster shot every five to ten years. And don't forget your yearly **flu shot:** Pneumonia often strikes as a complication of influenza.

Lifestyle Changes

Getting pneumonia may make you immune to one strain of microorganism, but there are hundreds more that can still attack. Maintaining a healthy lifestyle can help prevent reinfection with pneumonia (or with colds and flu that can lead to pneumonia) and reduce severity of symptoms you do develop. Follow some commonsense guidelines: Eat a nutritious diet, maintain a healthy weight, exercise regularly, get the sleep you need, and wash your hands frequently. Above all, stay away from cigarettes.

To speed your recovery: **Rest in bed** until your fever disappears. **Drink lots of fluids**—at least eight glasses of water or other liquids per day to help thin mucus. **Inhale steam. Use a heating pad** on your chest for 10 minutes at a time, as needed. Make sure it's on a low setting and not directly on your skin.

Procedures

If you're having trouble breathing, your doctor may give you **supplemental oxygen** to breathe through a face mask or nose tube. It's rare that someone with pneumonia requires a mechanical ventilator, a machine that assists breathing.

The only pneumonia complication requiring a surgical procedure occurs when fluid builds up in the area between your lungs and your chest wall (the pleural space). If this happens, your doctor may perform a **thoracentesis,** in which a needle is inserted through your chest wall and fluid is drained so you can breathe more easily.

Premenstrual syndrome

If misery loves company, PMS sufferers are an empathetic crowd. But by taking a proactive approach to this recurring condition—starting with diet and exercise—you may be able to eliminate the physical and emotional toll it takes.

What is happening

If you're one of the approximately 75% of American women who have premenstrual syndrome (PMS), you know it's hardly the joke TV comedians make it out to be. Every month, you really do feel crabby, crave that whole box of chocolates, and suffer from breast tenderness, bloating, cramps, weight gain, or headaches—and sometimes all at once. The discomfort may last from a few hours to several days. Or it may begin a week or two before your period and stop abruptly when the bleeding starts. Because PMS can elicit some 150 different symptoms, there's really no typical case. While most women find it annoying rather than disabling, an estimated 3% to 8% have truly severe symptoms, suffering from a variety of physical problems as well as serious depression—a condition called premenstrual dysphoric disorder, or PMDD.

Research remains inconclusive about the cause of PMS. Many experts blame an imbalance of female hormones estrogen and progesterone, which may interfere with brain chemicals that control mood and pain. Others suspect low levels of serotonin, a brain chemical associated with emotional well-being. Additional culprits may include nutritional deficiencies, fluid and sodium retention, low blood sugar, and a heightened stress response. No one theory offers a satisfactory explanation for all women. There's a natural limit to PMS: Symptoms, which usually strike in the mid-20s, generally subside after age 35. They disappear completely with menopause.

Treatments

Many women accept PMS as an unfortunate fact of life: A 1999 survey found that those who suffered most were the least likely to seek treatment, believing nothing could be done. Yet PMS is very treatable. If your symptoms are on the mild side, adopting a healthier lifestyle may be all it takes to make you feel better. You'll likely require some pharmaceutical help for moderate or severe PMS or PMDD. Once you find the right therapy, you should be virtually free of symptoms after three menstrual cycles.

Lifestyle Changes

One easy way to begin controlling your PMS symptoms is to adopt a low-fat, high-fiber **eating program** light on junk food and heavy on fresh produce, whole grains, and legumes. Whole foods tend to be high in complex carbohydrates, which relieve irritability by

LIKELY First Steps

- **A healthy diet** to reduce bloating and curb cravings.
- **Stress reduction** through regular exercise and mind-soothing techniques.
- **Vitamins and other nutritional supplements** to balance body chemistry.
- **Analgesics** to ease aches and relieve bloating.
- **Antidepressants** for PMDD or if lifestyle measures fail to lift PMS-related depression.

QUESTIONS TO Ask

- If I'm depressed only some of the time, why do I need an antidepressant?
- Could I be suffering from seasonal affective disorder?
- Will PMS or any treatment for it make it harder for me to conceive?
- Do you think a special PMS clinic or support group might help me?

TAKING Control

- **Keep a symptoms diary** for at least a few months. Chart how you feel and when, as well as dates when your period starts and ends. This will show the cycle of your symptoms and help your doctor eliminate other possible causes. Problems are often due to another ailment, such as pain linked to menstruation (dysmenorrhea) or seasonal affective disorder (SAD).

- **Don't eat meat.** A 2000 study found that women who ate a low-fat vegetarian diet for two menstrual cycles had less pain and bloating than meat eaters. Try replacing red meat with salmon, tuna, or other oily fish rich in the omega-3 fatty acids that can help relieve menstrual cramps and possibly related depression.

- **Try cognitive-behavioral therapy.** If you suffer from depression or feelings of hopelessness due to PMS or PMDD, a psychotherapist can help you master techniques for solving problems, managing obstacles, and restructuring priorities. The therapist will give you new ways of thinking about your condition so you can overcome pessimistic thoughts and regain a sense of control.

- **Be wary of certain PMS clinics.** If a clinic insists on expensive preliminary lab work, charges high fees payable in advance, pushes one treatment for all patients, or offers a fast diagnosis and quick fix, look out. Choose one that's run by a physician you trust and that tailors treatment specifically to you.

Treatment options

Lifestyle changes	
Eating plan & exercise	Good diet, regular aerobics key for relief.
Stress reduction	Yoga, meditation, visualizations, for tension.
Improved sleep habits	Can prevent PMS-related insomnia.
Natural methods	
Vitamins & minerals	To start, calcium, magnesium, vitamin B_6.
Progesterone cream	Produces a mild sedative effect.
Medications	
Pain relievers	Analgesics; bromocriptine for breast pain.
Diuretics	Try Aldactone for bloating.
Oral contraceptives	To keep hormonal fluctuations in check.
Antidepressants	Sarafem, other SSRIs, for serious depression.

raising blood levels of tryptophan. This amino acid converts to the mood-elevating hormone serotonin. Munching on fresh fruits and whole-grain breads may also curb an unhealthy appetite for sugary treats or salty snacks—foods that often lead to water retention or a bad mood. You'll also need to beware of caffeine. While coffee, tea, and colas can increase urination, they can also increase irritability and sleep problems.

In addition to diet, **regular exercise** also helps reduce many PMS symptoms. At the very least, aim for 30 minutes of aerobic exercise—walking, swimming, cycling—three times a week. Try some **stress-reduction techniques**—yoga, guided imagery, meditation—to help you relax and cope with any emotional symptoms. And don't forget the ultimate in relaxation: **sleep.** (*See Insomnia, page 188, for ways to regulate your sleep habits.*)

Natural Methods*

In addition to making lifestyle changes, many women with PMS have had success using these natural products, as well as the herbal remedies mentioned in the box opposite:

- **Calcium.** In a study from Columbia University, PMS patients who took 1,200 mg of supplemental calcium daily for three months reported a 48% reduction in such PMS symptoms as breast tenderness, bloating, headaches, and moodiness.
- **Magnesium.** During the last two weeks of your menstrual cycle, magnesium levels fall. That may increase water retention, headaches, and irritability. Try taking 250 mg of this mineral twice a day, every day, with food.
- **Vitamin B_6.** Some studies find B_6 works for PMS headaches, fatigue, depression, and breast pain; others don't. Just 50 mg

Herbal Remedies* for PMS

If you want to use herbs for PMS symptoms, allow three months for noticeable benefits. Be sure to tell your doctor.

- **Chasteberry (vitex)** helps normalize the ratio of progesterone and estrogen, providing relief for irritability, depression, and bloating. Avoid using it with oral contraceptives or bromocriptine.

- **Evening primrose oil** contains gamma-linolenic acid (GLA), an essential fatty acid (EFA), which reduces cramping by interfering with production of inflammatory hormone-like chemicals called prostaglandins. It may relieve bloating, breast tenderness, and irritability.
- **St. John's wort,** used for mild to moderate depression, appears to boost levels of serotonin, which controls moods and emotions. Avoid using it if you're on antidepressants or oral contraceptives.
- **PMS herbal combinations** provide a number of helpful herbs in one convenient capsule. Some products also contain the vitamins C, E, and B, plus magnesium.

twice a day can be effective. Avoid high doses: 200 mg or more for an extended period can cause nerve damage and irritability.

- **Natural progesterone cream.** This is synthesized progesterone, a mild sedative. Look for a 2% progesterone cream, such as Pro-Gest, with at least 400 mg of progesterone per ounce. Apply about ½ teaspoon twice a day, following label directions, during the two weeks before your period.

Medications

For mild PMS aches and pains, **OTC pain relievers** such as aspirin, ibuprofen (Advil), or naproxen (Aleve) often work fine. You can also try a specialized product such as Midol, Pamprin, or Premsyn, which contains acetaminophen along with a diuretic and/or antihistamine. For severe breast pain, ask your doctor about a prescription **dopamine agonist** called bromocriptine (Ergoset, Parlodel). It reduces the levels of the hormone prolactin, which controls lactational changes in your body, but it can sometimes cause side effects.

If you have bloating that doesn't respond to dietary measures, a prescription **diuretic** may help eliminate water and sodium. One of the best is spironolactone (Aldactone). Unlike other diuretics, it doesn't deplete potassium, which can lead to heart rhythm disturbances. If hormonal fluctuations are your problem, you may be given an **oral contraceptive** that contains both progestins (natural or synthetic forms of progesterone) and estrogen. A new combination contraceptive called Yasmin contains both estrogen and drospirenone, a substance similar to natural progesterone. It regulates mood swings and may relieve the severe emotional distress of PMDD.

Also useful are antidepressants called **selective serotonin reuptake inhibitors (SSRIs),** such as sertraline (Zoloft) and paroxetine (Paxil). They increase mood-elevating serotonin. Fluoxetine (Sarafem) was the first SSRI approved by the FDA for treating PMDD as well as PMS. Sarafem is taken right before your period (it's actually the same drug as Prozac, sold under a different name).

Natural methods are not subject to the same testing and regulation as prescription medications. Please seek your doctor's advice and use caution.

Promising DEVELOPMENTS

- One day soon, you might literally be able to sniff your PMS symptoms away. A new nasal spray called **PH80**, a few years away from release to the market, stimulates nerve receptors just inside your nasal passages. They send impulses to the hypothalamus, the area of your brain that regulates reproduction, stress, and emotions. Earlier research indicated PH80 had a positive effect on reducing anxiety, and scientists are optimistic that it may one day provide a safer, easier-to-use alternative to SSRIs for treating PMS/PMDD mood swings and depression.

FINDING Support

- For general information and treatment strategies for PMS, check out www.familydoctor.org, the website of the American Academy of Family Physicians.

- Compare notes and share experiences with other women who have PMS at www.feelgoodcounseling.com.

Prostate cancer

Early detection with PSA blood testing is changing the outlook for men diagnosed with prostate cancer. When the tumor is still confined to the prostate gland, it is highly curable with surgery or radiation therapy.

LIKELY **First Steps**

- Develop a **thorough understanding** of all available therapies, including surgery and radiation.
- If a procedure is needed, seek out the **most experienced doctor** for your treatment, whether a urologist or a radiation oncologist.
- Continue to work with your doctor to **map your strategies** for a cure.
- **Mobilize support** with family, friends, a counselor, or a support group.

QUESTIONS TO **Ask**

- What is my PSA? What is my Gleason score?
- What is your best estimate of the aggressiveness of my cancer? What is its stage?
- Am I a good candidate for watchful waiting, or do I need prompt treatment?
- How many surgical/radiation procedures do you perform weekly? What are your cure rates?
- What are the side effects of each treatment?
- Am I a good candidate for "seed" therapy?
- Should I travel to a large institution that specializes in treating prostate cancer?

What is happening

The diagnosis of prostate cancer may fill you with fear and the feeling that you have to do something immediately. Luckily, because most prostate cancers are slow-growing, time is on your side. When cancer is detected early, you have time to learn about how aggressive it is, then properly assess appropriate treatment strategies with your doctors (of urology, radiotherapy, oncology). Understanding the benefits of each doctor's approach will better equip you to make an informed decision about your next steps.

The prostate, a walnut-sized gland near the neck of the bladder, produces part of the fluid for semen. Prostate cancer is the unchecked growth of abnormal cells within the gland. Researchers don't know why cells become cancerous, but a fat-rich diet and the male hormone testosterone are suspected. Undetected cancer may spread through the capsule containing the tumor and invade nearby nodes and the bladder. Or cells may be carried by the bloodstream to the bones or elsewhere. If this occurs, the cancer is no longer curable. It can be controlled for some years with hormonal treatment, radiation, chemotherapy, and newer therapies under investigation. Your treatment is based on the stage of the cancer at diagnosis. Classifications below focus on the extent of the tumor (T1 to 4), and whether it's in the nodes (N) or has metastasized (M).

STAGES OF PROSTATE CANCER

Stage	Spread	Options
T1	Within prostate, and only detectable by a PSA blood test.	Watchful waiting, radical prostatectomy, radiation.
T2	Within gland and detectable by digital rectal exam.	Radical prostatectomy and/or radiation.
T3-4	Cancer has spread just beyond the prostate gland.	Radiation therapy and/or hormone therapy.
N	Cancer has spread beyond the prostate into one (or more) lymph nodes.	Hormone therapy and/or experimental therapies.
M	Cancer has spread to the bone or other locations in the body.	Experimental therapies, radiation, and medication for pain.

Treatment options

Lifestyle changes

Watchful waiting	Regular exams, blood tests, for very early stage.
Find support	Helps deal with emotional and practical issues.
Rethink your habits	Limit red meat and alcohol; meditation.

Procedures

Surgery	Radical prostatectomy removes gland/nodes.
Radiation	Various forms; used with and without surgery.
Brachytherapy	Radioactive "seeds" implanted in gland.

Medications

Hormone therapy	Blocks androgens, to inhibit tumor growth.

Prostate cancer is the most common cancer in men and, following lung cancer, the major cause of cancer death among American men. Each year an estimated 189,000 new cases are diagnosed in the United States, with 30,000 men expected to die of the disease. The likelihood of developing prostate cancer increases with age: The average age of diagnosis is 72. Thanks to the developed prostate-specific antigen (PSA) blood test, however, doctors are commonly finding prostate cancer at the earliest stage, and their ability to cure it at this time is much better than in later stages.

Treatments

Prostate cancer rarely produces symptoms, so the first indication of the disease is often found during a routine digital rectal exam, or DRE (*see page 360*), or a PSA screening test (*see page 364*). When detected early, prostate cancer can usually be cured with either surgery or one of a variety of radiation therapies.

Lifestyle Changes

If your cancer is confined to the prostate gland and surgery shows it has not gone beyond the thick envelope of tissue encasing it (called the prostate capsule), ask your doctor if **watchful waiting** is an option you should consider. Also called expectant management or the "wait- and-watch approach," this type of therapy does not include immediate medical or surgical treatment. Watchful waiting is best suited for men who have small, low-grade, slow-growing tumors, with Gleason scores between 2 and 4 (*see box at right*). It may also be a good treatment strategy if you are elderly, too weak to tolerate surgery or radiation therapy, or have an additional and more serious medical condition. Instead, your doctor will carefully monitor your status with DREs and PSA tests every 6 to 12 months. If your PSA levels rise, you must then determine what you want to do next.

TAKING Control

- **Talk over your options.** Don't be embarrassed. The best treatment evolves when you involve family members and various physicians in the discussion.

- **Take your time to decide.** In most cases, prostate cancer is slow-growing, leaving you time to plan a counterattack.

- **Find a pro.** Especially when opting for a radical prostatectomy, choose an expert in the field with an established track record.

- **Join a local support group.** Contact a nearby hospital or the local US TOO chapter (Support Hotline: 1-800-808-7866) or a local Man to Man group (1-800-ACS-2345). You will find peers who truly understand your dilemma and may have tips, suggestions, and advice for handling your concerns.

Understanding Your Gleason Score

Your pathologist will use your biopsy sample to determine a Gleason score, a figure from 2 to 10 that grades how cancerous your cells appear. A score of 2 to 4 indicates a low risk that your cancer will grow and spread; 5 to 6 shows an intermediate risk; and 7 to 10, a high risk. Your Gleason score, along with your PSA level, cancer stage, and age, are used to determine the best treatment for you.

Promising DEVELOPMENTS

- A particularly exciting approach in counteracting metastatic cancer is the use of **monoclonal antibodies.** These special injectable proteins zero in on prostate cancer cells in the blood and destroy them. Ongoing clinical trials in New York City look quite promising.

- Erectile dysfunction (ED) is a common side effect of both radical prostatectomy and radiation therapy. Viagra has helped many men with ED restore their erections. Two **additional Viagra-like medications,** rardenafil (Levitra) and Tedelafil (Cialig) have received FDA approval.

- Researchers have identified a gene (MSR1) that appears to be linked to prostate cancer. This very preliminary research is encouraging, suggesting that **immunotherapy** (in the form of a vaccine) may eventually fight metastatic (spreading) cancers.

You don't have to fight prostate cancer by yourself. To get the emotional support you need and keep abreast of the latest treatment developments, join a local **support group.** These male communities typically share information and personal stories and bolster spirits. **Altering your daily habits** may also yield promising changes in your survival outlook. Well-known heart disease guru Dr. Dean Ornish has reported on an ongoing research study of men's lifestyles. Those who switched to a vegan diet, eliminated alcohol, performed three hours of aerobic exercise a week, meditated daily, and attended support group meetings saw a drop in their PSA levels in the first year. The unanswered question is whether survival is better with this lifestyle regimen. Less fat and more exercise has multiple benefits, although adherence to the extreme regimen can be difficult.

Procedures

For early-stage prostate cancer, one good option may be **nerve-sparing radical prostatectomy.** The surgery's objective is total removal of the prostate gland, and if cancerous, the lymph glands in the pelvis. During the procedure, the surgeon will avoid nerves involved in bladder control and erections, although temporary incontinence and erectile dysfuncti on may occur. With an experienced surgeon, total cure rates can be as high as 90%. Erectile ability and bladder control will be restored over time.

Another treatment option is **radiation therapy.** If you go this route, high-energy x-rays will be used to destroy cancer cells and prevent them from growing and migrating. If the cancer has not spread (metastasized), radiation can be used instead of surgery to destroy malignant cells. In some situations, radiation may be rec-

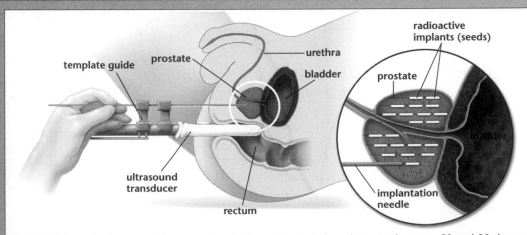

"SEED" THERAPY (BRACHYTHERAPY) FOR PROSTATE CANCER

Best used for early-stage prostate cancer, brachytherapy involves implanting radioactive "seeds" into the prostate using an ultrasound transducer for guidance (*above left*). The seed material varies: Some doctors prefer iodine, others use palladium. The number of implanted seeds ranges between 50 and 80 depending on prostate size. The seeds emit radiation for up to a year, destroying cancerous tissue in the prostate while sparing healthy tissues nearby. The seeds don't have to be removed after they stop functioning.

ommended after surgery and to treat a recurrence.

Radiation can be delivered using different techniques, including external beam radiation therapy (EBRT) or the newer refinements: three-dimensional conformal radiation therapy (3D-CRT) or intensity-modulated radiation therapy (IMRT). You will receive approximately five minutes of treatment, five days a week for seven to eight weeks, with any of these, from a special machine that aims radiation at your prostate. Long-term side effects are minimal but can range from bladder and rectal problems to erectile dysfunction.

If you choose **brachytherapy** (also known as "seed" therapy), rice-sized radioactive pellets are implanted inside your prostate using a sterile needle guided by ultrasound or MRI (*see illustration opposite*). Side effects are rare, but may include diarrhea, rectal bleeding, incontinence, and erectile dysfunction. You're a good candidate if you have early-stage prostate cancer, a low risk of disease outside the gland, a PSA of less than 10 ng/ml, and a Gleason score of 6 or less. The procedure can often be done on an outpatient basis, typically in about an hour. When compared to other, more time-consuming procedures, seed therapy can seem enticing. You must weigh the convenience of the treatment against the uncertainty over whether you're getting a definitive cure, however, as the disease's cure rate drops to as low as 60% over a decade.

Medications

Androgen-deprivation therapy (ADT) may be used to treat prostate cancer that has metastasized to other sites, block the production or effect of the male hormone testosterone, and slow tumor growth. ADT may be recommended before surgery or radiation, or to shrink prostate glands too large to be eligible for brachytherapy. The most effective method of reducing testosterone is a **bilateral orchiectomy,** surgical removal the testes.

Outlook

With the advent of regular PSA testing, many prostate cancers are now detected much earlier, making the long-term prognosis for

▶ **AT BIRTH, THE PROSTATE IS THE SIZE OF A PEA. It reaches walnut size by age 20. When a man turns 40, the prostate often begins to grow again, doing one of three things: It enlarges with no symptoms; it enlarges and then compresses the urethra (the tube carrying urine from the bladder through the prostate), often affecting urination; or it becomes cancerous.**

FINDING Support

■ The National Cancer Institute provides information about therapies, caregivers, and clinical trials (1-800-4-CANCER or www.nci.nih.gov).

■ Consult the American Cancer Society for cancer news and local support groups (1-800-ACS-2345 or www.cancer.org).

■ The National Prostate Cancer Coalition is a grass-roots group that fields questions about treatment, support, and how to push for more government support for prostate cancer research (1-888-245-9455 or www.pcacoalition.org/home.htm).

Prostate enlargement

A common sign of aging, an enlarged prostate eventually shows up in most men. The good news is that it doesn't signal prostate cancer, it doesn't lead to cancer, and you need to treat it only if you are bothered by frequent trips to the bathroom.

LIKELY **First Steps**

- **Wait and watch.** With mild symptoms, this may be the least bothersome approach.

- **Consider saw palmetto.** After getting the okay from your doctor, give this herb a try for several months.

- **Take medications** to help relieve your discomfort.

- **Investigate minimally invasive procedures.** Problems could be solved in less than 30 minutes.

- **Use TURP surgery as the last resort.** Ask your doctor if this procedure would be good for you.

QUESTIONS TO **Ask**

- What are the chances my symptoms will improve with or without therapy?

- How long will the effects of the treatment last?

- What are the risks of complications for this therapy?

What is happening

There's no cause to panic if your doctor has told you that your prostate is enlarged and you have a condition called benign prostatic hyperplasia, or BPH. "Benign" means that your prostate is not cancerous. "Prostatic" refers to your prostate, the walnut-sized gland below your bladder that supplies fluid for your sperm. "Hyperplasia" means an "excessive growth of cells." In short, you have a noncancerous enlargement of your prostate gland, the most common prostate problem. Like gray hair and sagging skin, BPH is simply part of the male aging process.

BPH symptoms occur because the urethra, the tube that drains urine from your bladder, passes through the prostate gland to your penis. When the prostate enlarges, it compresses the urethra and makes urination difficult, too frequent, and slow. No one knows exactly why the prostate enlarges, but it typically happens after about age 50. The main culprit seems to be the hormone dihydrotestosterone (DHT), which the body converts from the male hormone testosterone at an increased rate as you age. This increase in DHT is thought to trigger proliferation of prostate cells, leading to BPH.

Because researchers are not sure what causes it, doctors can't prevent BPH or eradicate it once it becomes a nuisance. Although it's often very irksome and inconvenient, an enlarged prostate is not life threatening. Symptoms—which include a frequent, urgent need to urinate day and night, a "stopping and starting" urine flow, difficulty starting urination, dribbling, or a feeling you can't fully empty your bladder—need to be treated only if they interfere with your quality of life. BPH symptoms are common in about 1 man in 4 by age 55. If you make it to your 80th birthday, 9 out of 10 of your contemporaries will also have the ailment to some degree.

Treatments

The goals of BPH treatment are to improve urinary flow and reduce symptoms. Urologists have never before had so many effective treatment options at their disposal. Whether or not you want to deal with your BPH is entirely up to you. The most important question you can ask yourself is: Do the symptoms caused by my BPH justify taking medication every day or the inconvenience of an invasive procedure? Discuss your options with your urologist, then

Treatment options

Lifestyle changes

Watchful waiting	Have annual checkup; monitor symptoms.
Avoid caffeine	It promotes frequent urination.
Reduce evening fluids	May help you sleep through the night.

Natural methods

Saw palmetto	Give it 2 to 3 months; try different brands.

Medications

Alpha-blocker	Quick-acting, but may cause dizziness.
5-alpha reductase inhibitor	Only for large (40+ gram) prostates.

Procedures

Heat therapies	Outpatient procedures to vaporize BPH tissue.
Surgery	TURP, reserved for major obstruction.

TAKING Control

- **Go to a specialist.** To benefit from the latest treatments, see a urologist. Urologists specialize in the diagnosis and treatment of BPH and other prostate disorders.

- **Say no to zinc.** No evidence supports the use of zinc in BPH management. This message has not really sunk in with many men who are fooled by marketing hype for over-the-counter prostate products. Countless men take zinc supplements in hopes of getting relief from BPH symptoms, even though zinc is not absorbed by the prostate gland and is quickly excreted.

Promising DEVELOPMENTS

- Researchers are testing a new minimally invasive treatment that uses **specially prepared alcohol injections** to shrink the bulk of the prostate. This facilitates urine flow and allows the bladder to empty more quickly and completely. Still considered experimental, this novel approach could one day prove to be a cost-effective option for men who do not experience any improvement in their lower urinary tract symptoms after traditional medical therapy.

decide for yourself. Your decision should be based on your medical history and how much your symptoms bother you.

To evaluate how well a particular treatment is working, your urologist may have you fill out an International Prostate Symptoms Score sheet before you begin the therapy, and again a month later. You'll be asked to rate your BPH symptoms and your answers to the seven questions will be scored. A score of 7 or less means your symptoms are mild; 8–19, moderate; and 20–35, severe. A copy of this self-assessment can be found at www.urologix.com/patient/auatest.html.

Lifestyle Changes

If your symptoms are relatively mild, you may want to simply monitor your condition and see if they stay the same, improve, or worsen. This no-drug, no-procedure course of action, widely called **watchful waiting,** is not designed to see how long you can go without a treatment you really should have (*see box, page 264*). It's an admission that your symptoms aren't all that bad and that you're better off taking a hands-off approach. Be sure to check with your doctor at least once a year to make sure you're not developing complications that may harm your kidneys or bladder. In the meantime, actions you can take to improve your symptoms include:

- **No caffeinated drinks after 5 PM.** Caffeine causes you to urinate, which can be very annoying in the middle of the night.
- **Limit or eliminate fluid intake** between dinner and bedtime.
- **Avoid OTC antihistamines and decongestants.** These can worsen BPH by preventing muscles in the bladder and prostate from relaxing to let urine flow out.

COOLED THERMOTHERAPY

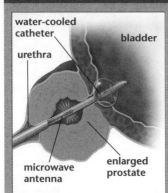

water-cooled catheter

bladder

urethra

microwave antenna

enlarged prostate

During this procedure a catheter containing a tiny microwave antenna is inserted deep into the prostate through the urethra. Microwave energy then destroys excess prostate tissue blocking the urethra, while cool water circulates through the catheter to protect the urethra from the heat.

Natural Methods*

Some men find **saw palmetto** very effective for BPH (*see box opposite*). Discuss this option with your doctor, and try the herb for two to three months. If symptoms don't improve in that time, you may need medical or surgical treatment.

Medications

Drugs for relieving BPH symptoms fall into two categories: alpha-blockers and 5-alpha reductase inhibitors. Medications can't cure BPH. Once medication is stopped, BPH symptoms return in most men.

Alpha-blockers were designed to treat high blood pressure by reducing tension of muscles in blood vessel walls. By coincidence, the so-called nonselective drugs (Hytrin, Cardura) also relax smooth muscle tissue within the prostate. A selective alpha-blocker (marketed as Flomax) was developed to target the smooth muscle of the prostate. Taken daily, an alpha-blocker may increase urinary flow and relieve symptoms of urinary frequency and nighttime urination (called nocturia). Possible side effects include dizziness upon standing (less so with selective alpha-blockers), fatigue, and headaches.

The only **5-alpha reductase inhibitor** drug is finasteride (Proscar). It works by reducing the size of the prostate and improving urinary flow. Finasteride can shrink the prostate by as much as 30% but takes time if it works at all. This medication is useful only if you have a large prostate (more than 40 grams as determined with a digital rectal exam). Finasteride also has limitations: It takes three to six months to work, must be taken daily, and has only moderate ability to improve symptoms. You may find ejaculatory volumes are reduced and may develop erectile dysfunction with long-term use of the drug. These side effects disappear when the drug is discontinued. Finasteride also lowers PSA levels (*see page 364*) by 50% after six months, so your doctor will have to adjust your PSA value to assess your prostate cancer risk.

If your symptoms are significantly unchanged after trying medications, you have three options. Keep taking the medicine. Have a minimally invasive therapy, or undergo surgery (a transurethral resection of the prostate).

Procedures

Newer, minimally invasive **heat therapies** provide excellent outcomes. A nonsurgical procedure called **transurethral needle ablation (TUNA)** uses low-level radio frequency waves to burn away extra tissue blocking the flow of urine. TUNA requires local anesthesia and takes less than an hour. Most men can return to their normal activities within 24 hours. Another option is innovative microwave technology called **Cooled ThermoTherapy** (*see illus-*

Natural methods are not subject to the same testing and regulation as prescription medications. Please seek your doctor's advice and use caution.

Treating BPH with Saw Palmetto

A growing number of American men are turning to natural therapies to treat their BPH. Routinely prescribed in Europe, complementary BPH medications (plant extracts or botanicals) have, until recently, been largely ignored by the medical establishment in the United States due to a lack of good clinical studies confirming their effectiveness. One exception, however, is the herb saw palmetto, botanically known as *Serena repens*.

A study published in the journal *Urology* reported that saw palmetto pills (160 mg taken twice daily) might be an effective BPH treatment. Men in the study who took saw palmetto experienced significant improvement in symptoms.

Saw palmetto is available in most pharmacies and health food stores. It's best to choose supplements made from extracts standardized to contain 85% to 95% fatty acids and sterols.

If you're interested in going the herbal route, buy the least expensive brand of saw palmetto and use it for several months. If no improvement occurs, try another brand. If, after three or four months on the herb, your symptoms have not improved, standard prescription medications or surgery may be indicated for you. Check out www.consumerlab.com/results/saw palmetto.html for an overview of the leading commercial saw palmetto products.

tration opposite), which offers safe and lasting treatment that can be more effective than medication and less invasive than surgery. Performed in a doctor's office or on an outpatient basis, Cooled ThermoTherapy, once called **transurethral microwave thermotherapy (TUMT),** costs significantly less than surgery or years of medication. The half-hour procedure uses microwave energy to heat and destroy enlarged prostate tissue, while a unique cooling system protects healthy, sensitive tissue nearby. You should have relief from symptoms 4 to 12 weeks after treatment.

Surgery is considered if your symptoms have not improved after other treatments. **Transurethral resection of the prostate, or TURP** (pronounced "terp"), is considered the "gold standard" of BPH treatment, the one to which other therapeutic measures are compared. TURP involves removing the inner core of the prostate with an instrument called a resectoscope that's passed through the urethra into the bladder. A wire attached to the resectoscope removes prostate tissue and seals blood vessels with an electric current. A catheter remains in place for one to three days, and a hospital stay of one to two days is generally required. There is often little or no pain with TURP, and you can expect full recovery within 3 weeks of surgery.

In the past, TURP was the only BPH treatment available, but those days are long gone. Most men benefit from TURP, but it's less commonly performed due to the potential for pain and suffering. There is also a high risk for bleeding, a minimal but serious risk for incontinence, and a small risk of erectile dysfunction. In short, it's a lot more invasive than the newer therapies now recommended.

▶ **Does diet make any difference with BPH?**

It may. Researchers are beginning to point a finger at high-fat, junk food diets lacking in fruits and vegetables as a cause of BPH. When men don't consume enough fresh fruits, vegetables, and whole grains, they may lose out on these foods' unique ability to fight off free-radical molecules that damage the prostate and may cause it to enlarge.

FINDING Support

■ Selected portions of *The Johns Hopkins Prostate Bulletin* are found at www.hopkinsprostate.com. At this site you can read about the latest advances in BPH research and treatment.

Prostatitis

When not linked to bacteria, prostate inflammation can be a mysterious and baffling complaint, frustrating patients and physicians alike. It's up to you to work with your doctor to find a therapy—or combination of therapies—that works well for you.

LIKELY **First Steps**

- **Find out** if bacteria are playing a role in the ailment.
- **Oral antibiotics** for acute and chronic bacterial cases; possibly even for chronic nonbacterial cases.
- **Self-help measures** for symptom relief. Keep trying until you find what works.

QUESTIONS TO **Ask**

- What success have you had treating prostatitis?
- If I have to use oral antibiotics for months, what can I do about their side effects?
- What do I do if antibiotics stop working?
- Can my prostatitis be transmitted by sexual contact?

Promising DEVELOPMENTS

- Some researchers believe that prostatitis is an autoimmune disorder like rheumatoid arthritis: The immune system launches an inappropriate and excessive attack on the body and destroys normal body tissues. The good news is that **national research trials** now underway, aim to define the disease, find its causes, and determine effective treatments.

What is happening

Prostatitis, or inflammation of the prostate—the walnut-sized gland located below your bladder—is a common medical name for several related conditions that lead to more than 2 million doctor visits annually. What these ailments have in common is pain and discomfort in the pelvic area, lower back, and groin; a burning sensation while urinating; and a frequent urge to urinate.

Diagnosing prostatitis can be difficult. You may need to see more than one doctor to find out what ails you. While this condition is not always curable, most prostatitis can be treated. Most forms are not contagious, and you can continue to have an active sex life without fear of passing the disease to your partner. Most important, prostatitis does not mean a greater risk for developing BPH or prostate cancer. While the ailment is not life-threatening, it can be uncomfortable until symptoms are under control.

The National Institutes of Health classifies three types of prostatitis. **Acute bacterial prostatitis** represents only 5% of cases and is easiest to treat. Symptoms come on quickly: severe pain between scrotum and anus (perineum), aggravated during a bowel movement, and painful urination with frequency, burning, and sometimes blood. Acute bacterial prostatitis responds well to antibiotics and symptoms resolve almost as quickly as they arrived.

Chronic bacterial prostatitis develops when antibiotics fail to kill all the bacteria responsible for acute bacterial prostatitis. Treatment generally means a fairly prolonged course of antibiotics. You'll need to be checked several times to verify that the infection is gone.

Chronic nonbacterial prostatitis (or noninfectious prostatitis) is the most common form of the condition and the most difficult to treat. Theories abound as to why it occurs, but none have been confirmed. Symptoms include pain in the perineum, difficult urination, and chronic pelvic discomfort, described by some men as the sense of "sitting on a golf ball." This form of prostatitis can disappear for weeks or months at a time. Doctors try a variety of therapies to treat it—antibiotics, prostate massage, dietary recommendations—but no single therapy works for every man.

Treatments

Seeing several doctors about chronic prostatitis is not unusual. No one therapy offers a cure or guarantees long-lasting relief. Many

Treatment options

Lifestyle changes

Apply hot or cold	If it feels good, keep doing it.
Dietary changes	May ease pain; drinking more water is key.

Medications

Oral antibiotics	May be prescribed for weeks.
Aspirin/NSAIDs	To relieve painful symptoms.

men find that a combination of therapies, especially lifestyle changes, is their best bet. On the other hand, antibiotics are extremely effective against the bacterial forms of prostatitis.

Lifestyle Changes

When you have chronic nonbacterial prostatitis, be prepared to try different remedies until you find one that brings some relief.

- **Take a warm bath** once or twice daily to relieve the pelvic pain.
- **Try cold.** Sitting on an ice pack may be comforting.
- **Give a "donut" a try.** This inflatable device, sold at most pharmacies, may help ease discomfort.
- **Make dietary changes.** Avoid spicy and greasy foods. Stay away from alcohol and caffeine or reduce your intake.
- **Regular ejaculation** may help, apparently by emptying the prostate of accumulated prostate fluid.
- **Drink plenty of fluids.** This helps prevent constipation, increase urine flow, and reduce discomfort during bowel movements.
- **Consider quercetin.*** A study reported that 82% of men who took the antioxidant quercetin (in onions, apples, tea, red wine, and supplements), had an improvement in their chronic prostatitis. They took 500 mg twice daily for a month.

Medications

Bacterial prostatitis requires at least 6 weeks of antibiotic therapy, usually with a broad-spectrum **antibiotic,** such as Cipro, Augmentin, Avelox, or Bactrim. This is longer than the typical 5- to 10-day course for other ailments because it is difficult for bacteria-killing levels of the drug to accumulate within the prostate. Be sure to take the full course of your prescription: Stop too soon and the infection may well come back.

While men with nonbacterial prostatitis don't have signs of infection, antibiotic treatment gives some relief. If urinating is difficult, the medications used for benign prostatic hyperplasia (prostate enlargement, or BPH) may help. These include terazosin (Hytrin) and doxazosin (Cardura), which are also used for hypertension, as well as finasteride (Proscar). **Aspirin** or other nonsteroidal anti-inflammatory medications (NSAIDs like ibuprofen) can be effective for occasional pain relief.

TAKING Control

- **Work with a urologist.** These specialists have more experience with chronic prostatitis than most family doctors.

- **Try self-help measures.** Your goal is to find symptom relief to improve your quality of life. No one therapy works best for everyone. If a particular treatment fails to improve your symptoms, try something else immediately.

- **Ask your doctor for a prostate massage.** This old treatment is still used by some patients. The doctor will insert a lubricated gloved finger into your rectum and vigorously massage or rub the prostate in an attempt to empty any clogged ducts within the gland that may be contributing to your pain. Some men feel better for weeks afterward.

- **Rate your improvement.** The Chronic Prostatitis Symptom Index is a nine-question self-grading quiz you can take on a regular basis to see if you are getting better. Go to www.prostatitis.org/symptomindex.html.

FINDING Support

- The Prostatitis Foundation keeps track of the latest treatment developments and tells you what works and what doesn't. It also allows you to share your experiences with others afflicted with the ailment (1-888-891-4200 or www.prostate.org).

Natural methods are not subject to the same testing and regulation as prescription medications. Please seek your doctor's advice and use caution.

Psoriasis

If you thought you'd never wear shorts again because of your blotchy, flaking skin, take heart. You—and 5 million other Americans with psoriasis—will be glad to hear that treatment options for this unsightly condition have doubled in recent years.

LIKELY First Steps

- **Sunbathing, treatment baths,** and **moisturizers** to soothe irritated skin.
- **Topical medications** and **shampoos** to treat mild or moderate cases.
- **Oral medication** for more severe cases.
- **Light therapy,** if necessary, from artificial sources.

QUESTIONS TO Ask

- When can I expect to see some improvement?
- How far is my psoriasis likely to spread?
- I'm trying to conceive. Which psoriasis drugs are unsafe for me?

What is happening

This chronic skin disease isn't easy to ignore: Its raised red patches covered with silvery scales itch (fittingly, psoriasis comes from the Greek for "itch"). Your self-image may suffer if it spreads. (The fact that ads once referred to "the heartbreak of psoriasis" isn't surprising.) The condition occurs when production of new skin cells outpaces the rate at which old ones are shed. As a result, live cells accumulate in raised areas covered with whitish flakes of immature skin cells (or plaques). Researchers say this rapid cell turnover relates to an inherited immune system disorder that can be activated by stress, cold weather, infection, or an abrasion.

Plaque psoriasis often appears on elbows, knees, palms, soles, the lower back, and the scalp. Less common forms of psoriasis include: guttate, with teardrop-shaped spots; pustular, with pus-filled skin lesions; inverse, appearing in skin folds; and erythrodermic, with widespread skin scaling and inflammation. Psoriasis flares up periodically and can persist for long periods before going into remission. Although it occasionally covers large areas, this condition is usually mild and manageable. Nearly one-third of patients develop psoriatic arthritis.

Treatments

There is no cure for psoriasis, but you can control it and minimize its symptoms. Milder cases usually respond well to OTC and prescription topical drugs and shampoos, in addition to sunlight. For more severe cases, you'll need oral drugs and specialized light therapy. Most doctors use a combination of treatments, and you may need to experiment to find the mix that best suits you.

Lifestyle Changes

The first relief for your psoriasis is as close as your yard or rooftop: Expose affected areas to **sunlight,** but not sunburn, for 15 to 30 minutes a day. This brings improvement within six weeks in about 80% of people who try it. (Be sure to protect unaffected areas with sunblock.) **Soaking in a bath solution** enhanced with coal tar, Dead Sea or Epsom salts, or colloidal oatmeal (Aveeno) can soften scaly buildup. As soon as you get out of the tub, apply a heavy **moisturizer,** such as Cetaphil, Eucerin, or petroleum jelly, to soften and soothe your skin. Your doctor may also recommend **watertight (occlusive) tapes,** especially if you have psoriasis-related cracks on your palms and soles.

Treatment options

Lifestyle changes

Sunlight (not sunburn)	Brings relief in 80% of cases.
Bath soaks	Various products help soften scaly buildup.
Moisturizers	Apply after bath to soothe skin.

Medications

Topical medications	Salicylic acid, coal tar, corticosteroids.
Medicated shampoo	Also steroid foam; stops scalp flaking.
Oral medications	Immunosuppressants, oral retinoids.

Procedures

Light therapy	Ultraviolet B or PUVA (with psoralen).

Medications

Most psoriasis requires medication. To begin, a **topical formulation** (cream, gel, ointment) can help. Try OTC salicylic acid (Hydrisalac) to dissolve scales, or coal tar gels to slow skin cell growth. Prescription topical corticosteroids can reduce more severe inflammation. (An occlusive tape, called Cordran Tape, has corticosteroids in it.) Daily use of a topical corticosteroid such as halobetasol (Ultravate), is a common regimen for more severe psoriasis. After the patch clears up, apply just on weekends. You can also combine weekend steroid use with weekday use of calcipotriene (Dovonex), a form of vitamin D_3.

For scalp psoriasis, try a **medicated shampoo** such as coal tar (Denorex Medicated) or anthralin (Dritho-Scalp). Both stain, and anthralin can irritate normal skin, so use them carefully. Tazarotene (Tazorac) or salicylic acid shampoo (DHS Sal) may slow flakes, too. There's also a fast-acting but expensive steroid foam.

For severe psoriasis, an oral **immunosuppressant drug** such as cyclosporine (Neoral) or methotrexate (Rheumatrex) may be needed. Once it begins working, an **oral retinoid** (vitamin A derivative), usually acitretin (Soriatane), is added. The immunosuppressant is then gradually withdrawn and a low-maintenance dose of Soriatane continued. Doctors also recommend rotational therapy—switching approaches after a couple of years—to prevent serious side effects or resistance to a drug's benefits. Immunotherapy agents have been approved for treatment of moderate to severe psoriasis.

Procedures

With moderate to severe psoriasis, you'll need **light therapy** with ultraviolet B (UVB) rays at your dermatologist's office, a hospital, or with a home unit. For more severe psoriasis, a special therapy called **PUVA** combines the oral drug psoralen with deeper-penetrating ultraviolet A (UVA) rays. Such treatments are very effective but can up your skin cancer risk.

TAKING Control

- **Be aware certain drugs can make your psoriasis worse.** Lithium, antimalarials, and such heart drugs as ACE inhibitors and beta-blockers are the worst offenders.

- **Winterize your program.** Winter's dry, cold air can mean more psoriasis. Be careful not to scratch; it can make lesions worse. Instead, slather on moisturizer more thickly, applying it while your skin is damp, and get some sun (using sunblock, of course). What better excuse for that tropical vacation?

- **Try meditation or relaxation techniques** if your psoriasis flares up under stress. They can help you deal with life's pressures.

Promising DEVELOPMENTS

- **A psoriasis vaccine** is in the works in New Zealand. It contains organisms called *Myobacterium vaccae* that have been killed with heat treatment. They appear to "turn off" immune system cells that attack the skin. In a preliminary test of 24 patients, psoriasis disappeared in 25% and improved in 50%, with benefits lasting as long as 18 months. Larger trials are now underway.

FINDING Support

- For the most recent information on psoriasis treatment, as well as information on clinical trials, contact the National Psoriasis Foundation in Portland, OR (1-800-723-9166 or www.psoriasis.org).

Restless legs syndrome

Up to 15% of Americans are familiar with an irresistible urge to move their legs that keeps them awake at night. Interestingly, lifestyle changes—and drugs if needed—will help banish those sleepless nights and even those groggy, grumpy tomorrows.

LIKELY First Steps

- **Massage, heat, or cold** to stop RLS symptoms.
- **Regular exercise** and **warm baths** to head off RLS.
- **Iron** or **other supplements,** if needed, to correct any deficiencies.
- **Medications** to relieve more severe cases.

QUESTIONS TO Ask

- Is my mild restlessness going to get worse?
- Is RLS a sign of more serious medical problems?
- Will I have RLS for the rest of my life?

What is happening

You're in bed ready to go to sleep, but your legs have other ideas. They want to kick, stretch, do anything but rest. Restless legs syndrome (RLS), more colorfully described as "the gotta-moves" or "Elvis legs," usually affects the area between the ankles and knees. The feet, thighs, arms, or trunk may also be involved. It's more noticeable if you're lying down or sitting for long periods, especially at night. In milder cases, there's a pulling, crawly feeling, or sensation of pins and needles that goes away when you move. More serious RLS is painful, can last for hours, and interrupts sleep repeatedly, leaving you dragged out. RLS is a neurological, not a muscular, disorder. The cause is most likely low levels of the brain chemical dopamine, which keeps nerve cells functioning smoothly. RLS tends to run in families and frequently develops during pregnancy.

Treatments

Restless legs syndrome is no walk in the park, but you have a number of treatment options. For mild symptoms, simple lifestyle changes may do the trick. When such remedies don't work, you'll want to have your physician rule out medical causes, such as kidney problems, diabetes, or vitamin or mineral deficiencies, then move on to medications that can help your legs give you a rest.

Lifestyle Changes

When your legs are agitating, the best thing to do is **move** them: walk around, stretch, do deep-knee bends. **Massage** or **acupressure** on the legs can further dissipate the creepy-crawly feeling. A **heating pad** or **cold compress** may also relieve restlessness. Finally, consider some **distraction**—a good novel, late-night TV show, or relaxation tape. You can also help prevent a future round of nighttime RLS by trying some of the following to see what works for you.

- **Get moderate exercise.** Some people find a stationary bike or treadmill workout before bed leads to a less restless night. Others sleep better if they stop exercising six hours before bedtime.
- **Warm yourself up.** Try a bath about 90 minutes before bedtime, and keep your legs and feet warm in bed.
- **Clean up your sleep habits.** Keep your bedroom cool. Go to bed and get up at the same time every day.
- **Steer clear of common irritants.** Caffeine, alcohol, and cigarettes can all provoke RLS or make it worse.

Treatment options

Lifestyle changes

Moderate exercise	Helps legs relax.
Warm bath	Take one 90 minutes before bed to calm nerves.

Natural methods

Supplements	Iron or other supplements for deficiencies.

Medications

Dopaminergics	Quiet leg restlessness.
Anticonvulsants	Blunt leg pain.
Benzodiazepines	Help you sleep through any restlessness.

Procedures

TENS	Electrical stimulation improves sleep.

Natural Methods*

Extra iron may remedy your symptoms if your iron levels are low, a common problem in RLS. The B-complex vitamins, as well as magnesium, vitamin E, and calcium, may also be useful. Before trying these, ask your doctor for a blood test to find out if you're low in any key nutrient.

Medications

Four types of prescription drugs are commonly used to treat RLS. (The FDA hasn't sanctioned any medication specifically for RLS, but drugs approved for other purposes often help.) Your doctor's first choice may be a **dopaminergic agent,** such as levodopa/carbidopa (Sinemet, Atamet) or pergolide (Permax). These are usually used to quiet the tremors of Parkinson's disease, but can quell restless legs too. (Don't worry, RLS doesn't lead to Parkinson's.) Another option is an **anticonvulsant,** such as gabapentin (Neurontin), which blunts restlessness and pain. Some people get relief with a **benzodiazepine** such as clonazepam (Klonopin). This mild tranquilizer will help you sleep through the "funny" RLS feelings. **Narcotics** are usually reserved for severe symptoms. These potent medicines, including propoxyphene (Darvon, Darvocet) and oxycodone (Percocet), reduce symptoms, but may cause side effects or drug dependence.

Procedures

Your doctor may also recommend **transcutaneous electrical nerve stimulation (TENS).** In this procedure, electrodes are attached to pads placed on the skin; the TENS machine then emits mild electrical impulses that feel like a massage, overriding pain or discomfort. Using it for 15 to 30 minutes before you turn in can substantially increase your chances of restful sleep.

Natural methods are not subject to the same testing and regulation as prescription medications. Please seek your doctor's advice and use caution.

TAKING Control

- **Inventory the medications you take.** A number of common medications can cause RLS, among them over-the-counter cold and allergy products, nausea drugs, and calcium channel blockers. Even drugs you take for RLS (tranquilizers, antidepressants, and levodopa) sometimes make symptoms worse.

- **Check out less likely treatments.** If other therapies haven't worked for you, ask your doctor about the antihypertensive drug clonidine (Catapres) and SSRI (selective serotonin reuptake inhibitor) antidepressants such as fluoxetine (Prozac). They bring relief to a few and could prove to be your ticket to slumberland.

- **Speak up if your medicine lets you down.** If the medication you've been taking stops working, let your doctor know. This phenomenon is common in RLS, and switching to a different prescription may bring you needed relief.

FINDING Support

- For information on restless legs syndrome and conversation with others who have this disorder, the Restless Legs Syndrome Foundation (www.rls.org) sponsors a website, support groups, and a chat room that's open all night. You can also contact the foundation in Rochester, MN, by calling 1-877-463-6757.

- The National Sleep Foundation is your best source for ideas on developing sound sleep habits (www.sleepfoundation.org).

Rheumatoid arthritis

Painful, tender joints can make even the simplest activities difficult for those with this inflammatory disease. Recently, pharmaceutical breakthroughs have revolutionized RA treatment, enabling many to again lead active and productive lives.

LIKELY **First Steps**

- **Anti-inflammatories,** such as NSAIDs (including COX-2 inhibitors) to ease pain.
- **Steroids,** such as prednisone, to control more serious cases of inflammation.
- Early treatment with a **DMARD drug**, such as methotrexate, to slow the disease's progression.
- **Biologic response modifiers,** such as Enbrel, Humira, or Remicade, alternatively or in combination with other drugs, to halt the disease's progression.
- Lifestyle measures such as **low-impact exercise** or **water aerobics,** as well as **plenty of rest.**

QUESTIONS TO **Ask**

- What type of rheumatoid arthritis do I have—mild or severe? Are my symptoms likely to keep getting worse?
- How long will I need to stay on medications?
- Will changing my diet help?
- Can I get pregnant while being treated?
- Are all my symptoms related to my illness, or are some a side effect of the medications I'm taking?
- Do I need to go on disability?
- Will I need joint replacement surgery?

What is happening

In healthy joints, the surfaces of bones and the cartilage that cushions them glide smoothly against one another, allowing easy, pain-free movement. But for the 2 million Americans with rheumatoid arthritis (RA), the cartilage becomes inflamed and breaks down, causing pain, stiffness, and swelling. If the disease progresses, bones and ligaments can permanently wear away. The heart, lungs, muscles, and skin can become damaged. There's an increased risk for blood or lymph cancers.

Unlike the simple joint wear and tear of osteoarthritis, rheumatoid arthritis arises from an immune system gone awry, which mistakenly attacks healthy joint tissue. Nobody knows what triggers this. Scientists speculate it may be the result of an infection, perhaps combined with genetic factors that make you susceptible to the disease. During a flare-up, white blood cells collect in your joints and mount an inflammatory attack, secreting substances called cytokines that join the battle. One form of cytokine is a destructive protein called tumor necrosis factor (TNF); another is interleukin-1. In response, cells in the besieged joint release defensive chemicals called prostaglandins. They cause the joint to become red, sore, and swollen. This is the basic inflammatory process, although some forms of RA are milder than others.

Treatments

The most important aspect of rheumatoid arthritis treatment is stopping the joint inflammation. The past decade has seen dramatic changes: New medications can now halt inflammation and progression of disease. Self-care measures are also important, and selected surgical and nonsurgical treatments may be helpful for advanced disease. There are so many options to choose from, so talk with your doctor about which ones may be right for you. While none is a cure, some may offer long-term relief.

The least aggressive medicines, such as aspirin, have traditionally been used first. If they didn't work, progressively stronger medications—with more severe side effects—were tried. Now doctors start with aggressive therapies to quell inflammation and halt the disease at an early stage, before damage is severe. Such treatment may be particularly beneficial for those with more serious disease. Just remember: You will have "good days" and "bad days" and even long periods when the condition seems to quiet down altogether.

Treatment options

Medications

Pain relievers	OTC or prescription NSAIDs for quick relief.
Corticosteroids	For severe flare-ups/recurrences.
DMARDs	Methotrexate and others, for inflammation.
Biologic response modifiers	Forestall progressive joint deterioration.
Immunosuppressants	Oral, intravenous, or by injection.

Lifestyle changes

Paraffin baths	Particularly good for hand pain.
Exercise/spa therapy	Walking, cycling, tai chi, water therapy.

Natural methods

Supplements	For inflammation and pain.

Procedures

Prosorba therapy	Blood filtration if drugs don't work.
Surgery	Joint replacement if major deterioration.

Medications

Many new drugs have become available in recent years. The key is to find the right one for you. A simple **pain reliever,** such as aspirin or another OTC or prescription nonsteroidal anti-inflammatory drug (NSAID), such as naproxen, ibuprofen, or indomethacin, often provides prompt relief. NSAIDs are available as pills and in pain-relieving creams. A newer class of NSAID called COX-2 inhibitors modulate inflammation-causing prostaglandins and may cause fewer side effects. COX-2s include celecoxib (Celebrex), rofexocib (Vioxx), and valdecoxib (Bextra). If NSAIDs are not strong enough to control the inflammation, you may need more potent drugs.

Although they may have serious side effects (*see box, page 274*), some of the best drugs to control rheumatoid inflammation fast are powerful anti-inflammatory **oral corticosteroids.** One way to minimize the side effects of prednisone, a commonly prescribed steroid, is to take it when your body naturally produces it—early in the morning, between 5 AM and 7 AM. Steroids may also be injected directly into joints for relief of flare-ups. This practice should be minimized because it may ultimately damage joints.

Stronger disease-fighting drugs are often started quickly to protect joints and organs from long-term damage. These medicines are called **DMARDs, or disease-modifying anti-rheumatic drugs.** Most commonly prescribed is methotrexate (Rheumatrex). Originally developed as a cancer drug, methotrexate in low doses eases pain and other symptoms by switching off underlying inflammation. Others include sulfasalazine (Azulfidine); injectable or oral gold; hydroxychloroquine (Plaquenil); penicillamine (Cuprimine,

TAKING Control

■ **Assemble a medical team.** A rheumatologist (a physician who specializes in arthritis) may be particularly valuable in tailoring a state-of-the-art treatment program that's right for you. You also need a primary care physician to monitor your overall health, a physical therapist to help keep your joints flexible, and an occupational therapist to offer tips on making the most of your life at home or at work.

■ **Be careful about drug combos.** Don't take prednisone and an NSAID together—this can increase your risk of developing a stomach ulcer.

■ **Start treatment early.** A study in the *Journal of Rheumatology* found that those with early rheumatoid arthritis who delayed treatment by nine months continued to feel worse (even three years later) than those who began therapy promptly. Early treatment is key to reducing damage and the need for more costly treatments, including surgery.

■ **If you smoke, quit.** Studies show that smoking can make symptoms worse. If you undergo joint replacement surgery, smoking can prolong your recovery.

▶ **SALMON AND OTHER OILY FISH are rich in omega-3 fatty acids that have anti-inflammatory properties and may help relieve symptoms of rheumatoid arthritis. Eat fish twice a week or try fish oil capsules.**

Promising
DEVELOPMENTS

■ Medications for rheumatoid arthritis don't just make you feel better, they may also save your life. Researchers at the University of Kansas Medical Center have reported that those taking the arthritis fighter **methotrexate** were 60% less likely to die prematurely, particularly from heart attack, than those not taking the drug. The scientists suspect that the benefits, if proven, may be due to the medicine's inflammation-blocking effects. Inflammation is increasingly suspected as a culprit in heart attacks and strokes.

▶ **ACUPUNCTURE MAY OFFER RA BENEFITS. A small British study showed less discomfort in rheumatoid arthritis sufferers after a treatment. Some patients were able to reduce their use of pain medications from an average of 17 tablets a week to just 6.**

Depen); and the immune suppressant cyclosporine (Sandimmune, Neoral). Leflunomide (Arava) eases inflammation by blocking the action of the protein interleukin-1. Arava increases the risk of serum infections. DMARDs are sometimes given in combination.

You may also benefit from a new class of arthritis drugs called **biologic response modifiers.** When used early, they forestall progressive joint erosion. These include infliximab (Remicade), which is infused by IV every four to six weeks in a doctor's office, etanercept (Enbrel), which you can learn to self-inject twice a week at home, and adalimumab (Humira). All these block the inflammatory cytokine tumor necrosis factor (TNF) and are sometimes called **TNF blockers.** Another biologic response modifier called anikinra (Kineret) may also help. In tests, patients felt better after taking these drugs. Some had complete relief of certain symptoms. Using these drugs with methotrexate or other DMARDs may be even more effective. For very severe flare-ups and recurrences, powerful **immunosuppressants,** such as azathioprine (Imuran), chlorambucil (Leukeran), or cyclophosphamide (Cytoxan), may be given. These medications suppress the overall immune system but can be very toxic.

With any of these drugs, you may feel better after several weeks, but treatment is usually continued long-term. Your dose may be reduced over time, or you may be given new drug combinations.

Lifestyle Changes

Despite the seriousness of this condition, you can take certain steps to help yourself feel better.

■ **Low-impact exercise** may have benefits. Try walking, cycling, or learn the slow, graceful movements of tai chi.

■ **Spa therapy,** with natural hot spring water, has long been used to relieve rheumatic complaints. Research confirms that warm-water exercise programs can be beneficial; optimal water temperature is 83° to 88°F. Gentle massage performed by a professional can also relax muscles and maintain flexibility.

Rheumatoid Arthritis Drugs: Know the Risks

Drugs effective against rheumatoid arthritis can have serious side effects.

NSAIDs such as aspirin and naproxen, can cause stomach ulcers, internal bleeding, and liver and kidney problems. They're estimated to contribute to tens of thousands of deaths each year. The newer **COX-2 inhibitors,** such as Vioxx, Celebrex, and Bextra appear to be more stomach-friendly, but studies show that Vioxx increases heart attack risk by 50 percent compared to Celebrex.

Methotrexate, like other **DMARDs,** has side effect risks, including liver problems. One consumer group called for a ban on Arava due to concerns over potentially fatal liver damage.

Some people taking the **TNF blockers** Enbrel and Remicade develop serious, even deadly infections. Using the lowest possible dose may minimize problems. Taking drug combinations may also reduce risks, since lower dosages can be used. However, drug cocktails also present new, unforeseen dangers.

Side effects of the **corticosteroid prednisone** are legendary. They include cataracts and glaucoma, gastric bleeding, osteoporosis, thinning of the skin, swollen facial tissues and weight gain, increased diabetes risk, even destruction of the hip.

Bottom line: Work closely with your medical team. Take an active role in your treatment. Know about your drugs. Monitor symptoms closely. Make lifestyle adjustments, and listen to what your body is telling you.

Juvenile RA

Some 50,000 children in the United States have the disabling inflammatory disease called juvenile rheumatoid arthritis, or JRA (in adults it's known as Still's disease). JRA often appears in toddlers and young teenagers, though it can begin at any age. It may begin with a fever and shaking chills, followed by a pink rash on the thighs or chest, swollen glands, and painful and swollen joints.

Aspirin, in high doses, is usually the first line of attack. Your doctor may then prescribe a DMARD, such as methotrexate, gold injections, or sulfasalazine (Azulfidine), which help about two-thirds of kids. One of the newer biologic response modifiers may be tried. Steroids such as prednisone are not normally used for children because they can stunt growth. Steroid injections directly into the joints, however, may allay occasional flare-ups. Many cases of JRA disappear by adulthood.

- **Melted paraffin baths** can be effective in easing hand stiffness and pain, especially prevalent early in the morning. Paraffin bath kits, available commercially, make the procedure easier.
- **Plenty of rest** is necessary, particularly during flare-ups, to preserve energy and optimize your ability to cope.
- **A diet rich in fruits and vegetables** that contain the antioxidant vitamins C and E may protect the joints from damage (although no foods can cure rheumatoid arthritis). Zinc, found in meats, eggs, dairy, seafood, and nuts, also has antioxidant properties.

Natural Methods*

Evening primrose oil (1,000 mg three times a day) has anti-inflammatory properties that may soothe sore joints. **Boswellia** (150 mg three times a day) has long been used in India to reduce inflammation. Cayenne creams with **capsaicin** can be applied to affected joints three or four times a day. A **food elimination diet** (*see page 27*), to identify the foods that trigger your symptoms, is advocated by nutritionally-oriented physicians to curb painful symptoms.

Procedures

A novel blood-filtration procedure called **prosorba (protein-A immunoadsorption) therapy** may benefit those who have not responded to medications. Blood is drawn from one arm, filtered through a special cylinder that pulls out inflammatory substances, then returned through your other arm. Sessions are once a week for 12 weeks. You should start feeling better soon after your last treatment, and benefits may continue for a year and a half. Only if deterioration is severe will **surgical procedures,** such as hip, knee, or finger joint replacement, be necessary (*see page 38*).

Natural methods are not subject to the same testing and regulation as prescription medications. Please seek your doctor's advice and use caution.

▶**When will I feel better?**
Your first RA flare-up can be frightening: It seems as if your joints have become swollen and painful in just a few days. You will quickly discover that aspirin and other NSAID pain relievers give relief in a matter of hours, but don't delay seeking medical advice and initiating a treatment plan with your doctor. Medications are now available to actually change the course of the illness, rather than just treat symptoms. It may take a month or so before you notice less pain, inflammation, and morning stiffness, but the relief may last a long time.

FINDING Support

- The Arthritis Foundation offers free brochures on treatment options and local courses, exercise classes, and other programs. Call 1-800-283-7800, or find a chapter near you at www.arthritis.org.

- Sock aids, button hookers, bathtub rails, orthotics. The federally funded ABLEDATA (1-800-227-0216 or www.ABLEDATA.com) offers unbiased advice on finding thousands of assistive and rehabilitation devices to facilitate independent living. Medicare (on the web at www.medicare.gov) can also locate resources to help you pay for equipment you might need.

- The American College of Rheumatology can help you find an expert in treating joint pain. Visit www.rheumatology.org, then click on "Find a Rheumatologist."

Rosacea

After the hormone storms of adolescence, most adults consider complexion problems a thing of the past. Then along comes the flush and sting of rosacea. Your skin can regain its normal, healthy glow, however, with the right drugs and lifestyle changes.

A B C D E F G H I J K L M N O P Q **R** S T U V W X Y Z

LIKELY First Steps

- **Topical drugs** to reduce redness and blemishes.
- **Identifying triggers** and making lifestyle changes to avoid them.
- **Oral antibiotics** or **anti-acne medicine** for more advanced cases.
- **Laser surgery** or other procedures if needed.

QUESTIONS TO Ask

- If I have to be on oral antibiotics long term, what can I do about handling their side effects?
- Do I have to give up my tropical vacation and other under-the-sun activities?
- Will I develop acne scars or bumps and a big nose?

What is happening

Your rosacea probably started innocently enough, as a simple tendency to blush easily. Then came the harder-to-ignore signs: persistent facial flushing, visible spidery blood vessels, an uncomfortable stinging in your face—all typical early symptoms. If your rosacea has progressed, you've probably also noticed small red bumps (papules) and pus-filled blemishes (pustules) on your face. A few people develop severe rosacea, with its overall facial inflammation, growth of excess skin tissue, or enlarged nose (called rhinophyma, mostly found in men). Half of those with rosacea also develop a burning or gritty feeling in their eyes.

While experts agree that rosacea is caused by dilated blood vessels in the face, they've been unable to pinpoint the precise reason why the dilation endures. Rosacea triggers vary from person to person, but certain situations in daily life can be counted on to set the inflammatory process in motion: hot drinks, alcohol, spicy foods, caffeine, stress, bright sunlight, extreme heat or cold, wind, or vigorous exercise. Medications, especially niacin and blood pressure drugs, are common culprits as well. Some cases are associated with the hormonal changes of menopause.

Rosacea is a chronic condition that tends to progress gradually, with flare-ups and periods of remission. Most common in women between ages 30 and 60, it tends to run in families and favors the fair-skinned. The "curse of the Celts," it's been called.

Treatments

There is no cure for rosacea, but faithfully using the right treatments can help clear your skin and keep symptoms from recurring. The best results usually come from a topical antibacterial drug, often when combined with an oral antibiotic. It's important to detect and avoid what sets off your flushing. In advanced cases, laser surgery, dermabrasion, and other surgical techniques have a good track record for repairing damaged skin.

Medications

For mild cases, rosacea treatment usually starts with a cream, gel, or lotion, most likely the **antibacterial drug** metronidazole (MetroGel), or the **topical antibiotic** erythromycin, which appears to work by reducing inflammation rather than by killing germs. The antibacterial sodium sulfacetamide (Klaron) can often benefit

Treatment options

Medications	
Topical drugs	Benefits seen in 3 to 9 weeks.
Oral antibiotics	Best for moderate to advanced rosacea.
Lifestyle changes	
Avoid triggers	The key to preventing flare-ups.
Cleansing regimen	Gentle routine; mild unscented soaps.
Eye care	Wash eyelids; use artificial tears.
Procedures	
Cosmetic surgery	Laser, debulking, dermabrasion, electrosurgery.

those who are not allergic to sulfa drugs. Topical drugs can take three to nine weeks to show improvement, so have patience and stick with it.

Treating more advanced rosacea is an inside job: **Oral antibiotics** such as tetracycline and erythromycin, or the **acne drug isotretinoin** (Accutane) work more quickly than topical preparations. Some antibiotics prevent eye damage. Once oral medications get rosacea under control, most people can manage symptoms successfully with just a topical drug.

Lifestyle Changes

The right lifestyle choices are the key.

- **Avoid what makes you red.** This might mean shunning spicy foods or alcohol, staying out of the noonday sun, letting hot drinks cool, or covering your face with a scarf when it's cold or windy.
- **Reduce stress.** Anxiety can trigger rosacea, so consider ways to keep yours to a minimum. A daily walk may help.
- **Use mild soaps.** Wash your face gently (no scrubbing) with a mild, fragrance-free cleanser. Pat—rather than rub—it dry.
- **Choose cosmetics carefully.** Anything you apply to your face should be alcohol-free, nonoily, and noncomedogenic (not pore-clogging). You can conceal redness with green-based makeup.
- **Wash your eyelids daily** if your eyes are affected. Use a commercial eye wash or a drop of baby shampoo diluted in water. Rinse thoroughly. If your eyes are very dry, you can get relief with artificial tears.

Procedures

A plastic surgeon or dermatologist can remove unsightly dilated blood vessels with **cosmetic surgery techniques,** using a laser or an electric needle. Excess skin tissue can be removed via surgical debulking, dermabasion, electrosurgery, or laser treatment. (*For more information on these techniques, see Acne, page 20, and Wrinkles, page 337.*)

TAKING Control

- **Become a sleuth.** People react differently to common rosacea triggers. To identify your personal flushers, keep a diary of episodes and what preceded each one.

- **Chill out.** If heat is a rosacea trip wire for you, keep the temperature on the cool side at home. Dress lightly. Take warm (not hot) showers. Take frequent sips of ice water as you exercise. Keep your (fragrance-free) facial moisturizer in the refrigerator so it cools your face when you apply it.

- **Avoid topical acne drugs.** Most topical medicines for teen-style acne (acne vulgaris) don't work for rosacea. They may make it worse. (Acne is caused by hormones and bacteria, while rosacea is a vascular disorder.)

- **Try cold-water soaks.** During flare-ups, press a cloth soaked in cold water against your face. Hold it in place for 10 minutes to constrict blood vessels.

▶ **THANKS TO W.C. FIELDS and what he called "gin blossoms" on his bulbous nose (caused by advanced rosacea), many people believe rosacea indicates alcoholism. Not true. Alcohol triggers flare-ups in some people, but many people with rosacea are teetotalers.**

FINDING Support

- For good information on treatments for rosacea, get in touch with the National Rosacea Society in Barrington, IL (1-888-NO-BLUSH or www.rosacea.org).

Shingles

Perhaps you thought that you were off the hook when your chicken pox cleared up way back when. But the very same virus can come back—with a vengeance—as shingles. Today, antiviral drugs and good home care can ease the pain and discomfort.

LIKELY **First Steps**

- **Antiviral medication** within 48 to 72 hours to shorten the virus' duration and prevent complications.
- **Pain relievers** to reduce shingles discomfort.
- **Topical lotions** to calm the itchy rash.
- **Specialized drugs for pain** if PHN develops.

QUESTIONS TO **Ask**

- My pain is a "10." What can I realistically expect from pain medication?
- Might I have an undiagnosed illness that triggered my shingles?
- How likely is it that shingles will spread to other parts of my body?

What is happening

Shingles (or herpes zoster) is a reawakening of the virus that once gave you chicken pox (varicella zoster). For most people, the virus lies dormant, often forever, in the nerves near the spinal cord. In 10% to 20% of adults, it mysteriously "wakes up," causing a painful, blistery condition called shingles (*see illustration below for its progression*). Why this happens is anyone's guess, but a weakened immune system seems to be key—from an illness, emotional stress, the use of immunosuppressant drugs, or even the natural aging process (many of those who get shingles are over age 60).

In about one-fifth of people with shingles, the discomfort persists for months after blisters disappear. Called post-herpetic neuralgia (PHN), this pain is the result of damage that the virus inflicted on your nerve cells. PHN discomfort can range from a continuous ache to severe shooting pain, leaving many people extremely sensitive to even a light touch. The good news is that most PHN sufferers eventually achieve near-complete pain relief.

Treatments

When it comes to the pain and itchiness of shingles, medications are the mainstay that bring relief: Antiviral drugs shorten the disease's stay. Analgesics relieve pain, and topical lotions or creams

HOW SHINGLES PROGRESSES

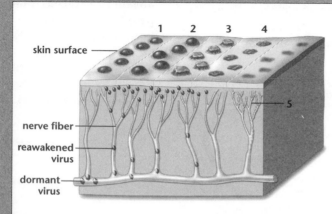

skin surface

nerve fiber

reawakened virus

dormant virus

After the chicken pox disappear, the varicella virus lies dormant in nerves near the spine. Once reawakened, it migrates along a nerve fiber to the surface of the skin, where it causes a burning or tingling sensation (**1**). Two to five days later, a red rash that produces itchy, fluid-filled blisters appears (**2**), usually in a swath on one side of your body. The bandlike pattern matches the distribution of the particular nerve affected by the virus. Over the next week or so, the blisters fill with pus, may break open (**3**), and finally crust over (**4**). After the rash disappears, the virus-damaged nerves can cause an extremely painful condition called post-herpetic neuralgia (**5**). It can last for months.

Treatment options

Medications

Antiviral drugs	Taken early, reduce severity of condition.
Pain relievers	OTC drugs; prescription for serious pain.
Topical medications	To relieve bothersome itching.
Specialized painkillers	For acute and chronic (PHN) pain.

Lifestyle changes

No scratching	To prevent infection.
Cold soaks	To soothe itchy blisters.

Procedures

TENS	Electrical stimulation to ease nerve pain.
Epidural block	Injections into nerve membranes.

soothe itchy skin. If you then develop PHN, your doctor will use a variety of treatments, beginning with painkillers. In severe cases, a spinal block may be needed to knock out the pain.

Medications

Your first step is to take an **antiviral medication** ASAP—within 72 hours of the rash's appearance for best results. These recently developed drugs block the spread of the virus and can significantly reduce your chance for getting PHN. Their best selling point may be that they can dispatch shingles in seven to 10 days; untreated, shingles can take two to four weeks to run its course. Most commonly prescribed is an original antiviral, acyclovir (Zovirax), requiring five doses a day. You might ask about newer drugs—famciclovir (Famvir) and valacyclovir (Valtrex)—which require only three daily doses.

You'll also need a **pain reliever.** If you have only mild discomfort, you may require only an OTC analgesic (aspirin, acetaminophen, ibuprofen). If you're in more serious pain, your doctor will prescribe something more powerful, such as codeine, propoxyphene (Darvon), or hydrocodone (Vicodin). For the blisters, **topical medications** can relieve itching and keep infection at bay. Apply calamine lotion, or wipe the area with a towel moistened with zinc sulfate (0.025%) or Burrow's solution (aluminum acetate). If your blisters become infected, see your doctor for an **antibiotic.**

The subsequent pain of PHN calls for stronger guns. One good option is a prescription **topical anesthetic,** such as the lidocaine patch (Lidoderm). Capsaicin cream (Zostrix), derived from the substance that makes chili peppers hot, has the same effect, but can take up to six weeks to be fully effective. Be sure to wait until your blisters have completely healed before using these creams.

Antidepressants or anticonvulsant drugs both have a solid history as effective pain therapies. **Tricyclic antidepressants,** taken in

TAKING Control

■ **Insist on real pain relief.** Although temporary, the pain of shingles can sometimes be intense. If your doctor implies you should "learn to live with it," find another doctor. A pain specialist may be your best bet.

■ **De-stress to decrease PHN pain.** Studies show you'll calm down and reduce your pain by practicing meditation, deep breathing, or progressive muscle relaxation. Visit a skilled practitioner of hypnosis, biofeedback, or acupuncture. They can help you achieve similar results.

■ **Stay away from people who haven't had chicken pox.** Shingles is not contagious, but you can give chicken pox to children and adults who have never had the varicella virus or the chicken pox vaccine.

▶ **My doctor just told me I have shingles, but it looks like poison ivy to me. How can my doctor tell?**

Lab tests can confirm your diagnosis. Your doctor can generally diagnose shingles by the way your blisters are distributed. Poison ivy and other conditions cause lesions in erratic patterns on both sides of the body. A shingles rash follows a bandlike formation on one side. This helps explain the condition's unusual name: Shingles comes from the Latin cingulum, which means "girdle" or "belt."

The Eyes Have It: Ophthalmic Shingles

The shingles virus can infect nerves of the eyes, creating a potentially serious condition called ophthalmic shingles. If blisters appear on your nose or forehead or if your eyes hurt, call an ophthalmologist right away.

Along with eye pain, ophthalmic shingles can produce blurred vision and sensitivity to light. The acutely painful phase can last several weeks. More seriously, it can lead to corneal scratching or scarring, inflammation of the iris and surrounding blood vessels, and impaired vision. In severe cases, ophthalmic shingles may cause blindness.

Treatment for ophthalmic shingles focuses on oral antiviral medications and pain relievers. You may also be given antiviral or antibiotic eyedrops.

Despite the serious complications ophthalmic shingles can cause, chances are that you will get through an outbreak with no serious problems. As with all types of shingles, the sooner you get treatment, the better off you'll be. If you start on an antiviral medication right away, ophthalmic shingles should clear up in a few weeks with no lasting effects.

Promising
DEVELOPMENTS

■ The **Shingles Prevention Study** is a large, five-year trial sponsored by the National Institutes of Health, testing whether a vaccine will prevent shingles in people ages 60 and older who have had chicken pox. To learn more about the study, search www.clinicaltrials.gov for "shingles."

FINDING Support

■ The National Institute of Neurological Disorders and Stroke, in Bethesda, MD, offers news and information about treatment and research, and literature on shingles and other neurological disorders (1-800-352-9424 or www.ninds.nih.gov).

■ The American Pain Foundation in Baltimore, MD, can help you find a pain management expert in your area. The group also specializes in providing support and advocacy for pain sufferers (1-888-615-7246 or www.painfoundation.org).

one-tenth the dose needed for depression, can block brain chemicals involved in pain perception. For PHN, nortriptyline (Pamelor, Aventyl) and amitriptyline (Elavil) are commonly used. **Anticonvulsant drugs** can help reduce pain by quieting overactive nerves. A relatively new drug in this class, gabapentin (Neurontin), has had good success in treating PHN. For severe pain, your doctor may prescribe **opioids,** such as oxycodone (OxyContin), alone or in combination with other drugs.

Lifestyle Changes

A number of simple strategies can help you get through a case of shingles. Try the following:

■ **Don't scratch** (no matter how much you want to). If you break the blisters, you risk infection. Keeping the blistered areas clean with soap and water will fight bacteria too.

■ **Cover your blisters** to protect them. Loosely place gauze over the area during the day. While you sleep, gently wrap a wide elastic sports bandage around the gauze dressing to keep it in place.

■ **Apply cold, wet compresses** or ice packs to itchy areas, or soak in a lukewarm bath laced with an Aveeno oatmeal product or cornstarch. Stay away from heat, which can intensify itchiness.

■ **Wear loose, breathable apparel.** This will prevent clothes from rubbing against your irritated skin.

Procedures

You might lower the volume on your pain with **transcutaneous electrical nerve stimulation (TENS).** This technique delivers low-level electrical pulses to nerve endings via electrodes on your skin. This stimulates production of endorphins, your body's natural painkillers. If your pain is so severe that it's affecting the quality of your life, consult your doctor about an **epidural block,** injections of local anesthetics or steroids into the membranes surrounding your nerves. In a 2000 study, more than 90% of those given such injections reported good to excellent pain control. Injections of antiviral drugs plus steroids are another effective option for difficult cases.

Sinusitis

Right now, one in seven Americans suffers from sinusitis, and the number is growing. The good news is that easy-to-follow at-home treatments can produce welcome relief, and plenty of symptom-specific medications can really help.

What is happening

If your cold, flu, or allergy simply won't quit, it may have transformed itself into sinusitis, an infection of the sinus cavities. The sinuses are four pairs of air-containing spaces in the front of your skull (*see illustration below*). They are connected to your nasal passages through narrow passages whose tiny openings called ostia normally let mucus drain and air flow in and out. When you have an allergy or a respiratory infection like a cold, the lining of your sinuses can swell and block these passages. The blockage traps mucus in your sinuses, where it builds up and thickens, inviting normally harmless bacteria to multiply.

When this happens you'll feel it. Sinusitis' calling card is thick, yellowish-green mucus, a sense of pressure in your face, a headache, and difficulty breathing through your nose. You may also have pain in your upper teeth, a persistent cough, a low fever, and/or fatigue.

If this is your first sinus infection, or you get them only rarely, you probably have **acute sinusitis.** This is usually caused by the bacteria *Streptococcus pneumoniae* or *Haemophilus influenzae*; with treatment, it lasts about three weeks. If your sinus infection

LIKELY First Steps

- **Steam inhalation, sinus irrigation,** and **drinking plenty of fluids** to thin mucus and reduce nasal swelling.

- **Analgesics, decongestants, cough suppressants,** or **expectorants** to relieve specific symptoms.

- If required, **antibiotics** to fight an acute bacterial infection.

- If nothing is effective, or you have a sinus blockage, **surgery** may be necessary to clear sinus passages.

QUESTIONS TO Ask

- Is there a chance that my "sinus headaches" could really be migraines?

- Could my recurrent sinus infections be caused by an obstruction in my nasal passages?

- I use a steroid nasal spray, but it irritates my nose. Are there any alternatives that would work for me?

- Would simply treating my hay fever cure my sinusitis? Should I be seeing an allergist?

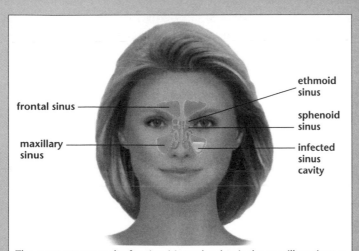

LOCATING THE SINUSES

frontal sinus

ethmoid sinus

sphenoid sinus

maxillary sinus

infected sinus cavity

The most common site for sinusitis to develop is the maxillary sinuses, located behind your cheekbones. Infection can also occur in the frontal sinuses (above your eyes), the ethmoid sinuses (between your eyes), or the sphenoid sinuses (behind your nose).

TAKING **Control**

■ **Reduce your stress level.**
Studies show that stress
and anger can weaken the
immune system, and a weakened immune system con-
tributes to the frequency and
severity of sinus infections.
Learn to defuse your stress
with meditation and other
relaxation techniques.

■ **Take precautions when
you fly.** Changing air pressure during takeoffs and
landings forces mucus into
your sinuses. Chew gum
or swallow often, or use
an OTC nasal spray during
these times to reduce sinus
pressure.

■ **Learn to blow the right
way.** Even if you're totally
congested, never blow your
nose forcefully. Inhale
through your mouth, then
blow gently through one
nostril at a time. Press the
other nostril closed as you
do so. If your nose gets raw,
use a little petroleum jelly
inside and below the nostrils.
(*For more on nose blowing,
see Colds, page 84.*)

■ **Sniff some eucalyptus oil.**
Putting a few drops of eucalyptus oil on a tissue and
sniffing it periodically during
the day can relieve swollen
nasal tissues. When inhaled,
eucalyptol, the oil's key
medicinal ingredient, tightens
and thus soothes inflamed
mucous membranes.

■ **Create an irritant-free
zone.** If dust or pollen aggravates your sinusitis, turn your
bedroom into a sanctuary.
Remove carpeting and drapes.
Keep the room well dusted,
wash linens weekly in hot
water, and bar the door
to pets.

Treatment options

Lifestyle changes

Steam inhalation & sinus irrigation	Keeps mucous membranes moist and mucus thin; electric steam inhaler good for chronic.
Lots of clear liquids	Choose water, tea, or broth to thin discharge.
Exercise	Can boost immune system.

Medications

Antibiotics	For acute: Amoxicillin usually first choice. For chronic: Only if bacteria is cause.
Analgesics	Soothes sinus pain and reduces fever.
Decongestants	Nasal spray: Only under doctor's orders. Oral: Limit use to 3 or 4 days.
Cough medicines	Suppressants or expectorants as required.

Procedures

Nasal endoscopy & CT scan	To detect underlying problems in chronic.
Sinus surgery	Last resort for chronic.

Natural methods

Spicy foods	Good for making mucus flow.

continues for two months or longer, despite treatment, the diagnosis is probably **chronic sinusitis.**

While chronic sinusitis may result from a hard-to-treat bacterial infection, damaged mucous membranes from unsuccess-
fully treated acute sinusitis may also play a role, or it may be the
result of polyps or cysts—small benign growths—in your nasal
passages. A blockage could result from a deviated septum, a common structural abnormality in which the septum (the bone and
cartilage in the center of the nose) is crooked. Hay fever and
asthma (both associated with allergies), contribute to chronic
sinusitis as well (in fact, about 70% of people with chronic sinusitis also have allergies). For some people, sinusitis is worsened by
sensitivity to certain foods, such as dairy products or wheat. Evidence has shown that some types of chronic sinusitis are triggered by an immune response to fungi naturally found in the
nose (*see box opposite*).

Treatments

Because about half of acute sinus infections eventually clear up on
their own, your doctor may want to take a wait-and-see approach
for a few days before prescribing an antibiotic. During this time,
there are a number of self-care measures—from inhaling steam to
simply reducing stress—you can try at home.

While bacterial sinusitis can make you feel temporarily miserable, complications are rare. However, swelling around an eye, impaired vision, a high fever, or a change in mental status, is a sign that the infection has spread. You should go to an emergency room immediately.

Treating chronic sinusitis is more complex because of all the potential underlying causes. Antibiotics and aggressive self-care measures are usually tried first, though they won't work if a polyp is causing your problem. If your condition persists, you'll probably be referred to an ear, nose, and throat specialist (otolaryngologist).

Lifestyle Changes

You can do many things on your own to thin mucus and unclog your blocked sinus passages. Perhaps the easiest method is **steam inhalation.** Simply boil some water, pour it into the basin, and add a teaspoon of Vicks VapoRub. Then place a towel over your head and the basin. Slowly inhale the steam for 10 minutes, morning and evening. Have tissues handy to blow your nose, but don't blow too vigorously. This can force infected mucus deeper into your sinuses.

Another method that loosens mucus and reduces swelling in the nasal passages is **sinus irrigation** with a saline solution. You can use an ear-bulb syringe or a more unusual device called a neti pot, which is available at health food stores (*see box, page 285*). Irrigate at least three times a day for acute sinusitis and once or twice a day for a milder condition.

It's also important to **drink plenty of clear liquids**—8 to 10 glasses a day—to keep nasal discharge thin. Warm beverages can be quite soothing, and the steam from a cup of hot tea or chicken broth will temporarily open your nasal passages.

Even though you might not feel like working out when you have sinusitis, **exercise** can stimulate the flow of mucus and boost production of infection-fighting white blood cells. So take a brisk walk, go for a bike ride, or choose any other aerobic activity you like, but don't do exercises (like toe-touches) where you lower your head. This will increase sinus pressure. If exercise worsens your congestion, stop working out.

Medications

For acute bacterial sinusitis, a variety of **antibiotics** work quite well. The drug your doctor initially prescribes will probably depend on which strain of bacteria is the common culprit in your geographic area. (Because reports from local hospitals provide this information, your mucus won't need to be tested.) Amoxicillin, a broad-spectrum antibiotic with a proven track record in treating this infection, is most doctors' first choice unless you have an allergy to penicillin. Other effective antibiotics include amoxicillin/clavulanate (Augmentin), cefuroxime (Ceftin), loracarbef (Lorabid), cefprozil (Cefzil), levofloxacin (Levaquin), and sparfloxacin (Zagam).

It Could Be Fungi

Until recently, microorganisms called fungi were thought to cause only a small percentage of chronic sinusitis. Remarkably, a 1999 study by Mayo Clinic researchers found fungi in the mucus of 202 of the 210 people studied. (*Aspergillis* is the fungus most commonly identified with chronic sinusitis.)

Further research found that nearly the same percentage of the general population has fungal growths in their sinuses. The difference is that in patients with chronic sinusitis, an immune system attack on the fungus causes the nasal passages to become inflamed and congested.

Treatment of allergic fungal sinusitis usually involves sinus surgery, then drug therapy with allergy shots, nasal steroids to control inflammation, and antihistamines (Claritin, Allegra) and antileukotrienes (Singulair) to control the allergic response.

How best to clear up fungal sinusitis is under debate. Doctors are investigating two possible options: treatment to get rid of the fungus and treatment to prevent the immune system from attacking the fungus. In the meantime, sinus irrigation with oral or topical antifungals has proved successful for some. For others, sinus surgery may be required to clear away any dead and infected tissue.

A
B
C
D
E
F
G
H
I
J
K
L
M
N
O
P
Q
R
S
T
U
V
W
X
Y
Z

▶**I've never had sinusitis before. Am I going to get a lot of these infections in the future?**

Probably not. Most attacks of acute sinusitis are just complications of an especially bad cold where thickened mucus in the sinuses becomes infected by bacteria. Once antibiotics have cured your infection, there shouldn't be a problem with recurrence.

▶**My doctor prescribed antibiotics for three weeks. Why do I have to take them for so long?**

Your sinuses are like caves within your skull. They receive a relatively small supply of blood (as compared with your lungs or kidneys). Since the antibiotics are carried to the infected sinuses through your bloodstream, you need to be on these drugs for at least 10 to 14 days for the medication to have its full effect.

▶**If the infection is in my sinuses, why am I coughing so much, especially during the night?**

When you lie flat, your sinuses start to drain down the back of your throat. A very small amount of mucus can cause a truly agonizing tickle that makes you cough. Before going to bed, take some cough syrup containing dextromethorphan (DM) or codeine and you may sleep better. Elevate the head of your bed by 45 degrees (use bricks or fat books under the legs) to promote sinus drainage. If only one side of your head is involved, sleep on your side, with the congested side up.

To be effective, an antibiotic must generally be taken for at least 10 days. Some doctors even prescribe a full two weeks to reduce the risk of relapse. You'll probably start to feel better after just four days—and the infected yellow mucus will begin to clear up—but don't stop taking the drug. If you do, the infection won't be wiped out, and you could end up with chronic sinusitis. If your symptoms don't start to disappear after four or five days, call your doctor. Most doctors are now prescribing a corticosteroid nasal spray along with antibiotics to reduce swelling in the nasal passages.

Other medications can be taken alone or with antibiotics to treat specific symptoms and speed recovery. For example, **over-the-counter analgesics** such as NSAIDs (aspirin or ibuprofen) or acetaminophen soothe sinus pain and headache, and **nasal or oral decongestants** reduce swelling of the sinus linings and help you breathe more easily. Popular OTC decongestants include Sudafed and Drixoral, which contain pseudoephedrine, and Afrin, Dristan 12-Hour, and Neo-Synephrine 12-Hour, which include oxymetazoline. Be sure to consult your doctor before trying a decongestant spray; in some cases, it can make congestion worse. Always limit use to three to four days to prevent a rebound effect: As the decongestant wears off, it may actually *cause* swelling in your nasal passages.

In addition, certain other drugs can be effective:

■ **If you have a nagging cough** and are losing sleep from postnasal drip, you might want to try a **cough suppressant** with dextromethorphan (Robitussin DM and Vicks 44). If your cough is severe, ask your doctor to prescribe a cough suppressant with codeine (Promethazine VC/Codeine, Phenergan with Codeine).

■ **If you need to loosen mucus,** an **expectorant** that contains the mucolytic (mucus thinner) guaifenesin, the active ingredient in Robitussin and Glycotuss, can help. Stronger versions (Fenesin, Humibid) are available by prescription.

■ **If an allergy is triggering your sinusitis,** your doctor may recommend OTC **antihistamines** containing the drug diphenhydramine (Benadryl-25, AllerMax) or a prescription **corticosteroid nasal spray** (such as Beconase or Nasacort) to reduce inflammation. Some nonsedating prescription and OTC antihistamines available are Allegra and Claritin. Don't use either if you have bacterial sinusitis. They can thicken mucus, making a bacterial infection worse.

■ **If you have chronic bacterial sinusitis,** you may require intense treatment with **a more potent antibiotic** such as clarithromycin (Biaxin) or cefadroxil (Duricef). You'll have to take the drug for three to eight weeks. Your doctor may also recommend that you use a corticosteroid nasal spray, as well as the expectorant guaifenesin and an oral decongestant. This powerful combo works for many people.

Procedures

If your sinusitis doesn't clear up after a couple of months of antibiotics along with good home care, your doctor may recommend that

Sinus Irrigation: How to Use a Neti Pot

Made of ceramic or plastic, a neti pot looks like a small watering can with a narrow spout. It has been used for centuries in India to cleanse nasal passages and enhance breathing during yoga sessions. Integrative physicians often recommend neti pots for irrigating the sinuses.

Making the saline solution

To use a neti pot, make a saline solution by mixing ⅓ teaspoon of noniodized table salt and a pinch of baking soda in 1 cup of lukewarm water. Pour only half of the liquid into the neti pot at one time.

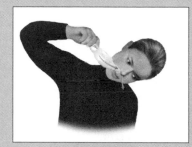

Doing the irrigation

1. Place the spout of the pot into one nostril, making a firm seal so it doesn't drip.
2. Stand over a sink, then tilt your head to the side and down, away from the spout.
3. Pour the saline solution into the nostril. Shortly, the liquid will come out of the other nostril (*see illustration above*).

4. Once the solution has drained, blow gently into a tissue to clear your nasal passage.
5. Repeat steps 1–4 with the other nostril, using the remaining solution.

Tips
- Keep breathing through your mouth as you pour. This prevents the solution from draining from the back of your nose into your mouth and throat. This gets easier with practice.
- If the saline solution stings your nostrils, dilute the saline strength by half, then gradually work back up to full strength.

---

you see an ear, nose, and throat specialist for **nasal endoscopy,** a nonsurgical procedure under a local anesthetic. The doctor will use a flexible, lighted telescope-like device called an endoscope to visually inspect your sinuses, then extract a sample of the infected mucus. This procedure detects small abnormalities in the sinuses and helps the doctor determine why the medications are ineffective.

In some cases of chronic sinusitis, your doctor may order a **computed tomography (CT) scan.** This sophisticated x-ray helps find infection hidden in the deeper air chambers. Depending on the results, **sinus surgery** may be recommended. The surgery uses a tiny fiberoptic scalpel that does not scar and can drain your sinuses, remove any polyps or cysts, or widen the openings into your nasal passages (a procedure known as **functional endoscopic sinus surgery, or FESS).** Most sinus surgery is done under general or local anesthesia. You'll go home the same day. Although surgery is never a guaranteed cure for sinusitis, studies show that the majority of people who have it report fewer symptoms.

Natural Methods*

For temporary relief from congestion, try **spicy foods.** Chili peppers and cayenne pepper contain capsaicin, a powerful compound that breaks up mucus. Mustard and horseradish, which contain the natural chemical allyl isothiocyanate, can act in a similar way. Fresh ginger is a natural antihistamine. Experiment to see which foods unstuff you best.

*Natural methods are not subject to the same testing and regulation as prescription medications. Please seek your doctor's advice and use caution.

Promising DEVELOPMENTS

■ For people with allergy-related sinusitis, some doctors are trying **leukotriene receptor antagonists,** drugs commonly used for asthma. These nonsteroidal drugs, which include montelukast (Singulair) and zafirlukast (Accolate), work by blocking leukotrienes, substances that worsen asthma symptoms and possibly those of allergies as well. Researchers believe relieving the underlying allergy will also help to treat the sinusitis.

FINDING Support

■ For the latest research findings on treatments for sinusitis, contact the American Academy of Otolaryngology, Head and Neck Surgery, in Alexandria, VA (703-836-4444 or www.entnet.org).

Skin cancer

Most of the 1.3 million Americans diagnosed with skin cancer every year do fine, thanks to a nearly 98% cure rate for basal cell and squamous cell carcinomas. Now more options are appearing for less common (but potentially deadly) melanomas.

LIKELY **First Steps**

- **Surgery** or other lesion-eliminating procedures (curettage and electrodessication, Mohs surgery, cryosurgery).

- For skin cancers that have spread beyond the skin, **chemotherapy, radiation therapy, photodynamic therapy, immunotherapy.**

- Sun protection, regular skin exams, and other **lifestyle measures** to help detect new problems early and prevent recurrences.

QUESTIONS TO **Ask**

- What number sunblock is the best for my skin type?

- Given my history, how often should I schedule a checkup with a dermatologist?

- What are the chances that my melanoma has been misdiagnosed?

What is happening

The skin is composed of many different types of cells—basal cells, squamous cells, melanocytes, others—that naturally grow and slough off over time. A diagnosis of skin cancer means some of these cells have become abnormal (or mutated) and are starting to reproduce out of control. This happens largely as a result of accumulated sun damage, although other factors, such as skin type, genetics, and environmental exposure, are also involved.

Affecting one of every eight Americans, **basal cell carcinoma** is the most prevalent form of skin cancer. It occurs in the skin's top layer (called the epidermis). The cells gather into clusters and replicate, growing slowly and forming painless, translucent bumps. Most appear on the face, although any part of you exposed to the sun is vulnerable: ears, neck, back, chest, arms, legs. It's rare, however, for these cancers to grow deep into the skin or spread to internal organs.

Squamous cell carcinoma also starts in the epidermis. Its earliest precancerous form is often actinic keratosis lesions, or sun spots (*see box, page 288*). Squamous cell cancer may begin as raised, reddish lumps, which sometimes become open sores (ulcerate). It's relatively unusual for this type of cancer to spread beyond the skin, but it can be deadly if it does. You're at increased risk for a more involved type of squamous cell cancer if the lesion develops on the penis or the vulva as a sequel to an infection with certain strains of genital warts.

Far less common but more dangerous is **malignant melanoma.** This cancer arises from melanocytes—cells that produce melanin, the pigment that gives color to skin, hair, and eyes. Melanin is concentrated in most moles and also acts to protect your skin from the sun's ultraviolet (UV) radiation, giving you a tan as a defense mechanism. Melanocytes that reproduce too quickly and appear as irregularly shaped, light-brown to black blemishes, signal trouble. This can occur within an existing mole, on unblemished skin, or, rarely, in the eye or under nails. Left unattended, a melanoma will penetrate deep into the skin and may spread (metastasize) via the lymphatic system or the bloodstream.

Treatments

The purpose of skin cancer treatment is to halt further growth of any malignancy. The specific approaches that your doctor will use are

Treatment options

Procedures

Surgical excision	Literally cutting out problem tissue.
Cryosurgery	Liquid nitrogen to freeze and kill cells.
Laser therapy	Beam of light burns off superficial cells.
Radiation	X-ray treatment for metastasized lesions.
Photodynamic therapy	For basal and squamous cell cancers.

Medications

Imiquimod	Aldara for basal and squamous cell cancers.
Chemotherapy	Immunotherapy, vaccines, perfusion.

Lifestyle changes

Avoid UV rays	Stay out of the sun and protect against it.

tied to your particular type of lesion. For most basal cell and squamous cell cancers that have not spread, the strategy is the same: Destroy the lesion by burning, freezing, or scraping it off. Usually not painful, these procedures are done in a doctor's office after numbing the site with a local anesthetic.

For basal cell or squamous cell cancers that have spread, nonsurgical techniques (medication, radiation, or other therapies) are generally used. In choosing the appropriate treatment, you and your doctor will weigh factors such as where the lesion is, how deep it is, and how quickly it's growing. Before treatment begins, make sure your diagnosis has been confirmed with a biopsy, a laboratory analysis of the excised tissue.

A malignant melanoma that's caught early, as a "local" cancer, is removed surgically. Your prospects for a full recovery are excellent; nearly 95% of superficial malignant melanomas can be cured. But once the cancer has penetrated deeper (even just a couple of millimeters down or into your lymph nodes), the strategy changes dramatically. Melanoma can spread quickly and prove fatal. While melanoma accounts for only 4% of skin cancer diagnoses, it's responsible for 80% of skin cancer deaths. Cutting out the cancer is still crucial, but so are chemotherapy or radiation, which may slow down the tumor and ease discomfort. Once a melanoma has spread, "cures" are rare, so early detection and removal are key.

In very rare cases, a melanoma spontaneously disappears when the immune system mounts a strong resistance. Researchers, witnessing this fierce stand, are exploring the value of immunotherapy drugs, therapeutic vaccines, and other strategies to stimulate the immune system of patients with malignant melanoma. Early results of these novel therapies show promising results and safety in the treatment of malignant melanoma.

TAKING Control

- **Push for an appointment.** If there's something suspicious on your skin, be proactive about getting it checked, and if necessary, removed. See a skin doctor (dermatologist) specializing in skin cancer if you can.

- **Give up the tanning parlor and sun lamp.** Neither is safe. A recent study found that people who used any type of tanning device have a 2.5 times greater risk for squamous cell cancer and a 1.5 times greater risk for basal cell cancer.

- **Reach out.** A diagnosis of skin cancer, especially a malignant melanoma, can be frightening. Talk with your doctor. Look to friends, family, and support groups. De-stress with exercise and yoga.

- **Question Internet info.** A study from the University of Michigan found many popular melanoma websites are simply wrong about diagnosis and treatment options.

- **Sign up for a clinical trial** if your melanoma is advanced. It's a chance to benefit from new treatments (see "Finding Support," page 290).

- **Catch the next one early.** Every month, use a mirror to examine every inch of your skin. Have someone check hard-to-see places. Call the doctor about alterations in lesion shape, color, or size. A Cancer study found that 57% of nearly 500 melanoma patients detected the cancer on their own.

- **Tell family members** to get screened regularly, especially if you've had a melanoma. Your cancer means they're at increased risk as well.

Actinic Keratoses

These precancerous growths, typically small, warty spots, are often called "sun spots" (solar keratoses) because they're directly related to sun damage. They can develop into squamous cell cancers. Your doctor will watch the area for suspicious changes, then excise the lesion, freeze the growth, or recommend the cream Efudex to stop cell proliferation.

Multiple lesions have been successfully treated with photodynamic therapy. Laser resurfacing and chemical peels are less popular options. The government is sponsoring research on the arthritis drug Celebrex, to see if it can prevent actinic keratoses from becoming cancerous.

Promising DEVELOPMENTS

■ Experimental drug treatments for malignant melanoma are showing some promise. Thalidomide and drugs similar to it have shown promise in improving the immune system's ability to delay progression of a malignant melanoma. Another treatment, **gene therapy,** creates changes in the melanoma cells themselves. (Cells are removed, subjected to genetic material that alters them slightly, and then infused back into the body.) The immune system is then prompted to kill the cancer.

Procedures

The treatment method chosen for a particular cancerous lesion will depend on its biopsy and diagnosis.

For basal cell cancer. One of the most common approaches is **surgical excision,** which involves cutting out the abnormal growth and closing the area with stitches. Laboratory analysis can then determine whether the edges of the excised tissue (margins) are free of cancerous cells. Excision is slightly less likely to be linked to a recurrence than if the tissue is "destroyed."

Depending on the type of lesion and its location, your doctor may recommend **curettage and electrodesiccation.** In this technique, the cancer is scraped away with a sharp, ring-shaped instrument called a curette. An electric wand is used to cauterize the base of the growth. The procedure is only as effective as the operator's skill, so try to find a doctor who has done it hundreds of times. Three cycles of treatment are typically needed. You'll probably be left with a broad, pale scar.

For lesions on the head and neck, where scarring can be a real cosmetic issue, **Mohs micrographic surgery** may be your best option. It's also valuable for skin cancers that are likely to (or have already) reappeared despite conventional treatments, for lesions with scar tissue that have nondefined edges, and for cancers that are growing fast or uncontrollably. Invented in the 1930s by Dr. Frederic E. Mohs, the procedure involves removing a tumor gradually, layer by layer. Each section is processed in the doctor's office and examined on the spot under a microscope. Removal continues until a cancer-free layer of tissue is reached. Mohs offers the highest cure rates and the least tissue loss; an important consideration for cancers that have developed on the face (eyelids, lips, temples, nose, ears). Cure rates for basal cell cancers treated with Mohs are as high as 99%. Be sure to find a dermatologist specifically trained in this specialized type of surgery.

Another option for small basal cell cancers on the head and neck is **cryosurgery.** In this procedure, liquid nitrogen is applied to an abnormal growth to freeze and kill the malignant cells. The dead tissue falls off as the area thaws. You might feel slight pain and have swelling for a while, and more than one freezing may be needed. Eventually a white scar may form in the area that has been treated. With **laser therapy,** a narrow, concentrated beam of light is used to remove or destroy cancer cells. This technique is used only for very superficial skin cancers.

For advanced basal cell cancer. If a basal cell cancer has grown significantly and is proving very difficult to treat, your doctor might recommend x-ray **radiation.** Some doctors recommend radiation following surgery to ensure that every last cancer cell is destroyed. Radiation is used slightly more often for squamous cell cancers than for basal cell growths because the former carry a greater risk of serious illness at all stages.

For squamous cell cancer. The preferred treatment approach is **simple excision** with a scalpel, though some small, superficial lesions can be successfully treated with **curettage and electro-desiccation.** Another option is **cryotherapy.** Lesions on the lips, ears, nose, or other sensitive facial areas, as well as aggressive tumors and lesions that have reappeared, are best treated with **Mohs surgery.** Although not yet widely available, a specialized technique called **photodynamic therapy** is often a good choice for treating multiple superficial basal cell cancers or a squamous cell cancer. The technique involves applying or ingesting a chemical that makes skin cells sensitive to a precise color of laser light. When applied, the laser instantly destroys only the cancerous cells.

For malignant melanoma. You'll need to have a **surgical excision** of the growth itself, along with (typically) at least a half inch of normal surrounding skin cut out as a safety precaution. This is done to thwart the growth of any lingering cancerous cells. If you have had a relatively superficial melanoma removed, the wound will take one to two weeks to heal. Avoid heavy exercise during this period so the incision can heal properly.

If there's any chance that malignant melanoma has traveled to your lymph nodes, the surgeon will remove the nodes for examination. Taking out the nodes may help prevent the cancer from spreading throughout your lymphatic system. If the cancer has already spread, surgically removing the nodes may ease pain and increase your chance of survival. **Radiation** may help relieve discomfort with metastatic melanoma, but won't destroy it.

Medications

For basal cell carcinoma, prescription creams such as fluorouracil (Efudex, Fluoroplex) are used with caution because cancer can still spread under the healed surface of the skin. Many experts are now placing hope in a cream called **imiquimod** (Aldara), normally used for genital warts. In pilot studies, this cream has successfully cleared up superficial basal cell cancers in about 90% of patients.

Medications aren't needed to treat thin melanomas (typically less than 1.5 mm thick), but if the cancer has spread, you'll want to consider **chemotherapy** to stop the growth and ease discomfort. Just remember no drug is a "cure" and any can cause side effects. Some drugs are given intravenously, others are taken orally. Dacarbazine (DTIC) is commonly used, although a combination of DTIC, carmustine (BCNU), cisplatin, and tamoxifen is becoming popular. Researchers worldwide are constantly testing new blends.

If your melanoma is advanced, you might want to find out about the developing field of **immunotherapy** (also called biological therapy). This drug strategy enlists the help of interferon-alpha (Intron-A), interleukin-2 (IL-2), and tumor necrosis factor (TNF). These chemicals occur naturally in your body and are produced in part by your white cells. When manufactured outside the body, these agents can be injected in drug form to stimulate your immune system to vigorously fight the melanoma tumor.

Clinical trials report long-term remission (sometimes for years) in about 6% of people taking Intron-A and IL-2, but many

▶**Can a squamous cell skin cancer spread to another part of my body?**
It's unlikely but possible. "Squamous" describes the type of cell associated with the tumor: flat and scaly. Cancers can develop in places that naturally contain squamous cells, including the lining of hollow organs such as the bladder and lung and the passages of the respiratory, digestive, and genitourinary systems. Squamous cell skin cancer is by far the most common form.

▶**What can I put on my skin to minimize scarring after a lesion is excised?**
Try breaking open a vitamin E gelcap and spreading the oil over the wound once it has scabbed. Gently massage in some oil every day. This may help lessen redness and accelerate healing. Applying silicate gel may also help.

▶**Are there any natural methods* I can use to treat malignant melanoma?**
Alternative medicines promoted for treating advanced melanoma and other cancers include cow and shark cartilage, Laetrile, coenzyme Q_{10}, and mistletoe. None has proved effective or definitively safe.

▶**IT'S A MYTH that pulling hairs from moles will make them cancerous. Plucking the hairs with a tweezer might irritate the mole, but that's about all.**

*Natural methods are not subject to the same testing and regulation as prescription medications. Please seek your doctor's advice and use caution.

Defend Against Those Deadly Rays

If you have a skin cancer now, there's a good chance it's probably due to sun exposure (and bad sunburns) you got as a child: About 80% of sun damage occurs before age 18. Here are some strategies to defend against future damage.

Sunscreens
At least 20 to 30 minutes before going outside, put on a broad-spectrum (UVA and UVB) sunscreen. Use a product rated SPF 15 or higher if you burn easily or will be on reflective surfaces (snow, sand) or at high altitudes in intense sun. Reapply often (every 90 minutes or so) while you're outside. Put on more after exercising or getting out of the water.

Sunblocks
Very effective, these products contain zinc or titanium oxide, which dries to a white film. Use enough (at least 2 ounces for an adult) to achieve the protection advertised on the label. Reapply as you would sunscreen.

UPF Factor
In sunstruck Australia, garments are given an Ultraviolet Protection Factor (UPF). The UPF is based on the degree that light penetrates a garment, as well as its thickness (density). The higher the UPF, the better the garment's sun protection.

Your standard white cotton T-shirt, for example, has a UPF of 7, while a pair of dark blue jeans has 1,000. When swimming, opt for sunscreen instead of the T-shirt; cotton fabrics lose up to 50% of their sun-protective capacity when wet.

Laundry
To increase a garment's sun-blocking quality, wash and dry it repeatedly to draw the fibers together.

You can also wash sunblock right into the fabric. Some laundry additives, such as RIT Sunguard, contain the colorless dye Tinosorb, which is designed to increase the UPF rating of cotton garments to at least UPF 30 with one washing.

FINDING Support

Several foundations and medical associations operate websites and can also mail you material. Among the best:

- The Skin Cancer Foundation in Manhattan (1-800-SKIN-490 or www.skincancer.org).

- The American Academy of Dermatology has a website, www.aad.org, so does the the American Society for Dermatologic Surgery, www.asds-net.org (or 847-956-0900).

- For information on joining a clinical trial that is testing new treatments, call the Cancer Information Service at 1-800-4-CANCER.

- If you have melanoma, look for support at such places as the Melanoma Patients' Information Page website (www.mpip.org).

refinements are still needed. The agent most commonly used—interferon-alpha—boosts survival only modestly. It can be highly toxic (many liken side effects to a bout of flu).

Experimental work in combining immunotherapy with **anti-melanoma vaccines** has generated great excitement. Unlike flu vaccines, such drugs are not given to prevent the disease, but to keep it from getting worse. The injection contains fragments of melanoma cells called antigens, which are little flags on the cell surface that signal they are foreign invaders. By bombarding the body with these antigens, it's hoped the immune system will launch its own attack on the melanoma cells. While there's no vaccine on the market just yet, clinical trial successes are generating high expectations for this treatment approach.

For a melanoma that has spread or reappeared on an arm or leg, ask about **chemotherapeutic regional perfusion.** In this technique, drugs are infused into affected areas, sparing most of the body a toxic reaction to chemotherapy.

Lifestyle Changes

Take care to **avoid UV rays** in any way possible (*see box above*). Two smart moves you can make are to check your own skin frequently for suspicious changes and schedule regular **skin checks with a dermatologist.**

The bottom line: The earlier you catch a skin cancer, the greater your chances of eliminating it with minimal scarring, and in the case of malignant melanoma, staying alive.

Sleep apnea

Nights are hardly restful if you have sleep apnea, a chronic and sometimes danger-ous condition in which your breathing literally—and repeatedly—stops during sleep. A few lifestyle changes, and a simple machine, may be all you need to control it.

What is happening

It's estimated that some 18 million Americans have sleep apnea, yet fewer than 1 million know it. Here's why: If you have sleep apnea, you'll breathe normally during the day. It's only at night, when you fall asleep, that your breathing stops—sometimes for 10 seconds, sometimes for a minute or more. You may snore loudly or even strug-gle for air when the level of oxygen in your blood starts to fall. In response, you wake only briefly—so briefly that you don't remem-ber it the next morning—then immediately fall back to sleep. This cycle can repeat itself many times a night (as frequently as 100 times an hour in some cases), preventing deep sleep and leaving you exhausted the next day.

The consequences go beyond a little fatigue. Those with sleep apnea are two to three times more likely to have car accidents than those who sleep normally. The buildup of carbon dioxide in your blood can put you at risk for high blood pressure and other health threats, including heart attack or stroke.

The most common form of the disease, **obstructive sleep apnea (OSA),** occurs when tissues in the airway relax and "collapse" dur-ing sleep, blocking the flow of air (*see illustration at right*). The seri-ously overweight are particularly prone to this condition, as are men and those over age 65. If you sleep on your back or are blood-related to someone with sleep apnea, you have an increased chance of developing it. Far fewer people have another form, called **cen-tral sleep apnea (CSA).** It has the same symptoms as OSA, but is thought to occur when the brain fails to send "breathing signals" to respiratory muscles.

Treatments

Once you've answered a few questions, your doctor will have a good idea whether or not you have sleep apnea, but you'll need a spe-cialized test to determine which kind of apnea it is. The main test for sleep apnea, polysomnography, takes place in a sleep labora-tory. For one or two nights, a technician monitors such things as your breathing pattern, oxygen levels, face and leg movements, and brain waves. These readings are studied to determine, scien-tifically, how well you're sleeping.

If you're like the vast majority of people with apnea, you prob-ably have the obstructive form. While you might need surgery to remove air-blocking tissue from your airways, most likely

LIKELY **First Steps**

- **Lose weight** by exercising more and eating a healthy diet. Obesity is the main cause of sleep apnea.

- **Avoid alcohol or sedatives at bedtime** to prevent the throat muscles from relaxing too much.

- **Sleep on your side or stomach,** not on your back, to keep airways clear.

- **Use a CPAP machine** to improve breathing during sleep (*see page 293*).

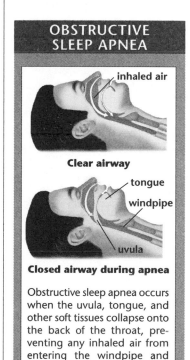

OBSTRUCTIVE SLEEP APNEA

inhaled air

Clear airway

tongue

windpipe

uvula

Closed airway during apnea

Obstructive sleep apnea occurs when the uvula, tongue, and other soft tissues collapse onto the back of the throat, pre-venting any inhaled air from entering the windpipe and lungs. To breathe, you must wake a bit from sleep.

QUESTIONS TO Ask

- Does my heavy-duty snoring mean I have sleep apnea?
- Will my apnea get worse if I ignore it?
- Is apnea the reason I can't stay awake until the end of a movie, or could I have another problem?

TAKING Control

- **Elevate the head of your bed** four to six inches using bricks or fat books. Doing so helps prevent heartburn, a common apnea trigger.

- **Get hay fever under control,** either by avoiding allergens or using nonsedating antihistamines to reduce congestion. Allergy symptoms often cause an increase in apnea and snoring.

- **Avoid a heavy meal** near bedtime. It can make breathing problems worse.

- **Watch out for LAUP.** Often recommended to decrease snoring, laser-assisted uvulopalatoplasty (LAUP) uses a laser device to eliminate tissue in the back of your throat. While it does work for snoring, LAUP does not eliminate sleep apnea. Since your snoring is gone after the procedure, you may not realize that you have apnea. This could be life-threatening for some, so ask your doctor whether you need an apnea test.

Treatment options

Lifestyle changes

Lose weight	Just a 10% loss can have great benefits.
Watch sedatives	Alcohol and sleeping pills increase apnea.
Change sleep position	Sleep on your side, not on your back.
CPAP machine	Keeps windpipe open; use every night.

Procedures

UPPP & ablation	Remove tissues surgically to widen airways.
Tracheostomy	For life-threatening cases only.

Medications

Antidepressant	Protriptyline can improve symptoms.
Sinus medication	Steroids and decongestants clear airways.

you'll be advised to make a few lifestyle changes and try a home device called a CPAP machine that makes it easier for air to get into your lungs.

Lifestyle Changes

Nearly everyone with sleep apnea needs to **lose weight.** Studies show that the frequency of breathing interruptions increases 32% for every 10% you're over your ideal weight. Looked at another way, losing just 10% of your weight could reduce apnea episodes by 26%. You'll also want to **avoid alcoholic beverages** and **sedating medications** (such as antihistamines or sleeping pills) in the evening. Both can relax your throat muscles and make them more likely to sag into your windpipe.

Another key suggestion for mild sleep apnea is to **sleep on your side or stomach,** not on your back. The reason is gravity: Sleeping on your back pulls on the upper part of your airway, encouraging the soft palate tissue to droop down and block air flow. One good way to stay on your side is to sew a tennis ball into a small pocket on the back of your pajamas or T-shirt. It will irritate you if you inadvertently roll onto your back.

Perhaps the most effective and widely used home treatment for obstructive apnea is an artificial breathing device called a **CPAP machine** (the letters stand for "continuous positive airway pressure"). Consisting of a bedside fan, connecting tube, and nasal mask (*see illustration opposite*), the device blows a steady stream of pressurized air into your nostrils. That helps keep your throat open during sleep. One key drawback is that you'll have to use the device for life: Your apnea will return as soon you stop. Regular CPAP users, however, report feeling much better, mainly because they're less tired and in a better mood during the day. Partners are happy, too, because they get some sleep for a change.

Procedures

Sometimes the CPAP machine, weight loss, or other lifestyle measures don't eliminate the problem. You may be diagnosed with severe sleep apnea or have a cardiac condition or frequent respiratory distress. In such cases, your doctor might recommend surgery.

One of the most widely used procedures for treating apnea is **uvulopalatopharyngoplasty (UPPP).** Despite its name, this is a fairly simple surgery in which tissue is removed from the uvula and other soft palate tissues at the back of your throat, including your tonsils, if you still have them. The goal is to widen your airway and reduce abnormal muscle movements that interfere with your breathing. While the procedure greatly reduces snoring, UPPP eliminates apnea in only about 50% of those who undergo it. A less invasive procedure is **radiofrequency ablation**, in which a surgeon uses radiowaves instead of a scalpel to destroy tissue at the base of your tongue. A number of treatment sessions are required, each taking about 20 minutes, for this procedure to work. Ablation is used only for mild obstructive apnea, but the success rate is high.

For many years, **tracheostomy** was the only treatment for sleep apnea. While nearly 100% successful, the procedure is recommended today only when apnea is life-threatening. It involves opening a permanent, quarter-sized hole in your windpipe and inserting a tube. The tube stays closed during waking hours so you can speak normally. You open it before bedtime, so air flows directly into your lungs, bypassing the obstructed airway.

▶**HEART ATTACK IS A SERIOUS RISK** If you have sleep apnea, but warning signs are easily missed. It's common with apnea to have perfectly normal heartbeats during the day, when most EKGs are performed. But once you're asleep, your heartbeat can slow dramatically during apnea episodes (and in some cases, stop completely for a few seconds). The heart, like any muscle, uses oxygen for fuel. Take away the fuel, and the heart muscle sputters to a halt. The good news is that heart irregularities may disappear for good, once apnea is properly treated.

Better Breathing with Better CPAP Masks

The CPAP machine is effective for treating obstructive sleep apnea, but many people won't use it or stop after a few months (statistics show that one in three users fails to continue). The problem may be that the face mask doesn't fit very well, so it's uncomfortable to wear. There are a number of solutions:

- **Style.** Discuss different headgear styles with your doctor. Experiment until you find a mask that fits properly. The hoses for most machines will fit any style of mask. You can also have a mask custom-fit to your face and head size.
- **Variety.** Buy more than one style of mask and rotate them to prevent skin irritation on

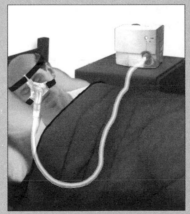

CPAP machine at work

your face. Some chafing can occur if you wear the same mask night after night. Even though some insurance companies won't pay for more than one mask, it may be a worthwhile expense.

- **Materials.** Try one of the newer masks made with gel-like materials. These cause less facial irritation than hard, plastic masks. Transparent masks are also available.
- **Inserts.** If you breathe primarily through your nose, you might be able to use what are called nasal "pillows" (flexible inserts that fit inside your nostrils) instead of a full-face mask.
- **Profile.** If you wear glasses and tend to fall asleep while reading or watching television in bed, consider buying a "low profile" mask that rides lower on your nose and doesn't interfere with your vision. That way you won't forget to put on your mask before falling asleep.

Snore No More: Tips That Work

It's easy to laugh at Dagwood Bumstead's sonorous snores in the comic strip *Blondie*. But snoring—which occurs when the soft tissues of your upper airways vibrate—isn't so funny in real life, especially for unfortunate partners who may find themselves wearing ear plugs or sleeping in another room. When you consider that the loudest recorded snore clocked in at 87 decibels—nearly as loud as a motorcycle—it's easy to see why people are desperate for solutions.

Most of the treatments for apnea—weight loss or CPAP, for example—also work for snoring. Here are some of the best ways to turn down the volume:

● **Stay off your back.** It's estimated that 60% of snorers snore most often when they sleep on their backs.
● **Drop a few pounds.** Obesity is a common cause of snoring. Excess fat accumulates (and then vibrates) in the neck and throat.
● **Add an extra pillow.** Raising your head slightly opens your airways.
● **Use nasal strips.** Sold in pharmacies, the strips (such as Breathe Right) hold your nostrils open and help prevent snoring.
● **Ask about splints.** Doctors sometimes advise snorers to wear a device called a mandibular advancement splint that looks like a mouth guard. It keeps the lower jaw from falling backward during sleep, which in turn stops your tongue from blocking the flow of air. A study in the *American Journal of Respiratory and Critical Care Medicine* reports that patients who used the splints had a 65% decrease in snoring.

Promising
DEVELOPMENTS

■ An experimental drug, dubbed **SR46349B,** may offer hope for treating sleep apnea as well as the subsequent morning-after fatigue. Preliminary studies suggest that the drug reduces snoring and increases the amount of time spent in deep, restorative sleep. It's thought to work by boosting levels of serotonin, a neurotransmitter that ferries brain signals to the throat. There's some evidence that it reduces airway obstructions as well.

FINDING Support

■ For the latest information on sleep apnea, contact the American Sleep Apnea Association (202-293-3650 or www.sleepapnea.org).
■ Another helpful organization is the National Sleep Foundation (202-347-3471 or www.sleepfoundation.org).

Other types of surgery may be required if you have a deformity of your lower jaw or a nasal obstruction such as polyps or a deviated septum (*see page 285*). If you are severely obese, your doctor may recommend gastric banding or bypass surgery to help you lose weight (*see page 240*).

Medications

Only a few drugs relieve apnea symptoms. Some can have serious side effects. Always use such medications under your doctor's supervision.

■ **Protriptyline.** This antidepressant (brand names Triptil, Vivactil) can increase tension in throat tissues and help keep them from sagging when you sleep. It also reduces the amount of rapid-eye movement (REM) sleep—the stage when most apnea episodes occur.
■ **Steroid nasal sprays.** These are typically used for sinusitis, but can help reduce inflammation and congestion that may contribute to apnea.
■ **OTC decongestants.** Good for relieving snoring and minor breathing difficulties due to mucus-clogged sinuses, decongestants (Sudafed, Drixoral) should be used for only a few days at a time. Some brands contain antihistamines, which can have sedating properties, making breathing problems worse.

Natural Methods*

Recently more patients (and sometimes their physicians) have turned to herbs and other alternative treatments for relieving dozens of medical conditions—*but apnea isn't one of them*. The potential health risks from apnea are so serious, in fact, that doctors advise everyone to use only mainstream treatments.

*Natural methods are not subject to the same testing and regulation as prescription medications. Please seek your doctor's advice and use caution.

Strains and sprains

If you are one of the 27,000 Americans who sprains an ankle every day or an over-zealous weekend warrior with a muscle strain, knowing what to do can make all the difference. Home care is the first step, but you may also need to see the doctor.

What is happening

Few injuries are as sudden and painful as a strain or sprain. When a muscle, tendon, or ligament stops functioning normally, you can be sidelined within seconds. A **strain** occurs when you twist or stretch a muscle (often referred to as a "pulled" muscle) or a tendon (the band that connects muscle to bone) beyond its limit. The muscle usually stays intact, although severe injuries can tear it, split it in two or shear it away from its tendon (sometimes the ripping makes a "popping" sound). A strain typically occurs after you lift something heavy the wrong way or overstress your muscles sprinting for a bus, swinging a golf club, or running to catch a Frisbee. Strains affect the muscles in your back, hamstrings (at the back of your thighs), calves, groin, or shoulders. They can also affect a previously injured muscle that has not been properly rehabilitated.

While a mild strain may not hurt much at first, a **sprain** usually causes intense pain right away. It happens when a joint is forced beyond its normal range of motion. One or more ligaments—the strong bands of connective tissue that attach bones at the joint and support them—get overstretched or torn. Sprains are generally caused by a sudden force, usually a falling or twisting motion, or a sharp blow to the body that yanks a joint out of its normal position. Your ankles are particularly vulnerable, though knees and wrists can also be trouble spots.

Treatments

Both strains and sprains are categorized—and treated—according to their severity. "Mild" sprains and muscle strains, which involve minimal pain and swelling and little loss of function, can often be treated at home. A "moderate" strain or sprain, which causes a good deal of pain and swelling and often bruising, should be x-rayed to see how bad the injury is. A "severe" injury, which means you can't move the body part or put weight on it, will probably require stabilization and even surgery if a ligament is torn.

You'll probably feel relief from a mild strain in a day or two. It should heal completely in about a week. A mild sprain can make it painful or impossible to move the joint normally for at least 10 days. For a moderate strain or sprain, three to six weeks of recovery may be required. Severe strains and sprains can take 8 to 12 months to fully heal. Once the swelling and pain

LIKELY **First Steps**

- **Rest, Ice, Compress, and Elevate (RICE)** the injured area.

- **Acetaminophen** for pain, **NSAIDs** (including **COX-2 inhibitors**) if there's swelling.

- **X-ray** for moderate to severe pain, to rule out a bone fracture or other serious problem.

QUESTIONS TO **Ask**

- Why do I need an x-ray?
- Will I recover fully?
- Should I start wearing a brace to protect this joint?
- Is it okay to run even when I'm in pain?

Stress Fractures

These microscopic breaks in a bone, usually in the foot, shin, or thigh, are overuse injuries often mistaken for sprains. The fractures are caused by the repeated impact of running or jumping. The pain is often mild at first, typically a dull ache that occurs during or right after exercise. When you continue the activity, the pain gradually increases. Stress fractures rarely break through the bone, so they don't require splints or casts, just rest.

- **Support yourself right.** If you're using a cane or one crutch for support when you have an ankle or knee injury, hold it on the uninjured side. This prompts you to lean away from—and lessen stress on—the injured side.

- **Follow the up/down laws.** Just like saints and sinners, the good go up and the bad go down. For the best stability when negotiating stairs, start with the uninjured "good" foot when ascending, and the injured "bad" one when descending.

- **Pack in the protein.** If you push yourself physically during a rehabilitation regimen, eat more protein to help repair muscles and ligaments. Choose healthful sources of protein such as poultry (without the skin), fatty fish such as salmon and mackerel (which contain potentially restorative omega-3 fatty acids), and soy foods (soybeans, tofu, soy milk).

- **Fall-proof your life.** Clear clutter from walkways, stairways, the yard and driveway, as well as the path to your bathroom (so you won't trip at night). In winter, salt icy walkways. Take your time getting out of taxis and crossing streets to avoid stumbling and tripping.

- **Stick to the 10% rule.** To prevent future muscle strains, regulate your activity level by following this golden rule: Don't increase your workout—whether it's adding mileage to a run or increasing the number of reps in the weight room—by more than 10% a week.

Treatment options

Lifestyle changes	
RICE method	Rest, Ice, Compression, Elevation early on.
Heat	Pads, packs, or baths, once swelling subsides.
Medications	
Painkillers	OTC or prescription, depending on severity.
Muscle relaxant	For spasms related to injury.
Corticosteroid injection	To reduce swelling in severe injuries.
Procedures	
Cast	Immobilizes injury to promote healing.
Surgery	For severe tears and other extreme injuries.
Natural methods	
Capsaicin cream	For relief of pain in mild strains and sprains.
Arnica/bromelain	To lessen pain and swelling.

subside, start some gentle stretching and strengthening exercises (*see box, page 299*), and make an appointment with a physical therapist (PT).

Lifestyle Changes

If your sprain or strain isn't severe, **rest, ice, compression**, and **elevation** (just remember the acronym **RICE**) are key for reducing swelling, slowing any internal bleeding, and reducing pain.

- **Rest.** For a day or two after the injury, avoid any activity that causes pain (and definitely stay away from sports). If you have an ankle or leg injury and must move around, use crutches, a sling, splint, brace, or other type of support to keep from reinjuring yourself. There are many products available; ask your doctor which is best for you.

- **Ice.** Just as important as resting is icing the area during the first 12 to 48 hours. This can blunt pain, lessen swelling, and speed healing in several ways. Cold tightens up (constricts) the blood vessels and limits the amount of blood and other fluids that can flood the injured area. Lowering the temperature of the skin over the affected area also calms any muscle spasms that might develop. Apply the ice for 10 minutes every two to three hours while you're awake. One way to do this is to put chipped or crushed ice in a heavy plastic bag, or wrap it in a towel and then run it gently over the injured area. A cooled gel pack also works, or in a pinch, a bag of frozen peas. All these conform to your body contours better than ice cubes. Immersing the injured area in ice water for a short time can also bring relief. While cooling is key, applying ice for too long (more than 10 minutes) can actually increase damage to your injury by lowering your skin temperature too far: At around 59°F, blood vessels start to widen rather than constrict. If the skin becomes red, hot, painful, or itchy, you'll know you've iced too long. Your skin should return to normal in four to eight minutes after you remove the ice.

- **Compression.** To protect the injured area and minimize swelling, ask your doctor about using an elastic wrap, air cast, splint, or specially designed boot. If the compression is too tight, it won't work.
- **Elevate.** Raise the injured area above heart level as often as possible. This allows gravity to draw blood and other fluids that can cause swelling away from the injury. It may take a couple of days before you see results, however. If you've sprained your ankle, prop your foot way up—toes above your nose.

Once the swelling has subsided, try **heat.** Use a hot compress or a heating pad, or take a hot bath or shower to increase blood circulation. If the swelling starts again, stop heat treatments and return to cold.

Medications

For moderate pain from a strain or sprain, try **acetaminophen** (Tylenol, Panadol), which is relatively gentle on the stomach. Because acetaminophen won't do anything for inflammation, it's not a good choice if you have swelling. For swelling (as well as pain) try a **nonsteroidal anti-inflammatory drug (NSAID),** such as ibuprofen (Advil, Nuprin), naproxen (Aleve), or aspirin. These OTC drugs don't promote healing and shouldn't be taken long term without checking with your doctor.

Sometimes OTC medications aren't enough. For a debilitating back strain, ask your doctor about a strong **prescription pain medication,** such as tramadol (Ultram), hydrocodone bitrate/acetaminophen (Vicodin), or the COX-2 inhibitor Celebrex. Adding a **prescription muscle relaxant,** such as cyclobenzaprine (Flexeril), can dramatically ease discomfort by stopping spasms. Most prescription painkillers and muscle relaxants should be used for a few weeks at most. If your injury is severe, a **corticosteroid injection** in the injured joint or the surrounding tissue may reduce pain and inflammation. Such injections aren't widely used for mild strains and sprains because they can delay healing. Relief might tempt you to use the injured joint before it's fully healed, making the situation worse.

Procedures

If you have a severe strain or sprain, your family doctor or a bone specialist (orthopedist) might treat it as if it were a fracture, applying a plastic or plaster **cast** for several weeks to immobilize the area and speed healing. **Surgery** is rarely needed for strains and sprains, but a ruptured ligament or a severe fracture (often mistaken for a sprain) does require surgery.

Make this Injury Your Last

Here are a few exercise pointers that can help lower your risk for future strains and sprains:

- Keep your weight down.
- Always warm up before exercising by riding a stationary bike or jogging in place for 5 to 10 minutes; warm muscles are less likely to tear. Do a few warm-up stretches, too, holding each one for between 10 and 30 seconds.
- Don't play sports when you're overtired or in pain.
- Be sure to wear properly fitted running shoes. Run on level surfaces.
- Apply ice post-exercise to minimize tissue irritation.
- Avoid re-injury by using a support, such as a brace or elastic bandage, on the weakened joint. Recent findings show that ankle bracing works better than taping the ankle.

▶ **How soon can I start playing sports again after an ankle sprain?**
Not until the joint has recovered its full range of motion. At that point, you'll have strength in all the surrounding muscles, your balance will be good, and you shouldn't experience pain or swelling when you play. Test your sports readiness with "the hop barometer": If you can't hop on the injured ankle three or four times without pain, you're not ready to get back in the game.

Promising
DEVELOPMENTS

■ Some doctors specializing in soft tissue injuries are experimenting with **prolotherapy,** also known as nonsurgical ligament reconstruction. A sugar water (dextrose) solution is injected into the area where an injured ligament or tendon attaches to the bone. This causes localized inflammation, which stimulates the flow of tissue-repairing blood and nutrients to the injury site. Although responses to prolotherapy vary, many people see results in four to six treatments.

▶ **TAKE CARE WITH COMMERCIAL ICE PACKS. Refreezable gel packs or self-freezing chemical packs get colder than regular ice. Move the pack around to prevent overexposure to the injured area (or wrap the pack in a thin towel). Throw the pack away if any holes develop; the chemicals can burn your skin.**

FINDING Support

■ To find out more about treating strains or sprains, or to find an orthopedic surgeon in your area, contact the American Academy of Orthopaedic Surgeons (1-800-346-2267 or www.aaos.org).

■ For more information on prolotherapy, check out the website www.prolotherapy.com.

About Tendinitis

Inflammation of a tendon, one of the fibrous cords that join muscle to bone, is called tendinitis. The injury is due to overuse from prolonged, repetitive movements, which irritate the tendon and make it swell. Common trouble spots are the elbows (tennis or golfer's elbow), shoulders, wrists, ankles (specifically, the Achilles tendon at the back of the ankle), and fingers (called trigger finger).

Treatment for tendinitis is similar to that for strains and sprains: Rest, ice, compression, and elevation, along with NSAIDs, followed by rehabilitation exercises (*see box opposite*). With tendinitis, it's especially important to resume activity gradually, incorporating gentle heat and stretching beforehand, and applying ice packs afterward. Most cases don't last more than two weeks. Repeated use of the injured tendon may lead to chronic tendinitis, characterized by scarring of the involved tissues and limited flexibility. Once the pain is gone, lift weights (very light ones at first) to strengthen the muscles around the tendon. The stronger the muscles, the less stress on the tendon. If inflammation persists, you might need a corticosteroid shot, or surgery if the tendon is torn.

Whatever the extent of your injury, most doctors recommend a regimen of **rehabilitative therapy** once the initial pain and swelling subside. This will strengthen muscles and tendons and prevent future injuries (the biggest risk for ankle sprain is having had one already). While you can do exercises on your own (*see box opposite*), you may prefer to work with a physical therapist, who can offer a range of rehabilitative techniques, including heat, electrical stimulation, ultrasound, and massage.

Natural Methods*

Many people swear by the cream form of **capsaicin,** derived from chili peppers, for relieving pain of mild strains and sprains. Capsaicin works by depleting the body's supply of substance P, a chemical component of nerve cells that normally transmits pain signals to the brain. Purchase a commercial product (sometimes called cayenne cream), and apply it three or four times a day for a few days after you're injured. **Arnica,** made from dried flower heads, is available as an oil, gel, or cream and can be gently rubbed into your swollen ankle or painful muscle. Use it externally in moderate amounts, but don't apply it to broken skin. **Bromelain,** a digestive enzyme derived from the pineapple plant, has a reputation for reducing swelling, bruising, and pain. Some studies indicate that it's as effective as NSAIDs. Take 500 mg three times a day between meals until you feel better.

*Natural methods are not subject to the same testing and regulation as prescription medications. Please seek your doctor's advice and use caution.

Exercises for Strains, Sprains, and Tendinitis

Exercises are key to treating strains and sprains and preventing future injuries. Once the swelling subsides and the pain isn't acute, several weeks of rehabilitation may be needed—possibly longer if your injury is severe. Don't resume preinjury activities until your doctor or a physical therapist (PT) gives you the green light. Starting too soon can lead to re-injury or chronic problems. The exercises that follow are for ankle sprains, hamstring strains, and a couple of forms of tendinitis. Ask your doctor or a PT about exercises for other injuries.

For hamstring strains

Start with the **standing stretch.** Place the heel of your injured leg on a fat book. Bend at the waist, and lean forward until you feel the stretch in your hamstring. Don't force it; stretch gradually.

After warming up your muscle, you can advance to a **prone knee bend.** Lie on your stomach with your legs straight behind you. Pull the heel of

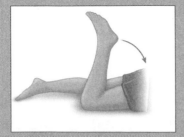

Prone knee bend

your injured leg toward your buttocks (using your hand to help, if necessary); hold this position briefly, then slowly release the leg down to the floor. Work up to three sets of 10 knee bends each.

For ankle sprains

For a sprained ankle, rehab can begin when swelling starts to subside, and you can tolerate pressure on the ball of your foot. Before beginning any exercise, warm the ankle by soaking it in warm water (this makes the joint more flexible).

Start with the **towel stretch:** Sitting with your injured leg out in front of you, draw a towel around the ball of your foot. Keeping your knee straight, pull the towel toward your body until you feel a gentle stretch in your calf. Hold 30 seconds. Relax. Repeat 3 times.

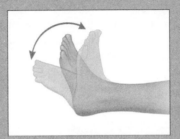

Alphabet range of motion

Once the swelling has gone down, try the **alphabet range-of-motion exercise.** Sit on the floor with your legs extended. Using the big toe of your injured leg as a pointer, trace the capital letters of the alphabet from A to Z (hold your big toe rigid to ensure that the motion comes from your ankle). Repeat once every hour while you're awake. You can also do this exercise while lying in bed with your foot propped on a pillow.

For tendinitis

For achilles tendinitis: Hamstring strains and Achilles tendinitis often go hand in hand. To stretch your Achilles tendon (the rope-like tendon that connects the calf mus-

cles to the heel), start with the towel stretch described under Ankle Sprains. When this exercise becomes too easy, try the **plantar fascia stretch:** Place the balls of your feet on the front edge of the first stair of a low staircase or on a fat book, toeing in

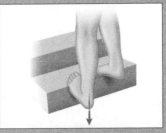

Plantar fascia stretch

slightly. Reach for the floor with the heel of your injured leg. Once you feel a stretch in your arch, stop. Hold the position for 30 seconds. Relax and repeat 3 times.

For tennis elbow: This injury, which can as easily result from housework as tennis, causes pain in the forearm.

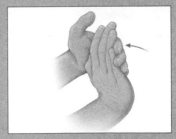

Wrist flexor stretch

Try the **wrist flexor stretch:** Extend your injured arm, with elbow straight and palm down. With the other hand, grasp the palm and fingers of the extended hand and pull back until you feel a stretch in your forearm. Do this 10 times, holding the position 3 to 5 seconds each time.

Stroke

Although stroke remains the third leading cause of death in the United States, many promising new drugs, devices, and therapies are being developed to boost survival rates and improve the quality of life for those who experience one.

LIKELY **First Steps**

- At the first signs of a stroke, **call 911,** or go to **an emergency room** right away.

- For a clot-related stroke, **medication** to dissolve the clot.

- Once stabilized, close **monitoring** in an intensive care unit for 24 to 48 hours.

- Post-stroke **rehabilitation** (physical, occupational, speech) to restore lost functions.

QUESTIONS TO **Ask**

- Will I ever be the same person again?

- Is there someone who can help make my home more "stroke friendly" after I get out of the hospital?

- Will I be able to return to work after my stroke?

- Do I have to worry about having another stroke when I have sex?

- After I recover, can I be tested to see if I can drive safely?

What is happening

A stroke occurs when oxygen-rich blood is suddenly unavailable to your brain. It's so much like when the heart is deprived of blood during a heart attack, a stroke is often called a "brain attack." Blockages, usually clots, inside tiny arteries in the brain cause **ischemic strokes.** A clot that forms in or near the brain in an artery narrowed by the buildup of cholesterol and other fatty substances is known as a **cerebral thrombosis.** One that forms in another part of the body, travels to the brain, and gets lodged there is known as a **cerebral embolism.** Ischemic strokes are treated very differently than **hemorrhagic strokes,** in which a vessel bursts, allowing blood to seep into the brain. While they are often more deadly, hemorrhagic strokes are far less common (*see page 302 for illustrations of all three types*).

Whatever the cause, when stroke cuts off blood supply, brain cells die. Parts of the body controlled by the affected part of the brain no longer function. This is often temporary, but can be permanent. Common results of a serious stroke include weakness, paralysis, numbness, problems with understanding and speech, and emotional difficulties. Because such damage can cause major disabilities, just getting through the day can become challenging. Strokes tend to affect only one side of the brain. If it's the side that controls speech, your ability to speak may be imperiled, even though your thoughts and emotions remain intact. If the stroke occurs in the part of your brain that controls movement, muscle activity on the other side of your body may suffer.

Treatments

Brain cells perish quickly when deprived of oxygen-rich blood. Irreversible damage can occur in as little as 30 minutes, so urgent treatment is essential when you (or someone else) appear to be having a stroke. The most effective treatments need to be started right away, ideally within the first few hours. Once you're at the hospital, doctors will determine if the stroke is ischemic or hemorrhagic and begin the appropriate treatment. A neurological exam, blood tests, CT and MRI scans, Doppler ultrasound, and arteriography can help distinguish one type of stroke from the other. If the stroke is ischemic, you'll get a drug to dissolve the clot and literally stop the stroke. If it's hemorrhagic, doctors will first try to lower your blood pressure to minimize bleeding. Then they may perform surgery (*see box, page 303*).

Treatment options

Medications	
Thrombolytics	First-line clot-busters, given at hospital.
Antiplatelets	Aspirin is a top choice to prevent future clots.
Thienopyridine	Ticlid or Plavix (if you can't take aspirin).
Specialized drugs	Antidepressants, stimulants, relaxants, Parlodel.

Procedures	
Physical therapies	Start PT and OT early to regain muscle control.
NDT	Enhances nerve function on damaged side.
Movement therapy	Improves limb mobility.
Speech therapy	Helps in forming words and sentences.
Endarterectomy	Cleans blocked artery to prevent future stroke.
Bypass (EC-IC)	Scalp artery rerouted; mixed results.

After the stroke, if you've had considerable brain damage, you'll have to stay in an intensive care unit so the functions of your brain, heart, and other organs can be monitored until your condition stabilizes. Life-support machines will supply oxygen, medicines, and nutrition. If your stroke caused relatively little brain damage, you might be able to go home in just a few days. However, you'll probably need daily rehab therapy in the hospital or a special stroke center. Recouping lost functions is one goal. Preventing a second stroke is another. Initially, the most dramatic improvements will occur after physical, occupational, or speech therapy. Disabilities lingering beyond a few months are harder to fix.

Medications

If you get to a hospital at the first signs of an ischemic stroke, you may be given powerful clot-busters called **thrombolytics**—the only drug therapy approved for an ongoing stroke. Thrombolytics dissolve existing clots, open blocked arteries, and restore blood flow to the brain. The main thrombolytic medication is called tissue plasminogen activator (tPA), though others are used and several are under investigation. If you arrive within three hours of the start of stroke symptoms, you'll get thrombolytics through a vein. Within six hours, they may be infused directly into a brain artery. In experienced hands, thrombolytics can dramatically reduce risk of permanent disability from a stroke. Thrombolytics affect blood clotting, so they also increase your risk of bleeding—which in itself can be dangerous. The bottom line is that most people get to the hospital too late for thrombolytic therapy. Only 2% of stroke victims ever receive tPA.

TAKING **Control**

- **Inspect your local hospital.** If you've had a stroke, you're at high risk for another. Familiarize yourself with services nearby. Does your hospital have a 24-hour stroke team? A stroke expert?

- **Make your family stroke savvy.** Do they know the major signs of stroke and when to call 911? Key alerts: one-sided weakness or numbness, vision loss, sudden balance problems, difficulty speaking or understanding, severe headache.

- **Review the rehab team's resume.** You want pros with extensive experience in treating strokes—as well as a hefty dose of patience and perseverance. An inspiring cheerleading squad is key.

- **Do a medications check.** Certain drugs can interfere with your recovery. Take all your medicine bottles to the doctor for review. Common culprits: anticonvulsants, antipsychotics, antianxiety medications, and blood pressure drugs.

- **Try biofeedback.** Physical therapy combined with biofeedback techniques has helped some stroke sufferers re-orient themselves to body sensations. If you have difficulty swallowing, for example, biofeedback training of key muscles may accelerate your ability to relearn this action. Working with the wrists and fingers shows similar promise.

- **Seek support** from family, friends, or an outside group. A stroke generates unique stresses, from dependence on others to mood changes. Don't try to deal with these problems alone.

Promising
DEVELOPMENTS

■ Surgeons are testing **mechanical devices** to open blocked brain arteries faster than clot-busting drugs. They're testing saline jets, ultrasound, laser energy, and snares and baskets to disrupt and dissolve clots.

■ Much brain damage caused by stroke is due to harmful chemicals which are released by dying brain cells and poison nearby tissues. So-called **neuroprotective agents,** designed to stop cells from self-destructing, stop the chain reaction by blocking certain brain chemical receptors.

■ Scientists have identified a new marker for increased stroke risk: **C-reactive protein (CRP).** This chemical indicates underlying inflammation. Measuring it may soon be part of basic blood tests. Drugs and healthy living can lower your CRP level.

If you're among the majority of stroke patients not receiving thrombolytics, you'll be started on an **antiplatelet drug** to prevent another clot from developing. **Aspirin** is a top choice. You're far less likely to die or suffer a disability if you start aspirin therapy within 48 hours of an ischemic stroke. Aspirin affects the blood's ability to form a clot, and this has two very positive benefits: Aspirin will make your current stroke less severe and will reduce your chances of developing another. If you've had a hemorrhagic stroke, take aspirin only on a doctor's recommendation.

Your doctor may recommend a drug that combines aspirin with another antiplatelet agent called **dipyridamole.** Named Aggrenox, the blend is more effective than aspirin alone for preventing a second stroke, especially if you're at high risk. While relatively safe, it's more costly than aspirin. Also slightly more protective against stroke than aspirin alone (and also somewhat costly) are **thienopyridine** drugs such as Ticlid and Plavix. If you don't respond to aspirin or can't tolerate it, antiplatelet medications might be recommended. The potent anticlotting drug warfarin (Coumadin) is sometimes prescribed, but bleeding risk is high.

Following a stroke, you may also need other medications to treat various complications. Depression is very common, and **antidepressants,** such as Prozac, Pamelor, and Elavil, can really be of benefit. They also help ease any crying episodes and increase your mental sharpness. A **brain stimulant** such as Ritalin may boost speech and motor skills when combined with physical therapy. The **muscle relaxant** baclofen can help with painful muscle spasms. When speech difficulties occur, **Parlodel,** a drug used for Parkinson's disease, can enhance the formation of sentences and multisyllable words.

DIFFERENT TYPES OF STROKE

1) Ischemic: Cerebral thrombosis

Area deprived of blood

Thrombus-blocked artery

2) Ischemic: Cerebral embolism

Area deprived of blood

Embolus-blocked artery

3) Hemorrhagic

Area of bleeding

Ruptured artery

A stroke happens in one of three ways. **1)** A thrombus (clot) can build up on a brain artery wall, causing a cerebral thrombosis. **2)** An embolus (usually a clot) can make its way to a brain artery and impede the blood flow, causing a cerebral embolism. **3)** A blood vessel within or on the surface of the brain can leak or rupture, causing a hemorrhagic stroke.

Hemorrhagic Stroke

The treatment for hemorrhagic stroke is similar to that for ischemic stroke, with two important differences. Anticoagulants and clot-busters aren't given with a hemorrhagic stroke, because they could worsen bleeding in the brain. Instead, medications focus on lowering blood pressure and minimizing blood flow from the ruptured artery. Second, surgery may be needed to remove accumulated blood and relieve pressure. (The skull allows little room for tissue to expand, so bleeding quickly raises pressure in a dangerous way.) Surgeons may remove blood clots in the damaged area. While surgery may save your life, it may leave you with severe neurological problems.

A common problem with hemorrhagic stroke is that blood vessels near the bleed can spasm and contract. This blocks oxygen to the brain, increasing potential stroke damage. To prevent this, your doctor may use a **calcium channel blocker** to relax the blood vessels. A novel means of administering the calcium channel blocker drug Cardene involves surgically placing 2 to 10 tiny drug pellets parallel to the affected artery and next to any blood clots. The journal *Stroke* reported in 2002 that doing this can virtually eliminate vessel spasms and their consequences.

Procedures

With speedy drug treatment, there's a good chance that problems such as numbness, weakness, and difficulties with speech, vision, and swallowing will improve on their own over the following weeks. Your powerful brain will also reassign tasks previously performed by non-damaged parts, but months of therapy may await you. Strokes are very individual, affecting different areas of each person's brain, so what you'll want from rehabilitation may be very different from someone else's needs. You may have to learn how to strengthen an arm and hand, while someone else may require speech therapy or help with swallowing. One or more of the following therapies may be right for you:

- **Physical therapy (PT).** It's best to start intensive rehabilitation as soon as your blood pressure, pulse, and breathing have stabilized— as early as two days post-stroke, if possible. The aim is to keep your muscles strong and prevent them from stiffening and developing tight contractions. Passive movements initiated by the therapist eventually give way to more active exercises on your part. Moving around may also prevent painful pressure sores.
- **Neurodevelopmental treatment (NDT).** Rehabilitation methods once taught people to compensate for lost function by working with their unaffected side and adding canes, braces, and walkers for support. Introduced by the British in the 1970s, NDT concentrates on enhancing residual function in nerves and muscles on the stroke-damaged side of the body.

▶**The stroke has made me wobbly. If I fall, will my brittle bones give way?**
You're right to be concerned about falling. Talk with your doctor about taking bisphosphonate drugs such as Fosamax, which increase bone density (and strength) and reduce the odds of fracture if you do fall. Physical therapy and aids around the house can help prevent treacherous spills during the post-stroke period.

▶**What about natural treatments*? Will they help?**
Acupuncture on scalp points that relate to the central nervous system seems to help damaged (but not destroyed) brain cells perk up and get back to work. When points on affected hands and feet are stimulated, acupuncture may jump-start lost sensation and motion. It can also relieve pain and stiffness of spastic muscles. The Feldenkrais method of "body education" for "relearning" movements helps with loss of nerve and muscle function or poor joint movement and balance. Hands-on therapies like Rolfing, and myotherapy can release muscle and nerve tension.

*Natural methods are not subject to the same testing and regulation as prescription medications. Please seek your doctor's advice and use caution.

▶**A PRE-STROKE WARNING. Brief episodes that result in temporary (24-hour) loss of function aren't true strokes. They're called transient ischemic attacks (TIAs) and often signal an impending stroke. One in five people who has a TIA will have a stroke within 12 months.**

Sidestep a Second Stroke

Once you've had a stroke, you're at high risk for another. Preventing recurrence is crucial. There's a lot you can do to increase your odds of a stroke-free future.

- **Stop smoking.** It nearly doubles your risk for stroke.
- **Get exercise.** Physicians encourage aerobic exercise three to seven days a week.
- **Watch your weight.** The less you weigh, the less pressure on the heart and vessels.
- **Know your blood pressure.** Check it regularly, and religiously take prescribed medicines for lowering it; hypertension ups stroke risk four- to sixfold.
- **Limit alcohol intake** to no more than seven drinks a week, no more than 1–2 per day.
- **Control stress** through exercise, yoga, or any other means that works for you.
- **Eat your way to health.** Flexible blood vessels, good circulation, and lower blood pressure are a few stroke-repairing benefits of eating nutritiously. Focus on citrus fruits, dietary fiber, crucifer-ous vegetables (broccoli, cabbage), calcium-rich dairy products, and fatty fish (salmon and tuna). Four ounces of fatty fish, two to four times a week reduces your risk for a clot-related stroke.
- **Control heart disease or high cholesterol.** Stick closely to your medication and treatment plan. Atrial fibrillation is a stroke risk factor requiring anticoagulants. High cholesterol leads to hardening of the arteries.

▶**DEMENTIA FOLLOWING A STROKE is often attributed to brain damage when depression may be to blame. Antidepressant medications and psychotherapy often can ease these problems.**

▶**FDA WILL BE REVIEWING carotid stents to open clogged carotid arteries. Patients at high risk of surgical complications would be good candidates for these less invasive devices.**

FINDING Support

- The National Stroke Association, located in Englewood, CO, has the latest information on treatment and prevention (1-800-787-6537 or www.stroke.org).

- For information on rehabilitation and products that can help you with a disability, contact the National Rehabilitation Information Center in Lanham, MD (1-800-346-2742 or www.naric.com). For more on specialized products to help with post-stroke daily living go to www.dynamic-living.com.

- **Constraint-induced movement therapy.** Researchers are finding this approach can help retrieve a person's ability to move a limb, even years after a stroke. In one study, stroke victims with right-side paralysis had their nonparalyzed arm immobilized, forcing them to use the paralyzed one. Most (11 of 13) participants experienced real improvement in their impaired arms, making daily basics such as brushing teeth and combing hair possible again.
- **Occupational therapy (OT).** During these sessions, the therapist helps you retrain your brain to control certain small muscle groups so you can resume daily basics (swallowing, using the toilet, cooking, writing). This helps not only your motor skills but also your independence and morale.
- **Speech therapy.** When you're having trouble forming words and sentences, but the thoughts are right there in your head, dramatic results can be realized with speech therapy. Pantomime, sign language, and pen and paper can also help get your point across.

Once you've had a stroke, there's little a surgeon can do. Brain tissue has died; even if a clot is removed, restored blood flow can't bring it back to life. There are times when surgery makes sense. If you've had a cerebral thrombosis (or a prestroke TIA) caused by an internal carotid artery blockage (responsible for about 9% of strokes), a **carotid endarterectomy** to clean out this large artery in the neck can reduce risk of a future stroke. It's commonly done if the artery is more than 70% blocked.

Mixed results have been had with a decades-old procedure called **extracranial-intracranial bypass (EC-IC),** in which surgeons reroute a healthy scalp artery to an area that was deprived of blood because of an artery blockage. There's hope that with new imaging techniques and refinements in surgery, this type of bypass will become safer and more effective. **Carotid angioplasty,** based on the same principles as angiography for heart disease, is being investigated as an EC-IC alternative.

Temporomandibular joints

Also known as TMD (or TMJ), this baffling and painful condition makes the hinges of your jaw ache, often when you wake up and when you chew or yawn. Sensible lifestyle changes are your best bet for easing the discomfort.

What is happening

Temporomandibular joint disorder (TMD) is a common, often mysterious affliction of the joints that connect your jaw to either side of your head just in front of your ears. By touching these spots as you open your mouth, you can feel the joints move. If you suffer from TMD, however, you don't have to use your fingers to find the spots: Pain will probably do it for you. You may also feel pain in your ears, neck, or shoulders, especially when you chew or yawn. Because the joints are so close to your ears, you might hear odd popping, crackling, or grating noises when your jaw moves. In more severe cases, you may even feel as if your jaw is unhinged, your upper and lower teeth are out of alignment, or your mouth won't open.

No matter how severe your symptoms are, don't panic. TMD is frequently a temporary problem that resolves itself over time. Unless your jaw pain is a rare case caused by arthritis, an anatomical problem, derangement of the bones due to disease or injury, or a birth abnormality, your symptoms are simply telling you that the muscles around your joints are tight and inflamed.

No one has discovered the underlying causes of temporomandibular joint inflammation, but its triggers are well known. These include emotional stress, a recent injury to the jaw, and bad postural habits, such as holding the handset between the side of your head and your shoulder when you talk on the phone or thrusting your chin forward when you work at a computer. You're also more likely to develop TMD if you grind your teeth when you sleep (*see box, page 306*) or if your teeth don't come together properly when you bite down, which dentists call a malocclusion. Even chewing tough foods like beef jerky or dried apricots can contribute. If you're female, you're at greater risk: Three times as many women as men complain about TMD symptoms to their doctors or dentists. Hormones may play some role in the disorder.

Treatments

When treating TMD, it's important to be *conservative*. Start with lifestyle changes that give your jaw a rest, and if needed, add OTC painkillers to reduce pain and inflammation. If your symptoms persist, prescription painkillers, muscle relaxants, or a mouth guard that keeps you from grinding your teeth can be useful. Only in severe cases should surgery be considered. If you're seeing a doctor who wants to operate, get a second opinion.

LIKELY First Steps

- **Resting the jaw** (soft foods, no gum chewing).
- **Heat or cold** to ease stress and discomfort.
- **Aspirin, ibuprofen, or naproxen** to reduce pain and muscle inflammation.
- **A visit to a dentist or doctor** for an evaluation if self-care measures don't work.

QUESTIONS TO Ask

- How long does an episode of TMD usually last?
- Does having one episode mean that I'll be more susceptible to TMD in the future?
- If my condition is due to stress, does that mean the pain is all in my mind?
- Could my TMD be due to arthritis or some other disease?

TAKING Control

- **Stop gnawing.** If you routinely bite your fingernails or chew on pencils, here's a good reason to drop a bad habit: Giving your mouth a rest is the best way to give TMD the boot.

- **Dispense with your pillow.** Until your jaw feels better, try sleeping on your back or on your side without a pillow. This will distribute your body weight more evenly.

- **Go to a pain clinic** if you don't get relief with self-help measures or medical treatments that your doctor or dentist recommends. Pain clinics, usually associated with hospitals or universities, are also a good source for second opinions for TMD treatments.

Not the Same Old Grind

Bruxism—grinding your teeth while you sleep—can contribute to TMD. Mainly it causes a host of other problems, including premature loss of your teeth, disrupted sleep, snoring, and potentially dangerous breathing pauses (sleep apnea). Tooth grinding occurs most often in the 19- to 44-year-old group and improves with age. Its cause is a mystery, but using alcohol, tobacco, or caffeine can be a trigger in some people, as can aggravation, stress, and anxiety. If you have this problem, psychotherapy and stress-reduction techniques like yoga, meditation, and moderate exercise may help.

Treatment options

Lifestyle changes

Soft foods	Less taxing for your jaw to chew.
Heat or cold	Applications reduce pain.
Stress reduction	Helps relax muscles in the jaw.
Correct posture	Alignment of head and neck relieves TMD.

Medications

OTC painkillers	NSAIDs ease pain and inflammation.
Prescription drugs	For severe and persistent TMD.

Procedures

Mouth guard	Prevents tooth grinding at night.

Natural methods

Alternative therapies	For body and mind; glucosamine for pain.

Lifestyle Changes

The first and best approach for easing the discomfort of TMD is to make simple changes in your day-to-day life. You may be surprised at how quickly your jaw responds. Here are a few things to try:

- **Eat soft foods until the pain goes away.** Stick with a "chewless" diet—mashed potatoes, scrambled eggs, yogurt. If you must eat meat or produce, run them through a blender. Don't eat anything that's bigger than bite-sized.

- **Apply heat or cold.** Both are equally helpful for reducing TMD pain and can be used interchangeably. A warm, moist compress is very effective, or try rubbing your jaw joint with a rough towel to bring blood flow to the area. An ice bag can do the trick as well.

- **Try not to yawn or chew gum.** Your jaw needs to rest. That means keeping your mouth closed and still. You might not even want to talk much until your symptoms start to go away.

- **Reduce stress.** Practice yoga, meditate, see a therapist, or do aerobics—anything that lessens the tooth grinding and jaw clenching you unconsciously do when you're sleeping.

- **Align your spine.** Although your jaw joint may hurt, your problem may start in your shoulders or neck. Correcting your posture can make a dramatic difference in the way you feel. Don't crane forward when you read, and don't carry shoulder bags that feel unusually heavy.

Medications

Drugs don't cure TMD but can sometimes help relieve its symptoms. If you're in pain, try OTC medications such as **acetaminophen** (Tylenol), or **NSAIDs** (nonsteroidal anti-inflammatory drugs), such as aspirin, ibuprofen, or naproxen, which reduce pain

Exercise Your Jaw—Gently

While certain doctors feel that rest, not exercise, is best for the jaw joint, there is evidence to show mild stretching can help alleviate pain. If any of these movements make your condition worse, stop immediately. Try 10 repetitions of each exercise:

1. Place one or two fingers on your lower front teeth and gently press down until your mouth is opened as wide as it can be without pain.

2. Place a palm or fist under your chin for a little resistance as you try to open your mouth.

3. Open your jaw slightly. Move it as far to the right as you comfortably can, then move it the same way to the left.

4. Open your jaw in front of a mirror, as wide as you comfortably can. Watch to make sure your descending chin remains centered relative to your face.

5. Turn your head as far as you can to the left, then the right.

6. Roll your head gently in a circle, right to left, left to right.

7. Tilt your head sideways, as if trying to touch your shoulder with your ear. Do this on both sides. Be careful not to inadvertently raise your shoulder instead of lowering your head.

---

and inflammation. If these aren't strong enough, ask your doctor about prescription NSAIDs, such as the **COX-2 inhibitors** celecoxib (Celebrex) or rofecoxib (Vioxx). A mild prescription muscle relaxant such as **diazepam** (Valium) may help. If your pain persists for more than six months, your doctor may prescribe a **tricyclic antidepressant,** such as amitriptyline (Elavil), which in very small doses can relieve muscle tightness and pain. Researchers are looking into the efficacy of injecting anesthetics into painful areas. Occasionally, a **corticosteroid** such as cortisone or prednisone can help, but should be used only if your TMD is related to rheumatoid arthritis.

Procedures

If you grind or clench your teeth as you sleep, you may get relief with a **mouth guard**. This plastic oral appliance, also called a splint or bite plate, fits over the upper or lower teeth to keep you from grinding. The FDA has approved a new appliance called an **NTI device.** For the two front teeth only, it's much less cumbersome than the old splint. Unless you need to set a broken jawbone, remove diseased tissue, or correct a dislocation in the joint, **avoid surgery.** Artificial jaw joint implants have proven especially dangerous. Some have been recalled because they break down and damage surrounding bone.

Natural Methods*

Chiropractic care can help if spinal misalignment is contributing to TMD. **Acupuncture** shows promise, and **biofeedback** is a standard therapy. Studies show that up to 70% of patients who are trained in biofeedback as part of their therapy will get rid of their TMD for good. A Canadian study also showed that 7 of 10 patients who used **glucosamine sulfate** (500 mg twice a day) had about a 40% reduction in pain.

Natural methods are not subject to the same testing and regulation as prescription medications. Please seek your doctor's advice and use caution.

▶ **Will my TMD go away if my bite is corrected?**
Some health-care professionals commonly recommend treating TMD with braces, crowns, and bridges to change and balance the bite. Or they may suggest grinding down your teeth to adjust your bite (called occlusal adjustment). For most people, these have little or no value, and they can have irreversible effects that you may not want. If your doctor or dentist recommends one of these procedures, get a second opinion before you make a decision.

FINDING Support

■ To find a specialist who can help with your problem, contact the American Dental Association in Chicago, IL (312-440-2500 or www.ada.org).

■ For up-to-the-minute information about TMD, get in touch with the National Institute of Dental and Craniofacial Research in Bethesda, MD (301-496-4261 or www.nidcr.nih.gov).

Thyroid disorders

Found in one in 20 Americans (nearly 13 million people), thyroid disorders affect the body's metabolism. When hormones produced by the thyroid gland get out of whack, a range of problems—from sluggishness to sleeplessness—can result.

LIKELY **First Steps**

- **Thyroid replacement hormone** in the form of daily oral tablets.
- **Period of adjustment** to fine-tune the dosage.
- **Regular checkups and blood tests** to monitor the gland and hormone levels.

QUESTIONS TO **Ask**

- Will I have to take medicines for the rest of my life?
- Is it worth trying natural thyroid hormone instead of the synthetic form?

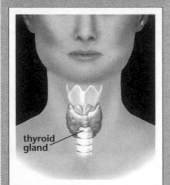

THYROID GLAND

The butterfly-shaped thyroid gland produces hormones essential for the proper maintenance and functioning of body cells. If the gland releases too much hormone, the body will speed up (hyperthyroidism); too little, and it will slow way down (hypothyroidism).

What is happening

Although small (only two inches across), the butterfly-shaped thyroid gland plays a huge role in controlling your body's basic metabolic rate, the speed at which essential chemical functions take place in your cells. The thyroid does this by secreting hormones that stimulate your tissues into using more oxygen, producing more protein, and generally working harder. If anything goes awry with this vital, double-lobed gland at the base of your throat (*see illustration below*), the resulting havoc is felt throughout your body.

Sometimes the gland puts out too much hormone, making all your systems rev up into overdrive. This disorder is known as hyperthyroidism (*see box, page 310*). More common, however, is its polar opposite, hypothyroidism, which occurs when the gland releases too little thyroid hormone. Because this natural chemical affects every system in your body, when there's not enough of it, everything s-l-o-w-s d-o-w-n. The predominant symptom, not surprisingly, is a sense of mental and physical sluggishness. Muscle aches, constipation, weight gain, dry skin and hair, and a feeling of being cold all the time often occur. Hypothyroidism is about four times more common in women than in men. It is a particular risk for postmenopausal women.

Common types of hypothyroid disease are caused by mild autoimmune disorders in which the thyroid is the sole victim of an attack by the body's immune system. (Hashimoto's thyroiditis is an example of this phenomenon.) Less often, the pituitary gland in your brain fails to produce enough thyroid-stimulating hormone (TSH), the chemical that prompts the thyroid to work. Hypothyroidism can develop when that happens. While hypothyroidism frequently runs in families, it also appears for no obvious reason. Sometimes an underactive thyroid will follow treatment for an overactive one (surgery may remove too much of the gland, or radiation can affect hormone production). If other hormones are disturbed elsewhere (as in pregnancy or menopause), hypothyroidism may result.

Treatments

Because hypothyroidism means your body is getting too little thyroid hormone, the goal of treatment is simple: You'll need to compensate for low thyroid levels by taking a replacement hormone. This daily oral medication will be necessary as long as the condition persists—in most cases, for the rest of your life. The trick is to adjust the dosage to your body's particular needs. Your doctor will

Treatment options

Medications

Levothyroxine	Hypo: Popular synthetic hormone, with T_4.
Natural hormone	Hypo: Animal derived, with T_3 and T_4.
Liotrix	Hypo: Synthetic form with T_3 and T_4.
Liothyronine	Hypo: Synthetic form of T_3, rarely needed.
Antithyroid drugs	Hyper: Decrease hormone production.
Radioactive iodine	Hyper: Destroys gland, reduces hormone.

Lifestyle changes

Diet	Hypo: High-fiber, low-calorie, iodine-rich. Hyper: Calcium to balance excess hormone.

Procedures

Surgery	Hypo and Hyper: To remove goiter. Hyper: To remove thyroid gland (rare).

Natural methods

Vitamins	Hypo: Bs to lower homocysteine levels. Hyper: C and Bs to help thyroid function.

TAKING Control

- **Stay on your medication.** No matter how good you feel, don't stop taking your medicine, or you'll start feeling droopy and sick again.

- **Consciously monitor how you feel.** If you're still chronically tired after taking the hormone for a while, you may not be getting enough. If you're restless or sweating, you may be getting too much. Either way, talk with your doctor.

- **Check your own thyroid.** Occasionally use your thumb and fingertips to press very gently along the front of your neck just below the Adam's apple. Feel for lumps and bumps, which may signal thyroid trouble.

- **Remind your doctor** about all the medications you're taking. A variety of prescription drugs, including estrogen, tamoxifen, and lithium, can affect thyroid hormone levels.

probably start you on a small amount of replacement hormone, then gradually increase your dosage as needed. Follow-up blood tests measuring TSH levels will help guide your treatment. If your hormone dosage is too low, your pituitary gland will be pumping out lots of TSH to try to get your thyroid working. As your dosage increases, your pituitary will pump out less and TSH levels will fall.

It usually takes a month or two to get the dosage exactly right. Then, every year, you'll need to get your TSH and other thyroid levels measured to be sure your dosage is still correct. If all goes well, you'll feel more alert and energetic in just a few weeks, and like your old self in several months. Be aware that if you stop your medication or alter your daily dosage, troublesome symptoms will inevitably reappear, and it can take weeks to get back in balance again.

Medications

If you have hypothyroidism, your doctor will most likely prescribe a synthetic thyroid drug consisting of a single hormone called T_4. The body converts this to an active form called T_3. Known as **levothyroxine**, this medication is available under several brand names, including Synthroid (the oldest and most widely prescribed), Unithroid, Levothroid, Levoxyl, and Euthyrox. Choose a brand and stay with it. Switching around is not advised, since small differences in potency between levothyroxine products may affect how you feel.

Some people, typically those who are older, lack enough of a certain enzyme that is key to the T_4 to T_3 conversion process. For them, a good alternative may be **natural thyroid hormone**, often referred

Are Generics OK?

Generic substitution for brand-name drugs is a valuable cost-saver, but it may not be a good idea for thyroid medications. Although generic preparations of levothyroxine have long been available, under current FDA rules generics will have to be taken off the market unless the manufacturers can prove they're interchangeable with brand-name products. Currently, with a generic, you may get a different manufacturer's product each time you fill your prescription. Your best bet is to find a name brand that works for you and stick with it.

Hyperthyroidism: An Overactive Thyroid Gland

Hyperthyroidism, in which an overactive thyroid produces too much hormone, is the mirror image of hypothyroidism. Instead of everything in your body slowing down, it speeds up. The predominant symptoms are nervousness and jitteriness, and eventually a sense of fatigue prevails. (Think of the effect on a car engine when the idle is set too high: It's a good comparison to what's happening in your body.)

Hyperthyroidism is five times more common in women and strikes most often between the ages of 30 and 40. Left untreated, it may cause a condition doctors term "thyroid storm," a life-threatening burst of thyroid overactivity marked by fever and extreme weakness, requiring emergency care.

● Graves' disease
Almost all hyperthyroidism is due to Graves' disease, a condition in which the immune system produces an abnormal antibody that excessively stimulates thyroid hormone production. Graves' disease may be accompanied by a **goiter** (a swelling in the neck), bulging eyes, and tremor of the hands. Another fairly common cause of hyperthyroidism is taking too much replacement thyroid hormone during treatment for underactive thyroid. Especially in women who have just given birth, the thyroid can become inflamed, causing a condition called **thyroiditis.** In this situation, a period of hyperthyroidism is followed by hypothyroidism. Usually, the latter is only a passing phase.

● Thyroid nodules
Nodules (adenomas) can also grow on the thyroid gland. They usually develop over many years and may occur alone or in clusters. Most are benign. Nodules must be checked regularly by a physician, who may order tests with radioactive iodine to indicate whether they are "hot" or "cold." Hot nodules can start producing excess thyroid hormone, necessitating treatment for hyperthyroidism. Cold nodules don't produce any hormone but should be monitored for cancerous changes. In rare cases, cancer occurs in a solitary nodule.

Treatment Options
Treatment for hyperthyroidism involves reducing the thyroid hormone production. This is accomplished with medications, radiation, or surgery.

● Medications
Your doctor may suggest one of two oral prescription **antithyroid drugs**—methimazole (Tapazole) or propylthiouracil—to decrease production of thyroid hormone. A **beta-blocking drug,** such as propranolol (Inderal), may be added to relieve symptoms such as shakiness and rapid heartbeat. Most doctors recommend that antithyroid drug therapy last for no more than a couple of years. After that, they usually propose radioactive iodine therapy.

● Radioactive iodine
Taken as a single oral capsule, radioactive iodine (I^{131}) is gathered up by the thyroid. It destroys part of the gland, reducing its hormone output. Eventually, this treatment results in permanent hypothyroidism, which is treated with daily thyroid hormone tablets. Radioactive iodine is not to be used by pregnant women, because it will destroy the thyroid of the fetus as well as that of the mother.

● Surgery
In some cases, part of the thyroid is removed surgically **(thyroidectomy).** This is often the choice during pregnancy, when the other forms of therapy can damage the thyroid of the developing fetus. It's also used when **thyroid cancer** is suspected. Hypothyroidism may result.

● Diet
Until your medication takes effect, you'll need extra protein, and vitamins and minerals (from fruits and vegetables) to keep key nutrients from being depleted by your hyped-up metabolism. Be sure to include such thyroid-fighting foods as **raw cruciferous vegetables** (broccoli, cauliflower, cabbage) and raw peanuts. Avoid iodized salt and iodine-rich foods. Eat **calcium-rich foods** or take supplements to counteract bone loss from excess thyroid hormone.

● Vitamins
Take a B-complex and vitamin C to promote healthy functioning of your thyroid and immune system.

● Eyedrops
Anyone whose hyperthyroidism is accompanied by bulging eyes should be closely followed by an ophthalmologist (eye specialist). You may need eyedrops for dry eyes, a change in your prescription if you wear eyeglasses, even surgery if your eyelids won't close completely.

to as Armour thyroid extract. This medication supplies both T_3 and T_4 and doesn't require the body to convert hormones. Natural thyroid hormone is derived from the desiccated (dried) thyroid glands of cows and contains some dose-to-dose inconsistencies. However, people who have taken it for years (and done well) are often loathe to change to a synthetic drug.

Many doctors prefer the newer synthetic thyroid hormone. **Liotrix** (Thyrolar), for example, supplies both T_3 and T_4 as natural hormones do, but doesn't pose the same risk of tablet-to-tablet variation in its hormone concentration. The synthetic forms also produce thyroid hormone levels that are easier to measure and track through standard blood tests.

If you take levothyroxine alone but just don't feel completely well, your doctor may suggest adding a synthetic form of T_3, called **liothyronine** (Cytomel, Triostat), to your regimen. This combination seems to work for a few select patients.

Lifestyle Changes

These self-care strategies can help manage your hypothyroidism:
- **Set a schedule.** Some experts say the ideal time to take your pill is first thing in the morning, at least 30 minutes before eating.
- **Get exercise.** Physical activity will stimulate your thyroid gland and help it absorb the hormone.
- **Eat high-fiber foods** if you're constipated, but don't overdo it: Too much fiber may inhibit absorption of thyroid hormone.
- **Choose low-calorie foods** to promote weight loss, but don't go on a severe diet: Too little food lowers metabolism even further.
- **Get enough iodine**—from iodized salt and foods such as shellfish and saltwater fish. This mineral helps the thyroid function.
- **Avoid thyroid-fighting foods,** so-called because they contain substances (goitrogens) that interfere with iodine absorption and suppress thyroid activity. These include raw cruciferous vegetables (such as broccoli, cauliflower, and cabbage), raw peanuts, and soybeans. It's safe to eat these nutritious foods, however—just cook them. Heat takes the fight out of them.

Procedures

A goiter, an enlarged thyroid gland that produces a bulge in the neck, can develop in some cases of hypothyroidism as well as hyperthyroidism. If you have a goiter that is interfering with breathing or swallowing, you may need **surgery** to remove it.

Natural Methods*

People with hypothyroidism tend to develop elevated levels of the amino acid homocysteine. This can be a risk factor for heart disease. **Vitamins,** specifically folic acid and B_{12}, will lower homocysteine levels. Taking a vitamin C and a B-complex capsule can improve thyroid function and help regulate your immune system.

Natural methods are not subject to the same testing and regulation as prescription medications. Please seek your doctor's advice and use caution.

Synthroid's Story

As the third most frequently prescribed drug in the country, Synthroid is widely used. Yet its name keeps appearing in headlines in a less than glowing light. What's the problem?
- The manufacturer (Knoll, bought by Abbott in 2001) refused to comply with the FDA's 1997 rule that it submit the drug for official approval. Knoll said Synthroid was "generally recognized" as safe and effective. The FDA refused to back down; the company applied for approval two weeks shy of deadline.
- During the standoff, the FDA claimed Synthroid had not been "reliably potent" and had a "long history of manufacturing problems," with recalls and violations.
- In 1997, consumers sued Knoll over its alleged suppression of a study showing Synthroid was not superior to other, less expensive brands of levothyroxine. Knoll settled the case for $135 million.

The bottom line: Synthroid now complies with regulations and remains a safe and effective form of thyroid replacement. It is still the favorite of physicians. If you're taking Synthroid, there's no reason to change.

FINDING Support

- For the latest word from physicians and scientists on thyroid disorders, contact The American Thyroid Association (703-998-8890 or www.thyroid.org).
- The Thyroid Foundation of America provides patient education (1-800-832-8321 or www.allthyroid.org).

Tinnitus

An estimated 50 million Americans suffer from ringing in their ears (or other noises in their heads) that characterize tinnitus. Today, researchers have a better understanding of this distracting disorder—and more effective ways to relieve it.

LIKELY **First Steps**

- **Doctor's visit** to rule out underlying medical causes.
- **Lifestyle changes** to minimize noise.
- **Hearing aid** or **tinnitus-masking devices** to reduce awareness of noise.
- **Supplements,** such as ginkgo biloba or niacin, to improve blood flow and nerve function.
- **Drugs** to help related depression and sleep problems.

QUESTIONS TO **Ask**

- Could a medication I'm taking be responsible for my tinnitus?
- Why does my tinnitus seem to come and go?
- Will this condition affect my hearing?
- Are there any activities that may worsen my tinnitus?

What is happening

Tinnitus comes from Latin meaning "ring like a bell," but the phantom noise you hear may also be buzzing, clicking, roaring, or hissing. It can be a constant, pulsating soundtrack in your head, or come and go in one or both ears. Its cause is a mystery, but it's more common in people who've been exposed to prolonged or intermittent loud noise. In young people, common sources are headphones, too-loud radios, and rock concerts. In older people, culprits are long-term exposure to loud noises (such as a job at a construction site) or simply the aging process. About 90% of those with tinnitus also have some hearing loss.

In some cases, unwanted sounds may result from an underlying physical problem, such as an ear infection, earwax buildup, an ear disease (Ménière's, for example), heart problems, or allergies. Once the ailment clears up, the sounds sometimes disappear. Tinnitus can also be caused by chronic stress and may be a side effect of certain medications or too much caffeine or alcohol. A less common form, called objective tinnitus, involves pulsating sounds that physicians can hear when they listen with a stethoscope. These sounds usually come from jaw movements or from the flow of blood in neck or head vessels. They can also be caused by blocked arteries.

Treatments

If ringing or other sounds in your ears don't go away, treatment usually begins by looking for an underlying cause, followed by a visit to an ear, nose, and throat specialist (an otolaryngologist) for further evaluation. Even when no cause can be found, lifestyle changes can give you relief. Special devices will also improve your hearing or mask the noise so you're less aware of it.

Lifestyle Changes

Try self-help techniques to keep your tinnitus from getting worse:
- **Reduce stress.** Situations that are stressful worsen tinnitus, and having tinnitus is stressful. Break free of this vicious cycle by relaxing with techniques such as meditation and deep breathing.
- **Shun stimulants** such as coffee, tea, colas, and nicotine. They can intensify symptoms by constricting blood vessels. Certain spices, chocolate, and red wine can also temporarily worsen tinnitus.
- **Be careful with certain medicines.** High doses of aspirin and other nonsteroidal anti-inflammatory drugs can cause ringing in the ears, as well as certain antidepressants, sedatives, and antibiotics.

Treatment options

Lifestyle changes

De-stress	Relaxation techniques can help.
No stimulants	Coffee, colas, et al. intensify symptoms.
Care with drugs	Aspirin and other drugs can cause ringing.
Avoid loud noise	Protect ears with earplugs.

Procedures

Hearing aid	Amplifies ambient sound.
Tinnitus masker	Produces pleasant sounds.
Blockage removal	Usually silences the noise.

Natural methods

Supplements	Support healthy hearing.
Biofeedback & acupuncture	Relieves stress; reduces intensity of sounds.

■ **Avoid loud noise.** Earplugs (foam rubber, silicone, or wax) work well to provide protection against the dangers of excessive noise.

■ **Reduce your salt intake.** Too much salt can decrease blood circulation and cause fluid to accumulate in your middle ear.

Procedures

If your tinnitus is associated with hearing loss, your doctor may prescribe a **hearing aid,** which often reduces or even stops the sound. Another option is a **tinnitus masker,** which produces pleasant sounds to drown out the noise. If tinnitus results from a blocked ear, **removal of the blockage** (such as earwax) usually silences the noise.

Natural Methods*

Natural treatments can make a real difference. **Vitamin B$_{12}$** helps the body manufacture myelin, a fatty substance that protects inner ear nerves. **Magnesium** promotes circulation to the brain and supports healthy auditory nerves. **Zinc,** aids healthy hearing, too. **Biofeedback** can help you reduce stress that may be contributing to your tinnitus. Some people claim **acupuncture** treatments help relieve the intensity of unwanted sounds.

Medications

Constant noise that can't be controlled may lead to depression or anxiety. If you feel down or overly stressed, tell your doctor. An **antidepressant** such as amitriptyline (Elavil) or fluoxetine (Prozac) may help.

*Natural methods are not subject to the same testing and regulation as prescription medications. Please seek your doctor's advice and use caution.

TAKING Control

■ **Check out Tinnitus Retraining Therapy (TRT).** A new approach available for tinnitus sufferers, TRT retrains your brain to process tinnitus sounds differently. This can make you less aware of them.

■ **Mask the noise.** Use a fan, ticking clock, tapes of nature sounds, or soft music. Open a window and concentrate on the rustling wind, street sounds, or chirping birds.

■ **Plan ahead for the sound.** Tinnitus usually gets worse in the evening, when the noises of the day stop. Try a tinnitus masker at this time. If tinnitus interferes with your ability to fall asleep, you might want to listen to music. Use a clock radio with an automatic shutoff.

Promising DEVELOPMENTS

■ There may soon be a way to turn off tinnitus. Researchers in Germany trained nine people with tinnitus in an **auditory technique** to distinguish between slightly different tones near the frequencies of the phantom noises they heard. After four weeks, their tinnitus was reduced by 35%. A full-scale clinical trial of this technique is under way.

FINDING Support

■ For up-to-date information on tinnitus or to find a self-help group, contact the American Tinnitus Association (ATA) in Portland, OR (1-800-634-8978 or www.ata.org).

Tobacco dependence

Smoking is the leading preventable cause of death in the United States, yet over 45 million Americans seem helplessly addicted to tobacco. You can up your odds of beating this life-threatening habit by combining several proven therapies.

LIKELY **First Steps**

- **Adopt a gradual with-drawal plan,** rather than going cold turkey.
- **Curb cravings** by eating better and exercising.
- Try a **nicotine replacement product** to ease withdrawal.
- Join a **support group** and get **counseling** to increase your chances of success.

QUESTIONS TO **Ask**

- How can I deal with stress without cigarettes?
- What can I do to prevent weight gain?
- Given what you know about me, my health, and my lifestyle, which replacement product do you think will help me most?

What is happening

You know you want to quit smoking and you know why: It's ever clearer that smoking will take a terrible toll on your health (if it hasn't already)—not to mention your pocketbook, your looks, and your social life. Then how come you're having so much trouble quitting? Studies show it time and again: Nicotine ranks as the world's most addictive drug, ahead of both cocaine and heroin. When you inhale tobacco smoke, the drug is absorbed immediately through your lungs into your bloodstream. If you use a cigar, pipe, or smokeless tobacco (in the form of chewing tobacco or snuff), it's absorbed through the mucous membranes of your mouth. Once it's in your bloodstream, after two or three pumps of your heart, you've got the most addictive drug on the planet in your brain. There it boosts key brain chemicals such as epinephrine, serotonin, and dopamine. That makes you feel more energetic, amazingly clearheaded, even euphoric.

As with all addictive substances, however, you'll need more and more nicotine to produce these same positive reactions. Go too long without your next "hit" and you enter withdrawal, becoming moody, lethargic, and confused. This drug dependence comes at a high price. Smoke and tar from tobacco contain more than 4,000 chemicals (including cyanide, benzene, and formaldehyde), many of which are definitely linked to cancer. Tobacco also increases your risk for other diseases, including heart attack and stroke, early menopause, osteoporosis, chronic respiratory ailments, and impotence. If that isn't enough to make you quit, keep the following facts in mind: Smoking is linked to one in seven deaths in the United States. In people between the ages of 35 and 70, the habit is blamed for one in three deaths!

Amazingly, when you do quit, your health will improve virtually within hours of your last cigarette (*see table, page 317*). Moreover, the longer you abstain, the greater your chances of never smoking again. Though 60% to 90% of smokers will relapse during their first year of tobacco-free living, only 15% do so during their second year, and a scant 2% to 4% after two years.

Treatments

Studies show that only a small number of people who try to quit tobacco without a concrete plan or the support of friends are able to stay off it permanently. You can improve your odds

Treatment options

Lifestyle changes

Don't go cold turkey	Quit slowly over a month or more.
Get support	Tell everyone you're quitting.
Limit alcohol	Drinking diminishes willpower.
Curb cravings	With healthy foods, exercise, and pastimes.

Medications

Nicotine replacement	Various products promote gradual quitting.
Antidepressant	Zyban reduces cravings and depression.

Procedures

Counseling	Find a specialist in smoking cessation.

Natural methods

Acupuncture	Proven useful to control addictive behavior.

dramatically by planning ahead and combining a number of different treatment methods. In fact, the "quit rate" from using a nicotine replacement product, such as the nicotine patch or inhaler, increases from 20% to 30% when you combine one or more of these products with counseling.

Lifestyle Changes

Rather than suddenly tossing your cigs into the trash and swearing never to smoke again—the famed "cold turkey" method—you can double your chances of success by **quitting in incremental steps** (*see box, page 316*). Choose a time when you're not overly stressed. It's also good to put your commitment in writing: Draft a "quit contract" indicating your start date, then sign it and give it to a friend or family member. Tell as many people as possible that you're quitting and ask for their help. Research shows that **social support** will significantly increase your success rate. During this time, avoid putting yourself in situations that can trigger your urge to smoke. During the first weeks, for example, stay away from places where others are likely to be smoking (and drinking). In fact, **limit alcohol** in general while you're trying to quit: It tends to reduce willpower.

Another key to success is to find new ways to **satisfy oral cravings.** Fill your fridge with low-calorie "bunny" foods, such as carrots, celery, and radishes. You can also chew sugarless or nicotine gum (*see "Medications," page 316*). If you're concerned about gaining weight, **start an exercise program.** Not only will it help keep the pounds off, it may also reduce those cravings. Keep your hands busy (pack-a-day smokers typically bring their hand to their mouth 400 times a day). Try computer games or such old-fashioned pastimes as knitting, sewing, or writing letters.

TAKING Control

- **Do it for your kids.** Children of smokers are 50% more likely to suffer asthma, bronchitis, and pneumonia than those of nonsmokers. Put your kids at the top of your list of reasons to stop.

- **Double your pleasure.** Every day you don't smoke, set aside the money you would have spent on cigarettes. At today's prices, it can quickly add up to a nice donation to a charity. This good deed will reinforce your commitment.

- **Get a scan.** In addition to the cholesterol screening and blood pressure tests you get at your regular checkup, ask your doctor to do an ultrasound of your arteries. Smokers who viewed images of their own plaque-clogged arteries were found to be four times more likely to quit.

Promising DEVELOPMENTS

- **Vigabatrin** (Sabril), a prescription drug used to treat epilepsy, may eventually help smokers. Used in low doses, it's thought to block nicotine-induced increases in dopamine, a brain chemical that gives you that pleasurable "nicotine" rush.

- Researchers are trying to develop a **vaccine** that will keep nicotine from reaching the brain, thus preventing the initial addiction. During experiments, scientists injected a single dose of nicotine into vaccinated rats and found that the amount of nicotine reaching the brain was reduced by two-thirds. Clinical trials with humans are not far off.

How to Quit in a Month

Follow this systematic withdrawal plan over four weeks, and with persistence, you'll have quit—hopefully for good.

- **Week 1:** Divide the number of minutes you're awake by the number of cigarettes you smoke in a day. For example, if you wake at 7 AM and hit the sack at 11 PM, you're awake for 960 minutes a day. If you smoke a pack a day (20 cigarettes), divide 960 (your waking minutes) by 20 (your daily cigarettes). Your answer, 48, equals the number of minutes you wait between smokes. Based on your answer, create a daily smoking schedule. Using the hypothetical answer from above, for example, you would smoke your first cigarette at 7 AM, your next at 7:48 AM, your next at 8:36 AM, and so on. You can smoke only at these intervals (set a timer if necessary). If you miss a set time, you must skip the cigarette.
- **Week 2:** Reduce the number of cigarettes you smoke by a third. Then recalculate the amount of time between cigarettes based on the new number.
- **Week 3:** Reduce the number of cigarettes again by a third. Recalculate the time between smokes based on the lower number.
- **Week 4:** Congratulations! You just quit. Toss your smoking paraphernalia—your cigarettes (or pipe tobacco, cigars, snuff), lighters, matches, ashtrays—in the trash. Now give yourself a reward.

As you gradually wean yourself from nicotine, expect to experience withdrawal symptoms as the brain chemical dopamine diminishes. You may feel moody, anxious, or depressed, particularly in the first two weeks. Exercise can help prevent these feelings, among a variety of other activities. Take a warm bath, meditate, read an upbeat book, or call a good friend. Many former smokers find deep rhythmic breathing helps by simulating the sensation of smoking (you can learn how in yoga classes).

Medications

While quitting tobacco without drugs is preferable, doctors recommend certain over-the-counter and prescription medications for those who've repeatedly tried and failed. The most popular are **nicotine replacement products,** which put low doses of nicotine into your blood without the cancer-causing contaminants. In fact, some people find that using two of these nicotine products at once (such as the patch and the inhaler) works better than one alone. Side effects are possible, so read instructions carefully and report any unusual symptoms to your doctor—regardless of which product you choose.

- **The nicotine patch.** Sold over-the-counter in varying strengths, the patch (Nicoderm CQ, Habitrol, Prostep, Nicotrol, Perigo) delivers a steady dose of nicotine through your skin. As the weeks progress, you wear the patch less often or switch to one with a lower potency. The patch won't counteract sudden cravings, because it takes two to four hours to deliver the drug. If you're a two-pack-a-day smoker, ask your doctor about using two patches.
- **Nicotine gum.** This OTC gum (Nicorette) allows you to gradually decrease the amount of nicotine you're getting while satisfying the need to have something in your mouth. You chew the gum until it releases the peppery-tasting nicotine, then tuck the gum between your gum and cheek, allowing the drug to be absorbed through the mucous membranes. Each piece lasts about 30 minutes. Most people chew 10 to 15 pieces a day at first, cutting that back to half after two weeks. Because the gum itself can be addictive, it's important to stop using it after you've quit tobacco.
- **Nicotine nasal spray.** Sold only by prescription, nicotine spray (Nicotrol) comes in a pump bottle, which shoots the drug directly into your nostril. By providing an immediate nicotine rush, the spray is a good solution for a sudden tobacco craving.
- **Nicotine inhaler.** The prescription inhaler (Nicotrol Inhaler) looks like a short cigarette with a plastic mouthpiece. It is intentionally designed to simulate the act of smoking. A replaceable cartridge inside the inhaler releases small amounts of nicotine when you draw on it.

Another nonnicotine aid for quitting is the **antidepressant** drug buproprion hydrochloride, marketed for depression under the name Wellbutrin and for smoking cessation as **Zyban.** How Zyban works is unknown, but it appears to alter brain chemistry that affects cravings and depression. In studies, Zyban combined with

BOOST WILLPOWER WITH HEALING POWER

The vast majority of smokers relapse during the two weeks immediately after quitting, when withdrawal symptoms are greatest. During this difficult time, try to focus on the positive things you're doing for your body. This timetable shows just how quickly your health improves after your last cigarette.

Time After Quitting	Health Benefits
Just 20 minutes	Blood pressure and pulse normalize.
8 hours	Blood levels of carbon monoxide and oxygen levels return to normal.
24 hours	Risk of heart attack drops.
48 hours	Nerve endings begin to regenerate, increasing your sense of smell and taste.
72 hours	Bronchial tubes relax, improving your lung capacity.
2 weeks to 3 months	Lung function improves by up to 30%.
1 to 9 months	Less coughing; fewer colds and sinus infections; more energy; and even greater lung capacity.

▶ **Is there a safe tobacco product?**

In a word: No. Studies show that people who switch from regular cigarettes to those that are low-tar, light, or low-nicotine not only inhale the same amount of carcinogens but may even increase their cancer risk by smoking more—and inhaling more deeply and more often. While cigars and pipes may appear safer than cigarettes because they contain less tobacco, cigar and pipe smokers are still 50% to 70% more likely to suffer lung cancer than nonsmokers. Smokeless tobacco is no better. Although you don't inhale it into your lungs, the chemicals in snuff and chew enter the mucous membranes in your mouth and upper airways, making you more likely to suffer cancers of the mouth, throat, and esophagus.

nicotine replacement has the highest quit rate. Using them together is more effective than either method alone.

Procedures

Counseling provided by a smoking cessation specialist or a psychologist trained in this area has been found to help more than 25% of those who quit. It is especially effective when combined with nicotine replacement. Such counselors give you tips on dealing with your new smoke-free lifestyle and teach you to control triggers that encouraged you to light up in the first place. Try to schedule four to seven 30-minute sessions early on.

Natural Methods*

No alternative treatments have been definitively shown to help you quit smoking. Many people swear by **acupuncture,** an ancient Chinese method in which thin needles are inserted at key points on your body. The acupuncturist may also attach tiny staples or small pellets to the edge of your ear. Pressing on these whenever you crave a cigarette. Doing so is thought to stimulate a part of the brain connected with addictive behavior. It appears to defuse your recurring urge to smoke.

*Natural methods are not subject to the same testing and regulation as prescription medications. Please seek your doctor's advice and use caution.

FINDING Support

- When a craving hits, don't wait it out alone. Call an anti-smoking hotline staffed by the American Lung Association (1-800-548-8252), the American Cancer Society (1-800-ACS-2345), or the National Cancer Institute (1-800-4-CANCER).

- Boston University offers 24/7 online support from ex-smokers at www.quitnet.com.

- To find a local acupuncturist, contact the National Certification Commission for Acupuncture and Oriental Medicine (703-548-9004 or www.nccaom.org). Be sure to ask the acupuncturist if smoking cessation is one of their specialties.

Tooth loss

The main cause of tooth loss is periodontal disease, a common but serious condition that's easily prevented. Even if you already have missing teeth, there are many new techniques—from dentures to implants—that can restore your natural smile.

LIKELY **First Steps**

- **Deep cleaning** to reverse periodontal disease.
- **Oral or topical antibiotics** to eliminate infection.
- **Brush and floss daily** for optimal gum health.
- **Plenty of dietary calcium** to increase bone strength.
- **Tooth implants** or **dentures,** if needed.

QUESTIONS TO **Ask**

- What kind of toothbrush is best for me?
- Will I lose my teeth because I have gum disease?
- Are there drugs that will help me keep my teeth?
- What can I do to strengthen the supporting bones?
- Am I a good candidate for dental implants?

What is happening

A few decades ago, nearly half of adults lost all or most of their teeth by age 65. Today, that number is down to 30%, and it's dropping all the time, thanks to better dental hygiene. While accidents account for some 3 million dislodged or knocked-out teeth every year, a serious gum infection called periodontal disease is the main cause of actual tooth loss (*see Gum Disease, page 146*).

Periodontal disease begins when bacteria that normally live in your mouth collect, then produce a sticky film called plaque. When not removed promptly, plaque hardens into a solid coating, called tartar, that irritates your gums. Plaque provides a rich environment for more bacterial growth, which triggers infections that damage the gums as well as the bone and connective tissues that hold the teeth in place.

You can't always prevent tooth-damaging accidents, but if you care for your teeth properly, you can almost always prevent periodontal disease and tooth loss. Even if you haven't seen a dentist in years and have loose or missing teeth, a variety of new techniques can restore your smile.

Treatments

There are two main approaches to tooth loss. The first and most important is to control periodontal disease. Even if you've had this condition for years, you can reverse it by getting a professional cleaning and spending more time on your teeth at home. For serious cases, an oral surgeon might have to remove damaged tissue and possibly reshape the underlying gum or bone to eliminate infection and prevent future problems.

The second approach is to replace lost teeth. Bridgework and dentures are always an option, but more and more people are opting for tooth implants. They're nearly as strong as the originals and can be customized to perfectly match surrounding teeth.

Procedures

To begin, if you have advanced periodontal disease, you'll probably need an extensive cleaning, called **cleaning and curettage.** Your dentist gives you a local anesthetic, then scours away tartar buildup on your teeth above and below the gum line. Damaged tissue is removed, and the surfaces of the damaged tooth roots are smoothed. The goal is to expose healthy tissue and get rid of rough surfaces that promote future tartar buildup.

Treatment options

Procedures

Deep cleaning	Removes tartar from teeth.
Implants or dentures	Replace lost teeth.

Medications

Antibiotics	Clear up oral infections.
Periostat	Strengthens tooth-to-bone attachments.

Lifestyle changes

Good oral hygiene	Prevents tooth loss.
Regular dental cleanings	Four times a year with periodontal disease.
Diet	High-fiber and calcium inhibit oral bacteria.

Natural methods

Black tea	Battles bacteria in the mouth.

If you have deep pockets underneath your gums even after cleaning, surgery is the next step. The most common procedure, **open flap curettage,** involves cutting open a small flap in the gums to expose the tooth and root. Damaged tissue is cleaned out, then the gum flap is sewn back into place. If the bone that supports your teeth has been badly damaged, it might have to be restored with a procedure called **bone grafting.** The surgeon inserts bone-graft material, which promotes new bone growth in the damaged area over the next several months. A relatively new procedure called **guided-tissue regeneration** is sometimes used in conjunction with bone grafting. A specialized, cloth-like material is applied to craters in the original bone. It prevents gum tissue from growing into the bone and allows healthy bone tissue to regenerate with the cloth as a wall.

If you've lost one or more teeth but the underlying tissue is healthy, you'll want to consider **dental implants,** artificial teeth that are surgically affixed (*see illustration, page 320*) in or on top of the jaw. It's a lengthy (and expensive) process, but implants are nearly as strong as natural teeth and don't require special care once they're in place.

If you've had severe periodontal disease, however, the gum and bone might not be strong enough to support implants. In this case, your best option is to wear **dentures.** If you're missing only one or two teeth, your dentist will probably create a **bridge,** a denture that anchors to the healthy teeth on either side. **Complete dentures** are used when all of the teeth in the upper or lower jaw are missing or weakened and must be replaced.

Periodontal disease doesn't always cause tooth *loss,* of course. You might notice one or more of your teeth getting looser, an uncomfortable condition that can cause a natural tendency to grind or clench at night. There's a good chance that your dentist can save the teeth

TAKING Control

- **Brush with Total.** This Colgate toothpaste is the only one approved by the FDA for treating gum disease, tooth decay, and plaque.

- **Rinse your mouth with Listerine.** After you brush, a quick swish-and-spit with this widely available mouthwash will help kill the bacteria that damage gums and teeth.

- **Drink plenty of water.** It flushes out food particles and promotes the flow of saliva—the body's way of cleaning out bacteria and plaque.

- **Schedule regular cleanings.** Twice a year is enough if your gums and teeth are healthy. If you have periodontal disease, get your teeth professionally cleaned every three months.

▶ **I'm plagued by persistent bad breath. Could that lead to tooth loss?**
Frequent bad breath is usually a sign of periodontal disease, so you'll want to see your dentist. In the meantime, there are a few quick ways to sweeten your breath. Start by drinking water. Sugarless gum will also boost saliva production. Also, take a few seconds to clean your tongue, using your toothbrush or one of the plastic tongue scrapers available at drugstores. Bacteria on the tongue are a common cause of bad breath. Breath mints will temporarily mask bad breath, but they can't prevent or treat it.

Watch Out for Smoke Damage

Even if you don't smoke, environmental tobacco smoke can threaten your teeth. Studies suggest that exposure to secondhand smoke can increase the risk of periodontal disease by 50% to 60% in nonsmokers. It's thought that tobacco smoke reduces the immune system's ability to combat gum infections. It also decreases the amount of oxygen in gum tissue, making it easier for bacteria to thrive.

Promising
DEVELOPMENTS

- The FDA has approved **Emdogain,** a drug that can reverse gum damage in those with periodontal disease. The drug, applied to the gums during surgery, contains amelogenin, a protein that promotes growth of new tissue. Patients may regain up to two-thirds of their gum tissue within 16 months—and all of it after three years.

- You may be able to go to the dentist without fear of pain, thanks to a new anesthetic patch recently approved by the FDA. Researchers at Ohio State University found that **DentiPatch,** which releases the numbing agent lidocaine into the gums, provides pain relief that penetrates deeper and lasts 45 times longer than traditional anesthetic gels. Patients who tried the patch experienced only half as much pain from needle sticks and less discomfort during deep cleanings.

by fitting you for a **retainer** to wear at night. It won't make your teeth stronger, but it will protect them from additional damage.

Medications

Antibiotics are an essential step in reversing periodontal disease and stopping the infections that weaken gums and bones. Antibiotic therapy is often used in combination with surgery. There's also good evidence that antibiotics can be used instead of surgery. One study, for example, found that applying doxycycline to the gums was as effective as cleaning and curettage. Another antibiotic option is Actiste, a thin thread that's impregnated with the antibiotic tetracycline. The thread is temporarily inserted between the tooth and gums, where it releases steady amounts of medicine over time. Research has shown that Actisite, combined with cleaning and curettage, reduces the need for tooth extractions or gum surgery by 88%.

The FDA has approved a new drug for periodontal disease, **Periostat**, which uses a low dose of doxycycline. It's an antibiotic, but killing germs isn't its main job. Rather, the drug blocks the action of collagenase, an enzyme that destroys the connective tissue that holds your teeth in place. With Periostat, you can expect to see gains in tooth-attachment strength of 50%.

Lifestyle Changes

Good oral hygiene—flossing every day and brushing twice a day with a soft-bristled toothbrush, using a bacteria-killing mouthwash, and rinsing your mouth with water after meals—is the best way to prevent tooth loss from periodontal disease. It's never too late to start: Studies suggest that caring for your teeth, along with **regular professional cleanings,** is often enough to reverse existing peri-

DENTAL IMPLANT

An implant can replace one or more teeth and support a partial or full denture. To be a candidate, you must have healthy gums and jawbones. It's a multistep procedure: First, the anchor is surgically implanted. It can take up to six months for the bone to grow around it. Once it's firmly attached, an abutment, or post, is added. In a couple of months, after gum tissues have healed, the artificial tooth crown is put on top.

What to Do for a Knocked-Out Tooth

Don't assume the worst if one of your teeth gets jarred loose or knocked out entirely. There's a good chance the tooth can be saved if you get to a dentist within 30 to 60 minutes. Here's what to do in the meantime:

- **Gently rinse the tooth** in warm, running water. Hold it by the top (the crown) to avoid damaging the root.

- **Try to reinsert the tooth in the socket.** Don't push—it should slip easily back into place. Gently bite down on a handkerchief to hold the tooth in place until you can get to your dentist.

- **Drop it in a glass of milk** if you can't nudge it back into its socket. This keeps the tooth moist. The protein in the milk will help keep the root alive.

- **Don't touch it if it's only been loosened,** but do call your dentist. Baylor College of Medicine researchers found that moving a loose tooth around causes more tissue damage than a hands-off approach. Once the tooth is partly healed—it usually takes one to two weeks—your dentist can easily push it back into its proper position.

---

odontal disease. You're also better off if you **don't smoke.** People who puff on cigarettes, cigars, or pipes are much more likely to lose their teeth than those who don't (*see box opposite*).

One of the most important aspects of a tooth-protection plan is to eat a healthful diet that includes plenty of **nuts and cheese.** These foods contain chemical compounds that inhibit the growth of tooth-damaging bacteria. You'll also want to have several daily servings of **calcium-rich foods,** such as milk or fortified cereals or juices. Calcium strengthens bones throughout the body, including those that support your teeth. Adults who get the least calcium in their diets are twice as likely to develop gum disease as those who get the most. Be sure to eat plenty of **high-fiber foods.** The fibrous tissues in fruits, vegetables, and other plant foods scour away plaque buildup and stimulate healthy gum tissue.

If you play active sports, do your teeth a favor and wear a **mouth guard.** Custom-fitted mouth guards made by a dentist tend to be the most comfortable, but it's fine to use the ones sold in sporting goods stores. Dentists recommend "boil and bite" styles. The mouth guard is softened in hot water, then placed in the mouth and shaped around the teeth for a comfortable fit.

Natural Methods*

A tasty way to protect your teeth is to drink a cup or two of **black tea** daily. This type of tea contains chemical compounds that suppress growth of bacteria and inhibit their ability to cling to teeth.

You can't have healthy teeth without a healthy immune system. One way to boost your immunity and prevent inflammation and tooth-damaging infections is to **reduce the stressors** in your life. Studies have shown that **regular exercise, yoga,** and **other relaxation techniques** can help prevent periodontal disease.

Natural methods are not subject to the same testing and regulation as prescription medications. Please seek your doctor's advice and use caution.

▶ **THE DISCOMFORT AND STRESS** of dental procedures can significantly increase your risk of heart attack. That's the conclusion of Italian researchers, who found that increases in heart rate and blood pressure due to stress can be life-threatening for those with serious heart disease. They advise heart patients to schedule dental visits first thing in the morning, and keep them brief to minimize stress. They also recommend that dentists use stress- and anxiety-reducing techniques when treating people who have heart disease.

FINDING **Support**

■ For more information about periodontal disease or replacing lost teeth, contact the National Institute of Dental and Craniofacial Research in Bethesda, MD (301-496-4261 or www.nidr.nih.gov).

Ulcers

Much of what we used to believe about peptic ulcers turns out to be wrong. In place of yesterday's bland diets (including plenty of milk), antibiotics and acid-reducing drugs are now the first line of attack against this common digestive ailment.

LIKELY **First Steps**

- **Antibiotics** to fight *H. pylori* bacterial infection.
- **Other medications** to reduce digestive acids and promote healing.
- Moderation in **diet** and other **lifestyle changes**.
- **Abstinence from alcohol** and **aspirin and other NSAIDs**, especially if ulcer is caused by these drugs.

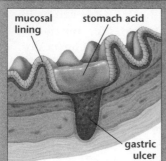

GASTRIC ULCER

mucosal lining

stomach acid

gastric ulcer

Stomach cross-section

A peptic ulcer that develops anywhere on the mucosal lining of the stomach is called a gastric ulcer. It occurs when the digestive tract's defense mechanisms break down, and the lining of the stomach becomes exposed to corrosive digestive juices, primarily hydrochloric acid and the enzyme pepsin. People with gastric ulcers typically experience pain 15 to 20 minutes after eating, when acidic juices begin to flow to digest the meal.

What is happening

A peptic ulcer is an open sore in the lining of your stomach or duodenum (the upper part of your small intestine). Its immediate cause is your own digestive juices—hydrochloric acid, an enzyme called pepsin, and other chemicals your stomach secretes to break down food (*see illustration below*). Even though these juices are as corrosive as battery acid, the linings of your intestine and stomach usually are protected by a layer of mucus and other defenses. If those defenses fail, you may get an ulcer, which most commonly announces itself with bouts of gnawing pain in your upper abdomen.

In 70% to 90% of cases, the culprit is the *Helicobacter pylori* bacteria. Many people harbor this organism, but experts believe certain genetic and lifestyle factors, as well as immune system abnormalities, can make *H. pylori* harmful for some individuals. The bacteria burrows into your stomach lining, wreaking havoc by thinning the protective mucus and causing inflammation. The second most frequent cause of ulcers is the long-term use of nonsteroidal anti-inflammatory drugs (NSAIDs), such as aspirin and ibuprofen, which disrupt the stomach's anti-acid defense system. Ulcers afflict about 1 in 5 men and 1 in 10 women at some point. In the United States, duodenal ulcers are the most common variety—three times more prevalent than peptic ulcers in the stomach.

Treatments

Not so long ago, an ulcer was generally viewed as a life sentence. Antacids and diet might have managed it, but it couldn't be cured. The prognosis changed dramatically in 1994, when the medical establishment accepted the key role played by *H. pylori*. If it's causing your ulcer, your doctor will treat you with drugs that eliminate the bacteria. Under this regimen, you should begin to feel better in just a few days. Your ulcer should heal fully within a month of killing off the bacteria. Sometimes a follow-up test is suggested to confirm that all the bacteria are gone. (*For ulcers caused by NSAIDs, see box, page 324.*)

Medications

H. pylori is one tough bug, so you'll need more than a single drug to wipe it out and repair the damage it has done. Nearly all drug regimens to treat ulcers begin with two **antibiotics,** taken together for 10 to 14 days. Your doctor may prescribe a broad-spectrum penicillin called amoxicillin with clarithromycin (Biaxin), a new macrolide

Treatment options

Medications

Oral antibiotics	Two are prescribed for greatest effectiveness.
PPIs/ H$_2$ blockers	Cut down on stomach acid secretion.
Bismuth	Protects against acid and bacteria.

Lifestyle changes

Eat & drink moderately	Keeps stomach pain at bay.
Avoid NSAIDs	Can cause and/or aggravate certain ulcers.

Procedures

Endoscopy	Detects and treats complications.

Natural Methods

Licorice	Deglycyrrhizinated (DGL) promotes healing.

antibiotic. (A cost-saving alternative is tetracycline, which also works well with amoxicillin.) Metronidazole (Flagyl) can also be paired with amoxicillin or clarithromycin. Antibiotics can cause intestinal queasiness. It's important to tough it out and to stay on them so your ulcer will heal completely.

Your doctor will probably also want you to take a drug that cuts down on the acid your body secretes. The preferred (and most expensive) medication of this type is a **proton pump inhibitor (PPI).** There are five PPIs: omeprazole (Prilosec), rabeprazole (AcipHex), esomeprazole (Nexium), lansoprazole (Prevacid), and pantoprazole (Protonix). All suppress acid production by turning off the molecular pumps that secrete acid into your stomach. A somewhat less effective (and less costly) alternative is an **H$_2$ blocker,** such as famotidine (Pepcid AC), cimetidine (Tagamet), or ranitidine (Zantac). These block the body chemical that triggers acid secretion. Prilosec is now available without a prescription.

Your doctor may also recommend a fourth drug, one that helps your intestinal lining protect itself against acid and bacteria. (Some doctors use this group of drugs instead of a proton pump inhibitor or H$_2$ blocker.) **Sucralfate** (Carafate) sticks to the ulcer and shields it from further damage; **bismuth** (Pepto-Bismol) coats the stomach lining with an antimicrobial substance. For short-term relief, you might take an **OTC antacid,** such as Maalox or Mylanta (aluminum and magnesium combinations), which neutralizes digestive acids. Check with your doctor or pharmacist first: Antacids can interfere with some prescription drugs if taken simultaneously.

Lifestyle Changes

Contrary to yesteryear's conventional wisdom, doctors now believe a bland diet is no help against ulcers, that frequent small meals are no better than three squares a day, and that milk stimulates rather than protects against acid secretion. What to do in the face of changing advice? Stick with the following sensible strategies:

QUESTIONS TO Ask

- Should I make any major changes in my eating habits?
- I've been taking a daily dose of aspirin to help me with heart disease. Should I continue to do so?
- Does having *H. pylori* put me at risk for stomach cancer?
- Will I need follow-up testing to make sure the ulcer has healed? How will I know the bacteria has been killed?

TAKING Control

- **Consider prepackaged therapy** if your drug regimen seems too complicated. In this approach, the medications you need to take are conveniently grouped together. One of these packages is Prevpac, which combines amoxicillin and clarithromycin (antibiotics) with lansoprazole (a proton pump inhibitor). Another is Helidac, which pairs tetracycline and metronidazole (antibiotics) with bismuth (a germ-fighter). Ask your doctor if one of these is right for you.

- **Speak up if your stomach still hurts.** If your treatment doesn't make your symptoms disappear, tell your doctor. Your ulcer may have failed to heal, or you may have an altogether different medical problem. *H. pylori* is a stubborn bacteria. About 10% to 20% of patients need a second course of antibiotics to beat it.

A
B
C
D
E
F
G
H
I
J
K
L
M
N
O
P
Q
R
S
T
U
V
W
X
Y
Z

▶**What's a bleeding ulcer?**
Up to 15% of people with ulcers have some bleeding. This is more likely to happen if NSAIDs, not H. pylori, induced the condition. If your bleeding is chronic and hidden, the only indications you may have are the symptoms of anemia, such as fatigue and shortness of breath. Let your doctor know if you suspect bleeding, even though it usually stops spontaneously. Severe bleeding is a different story. Signs are tarry or bloody stools and vomit with blood or what looks like coffee grounds. For this you'll need immediate emergency care. The bleeding can often be stopped with endoscopic treatment, in which a physician uses heat, electricity, or medications, delivered via a lighted telescope-like tube.

Promising
DEVELOPMENTS

■ An **oral vaccine** now in clinical trials has shown promise in immunizing people against *H. pylori*. Known as Helivax, the vaccine is being developed by Antex, a Maryland biotech company. If successful, it comes not a moment too soon. Some strains of the ulcer-causing bacteria are starting to show resistance to the antibiotics commonly used to treat them.

FINDING **Support**

■ For more information on ulcers and related diseases, contact the National Digestive Diseases Information Clearinghouse in Bethesda, MD (301-654-3810 or www.niddk.nih.gov).

Natural methods are not subject to the same testing and regulation as prescription medications. Please seek your doctor's advice and use caution.

NSAID-Induced Ulcers

Nonsteroidal anti-inflammatory drugs (NSAIDs)—aspirin, ibuprofen (Advil), naproxen (Aleve), and many others—are a boon to people with chronic pain conditions. They are also the second most common cause of ulcers, especially stomach ulcers. In fact, 15% to 30% of chronic NSAID users develop ulcers. To help:

● **Discontinue the offending NSAID.** NSAID-induced ulcers usually heal once the problem medication is stopped. If a complete break isn't possible, at least lower the dosage.

● **Switch to a different pain reliever.** Acetaminophen is better for the stomach, but it won't reduce inflammation. COX-2 inhibitors, such as celecoxib (Celebrex) and rofecoxib (Vioxx), are prescription NSAIDs, with less likelihood of hurting the digestive tract. Ask your doctor what's best for you.

● **Reduce acid** with proton pump inhibitors, H_2 blockers, or antacids. Bismuth or sucralfate protect the stomach as it heals.

● **Try misoprostol (Cytotec)** to prevent a recurrence if you must continue NSAIDs. This drug works by increasing levels of prostaglandin, a protective substance in your stomach lining.

■ **Eat in moderation.** Don't supersize your meals. Stretching your stomach can cause pain. Skip foods that make you feel worse.

■ **Choose foods rich in flavonoids,** which may inhibit *H. pylori*. These include cooked apples and onions, and cranberry juice.

■ **Watch what you drink.** Limit caffeinated beverages and acidic juices. Avoid alcohol: It irritates the stomach's mucosal lining.

■ **Don't smoke.** Smoking delays healing of ulcers because it stimulates the secretion of stomach acid.

■ **Avoid aspirin and other NSAIDs** unless needed for preventing blood clots. They eat away the body's natural protective barriers.

■ **Practice good hygiene.** *H. pylori* can be transmitted through stool, so always wash your hands after bowel movements.

■ **Reduce stress.** Being a Type A personality can keep an ulcer from healing. Look into relaxation techniques if stress is an issue for you.

Procedures

If you have complications, you may need an **endoscopy,** in which a long, flexible viewing tube is passed down your digestive tract and repairs are made. **Traditional surgery** is reserved for uncontrolled bleeding, a blockage (obstruction), or a deep ulcer that causes intestinal contents to spill into your abdomen.

Natural Methods*

Studies show that **deglycyrrhizinated licorice (DGL)**, a licorice derivative, has ulcer-healing properties. Chew one or two DGL wafers of 380 mg each about 30 minutes before each meal. Use them for about three months to maximize healing.

Urinary incontinence

When you've "gotta go" too often, or you just can't hold it in, inconvenience and embarrassment often follow. Take heart: There are numerous solutions—from exercises to medications—for the all-too-common curse of incontinence.

What is happening

Some 17 million Americans have urinary incontinence, but many never tell their doctors, either because they're too ashamed or they mistakenly think it's part of getting older. This is too bad, because there's a lot your doctor can do to control or cure this condition. Urinary incontinence is more often a problem for women than men: Pelvic floor muscles get strained during pregnancy and childbirth, and hormonal changes during menopause add to urinary urges. In men, incontinence may be due to prostate problems or surgery (*see Prostate Enlargement, page 262*). Other general causes include diabetes, medications, urinary tract infections, and structural problems.

There are two common types of incontinence. If you have a little leakage when you laugh, sneeze, or exert yourself (lifting something or running hard, perhaps), that's **stress incontinence.** Your urinary sphincter—the muscles that surround the urethra, which carries urine from the bladder—is weak and opens during "stress." If you have unpredictable, overwhelming urges to urinate and realize you might not make it to the bathroom, you've got **urge incontinence.** This begins as a condition called overactive bladder, an intense and too-frequent need to urinate. With urge incontinence, problems arise when muscles around the bladder abruptly contract, and suddenly you have to go. Your sphincter and pelvic muscles might be able to stop the flow, but your bladder is insisting on relief.

More severe types of incontinence are called overflow incontinence and total incontinence. People with these conditions often need special devices to hold urine overflow.

Treatments

For stress and urge incontinence, many people have success with lifestyle changes—pelvic floor muscle exercises (Kegels) and bladder training to improve control. Changes in diet and drinking habits may also help. Your doctor can recommend medications, and many surgical procedures are available.

Lifestyle Changes

The following everyday measures can help you better control this condition and may even eliminate the problem:

- **Learn Kegel exercises.** Good for stress and urge incontinence, these exercises strengthen the pelvic floor muscles that support the bladder. Begin by periodically contracting your pelvic muscles,

LIKELY First Steps

- **Get treated for any contributing condition** such as a urinary tract infection.
- Practice **Kegel exercises** or **bladder training.**
- Watch what and when you **eat and drink.**
- **Medications** to improve control.
- **Surgery** if other treatments don't help.

QUESTIONS TO Ask

- Could my incontinence be related to another health condition or a medicine I'm taking?
- Can I put a complete stop to my problem with exercises or bladder-control training?
- Could anything in my diet be contributing to my incontinence?
- Will this problem get worse as I get older?
- Is this a "warning sign" of a more serious health condition? If so, what other symptoms should I be watching for?

TAKING Control

- **Find a specialist.** If you have a serious problem, a urologist or urogynecologist (for women) can often identify the best approaches.

- **Keep a diary.** For three days, write down when you urinate, your feelings of urgency, when you have leaking, what you eat, and what you're doing when the problem occurs. This will help you uncover what might trigger your incontinence, and help your doctor choose the best treatment for you.

- **Cross your legs.** When you think you're going to sneeze or cough—causing involuntary leakage—this simple maneuver might stop the flow.

- **Join a support group.** Just talking to others who've suffered similar embarrassments can be comforting. It's also a good forum for exchanging helpful strategies.

Promising
DEVELOPMENTS

- The same drug that erases wrinkles may also help treat urge incontinence. In one trial, a safe concentration of **botulinum toxin (Botox)** was injected into the bladder to paralyze and relax sphincter muscles. Among patients with persistent incontinence problems, about two-thirds experienced significant improvement after undergoing this treatment.

Treatment options

Lifestyle changes

Kegel exercises	Strengthen pelvic floor muscles.
Bladder training	Increases intervals between bathroom visits.
Diet	Avoid food triggers; limit fluids at night.
Weight loss	Relieves pressure on bladder.

Medications

Antibiotics	Clear up urinary tract infections.
Drugs for stress form	Help keep urinary sphincter closed.
Drugs for urge form	Treat involuntary bladder contractions.

Procedures

Surgery	Often for bladder neck or urinary sphincter.

as tightly as possible when urinating, to stop the flow. (Women should also contract the vaginal area.) Then, practice tensing these muscles when you're not urinating. But don't hold your breath or squeeze your stomach, groin, or thigh muscles, which adds pressure to the bladder. Do the exercises daily, alternating a series of slow contractions (holding for 5 to 10 seconds) with rapid ones (holding for just a few seconds). Work up to sets of 10 to 15 contractions, repeating the exercise three times daily. Do Kegels when you're driving, standing on line, or sitting at your desk. No one will ever know. For women, your doctor may recommend practicing with graduated vaginal cones to further strengthen your muscles.

- **Try bladder-training** if you have urge incontinence. You begin by voiding at set intervals, such as every hour. Then, gradually increase the intervals until you can manage the normal three or four hours between bathroom visits.

- **Check for triggers.** Many foods can send you to the bathroom more often. These include carbonated drinks, caffeine, alcohol, citrus fruits and juices, tomato products, spicy foods, chocolate, sugar, honey, artificial sweeteners, and milk products. Try eliminating each in turn for 10 days. Note any improvements.

- **Lose weight.** If you're overweight, extra pounds can exert more pressure on the bladder, making an existing problem worse.

- **Stop smoking.** Nicotine irritates the bladder, so smokers are much more likely to have incontinence problems.

- **Limit evening fluids.** It's a good idea to drink normal amounts of fluids during the day (in fact, drinking too little fluid can irritate the lining of the urethra and bladder). Stop drinking two to four hours before you go to bed to prevent nighttime accidents.

- **Use protective devices** if you need them. Some women benefit from foam pads to catch leaks or "barrier devices" such as urethral shields or caps to block the urine. For men, there are specially designed condoms and drip collectors. For both sexes, a variety of disposable undergarments and underwear liners are available.

Medications

If lifestyle changes and exercises don't banish your problem, your doctor may want to treat it with medication. If you have a urinary tract infection (*see page 328*), you'll first be given **antibiotics** to clear it up.

For both stress and urge incontinence: Your doctor may prescribe a **tricyclic antidepressant,** such as imipramine (Tofranil) or doxepin (Sinequan). These medications relax the bladder, strengthen the urinary sphincter, and prevent involuntary bladder contractions. They work for both men and women. For postmenopausal women, various **topical estrogen products**—creams, ointments, rings (Estring), and patches—applied to the vagina are often recommended.

For stress incontinence: Your doctor will likely suggest **alpha adrenergic agonists,** commonly found in over-the-counter decongestants). These drugs strengthen the muscle that opens and closes the urinary sphincter.

For urge incontinence: You might be given an **anticholinergic drug,** such as oxybutynin (Ditropan) or tolterodine (Detrol), which inhibits involuntary bladder contractions. Certain **antispasmodics,** including flavoxate (Urispas) and dicyclomine (Bentyl), may help control urge problems. They help relax the bladder.

Drugs used to treat incontinence all have side effects. Be sure to tell your doctor how your medication affects you, so timing and dosages can be adjusted, if necessary.

Procedures

For more serious urge incontinence, doctors may recommend women try **transvaginal pelvic floor electrical stimulation.** This painless office procedure uses gentle electrical stimulation to strengthen muscles around the bladder and urinary sphincter. Another option is **sacral nerve stimulation (InterStim).** It involves sending electrical pulses from a small device implanted in your abdomen to sacral nerves in your lower back to stimulate nerves and control muscle spasms in the bladder.

There are many possible surgical procedures for structural problems. **Bladder neck suspension,** in which the bladder neck and urethra are sewn into their proper position, has an excellent success rate. If you have severe stress incontinence, you may be helped with a **sling procedure.** The surgeon attaches the urethra and bladder neck to the abdominal wall with a synthetic sling or one made from muscle tissue. If your urinary sphincter doesn't work well or at all, an **artificial sphincter** can be implanted. In some cases, you can instead get injections of collagen (or other material) to provide bulk around the urethra and help the sphincter close more tightly. Talk with your doctor about what's best for you.

▶ **Can biofeedback help?**
In a study of women who used electronic biofeedback equipment, 79% were able to control incontinence completely or showed a marked improvement. To relay electronic signals to a biofeedback monitor, a small "probe" is inserted in the vagina or rectum. When doing Kegel exercises correctly, the monitor rewards good performance with a beep or a flash of light. The study showed that biofeedback equipment helps improve control techniques.

▶ **Which drugs can cause incontinence?**
Among the most problematic medicines are diuretics prescribed for high blood pressure, certain antidepressants, antihistamines, calcium channel blockers for heart disease, and sedatives for insomnia. If you're taking any of these prescription drugs, talk with your doctor. Perhaps another medication can be prescribed instead.

FINDING Support

■ The Simon Foundation for Continence, in Wilmette, IL, gives you Internet access to discussion groups and authoritative information about treatment and research, with links to other sites (1-800-23-SIMON or www. simonfoundation.org).

■ For comprehensive medical information about health issues related to incontinence, www.urologychannel.com is an excellent source. Using your ZIP code, you can also get a list of nearby urologists.

Urinary tract infection

If this is your first UTI, you can take solace in the fact that you're not alone: One in five women suffers from a UTI at least once a year. Treatment may now be only a phone call away, and you could feel better in a single day.

LIKELY **First Steps**

- **Antibiotics prescribed in person or by phone** to combat bacteria.
- **Analgesics** to relieve urinary pain and burning.
- **Lots of fluids** to wash the infection from your system.
- For more complicated cases, a **doctor's visit** and **urine culture** to determine appropriate care.

QUESTIONS TO **Ask**

- Can a vaginal infection trigger a UTI?
- Is there a way I can tell if my kidneys are infected?
- Could my recurrent UTIs be due to an anatomical problem?

What is happening

A urinary tract infection (UTI) occurs when bacteria or other germs find their way up the tube that leads into your bladder (called the urethra), adhere to the cell walls, and start multiplying. Normally, urine helps flush away these occasional invaders, but once in a while, this natural policing system simply can't cope, and you find yourself in the throes of a UTI.

Most urinary infections are called "lower UTIs," meaning the germs have taken hold in your urethra (a condition called urethritis) or in your bladder (a condition called cystitis). If the germs travel further, an "upper UTI" can develop, affecting the narrow tubes (ureters) leading to the kidneys or even the kidneys themselves. This potentially serious infection is known as pyelonephritis.

Between 80% and 90% of UTIs are caused by *Escherichia coli* (*E. coli*), a bacterium usually confined to the colon and rectum that can spread from the anus to the urethra. Because a woman's urethra is relatively short, women are more prone to UTIs than men (whose much longer urethra in the penis makes it harder for the bacteria to travel to the bladder). After menopause, some women are increasingly susceptible to infection because of a lack of estrogen. When a man does get a UTI—typically because of infection from a urinary catheter put in while in the hospital or from an obstruction such as a urinary stone—therapy is generally lengthy and aggressive because of the risk of a serious prostate gland infection (*see Prostatitis, page 266*).

Treatments

The good news for uncomplicated bacterial UTIs, including cystitis, is that doctors will now often prescribe antibiotics over the phone, skipping the need for an in-office urine culture. The bad news is that so many strains of bacteria have become antibiotic-resistant, your initial drug may not work. A recent study of 75,000 UTI patients ages 15 to 44, for example, found that roughly 14% needed a second course of treatment within 28 days—regardless of which antibiotic they took initially.

So-called "complicated UTIs," which strike men and women equally, are a different story. These infections are more likely to occur if you have kidney involvement, are pregnant, have had a catheter put in, or have an abnormally structured urinary tract. Your doctor will want to carefully monitor you and aggressively

Treatment options

Medications

Antibiotics	First-line treatment; cure 85% of UTIs.
Anti-infectives	Next step if antibiotics fail.
Analgesics	Ease burning, cramps, and pain.
Antispasmodics	Relieve painful bladder spasms.

Lifestyle changes

Increase fluid intake	Flushes out germs; just avoid acidic juices.
Practice good hygiene	Helps prevent recurrences.
Avoid irritants	No hygiene sprays, scented douches, or petroleum-based lubricants.

Procedures

Surgical repair	Corrects anatomical problems; rarely needed.

Natural methods

Cranberry juice	Discourages bacteria from adhering to tissues.

treat any problem to prevent permanent damage or a system-wide infection. While uncommon, surgery for UTIs is extremely effective if anatomical problems are obstructing urine flow.

Medications

Although some doctors prescribe a one-day dose of an **antibiotic** for a routine UTI, you'll probably be given a minimum of three days on the combination drug TMP-SMX (trimethoprim-sulfamethoxazole), best known by its brand names: Bactrim and Septra. If your symptoms warrant it, your doctor may instead choose a class of potent antibiotics called fluoroquinolones (quinolones), which includes ciprofloxacin (Cipro), as well as norfloxacin (Noroxin), oflaxacin (Floxin), and gatifloxacin (Tequin), the newest member of the group. A recent study showed that a single dose of Tequin worked just as well for an uncomplicated UTI as a regular dose taken over three days.

If these standard treatments are ineffective, you may have to move on to the antibiotic cephalexin (Keflex) or, depending on the organism involved, to **anti-infective drugs,** such as nitrofurantoin (Macrodantin) or methenamine (Prosed). Whichever medication you take and however tedious it becomes, make sure you complete the entire course. If you don't, germs can fight back and find a way to resist the drug, making future UTIs harder to treat. Here are a few other drug pointers:

■ **If you still have symptoms after taking antibiotics** for a few days, you may need to give a laboratory urine sample. When the specific germ causing your problem is identified, your doctor can suggest customized medication and care.

TAKING Control

■ **Be wary of home tests.** Although widely available, home tests can be unreliable, and UTI symptoms always require a call to the doctor, regardless of what the test shows.

■ **Ask about long-term antibiotics.** If you have recurrent UTIs (three or more a year), continuous low-dose antibiotic therapy may be the answer. It's likely to be cheaper than treating each infection.

■ **Consider switching your birth control method.** Research shows that women who use diaphragms are more susceptible to UTIs. The reason: Spermicides containing nonoxynol-9, often used with diaphragms, can change the bacterial balance in the vagina, enabling *E. coli* to proliferate.

Promising DEVELOPMENTS

■ Now in development at the University of Wisconsin, a new **suppository vaccine** may ward off recurring UTIs when inserted into the vagina monthly. Made from 10 killed strains of *E. coli* and other germs, it prompts the body to fight bacteria in the vagina—and never gives germs a chance to travel to the bladder (or kidneys). Small trials have proved successful; larger ones are needed before the FDA approves the drug.

■ **If you tend to develop a UTI after sexual intercourse,** a single dose of antibiotics before or after sex may prevent the infection. Vigorous intercourse can sometimes bruise the urethra, making bladder infection more likely.

■ **If the pain of your infection is really getting to you,** try an **analgesic.** For mild cramps or stomach pain, over-the-counter NSAIDs (aspirin, ibuprofen, naproxen) or acetaminophen may do the job. If burning during urination is intense, your doctor might also prescribe phenazopyridine (Baridium, Eridium, AZO Standard, Pyridium). Limited to short-term use (two to three days), this drug mixes with urine and numbs the urethra to relieve the discomfort. It may also turn your urine a harmless orange.

■ **If you have what feel like bladder spasms**—waves of intense pain—tell your doctor. Prescription **antispasmodics,** such as flavoxate (Urispas), can provide relief.

Lifestyle Changes

You can do a number of things on your own to make UTIs less overwhelming. At the first sign of an infection, start drinking **plenty of fluids:** An eight-ounce glass of water once an hour during the day is a great way to flush germs from your urinary tract. Never try to "hold it" when you have to urinate. Delayed urination is a major cause of UTIs. Also, **keep your genital and anal areas clean.** Wipe from front to back to prevent bacteria around the anus from entering your urethra. Be sure to cleanse your genitals before and after sexual intercourse.

If your vaginal tissues are sensitive, **avoid potential irritants.** Feminine hygiene sprays and scented douches can aggravate the urethra, making it more susceptible to infection. If you're postmenopausal and have been experiencing vaginal dryness, consider using a water-based—never a petroleum-based—vaginal lubricant (Astroglide, Lubifax, K-Y Jelly) during sex.

Procedures

Some women have abnormally shaped urinary tracts that interrupt the flow of urine. Your doctor will likely investigate with an instrument called a cytoscope, which provides a way to examine the bladder via the urethra. **Surgical repair** might finally liberate you from UTIs.

Natural Methods*

Lab studies have discovered that cranberry juice prevents *E. coli* from adhering to the bladder walls. A 2001 Finnish study found that women prone to UTIs were half as likely to suffer a recurrence within six months if they drank an eight-ounce glass of cranberry juice every day. If possible, always purchase the unsweetened juice, available at health food stores.

*Natural methods are not subject to the same testing and regulation as prescription medications. Please seek your doctor's advice and use caution.

Uterine fibroids

If your doctor says you have a fibroid, it's not the end of the world. These common uterine growths are often problem-free. When you do need treatment, you have a number of uterus-preserving options beyond a traditional hysterectomy.

What is happening

Fibroids are rubbery masses of muscle and fibrous tissue that develop within or along the wall of a woman's uterus (womb). They come in multiples, vary greatly in size (from microscopic to up to 20 inches or so), and generate a range of symptoms. You may be completely unaware of their existence, or you may have the most common symptom—a heavy or prolonged menstrual period—potentially serious, because it can lead to anemia.

The pressure of large fibroids on nearby organs can also cause low back pain, abdominal cramping, pain during intercourse, difficult or increased urination, and constipation. By distorting your uterus, fibroids may also hamper your ability to become pregnant and increase the risk of miscarriage or heavy bleeding after giving birth. Once in a while, stalk-like (pedunculated) fibroid develops and gets twisted, causing its tissues to die. This painful condition, known as necrosis, usually calls for immediate surgery.

Between 20% and 40% of women over age 35 have uterine fibroids of significant size, and as many as 75% of African-American women have them. It's not known why fibroids form (although new research suggests genetics may be responsible). Once they do, the female hormone estrogen certainly spurs their further growth. Fibroids tend to enlarge during pregnancy, when estrogen levels increase, and shrink or disappear with menopause, when estrogen falls. On the bright side: If you've carried at least two pregnancies to term, or are athletic, you may be less prone to them.

Treatments

Fibroids are almost never life-threatening: They don't develop into cancer. Nor do they increase your risk of uterine cancer, so if you have only mild symptoms, you may initially want to opt for a wait-and-see approach. You'll still need regular pelvic exams and ultrasounds to monitor any growth, and you'll want to relieve symptoms with medications and self-care remedies. More troublesome fibroids—those that cause particularly painful menstrual periods or related pain or that could interfere with fertility or pregnancy—should be removed. At one time, the traditional treatment for fibroids was removal of the uterus, a surgical procedure known as a hysterectomy (*see box, page 333*). Today, there are a number of less radical procedures to consider first.

LIKELY First Steps

- **Anti-inflammatory drugs (NSAIDS)** to control pain.
- **Cut dietary fat,** which may stimulate fibroid growth.
- **Consider procedures** to treat problematic fibroids.

QUESTIONS TO Ask

- How many fibroids do I have? Where are they located?
- How will I know if they're getting bigger?
- Will fibroids affect my sex life?
- What are the odds my fibroids will regrow after surgery?

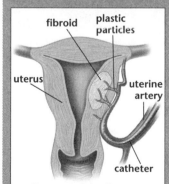

UTERINE FIBROID EMBOLIZATION (UFE)

fibroid · plastic particles · uterus · uterine artery · catheter

Cross-section of uterus

In this minimally invasive procedure, a catheter is inserted into the uterine artery. Tiny plastic or gelatin particles are injected into the artery to block blood supply to the fibroid in the uterus. Without blood, the fibroid withers away.

- **Schedule regular checkups.** An annual pelvic exam ensures early detection of fibroids; twice-yearly exams monitor existing ones.

- **Seek relief with heat.** If fibroids cause abdominal pain, apply a heating pad or hot-water bottle at least three times a week for an hour.

- **Soothe with moves.** Yoga exercises can help relieve feelings of heaviness and pressure from fibroids. Look for classes at your local Y or through a health club.

- **Put it in writing.** Track symptoms, noting periods and heaviness of flow or pain. Then discuss the data with your doctor.

- **Ask about endometrial ablation,** or removal of the uterine lining, if your chief complaint is heavy periods. *Be aware:* This procedure destroys fertility, and it won't help fibroids.

Promising
DEVELOPMENTS

- Two experimental techniques appear to wipe out fibroids. With **cryomyolysis,** a probe is passed through a small abdominal incision and freezes fibroids into submission. With **radiofrequency ablation,** a needle electrode is inserted to "cook" the growth with heat.

- Studies suggest the progesterone antagonist drug **mifepristone (RU 486)** shrinks fibroids and stops periods, but it isn't currently available in the United States. Also under scrutiny is a new drug, **pirfenidone,** which blocks growth factors that can affect fibroids.

Treatment options

Medications	
Anti-inflammatories	NSAIDs (Advil, Aleve) for pain and cramps.
Oral contraceptives	Reduce bleeding and spotting.
GnRH agonists	Often used presurgically to shrink fibroids.
Procedures	
Hysterectomy	Eliminates fibroids by removing uterus.
Myomectomy	Removes only fibroids; variety of methods.
UFE	Shrinks fibroids by cutting off blood supply.
Lifestyle changes	
Improve diet	Low-fat, high-fiber reduces fibroid growth.
Increase iron	Prevents anemia due to heavy menstrual flow.

Medications

If your fibroids are causing heavy, painful periods, regular doses of **nonsteroidal anti-inflammatory drugs (NSAIDs)** may bring relief. They reduce discomfort and curb the activity of prostaglandins, chemicals that stimulate uterine contractions. Good choices include ibuprofen (Advil, Motrin) and naproxen (Aleve). If you're truly plagued by heavy periods, **oral contraceptives** (Lo/Ovral, Norinyl, Ortho-Novum, Demulen) may help control the bleeding.

Because of the direct link between estrogen and fibroids, drugs that block this hormone can reduce bleeding and shrink fibroid growth. **Gonadotropin-releasing hormone (GnRH) agonists** accomplish this by releasing reproductive hormones, which signal ovaries to stop producing estrogen. The drugs come in a variety of forms, including leuprolide injections (Lupron Depot), nafarelin acetate nasal spray (Synarel), and goserelin acetate implants (Zoladex). These medications are generally prescribed only for short-term use, usually to shrink fibroids by about 50% before surgery. The downside: GnRH agonists can cause unpleasant side effects that mimic menopausal symptoms (hot flashes, vaginal dryness, irritability). If taken for more than six months, they can increase osteoporosis risk (strong bones need estrogen), and fibroids usually grow back once the drug treatment ends.

Procedures

If you've been told the only surgery for fibroids is a **hysterectomy** (*see box opposite*), it's time to become acquainted with other possibilities, especially because hysterectomy means you'll no longer be able to bear children. Although fibroids remain a top reason for a hysterectomy, other options exist. Only a hysterectomy offers a sure cure. Fibroids may eventually return following other procedures.

If you hope for a future pregnancy, you might choose a myomectomy. This surgical procedure removes individual fibroids either

Hysterectomy: Is It Right for You?

Until recently, hysterectomy was an almost automatic solution for fibroid problems. Surgically removing the uterus guarantees an end to fibroids. Today the operation is controversial, with many questioning its medical necessity when other options don't affect fertility. Still, fibroid treatment accounts for about a third of the 600,000 hysterectomies U.S. doctors perform each year.

Additional reasons for a hysterectomy include cancer of the endometrium, cervix, or ovary; chronic pelvic pain; severe endometriosis; chronic vaginal bleeding; and a prolapsed uterus.

Two types of hysterectomy are usually used for fibroids. One is **partial hysterectomy,** which removes the uterus through an abdominal incision, but leaves the cervix, fallopian tubes, and ovaries in place. The other is **total hysterectomy,** which removes the uterus and cervix, fallopian tubes, and ovaries, either by vaginal incision (if the fibroids are small) or by abdominal incision (if they're large). This procedure is often recommended for premenopausal women: Removing the ovaries eliminates the possibility of ovarian cancer.

A hysterectomy requires a hospital stay of several days. You can sometimes recover in just two weeks (particularly from a vaginal procedure, which is faster and less painful), or it may take up to two months.

You'll need to discuss the pros and cons of each possible treatment with your doctor. Be sure to seek a second opinion if hysterectomy is presented as your best—or only—option.

through your cervix (hysteroscopic myomectomy), in which case no incision is needed, through your abdomen (laparoscopic myomectomy), and sometimes through both (abdominal myomectomy). All require general anesthesia. Recovery from abdominal myomectomy takes up to six weeks, but you may bounce back from the hysteroscopic and laparoscopic procedures within two.

A newer, nonsurgical technique called **uterine fibroid embolization (UFE),** also called uterine artery embolization, works by stopping blood flow so fibroids wither away (*see illustration, page 331*). A specially trained interventional radiologist makes a tiny cut in your groin, then inserts a catheter through an artery to the uterus. The doctor then injects tiny plastic (or gelatin) particles to block blood supply to the fibroids. General anesthesia isn't necessary, although an overnight hospital stay is (many women suffer cramps, nausea, and fever a few hours after the procedure). If you choose to undergo UFE, you should be able to resume your regular activities in about a week. Its effect on fertility isn't yet known, and UFE is usually recommended only for women who are no longer fertile or aren't planning to become pregnant.

Lifestyle Changes

Nutritionists recommend a **low-fat, high-fiber** diet to help ward off a host of health woes. It's good advice for fighting fibroids, too. Research suggests that a steady diet of fats and red meat stimulates fibroid growth, whereas eating plenty of fruits and vegetables checks their development. Fiber-rich whole grains may also ease fibroid-related bowel difficulties. To pump up your iron stores and help prevent anemia related to excessively heavy periods, ask your doctor about taking an **iron supplement.** Good food sources of iron include lean meats (the less marbling, the less fat), poultry, dried fruits, and fortified cereals.

FINDING **Support**

■ To locate a gynecologist in your area, visit the website of the American College of Obstetricians and Gynecologists at www.acog.com.

■ For more information about uterine fibroid embolization, or to find an interventional radiologist, contact the Society of Interventional Radiology (SCVIR) (1-800-488-7284 or www.scvir.org).

■ The National Uterine Fibroids Foundation (NUFF), a nonprofit organization in Colorado Springs, CO, promotes education and research related to fibroid treatment (1-877-553-NUFF or www.nuff.org).

Varicose veins

You may think varicose veins are simply an unsightly fact of life that come with the onset of middle age. The happy news is that less-invasive, state-of-the-art techniques now reduce scarring and give you legs you'll gladly show off again.

LIKELY First Steps

- **Compression stockings** to help blood flow's fight against gravity.

- **Elevating the legs** to improve blood flow back to the heart. **Exercise** and **weight control** also promote good blood flow.

- **Herbal and nutritional supplements** to help reduce inflammation and swelling.

- **Surgical procedures** to remove or collapse "problem" veins.

QUESTIONS TO Ask

- Why do you think the technique you're recommending is the best therapy for my varicose veins?

- What kind of scarring can I expect from this procedure?

- What is the likelihood that my varicose veins will recur or that new ones will appear?

What is happening

Varicose veins aren't exactly shy. These bluish, ropelike veins sit just under the surface of the skin, usually on the back of your calves or on the inside of your thighs. Their protruding presence is not only unsightly, it can also be uncomfortable, causing aching or throbbing, or a heavy feeling in your legs. In advanced cases, your skin can itch and become discolored. Ulcers may form over a bulging vein. Also bothersome are spider veins, little webby starbursts of blue and red that often appear around your knees and ankles, but can also show up on your face. While spider veins, medically known as telangiectasia, are usually only a cosmetic problem, sometimes they can make your legs ache.

Varicose veins are due to a malfunction in your circulatory system. After blood has been pumped out to your extremities, it travels against gravity back to your heart, pushed along in rhythmic bursts by tiny valves inside the veins that open and close. When these valves malfunction or wear out, blood flows backward or pools in the veins. This causes varicose veins (*see illustration opposite*).

Varicose veins most frequently show up on your legs, but they can also appear on your feet. They eventually afflict about 50% of women. About 10% to 15% of men get them, too. Aggravating factors include obesity, pregnancy, long-term heavy lifting, and jobs that require you to spend a lot of time on your feet, such as nursing or sales work. People of Irish and German ancestry have a greater risk of malfunctioning valves, as do those who have a family history of varicose veins. Aging is definitely a factor, because the skin's connective tissue becomes less elastic as you get older. Spider veins can also be kick-started by hormonal surges, which are caused by puberty, pregnancy, and hormone replacement therapy.

Treatments

If you have varicose veins, consult your doctor about the best treatment. Don't delay: The earlier you intervene, the easier this condition is to treat. Many people can keep varicose veins from causing problems by making lifestyle changes, including wearing compression stockings, exercising, and taking certain nutrients and herbs. But if your varicose veins are painful or you're sick of always covering up your legs, a number of surgical techniques, including a new procedure using radiowaves, can help. For spider veins, lasers are producing good cosmetic results.

Treatment options

Lifestyle changes

Compression stockings	Support proper functioning of leg veins.
Exercise	Builds calf muscles and aids blood flow.
Don't stand too long	Standing contributes to varicose veins.

Procedures

Vein stripping	Surgically removes large veins.
Radiofrequency closure	Shrinks large veins.
Sclerotherapy and lasers	Treat spider veins.

Natural methods

Vitamins & herbs	Promote good vascular health.

Lifestyle Changes

You may be able to keep varicose veins under control and reduce the risk of getting additional veins by adopting some lifestyle measures. The following strategies are often quite helpful:

- **Wear compression stockings** to help nudge the blood back up to your heart. These knee-high stockings come in a range of sizes and must be fitted to the shape of your legs. You can get them at medical supply stores, or your doctor can prescribe them. Don't worry that they're fashion gone bad: They come in a variety of styles and colors. You may also benefit by having your doctor prescribe Velcro-closing elastic bands designed to go over the specific areas of the leg that cause you problems.

- **Elevate your legs** above your hips several times a day. Keep them there for 10 to 20 minutes. Try not to cross your legs when you sit.

- **Avoid constriction.** Toss out any girdles and other tight, binding garments (such as too-snug belts and too-tight shoes) that put undue pressure on veins anywhere in your body.

- **Get regular exercise.** Building up your calf muscles helps push blood back up to your heart. It's best to stick with low-impact workouts. Swimming and water aerobics are the best activities for varicose veins. The water acts as a giant compression stocking. If the water is cold, it's all the better to tone your muscles. Other good choices are walking (be sure to put on your compression stockings first) and easy bike riding.

- **Lose weight if you need to.** Excess pounds put extra pressure on your legs and veins.

- **Don't stand for long periods.** Standing makes it harder for blood to flow back up to your heart. If you have to stand for a long time, do heel raises and stand on tiptoe to stimulate your calves.

- **Resist the urge to scratch,** even when your veins bother you. Doing so may prompt a skin ulcer. Apply a moisturizing cream, or ask your doctor to prescribe something to soothe the itch.

TAKING Control

- **Beware of female homones.** The estrogen in birth control pills and hormone replacement therapy (HRT) can contribute to varicose and spider veins. If you're taking either of these, ask your doctor about alternatives.

- **Use a cover-up.** Varicose veins can be difficult to eradicate. If you can't get your limbs to look the way you'd like, try leg makeup or a self-tanning product.

- **Pick a trustworthy practitioner.** Lasering and using other techniques to eradicate veins can be tricky. Make sure your doctor has a good track record and is experienced in treating veins of your type.

- **Raise the foot of your bed** by two to four inches so you can sleep with your feet higher than your head. You can do this by placing blocks under the end of the bed. This helps blood flow back to your heart.

VALVE FAILURE

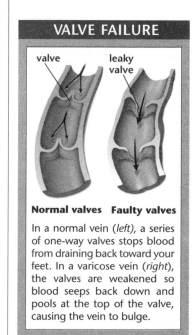

Normal valves   Faulty valves

In a normal vein (*left*), a series of one-way valves stops blood from draining back toward your feet. In a varicose vein (*right*), the valves are weakened so blood seeps back down and pools at the top of the valve, causing the vein to bulge.

FINDING Support

- For more information on varicose vein treatment, contact the American College of Phlebology, an organization of physicians from many specialties who treat venous disorders (510-834-6500 or www.phlebology.org).

- To find referrals to doctors in your area, get in touch with the American Society for Dermatologic Surgery. Call the consumer hotline (847-956-0900) or visit the website (www.asds-net.org).

Procedures

If the appearance of your veins bothers you or they are very uncomfortable, it's best to consult a specialist. General and vascular surgeons typically do major overhauls, such as removing large veins. Dermatologists specialize in spider and other smaller veins. Ask each specialist what the best procedure is for veins of your type. Check out the doctor's success rate with the treatment.

To remove large veins, a procedure called **vein stripping** is traditionally used. This involves opening the largest superficial vein, the saphenous, which extends from your groin to your ankle. Several small incisions are made, and a flexible wire is used to remove the vein. Don't worry that you'll be increasing the load on adjacent veins: The damaged vein has already lost its ability to function, and blood flow has been naturally rerouted. This treatment is most likely to prevent the appearance of new varicose veins. It also requires the longest recuperation (up to two weeks) and leaves the most scarring.

An alternative treatment for large veins near the surface of the skin is **ambulatory phlebectomy,** also called the stab avulsion technique. This mini-stripping procedure involves pulling out large veins through a series of small incisions. It has become increasingly popular because it requires only local anesthesia, causes less discomfort than vein stripping, and involves just one day of rest.

The newest, most advanced procedure for treating large varicose veins is called the **radiofrequency closure technique.** Doctors insert a tiny catheter through a slit in the skin and deliver radiowaves to the vein wall. The vein shrinks and seals shut. Many people choose this method because it causes minimal bruising and normal activities can be resumed immediately.

If you have spider veins or other small veins on your legs, your doctor may recommend **sclerotherapy.** The veins are injected with an agent designed to irritate them, causing the vessel to collapse and glue itself shut. Over time, the veins will be absorbed by the body and disappear. Effectiveness of this procedure is greatly improved with the application of a compression bandage afterward.

Although they can't be used for larger spider veins or varicose veins, **lasers** have revolutionized the treatment of small superficial spider veins on the face or legs. A laser is passed through a small tube inserted in the vein, and laser energy is applied. Many dermatologic surgeons are also using new polarizing scopes to see the veins in 3-D. That means they can zap your vascular firework display at its origin with enhanced accuracy.

Natural Methods*

To boost vein health, take a daily multivitamin that contains **vitamins C and E.** Several herbs are also helpful. **Gotu kola** works to tone surrounding tissues, keep veins flexible, and encourage blood flow. **Horse chestnut seed extract** (sold as Venastat) may reduce vein swelling and inflammation. It's often taken with **bilberry,** an antioxidant herb that appears to enhance blood flow and reinforce vein walls.

Natural methods are not subject to the same testing and regulation as prescription medications. Please seek your doctor's advice and use caution.

Wrinkles

Time, gravity, genes, and sun leave their mark on your face in the form of lines and wrinkles. You can choose to accept them as a badge of experience or banish them, at least temporarily, with an array of ever-evolving weapons.

What is happening

Between the ages of 25 and 65, your skin goes through a lot of changes. Cell division slows and the inner layer of your skin thins. The underlying web of elastin and collagen fibers loosen and uncouple, making your skin less elastic. Fat cells diminish, leaving your skin less plump. Aggravating all of this, sweat and oil-secreting glands wither, depriving your skin of its ability to retain moisture. Moods can leave their mark, too. Frowning or squinting etches vertical furrows between the eyebrows. A lifetime of laughter may engrave two deep parentheses around your mouth and a spray of crow's feet at the corners of your eyes.

Why are some people more lined than others? Genetic makeup and gravity play a role, but the biggest culprit is the sun. Even small exposures can damage critically important collagen fibers. The sun also releases rogue oxygen molecules called free radicals. They wreak havoc on cell membranes, helping create wrinkles. Air pollution and smoking both contribute to wrinkles as well.

Treatments

The treatment you select for your wrinkles will depend on how much you're willing to spend and the downtime you can spare for recovery. Over-the-counter and prescription creams often help hide fine wrinkles. Deeper wrinkles can be filled, zapped with a paralytic agent, or burned or peeled away. For the most dramatic results, you can opt for a facelift. Whatever you decide, you're likely to be footing the bill yourself. Almost no insurance plan covers wrinkle-removing procedures, except in unusual circumstances, such as skin cancer, that requires prophylactic skin-peeling therapy.

Lifestyle Changes

There are strategies you can employ to keep wrinkles from deepening and to slow down the rate at which they show up:

- **Use sunscreen.** Don't go out, even in winter, without slathering on sunscreen (SPF 15 or above) and wearing a wide-brimmed hat.
- **Stop smoking.** Or accept the fact that your wrinkles will get worse. Smoking is terrible for your circulation, thins the skin's outer layer, increases your cancer risk, and forms vertical "lipstick lines" when you purse your lips to smoke. Don't count on a facelift to help: In one survey, 40% of surgeons refused to operate on cigarette smokers because they are notoriously bad healers.

LIKELY First Steps

- **Avoid the sun,** and always **use sunscreen.**
- **Topical creams** to remove fine wrinkles.
- **Skin resurfacing** or **injections** for deeper wrinkles and scars.
- **Facelift** for a more youthful appearance.

QUESTIONS TO Ask

- Which of the new anti-aging therapies is right for my particular skin type?
- How long is the recovery from this procedure? Do I have to take time off from work?
- How many times have you performed the procedure you're suggesting? What are your complication and side effect rates?
- Will the cost of any of these procedures be covered by my health insurance?

TAKING **Control**

- ■ **Make sure your doctor is board certified** with an organization approved by the American Board of Medical Specialties. (The American Board of Plastic Surgery and the American Board of Dermatology are two examples.) Boards not affiliated with the ABMS require much less rigorous training and exam criteria.

- ■ **Request before-and-after pictures** of your doctor's patients who have had the cosmetic procedure you're contemplating. It's also a good idea to get the phone numbers of some of them so you can ask about their experience with the doctor and procedure.

- ■ **Dilute your prescription tretinoin (Retin-A) cream with a moisturizer.** This will not only save you money (a small tube of the medicine may cost more than $60), it will reduce side effects on your skin, including excessive dryness, peeling, redness, blistering, and extreme sensitivity to the sun.

▶**SOME DOCTORS TRY TO TALK PATIENTS into silicone injections for wrinkles, claiming that silicone lasts longer than collagen. Direct silicone injections are not approved by the FDA and are associated with traumatic, face-scarring inflammations and complications ranging from death to embolisms. If your doctor recommends silicone injections, find another doctor.**

Treatment options

Lifestyle changes	
Sunscreen	Protects against future skin damage.
De-stress	Gives skin a healthy "glow."
Medications	
Exfoliants	Remove top layer of wrinkled skin.
Procedures	
Skin resurfacing	Strips off damaged skin so new skin can form.
Implants	Fill in wrinkles and scars.
Botox	Erases wrinkles by relaxing facial muscles.
Facelift/eyelift	Surgery, for more dramatic results.

- ■ **Maintain a steady, healthy weight.** Any abrupt, rapid weight loss compounds shrinkage of the fat cells in your facial skin. That can leave you with baggy-looking skin.
- ■ **De-stress.** Stress leaves souvenirs on your skin in myriad ways. Although de-stressing through exercise, biofeedback, massage, yoga, acupuncture, and even psychotherapy can't elevate sagging tissue, it will make you look healthier and more refreshed.
- ■ **Exercise vigorously on a regular basis.** It not only strengthens and rejuvenates your body, it also helps your skin by revving up circulation. Facial exercises often worsen wrinkles by deepening expression lines.
- ■ **Use a little TLC on your face.** Wash with nonalkaline soap, gently pat dry, and moisturize right away. Occlusives, such as petroleum jelly, are ideal if you have dry skin: They prevent moisture from evaporating from your skin. Water-based moisturizers (which pull moisture up to the surface) are best for oily skin.

Medications

If you want to reduce fine lines and wrinkles, start with products that remove the top layer of skin and allow new skin to grow, a process called **exfoliation.** The best over-the-counter option is **alpha hydroxy acid (AHA).** Derived primarily from fruit and milk sugars (lactic and glycolic acid), AHA may reduce wrinkles by swelling your skin slightly. Exactly how it works is unclear, but because it strips off the upper layer of the skin, it makes your face much more vulnerable to the sun. Apply sunscreen often every day—even if you use AHA only at night.

For a more powerful and effective topical treatment, ask your doctor for a prescription for topical **tretinoin** (Retin-A, Renova). Used regularly, this cream reduces the incidence of large wrinkles, age spots, and surface roughness. It also makes the skin appear plump and glowing (which is why some women wear it under their makeup instead of just applying it at night).

Botox is the most popular cosmetic nonsurgical procedure in the U.S. today. Injections of Botox, or botulinum toxin (in purified and diluted form), work by stopping nerve impulses to injected muscles. Botox (made by Allergan) or Myobloc (produced by Elan Pharmaceutics), relax the muscles and stop your ability to squint or frown without causing numbness.

Physicians can inject Botox into various spots (*see illustration*) including horizontal lines on the forehead, crow's feet, lower eyelids, lines on the side of the nose,

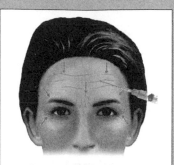

Arrows indicate injection sites

the region between the nose and the upper lip, and occasionally, the muscle bands on the neck. Botox cannot be used for the fur-

rows around your mouth, an area that must remain pliable so you can talk, eat, and pucker up.

Once in a while, physicians "miss" a targeted muscle with the syringe and a patient is left with a droopy eyelid. The desirable effects of the shots disappear in three to six months, as well as these unintended effects.

A Botox injection takes only a few minutes; you see results in one to seven days. Costs for a treatment vary, but average about $400. The injections generally aren't covered by insurance.

Procedures

If you want to erase deeper wrinkles, there are many options. One is **skin resurfacing.** All resurfacing procedures involve burning or stripping off the top layer of damaged, wrinkled skin and controlling healing so that fresh, new skin can form. Generally speaking, the deeper the treatment, the more dramatic the results.

Chemical peels help reduce wrinkles and light scarring. A chemical solution, available in a variety of intensities, is applied to the face. The stronger peels remove deeper wrinkles, but also leave your face red longer. In **dermabrasion,** a rotating brush removes the top layer of skin. This can reach deeper layers of skin than chemical peels and is especially effective at removing heavy wrinkles, disfiguring marks, and scars left by cystic acne. A gentler process, **microdermabrasion,** uses crystals to polish the skin. The results are like that of a mild chemical peel.

Laser resurfacing is popular because it not only eliminates wrinkles, it tightens the skin. Here's how it works: Laser pulses penetrate the skin, vaporizing the surface layer of skin and shortening collagen fibers to restore elasticity. The **carbon dioxide (CO_2) laser** is the most powerful for zapping deep wrinkles. The **erbium: YAG laser** is often used for shallower indentations. After surgery, your face will be swollen and raw for a week or more and can be red for one to four months. Two new technologies are also gaining fans. A procedure called **cold ablation** uses salt water and electricity to vaporize the shallow top layer of the skin while causing minimal damage to surrounding tissues. **Radiofrequency resurfacing,** which uses low radiofrequency energy, shows promise for reducing deep eye and mouth wrinkles with relatively little pain and a short recovery.

There are a variety of **implants** to fill in deep wrinkles and scars, but for any injectable substance, the effects aren't permanent. The procedure will have to be repeated. **Microlipoinjection** entails

Promising
DEVELOPMENTS

■ Until recently, nothing much aside from Botox injections and surgery could really wipe out wrinkles around your eyes. The FDA has granted permission to ICN Pharmaceuticals to market its **NLite laser technology** for lines and wrinkles around the eyes, as well as dermatological time lines elsewhere on the face. Unlike other lasers, the NLite can be controlled so it doesn't damage the delicate skin around the eye while it helps collagen replenish itself. More than one treatment may be required and full results (expect a 50% or so reduction of your crow's feet) aren't seen for 90 days. No anesthesia is required, and you can undertake your normal daily activities immediately.

Natural Erasers

There are a number of natural ways to keep tiny lines at bay. While not panaceas, these approaches are probably worth a try before resorting to more costly treatments.

- **Topical creams.** Regular use of a vitamin E cream with alpha tocopherol may help decrease the length and depth of facial lines. Creams with vitamin C may promote collagen production. Those with coenzyme Q_{10} may reduce crow's feet, and those with alpha-lipoic acid (ALA) or DMAE may help tone saggy skin.

- **Supplements.** Along with a daily multivitamin and a free-radical fighting antioxidant combination containing vitamins A, C, and E, consider short-term use of such skin-promoting supplements as L-glutamine, selenium, and acetyl L-carnitine.

- **Dietary changes.** Eating well is always good for your skin. But what to eat? Doctors' opinions vary, but if you believe Dr. Nicholas Perricone, author of *The Wrinkle Cure,* a diet rich in seafood (salmon in particular) and low in complex carbohydrates (no sugar, alcohol, bagels, and so on) can go a long way toward reducing the cellular inflammation he believes leads to wrinkles. Experiment and see.

FINDING Support

- For more information, visit the websites of the American Academy of Dermatology (www. aad.org) or the American Society for Dermatologic Surgery (www.asds-net.org).

About Eye Procedures

Your eyes usually show your age first, so many people make their initial foray into plastic surgery with an eye-tightening procedure called **blepharoplasty.** Incisions are made into the fold of the upper eyelid (and sometimes in the line under the lower lashes as well). Excess fat is sucked out and extra skin removed. This corrects puffy or drooping eyelids as well as bags and circles under the eyes. Results last from 5 to 10 years.

If you don't have much loose skin, you may be a candidate for a **transconjunctival blepharoplasty,** performed on both the upper and lower eyelids. In this procedure, the incision is made on the inside, and fat is removed from the membrane that lines the eyelids. The incision is sealed with dissolving stitches. It leaves no scars in the nasal area (unlike traditional blepharoplasty) and has a reduced risk of undesirable outcomes, such as pulling down the lower lid too far.

Either of these procedures can be combined with **Botox** or **laser resurfacing.** Some doctors even recommend Botox injections followed by laser resurfacing *instead of* blepharoplasty, suggesting they get better results.

"harvesting" fat from your buttocks, and after processing, injecting it into your face. **Collagen implants** using purified bovine (cow) collagen (Zyderm, Zyplast) are the most popular wrinkle plumpers in the U.S. **Dermalogen,** taken from cadavers, can also be injected into wrinkles. Doctors can even save the "leftovers" from various cosmetic surgeries such as facelifts, then reinject any remaining depressions or furrows with your own personal collagen. It's produced under the name **Autologen.** (If you're about to have a facelift, ask your doctor about this option.)

Synthetic strips of materials such as **Gore-Tex** can be inserted under deep wrinkles with the aid of tiny incisions. Ideally, this suppresses wrinkle formation much longer, but it's also riskier than injectables: The Gore-Tex sometimes migrates, and some people with these implants complain that they look unnatural. Another way to eliminate facial wrinkles is with **Botox,** popular injections of the botulinum toxin (*see box, page 339*).

If your problem is not so much fine lines but saggy skin, you may want to undergo a **facelift,** or rhytidectomy. The best candidate for a facelift has great facial bone structure and some remaining skin elasticity. There are a number of variations on this procedure (full, mid-face, lower) and many different approaches and techniques. Some incorporate less invasive (endoscopic) incisions or involve incisions made with lasers. Before making a decision, consult several surgeons. Ask how each would surgically make you look younger. If you want only your **eyes lifted,** there are several specialized procedures to choose from (*see box above*).

Part II
Everyday Complaints

Everyday
COMPLAINTS

This A-to-Z guide provides treatment information for common ailments that everyone deals with at some point. Most require basic over-the-counter medications or self-care measures; some will eventually disappear on their own. Everyday complaints can occasionally be a sign of a more serious disorder, so it's important to seek a doctor's care if any of these conditions (or other common health problems) persist.

Athlete's Foot

The most common fungal infection of the skin, athlete's foot (*tinea pedis*) typically begins between the toes, causing itching, scaling, and sometimes painful skin breaks. The fungi thrive in cramped, moist places, such as inside shoes and socks.

Medications
▶ The usual treatment is an over-the-counter antifungal cream, lotion, or powder containing an antifungal agent such as clotrimazole. Use creams on the soles of your feet and lotions or powders between your toes.
▶ Also effective are twice-daily, 20-minute soaks in an aluminum acetate solution, such as Domeboro.

Self-care Strategies
■ Keep your feet clean and dry, and change your socks every day.
■ Air your shoes after each use, and don't wear the same pair every day.
■ Go barefoot whenever you can. Opt for sandals or other well-ventilated shoes that allow your feet to breathe.

Duration of Treatment
Symptoms often clear up after 3 days of antifungal treament. Six or more weeks of treatment may be necessary, however, to completely resolve the infection and to prevent a recurrence.

When to Call the Doctor
■ If home treatment does not seem to be working within 4 weeks.
■ If an area becomes red and swollen; it's a sign of a more serious bacterial infection.

Blisters

These fluid-filled bubbles form on the skin in response to injury or irritation— often from ill-fitting shoes, sports equipment, or tools— but also from burns, frostbite, allergic reactions, and infections.

Medications
▶ The best treatment for most blisters is to simply leave them alone to heal themselves. You can keep a blister from breaking with a bandage or by placing a moleskin "doughnut" around it.
▶ If a blister breaks, wash it with soap and water, let it air dry, and apply an OTC antibiotic cream (such as Neosporin).
▶ If a blister swells from irritation and needs to be drained, carefully puncture it with a sterilized needle, leave the top skin layer in place, and cover with antibiotic cream and a sterile bandage.
▶ Topical hydrocortisone products (Bactine) or some calamine lotion may help if the blistered skin itches.

Self-care Strategies
■ Wear shoes that fit and socks that absorb moisture. Protect sensitive skin with gloves, talcum powder, moleskin, or petroleum jelly.

Duration of Treatment
Blisters that do not become infected usually clear up within a few days.

When to Call the Doctor
■ If a blister is large, caused by a burn, or is of unknown origin.
■ If a blister becomes infected (filled with pus) or is red or swollen.
■ If you have other symptoms, such as fever or fatigue.

Burns

Whether caused by heat, chemicals, or electrical current, a burn is classified by how deeply it penetrates. A first-degree burn may be a mild scald or sunburn. A second-degree burn goes deeper, and the skin becomes red and blisters. A third-degree burn, which destroys the skin and underlying tissues (yet because of nerve damage may not be painful), is a medical emergency. Go to a hospital immediately for treatment.

Medications
▶ Put first-degree and minor second-degree burns under cold running water or immerse the burn in a cold-water bath. Let the burn dry, and apply an OTC antibiotic cream. Be careful not to break any blisters. Cover the burn with sterile gauze pads held loosely with tape.

Self-care Strategies
■ Avoid exposing burned skin to sun or hot water.
■ Apply aloe vera gel or vitamin E cream to speed healing.

Duration of Treatment
Most first-degree burns heal within a few days; second-degree burns within 14 days.

When to Call the Doctor
■ If you are in doubt about the severity of a burn.
■ If a burn covers a large area, is very painful (as with severe sunburn), or develops blisters larger than a dime.
■ If the burn is caused by electricity: There may be minimal damage to skin, but considerable internal injury.
■ If there is pus, an unpleasant odor, or fever.

Canker Sores

These tiny, craterlike, painful lesions usually appear on the tongue or inside the lips or cheeks. They can be triggered by irritation—as well as by emotional stress and hormonal changes.

Medications
▶ For pain, apply an ice cube, rinse your mouth with salt water, use an OTC oral anesthetic with benzocaine, or take an OTC pain reliever.
▶ To aid healing, dab sores with a solution of 1 part hydrogen peroxide and 1 part water, or apply a liquid bandage (there are several brands).
▶ For severe sores, your doctor may prescribe an anti-inflammatory steroid gel, a paste with amlexanox (Aphthasol), or a tetracycline antibiotic mouthwash.

Self-care Strategies
■ Avoid foods that are acidic or spicy or that can irritate the tissues of the mouth.
■ Brush your teeth after every meal. Floss daily, and get regular professional cleanings.
■ Reduce stress.

Duration of Treatment
Canker sores usually heal in 5 to 15 days.

When to Call the Doctor
■ If sores cause severe pain or persist for longer than 2 weeks or so.
■ If sores recur frequently, which may signal an allergic reaction, poor immune function, or a vitamin deficiency.
■ If you have a fever of more than 101°F or swollen glands.

Cold Sores

The herpes simplex type 1 virus (HSV-1) causes these small, often painful sores around the mouth or nostrils. Many people have HSV-1, but only some get cold sores, which usually progress from a tingling sensation to a swollen red lump, and after a day or two, to a blister that bursts and crusts.

Medications
▶ Use an OTC antibacterial ointment to prevent infection.
▶ The OTC drug Abreva may reduce healing time.
▶ For frequent outbreaks, your doctor may prescribe an antiviral drug such as acyclovir (Zovirax). Valacyclovir (Valdrex) is approved for once-a-day use.

Self-care Strategies
■ Apply ice at the first sign of a sore to reduce swelling and discomfort.
■ Cold sore blisters are contagious. Avoid touching them or kissing anyone. Do not touch your eyes, which can become infected.
■ Cold sores can be triggered by sun exposure: Wear SPF 15 sunscreen or lip gloss on and around your lips.

Duration of Treatment
Cold sores usually clear up within 7 to 10 days.

When to Call the Doctor
■ If a cold sore persists for more than 2 weeks or if you develop a fever.
■ If you have several outbreaks during one year.
■ If your eyes hurt or are light-sensitive during an outbreak.

Conjunctivitis

This is an infection of the membrane that lines the eyeballs and inner eyelids (the conjunctiva). It causes a sensation of grittiness when blinking, discharge, itching and tearing. Conjunctivitis (aka pinkeye) can be due to a viral or bacterial infection, an irritation, or allergy.

Medications
▶ Both viral and bacterial conjunctivitis are highly contagious, so avoid touching your eyes, and wash your hands frequently.
▶ Prescription antibacterial eye ointment and eyedrops will clear up most bacterial conjunctivitis.
▶ If the cause is an allergy, apply cool compresses to your eyes and take an OTC antihistamine. Use eyedrops to reduce redness and itching. If this conditrion persists, your doctor may prescribe oral antihistamines or corticosteroid eyedrops.

Self-care Strategies
■ If there's discharge, bathe your eyes with warm water and a clean washcloth. Wash your hands afterward.
■ Do not use contact lenses or eye makeup. Do not share washcloths, towels, or eye makeup.

Duration of Treatment
Viral conjunctivitis usually clears up on its own in a week or so. A bacterial infection requires medication from your doctor.

When to Call the Doctor
■ If discharge or redness worsens, or the eye is painful.
■ If your vision is persistently blurry.

Cough

A protective reflex to clear the airways, a cough is usually the result of irritation, an allergy, or an infection such as a cold or the flu. However, a persistent cough could indicate a more serious condition, such as asthma, pneumonia, acute bronchitis, damage from smoking, and rarely, lung cancer, tuberculosis, congestive heart failure, or AIDS.

Medications
Treatment depends on the cause and type of cough. Consult your doctor about any cough that persists for 2 to 3 days without any obvious cause.
▶ If a cough from a cold is bringing up mucus, don't take a suppressant; an expectorant (Triaminic Cold & Cough) will help loosen the phlegm.
▶ For a dry, hacking cough, try a cough suppressant containing dextromethorphan (Sucrets 4-Hour or Vicks 44).

Self-care Strategies
■ To help control coughing caused by postnasal drip or irritation, suck on hard candy or a cough drop.

■ Avoid irritants, especially tobacco smoke.
■ Drink plenty of water to thin secretions. In milder cases, it reduces coughing as effectively as medicines.
■ Use a vaporizer or humidifier, especially at night.

Duration of Treatment
A cough usually subsides on its own.

When to Call the Doctor
■ If a cough is severe or accompanied by such symptoms as chest pain, green or yellow phlegm, coughed-up blood, or difficulty breathing.
■ If a cough from a cold or flu isn't gone in 3 weeks.

Diarrhea

The common type of diarrhea is characterized by unformed, watery stools and frequent bowel movements. It's often accompanied by intestinal gas, cramping, and nausea.

Medications
▶ Diarrhea actually helps rid your body of the irritants or infectious agents causing the upset, so wait several hours before taking medication.
▶ OTC products for simple diarrhea contain loperamide (Imodium A-D) and bismuth subsalicylate (Pepto-Bismol). Diphenoxylate hydrochloride (Lomotil) is an effective prescription drug.

Self-care Strategies
■ To prevent dehydration, drink as much clear liquid—water, broth—as your stomach will tolerate.

■ For severe diarrhea (defined as more than 10 watery bowel movements in 24 hours), drink an oral rehydration solution (½ teaspoon salt and 4 teaspoons sugar in a quart of water) or Gatorade to replace needed electrolytes.

■ Do not eat until you feel better, then consume only rice or rice cereal, clear liquids, or flavored gelatin.

Duration of Treatment
Most diarrhea is short-lived.

When to Call the Doctor
■ If you suspect diarrhea is caused by a medication.

■ If diarrhea lasts more than 48 hours (24 hours in a child under age 2) or is accompanied by severe abdominal cramping, fever, dizziness, or blood or pus in the stool.

■ If you have frequent bouts of diarrhea.

Fever

You're considered to have a fever if your body temperature is 100°F or above You may feel cold at first, then hot, then cold again, as your body strives to fight off infection or heal an injury.

Medications
▶ Fever is an effective immune system response to infection, so don't try to quell it too soon. If your fever is mild and no other problems exist, just drink fluids and rest.

▶ If your temperature goes above 102°F, an OTC painkiller can help relieve recurrent chills and lower your body temperature.

Self-care Strategies
■ If you're shivering, don't bundle up—that will only cause the fever to go up.

■ If you have a fever of over 103°F, soak in a tub of tepid water to help bring it down.

■ Drink lots of fluids; rest and sleep as much as possible.

Duration of Treatment
Most fevers go away in just a few days.

When to Call the Doctor
■ If you have a temperature above 104°F.

■ If your fever lasts more than 48 hours or is recurrent.

■ If an infant younger than 6 months has fever; or if a child under 1 year has a fever that lasts more than 24 hours.

■ If a temperature of 103°F or higher doesn't respond to home treatment within 2 hours.

Headache

The garden-variety tension headache—a dull, steady pain in the forehead, temples, back of the neck, or throughout the head—is caused by muscle contraction. (*For other types of headache, see pages 228–231.*)

Medications
▶ OTC painkillers (aspirin, ibuprofen, and acetaminophen) usually provide relief. If one type doesn't work, when it's time to take another pill, try a different kind.

Self-care Strategies
■ You can prevent headaches by reducing stress and tension: Take frequent breaks from desk and computer work, practice relaxation techniques, exercise regularly, and seek emotional support.

■ Once you have a headache, lie down and rest, or sit quietly with your eyes closed, breathing deeply.

■ Gently massage the muscles of your shoulders, neck, and head.

Duration of Treatment
Most tension headaches clear up quickly, although some can last for days at a time.

When to Call the Doctor
■ If you have frequent or long-lasting headaches.

■ If a severe headache comes on quickly.

■ If a headache occurs after strenuous exercise, which might indicate an internal head injury.

■ If headache is accompanied by dizziness, inflamed sinuses, fever and neck stiffness, slurred speech or confusion, or symptoms of depression.

Hemorrhoids

Also known as piles, hemorrhoids are swollen veins either inside the rectum or just outside the anus. They can cause discomfort or minor bleeding during a bowel movement.

Medications
▶ To help ease irritation and itching, you can use petroleum jelly, zinc oxide paste, hemorrhoid creams that contain lidocaine, hydrocortisone preparations, or cotton pads soaked with witch hazel.

▶ OTC suppositories may help ease discomfort, but should not be used repeatedly.
▶ Unless your doctor prescribes laxatives, don't take them. They may cause diarrhea and further irritation.

Self-care Strategies
■ Use an ice pack, or sit in a warm-water bath two or three times a day to relieve itching and discomfort.
■ If an internal hemorrhoid protrudes, push it gently back into the anal canal. You can do this while taking a shower.
■ Keep the anal area clean using moist, soft toilet paper or premoistened wipes.
■ Avoid constipation: Drink plenty of water. Gradually increase fiber in your diet, and exercise every day.

Duration of Treatment
A combination of medication and self-care measures usually relieves hemorrhoids in just a few days.

When to Call the Doctor
■ The first time you notice bleeding and suspect that you have a hemorrhoid.
■ If bleeding from a hemorrhoid continues for more than a week or if bleeding is occurring between bowel movements.
■ If there is constant pain or persistent bleeding.

Indigestion
This common eating-related condition involves pain or discomfort in the upper abdomen. Typical triggers are overeating, eating too fast, spicy or fatty foods, smoking, alcoholic or caffeinated beverages, painkillers or other medications, and stress or anxiety. (*See also Heartburn, page 161.*)

Medications
▶ Your doctor may prescribe medication if there's a problem with the digestive squeezing action of the stomach.
▶ Antacids are not recommended: Excess stomach acid does not usually cause or result from indigestion.

Self-care Strategies
■ Most indigestion can be solved by eating sensibly and slowly, staying away from known triggers, and taking time to relax.
■ Drinking chamomile or fresh ginger tea may help settle your stomach.
■ Walking after eating is good for the digestive process. Don't exercise vigorously until 3 hours after a heavy meal.

Duration of Treatment
A stomachache usually goes away in an hour or two.

When to Call the Doctor
■ If a stomachache lasts longer than 6 hours, or you have frequent indigestion.
■ If you have vomiting, a change in bowel movements, weight loss, or appetite loss.
■ If you suspect medication is causing the indigestion.
■ If indigestion is accompanied by shortness of breath, sweating, or pain radiating to the jaw, neck, or arm. This could be a heart attack.

Insect Bites and Stings
While annoying and painful, insect and spider bites and bee stings are usually harmless. In susceptible people, some stings and bites can provoke an allergic reaction so severe that the person goes into extreme, life-threatening shock.

Medications
▶ OTC anti-inflammatory drugs (aspirin, ibuprofen) can help relieve pain.
▶ To reduce pain and itching, use an ointment with a combination of an antihistamine, analgesic, and corticosteroid, or a spray containing a topical analgesic (Benadryl).
▶ If you've had an allergic reaction, carry an emergency kit (a syringe with epinephrine) whenever you are outdoors.

Self-care Strategies
■ Remove a bee stinger at once by scraping it out with a clean, sharp blade, a credit card, or long fingernail (don't pull the stinger, as that releases more venom). Wash the area with soap and water.
■ Run the sting or bite under cold water or apply an ice pack to it.
■ Apply a paste of baking soda, meat tenderizer containing papain, and water to relieve pain.

Duration of Treatment
Swelling usually subsides within 48 hours; itching may need to be treated over a somewhat longer period.

When to Call the Doctor

■ If there's any unusual reaction (such as trouble breathing or swallowing), call 911 or go to a hospital emergency room immediately.

■ If localized redness or swelling doesn't subside within 72 hours or a fever develops.

Motion Sickness

Uncomfortable and sometimes debilitating, motion sickness is the loss of equilibrium that results from riding in cars, boats, planes, or on amusement park rides. Dizziness, headache, nausea, and sometimes vomiting result.

Medications

The best treatment comes before you travel.

▶ OTC antihistamines such as cyclizine (Marezine), dimenhydrinate (Dramamine), and diphenydramine (Benadryl), and the antivertigo agent meclizine (Antivert) relieve symptoms of motion sickness; take them 30 to 60 minutes before traveling.

▶ A sedative or tranquilizer may help prevent air sickness.

▶ Your doctor may prescribe the antinausea drug scopolamine, which is delivered by a patch behind your ear. It lasts 72 hours.

▶ Special acupressure wrist bands (Sea-Band and others) that apply pressure to the inside of the wrist reduce symptoms in some people.

▶ Capsules containing dried ginger may prevent or relieve nausea. You can also try drinking fresh ginger tea.

Self-care Strategies

■ To maintain your equilibrium in a car or on a boat, focus on the horizon or some fixed, distant point.

■ In a plane or car, lean back, relax, and don't read.

■ Before travel, eat only small amounts. Avoid alcohol.

■ Don't sit in smoky spaces.

■ Dry crackers and a noncarbonated drink can help settle your stomach.

Duration of Treatment

Some people adapt to the motion. Others feel sick as long as the trip lasts.

When to Call the Doctor

■ If you're often bothered by motion sickness, get advice on prevention.

Sore Throat

The scratchy, burning sensation and redness of a sore throat is most often caused by a cold or flu virus. It may also be the result of a bacterial infection (most commonly "strep throat"), which must be treated with antibiotics.

Medications

▶ To ease sore throat discomfort, take an OTC painkiller.

▶ If a bacterial infection is suspected, your doctor will take a culture, and if it's strep, prescribe an antibiotic such as penicillin or erythromycin.

Self-care Strategies

■ Drink plenty of fluids, especially hot or very cold drinks.

■ Gargle with a solution made by mixing ½ teaspoon salt in a glass of warm water.

■ Suck on a lozenge or hard candy, or chew sugarless gum, to stimulate saliva.

■ Avoid tobacco smoke, and don't drink any alcohol.

■ Rest your voice at every opportunity.

Duration of Treatment

Most viral infections clear up in a few days or a week. For strep throat, be sure to take the antibiotic for the prescribed time, even if your symptoms have subsided.

When to Call the Doctor

■ If the sore throat is severe and you have a fever that is over 101°F.

■ If any kind of throat discomfort lasts more than 2 weeks.

■ Seek emergency care immediately if you have trouble swallowing liquids or difficulty breathing.

Toenail Fungus

The fungus may first appear as a small white or yellow spot on a nail. Eventually the nail becomes dry, thickened, or discolored. There may be scaliness on the surrounding skin.

Medications

See your doctor at the first sign of infection: A lab culture helps determine the best treatment.

▶ Ciclopirox, sold as Penlac Nail Lacquer, may be applied for up to 48 weeks.

▶ Oral antifungal medications such as itraconazole (Sporanox) and terbinafine (Lamisil) are usually effective, but must be taken for 3 to 4 months.

Self-care Strategies
The best defense is prevention: Follow the self-care strategies for Athlete's Foot (*see page 342*). In addition:
■ Don't share socks, shoes, nail clippers, or nail files with other people.
■ Use shower shoes or sandals in spas or pool areas used by others.
■ Don't attempt to dig out an ingrown toenail.
■ Disinfect pedicure tools with alcohol after every use, and air dry for 1½ hours.

Duration of Treatment
Even if treatment is effective, infection may recur and need to be treated again.

When to Call the Doctor
■ If you have an ingrown toenail or any portion of a toenail has become discolored or abnormally thick.
■ If any problem with your feet makes walking painful.

Warts
These benign skin growths are caused by certain strains of the human papilloma virus (HPV). They usually appear on hands and fingers, but also can grow on the bottoms of the feet (plantar warts), where they can be painful. As people grow older, they usually develop an immunity to the virus.

Medications
▶ Try an OTC salicylic acid treatment to remove a wart; be sure to protect the surrounding skin with petroleum jelly or a corn pad.
▶ Your doctor may recommend seeing a dermatologist to remove bothersome or painful warts. Methods include: freezing with liquid nitrogen, burning off with a laser, cutting off with a scalpel, or electrosurgery.

Self-care Strategies
■ One popular remedy is to tape a wart with waterproof or silver duct tape. Leave the tape on for a week and remove; repeat until the wart disappears.

Duration of Treatment
■ With salicylic acid, it can take many weeks before you see results.
■ Even when warts go away, they may recur.

When to Call the Doctor
■ If you or your sexual partner have warts around the genital/anal area.
■ If you have warts on your face.
■ If you are over age 45 and develop a wart or if you have a weakened immune system and develop any unusual skin growth.

Yeast Infection
Most women will experience the itching and burning of a yeast infection, which is an overgrowth of the *Candida albicans* fungus that normally lives in the vagina. Anything that upsets the balance of vaginal organisms—taking antibiotics or steroid medications, pregnancy, a weakened immune system, fatigue or stress, or poor hygiene—can trigger a yeast infection.

Medications
▶ Treatment with an OTC anti-yeast preparation inserted into the vagina is usually effective, but only if you actually have a yeast infection and not another form of vaginitis. See your doctor if OTC drugs don't help.
▶ An antifungal pill called fluconazole (Diflucan) is often prescribed. It is faster-acting than OTC products.

Self-care Strategies
■ Do not douche or use feminine sprays.
■ Wear "breathable" underwear. Avoid tight pants or sitting in a wet bathing suit.

Duration of Treatment
Vaginal medications are taken over several days; a fluconazole pill usually clears symptoms in 24 to 48 hours. Recurrent infections require longer treatment.

When to Call the Doctor
■ If you are pregnant and have symptoms of vaginal infection.
■ If you have recurring vaginal infections.
■ If your "yeast infection" does not respond to an OTC antifungal medication in 3 to 4 days.
■ If you develop any abdominal pain or a fever higher than 101°F.

Part III
Preventive Tests

Improving Your Odds

W hether you're perfectly healthy, dealing with an illness, or at high risk for developing one, regular checkups and specific screening tests are essential for spotting potential problems and staying well.

Without exception, experts will tell you that one way to effectively combat disease is to find it early and treat it promptly. Survival statistics for the major diseases bear this out. The problem is that you may not have overt symptoms—or even subtle warnings—that something is out of whack. That's why this book includes a section on preventive tests. The fact is, screening tests such as Pap smears, mammograms, colonoscopies, and standard blood work (along with regular checkups and immunizations) are your best chance at a personal early warning system. They're invaluable in helping your doctors spot and solve a problem before it gets out of hand. Having these tests at the right times ups your odds for enjoying a long, healthy life.

A recent government study, however, found that more than half of all Americans are not getting these essential tests as often as they should. The reasons are many: lack of insurance, fear of the results, confusion over which tests are needed and how often. It can be tough to figure out just what the best timetable is. Government agencies, professional health associations, and nonprofit groups all issue differing guidelines.

Among the most highly regarded are recommendations from the U.S. Preventive Services Task Force (USPSTF), a government-sponsored group of experts who have reviewed and updated evidence about common screening tests since the 1980s. While various medical specialty groups haven't always agreed with USPSTF findings (e.g., how often a man should have a PSA test for prostate cancer or a woman, a mammogram), USPSTF reports offer a good place to start.

Medical experts do agree that not everyone needs to have the same battery of tests. Your doctor will probably recommend only targeted screenings based on your age, sex, risk factors, and other medical conditions, rather than follow the sweeping guidelines that once lumped everyone into the same category.

8 Stats You Need to Know

To get a quick grasp of how you're doing health-wise, you should keep track of the following numbers (put them on your Palm Pilot if you have to). If you don't know what they are, start by calling your doctor for the results of your last physical.

- **Blood pressure:** Aim for "normal": 120/80.
- **Blood type:** A handy stat for emergencies.
- **Body Mass Index:** See page 355 to find yours.
- **Cholesterol levels:** Total, LDL, and HDL.
- **Dosages:** For all medications you're taking.
- **Resting heart rate:** Check when you wake up.
- **Target heart rate:** Need this when exercising.
- **Weight:** Step on the scale regularly.

About the Tests and Guidelines

On the following pages, you'll find information on what to expect from a routine physical as well as concise descriptions of more than 20 commonly recommended screening tests, ranging from blood pressure measurement to vision testing. Many of these tests are part of your routine physical, but some (such as a colonoscopy and mammogram) may require a specialist. Although modern screenings are less invasive than ever, some still pose real and serious risks. It's simply good sense to get a full explanation from a doctor, nurse practitioner, or other medical professional before undergoing any procedure. The chart on the opposite page offers a general timetable for various tests. If you've had a particular ailment or have a family history of one, you're considered "high risk" and will need more frequent testing.

ADULT PREVENTIVE SCREENING GUIDELINES

This information is based on widely respected recommendations.* For optimal health, however, you should set up a personal schedule with your doctor, based on your medical history and needs.

Test/Exam	When to Get Tested	If You're at High Risk
Routine		
Full Physical Exam and Medication Review	Every 2 years until age 50; yearly after age 50.	Every 6 months or more often at doctor's discretion.
Blood Pressure	Every 2 years if normal; more if borderline.	Daily to weekly self-monitoring.
Cholesterol Measurement	Every 5 years.	Every 3 to 6 months.
Glucose Measurement	Every 3 years after 45.	At doctor's discretion.
Hearing Tests	Every 1 to 2 years, especially after 75.	At doctor's discretion.
Hemoglobin (blood) Test	Every 5 years after 20.	At doctor's discretion.
Sexually Transmitted Disease Testing	Every year, if sexually active with multiple partners.	Every 3 to 4 months.
Stress Test	Baseline: Age 40 for men, 50 for women.	Every 6 to 12 months, if needed.
Vision Testing	Every 5 years; 1 to 2 years after 50.	More than once a year, if needed.
Cancer Detection		
Breast Cancer Exam a) Self-Exam b) Clinical Breast Exam c) Mammography	a) Every month after 20. b) Every 3 years, 20 to 40; yearly after 40. c) Every 1 to 2 years after 40; less after 70.	a) Every month. b) Every 6 months or more. c) At doctor's discretion.
Colonoscopy	Every 5 to 10 years after 50.	Every 1 to 3 years.
Digital Rectal Exam	Every year as of 50.	More frequently, if needed.
Pap Test and Pelvic Exam	Pap: Every 2 or 3 years if results are normal. Pelvic: Every 3 years, 18 to 39; yearly after 40.	Pap: Every 6 months. Pelvic: Annually.
Sigmoidoscopy	Every 3 to 5 years as of 50 with stool FOB.	Discuss with doctor.
Skin Cancer Exam a) Self-Exam b) Dermatologist-Directed	a) Every 6 months. b) Every 3 years 20 to 40; yearly after 40.	a) Monthly. b) Every year or more frequently.
Stool Test with Fecal Occult Blood (FOB) Test	Every year after 50.	Discuss more frequent testing with your doctor.
Testicular Self-Exam	Every month from 15 to 40.	Monthly starting at an early age.
Other		
Bone Density	At doctor's discretion.	Every 1 to 5 years; often over 65.
Genetic Testing	Any age.	Discuss with doctor if you have a family history of a specific disease.

*Derived primarily from guidelines issued by the U.S. Preventive Services Task Force, the American College of Physicians, the National Cholesterol Education Program, the American Cancer Society, and the National Cancer Institute.

Routine Physical Exam

Not so long ago, a routine physical was a fairly straightforward affair. Every year, you went to your doctor for a comprehensive battery of tests and an unhurried, hands-on examination, a practice long endorsed by the American Medical Association (AMA) for everyone over the age of 35. In the 1980s, the AMA changed its recommendation to a checkup every 5 years for those under 40 and every 1 to 3 years thereafter. Today, the AMA has stopped recommending a standard interval for a routine physical. Instead, it states that age, sex, general health, medical history, and other personal concerns dictate when you need one.

In fact, in this era of managed care and cost containment, it's unlikely that you'll receive the comprehensive annual checkup of yesteryear: It's simply too expensive for the relatively few results your doctor will obtain. Some tests that were common in the past, such as chest x-rays, electrocardiograms (ECGs or EKGs), complete blood counts, and urinanalyses, are no longer routinely recommended for healthy adults. These tests are still important, however, if you are at high risk for a particular condition, either because of symptoms, lifestyle, obesity, a personal or family history of the disease, or other reasons. Many preventive tests and treatments, such as blood pressure checks, cholesterol measurements, Pap smears, and vaccinations, are still cost-effective interventions for preventing disease.

About the Exam. Taking your medical history and giving you a routine physical exam offers your doctor a unique opportunity to assess your overall health. Periodic checkups are also a good time for you and your doctor to talk openly and build a partnership. You should discuss any health problems or lifestyle concerns you may have, and ask the doctor for specific tips on staying healthy. Among the components of a routine physical are:

- Review of specific symptoms you may have experienced since your last exam.
- Discussion of any known family predisposition to particular medical conditions.

- Complete physical examination with visual observation, hands-on palpation, and listening through a stethoscope (auscultation).
- Education about hygiene and other habits.
- Immunizations, as required, to prevent infectious diseases (*see box opposite*).
- Screening tests for early detection of illness.

How Is It Done? During a routine visit, your doctor will ask you questions, examine your body, order appropriate tests, prescribe treatment, and offer advice. A typical checkup includes many or all of the following components:

Questions about personal and family history. Especially on your first visit, your doctor will ask you at length about illnesses you've had in the past, about any medical problems that may be affecting your close relatives, and about lifestyle issues (stressors, unhealthy habits, diet) that are of concern. The history will also include a series of questions about the many different parts of your body, as well as questions about any allergies you may have and your mental health. Your doctor will also address any current health issues.

Physical exam. To assess your physical health, the doctor will probably:

- Measure your height and weight, which determines your Body Mass Index (*see page 355*).
- Take your pulse and blood pressure (*see page 354*).
- Listen to your heartbeat, the blood vessels in your neck, and breath sounds.
- Check your reflexes, joints and range of motion, spinal alignment, and balance.
- Feel for lymph nodes or swellings in the neck, armpits, groin, abdomen, and other areas.
- Palpate the thyroid at the base of your neck.
- Feel for any hernia in the groin region.
- Examine your skin, mouth, gums, and throat.

Mental health exam. You will be asked about your overall mood and whether or not you're having any problems with depression or anxiety. The doctor may perform tests to assess your memory.

Medications review. Your doctor will need to know about any medications you take. Be sure to mention all prescription and over-the-counter drugs as well as any vitamins, herbs, or other dietary supplements. If you are taking a number of medicines, bring them to your appointment in a paper bag for an annual "brown bag review."

Lifestyle concerns. The doctor will also bring up various lifestyle and safety matters, including the following:

- Do you smoke or use other tobacco products or illicit drugs?
- If you drink alcohol, how much?
- Are you sexually active?
- How much exercise do you get?
- What is your typical diet?
- How much sleep do you get?
- Do you wear a seat belt? A bike helmet?
- Are you regularly exposed to any toxins, such as solvents or asbestos?
- What has caused stress in your life since your last exam?

Additional tests. Your doctor will likely order a number of routine blood tests. These generally include the following:

- A complete blood count (CBC) to determine if you are anemic and if you have the normal number of red and white cells.

- A chemistry profile to check your blood sugar levels for signs of diabetes, as well as your liver and kidney function.
- A lipid profile to check levels of total cholesterol, LDL ("bad") and HDL ("good") cholesterol, and triglycerides, which comprise much of the fat stored in the human body.

Various other tests. A number of very targeted tests, which are detailed on pages 354–367, also may be performed or scheduled to screen for diseases or assess therapies. Your doctor or a nurse practitioner may perform the test directly or you may be referred to a specialist.

You'll Need a Physical More Often If . . .

▶ **You've been diagnosed with a medical condition. (The type of exam you receive, and how often, will depend on the nature of your illness and its treatment.)**

▶ **You're taking medications that require regular blood tests to check blood count and detect liver or kidney problems. (At doctor's discretion.)**

▶ **You have a potentially recurrent disease like cancer. (Your doctor will establish a schedule and routine that is right for you.)**

Vaccinations You May Need

Vaccines create immunity by boosting the body's natural immune response. Their benefits outweigh the risks in most cases.

Tetanus booster
Every ten years, you should get a shot to protect against tetanus (lockjaw), even if you're over 50.

Flu shot
Immunizations for the flu (influenza) are given each year in the fall before the start of flu season. You should get a flu shot if you are 65 or older or if you have a chronic lung ailment (such as asthma or emphysema), heart disease, diabetes, sickle-cell

anemia, or cancer. These conditions put you at high risk for flu complications. Younger adults may also benefit from a flu shot.

Pneumococcal vaccine
To prevent pneumonia and infections of the blood or brain, you should get a pneumococcal vaccine after age 65. You should also be immunized if you are under age 65 and have heart, kidney, liver, or lung disease, diabetes, Hodgkin's, or an immune system disorder. One shot usually gives lifelong protection; boosters may be recommended after 6 years for those at high risk.

Rubella vaccine
If you are a woman of childbearing age, you should be immunized against rubella (German measles). The shot is not recommended during pregnancy.

Hepatitis B vaccine
Children and infants are now routinely immunized against hepatitis B. Young adults and others at high risk should also be immunized.

Other immunizations
Special immunizations can protect against infectious diseases such as diphtheria, meningitis, typhoid, and chicken pox.

Blood Pressure Measurement

Optimal blood pressure for an adult is 120 systolic over 80 diastolic. Your blood pressure should be checked regularly to confirm that it hasn't strayed too far from these ideal numbers. If it rises very high (hypertension), you run a risk of serious health problems, such as heart disease and stroke.

About the Test. Blood pressure readings are expressed in millimeters of mercury (mm Hg). The first and higher number is the systolic pressure—the highest pressure exerted on your arterial walls as the heart contracts to pump blood out. The second, lower number is the diastolic pressure. That's the moment of lowest pressure, when the heart relaxes between contractions. (*See High Blood Pressure, page 170, for more information.*)

How Is It Done? The traditional way to measure blood pressure involves placing a cuff attached to a pressure gauge (sphygmomanometer) around your upper arm. The cuff is inflated with a hand-operated bulb pump. A stethoscope is inserted under the edge of the cuff, on the inside of the elbow. The cuff is then slowly deflated by squeezing the bulb. The numbers on the dial when the thumping sounds begin and end correspond to your systolic and diastolic pressures.

How Often Is It Needed? If you're healthy and your blood pressure is normal, you should have it tested every 2 years.

You'll Need Annual Testing If . . .

► Your blood pressure has been high-normal in the past (130 to 139 systolic with 85 to 89 diastolic).
► You're overweight or sedentary.
► You have a family history of hypertension.
► You're African-American.

You'll Need Weekly or Daily Testing If . . .

► Your blood pressure has been 140 or higher systolic, 90 or higher diastolic. This determines whether lifestyle measures and/or medications are working effectively.

Blood Pressure Monitors for Home Use

Checking your blood pressure at home can help you determine whether or not it's under control. Whichever monitor you buy, take it in to your next doctor's visit to make sure it's accurate. Be aware that stress, exhaustion, drinking caffeinated beverages prior to the reading, recent exercise, and other factors can alter readings. Four types of home monitor are available:

Aneroid manometer. This inexpensive unit relies on a stethoscope (sometimes built-in) and a handheld bulb pump to inflate and deflate the arm cuff. The reading, which is generally accurate, is displayed on a numbered dial. Check its accuracy after purchase, then annually. If your hearing is impaired or your hand dexterity poor, this monitor can be difficult to use.

Digital manometer. Powered by batteries, this monitor automatically inflates and deflates an arm cuff at the push of a button. The result is displayed on a digital screen. It's also available as a portable monitor that you wear for 24 hours and that automatically takes readings at regular intervals. This manometer is easy to use and recommended for those whose hearing or vision is impaired or who have wide variations in basic blood pressure levels.

Wrist manometer. This battery-powered cuff is placed on the wrist and automatically inflates and deflates with the push of a button; the result is displayed on a monitor. It's easy to use and conveniently small and portable, but readings can be inaccurate (especially the diastolic, or lower, number). To improve the reading, hold your wrist at heart level.

Mercury sphygmomanometer. Used for decades in doctor's offices, hospitals, and clinics, this monitor can also be used at home. It is accurate, but can be difficult to to handle (you'll probably need assistance). Because a small but real risk of mercury spill exists with this unit, you may prefer another type.

Body Mass Index

About the Index. In recent years, the Body Mass Index (BMI), which evaluates weight in relation to height, has become the medical standard for measuring weight and obesity. The BMI quickly determines (beyond the scales) if you are carrying too much weight. It can also be a predictor of heart disease, high blood pressure, diabetes, and other health problems related to excess weight.

How Is It Done? Your BMI is calculated using a complicated mathematical formula. To save time, most doctors use a quick chart like the graph at right. You can find your BMI yourself as well: Simply locate your weight at the bottom of the graph, go straight up to the line that matches your height, then find your BMI range. A "healthy weight" is a BMI of between 18.5 and 25. Between 25 and 29 is considered moderately overweight and above 30, severely overweight (or obese). For a man or woman who is 5'6" tall, that works out to a healthy range of 118 to 155 pounds, with obesity starting at 179.

How Often Is It Needed? If you need to lose weight, use this tool often to chart your progress.

A Note of Caution

▶ If your BMI is 30 or more, you may need medications and if you're more than 100 pounds overweight, surgery. (See Obesity, page 236.)

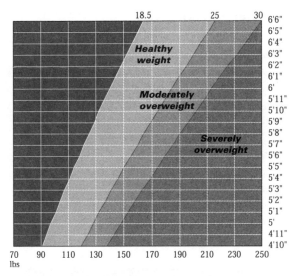

Bone Density Test

About the Test. A bone density test is used to measure bone mass, or how dense and strong your bones are. It helps determine your risk for broken bones (fractures), spinal abnormalities, and osteoporosis (bone-thinning disease) and assess your response to bone-building treatments.

How Is It Done? There are several types of bone density tests. The most accurate, called DEXA, uses x-rays to detect bone thinning, most commonly in the hip or spine. Portable office-based machines that use x-rays or sound waves can measure density in smaller bones such as the finger, wrist, heel, or shin. Your results are compared with peak bone densities expected in a young adult. A deviation from the norm of 1.0 to 2.5 is a warning sign that your bones are thinning. A score greater than 2.5 indicates osteoporosis.

How Often Is It Needed? Routine bone density testing is controversial, because it can be expensive. However, many experts now recommend that women 65 and older be routinely screened.

You'll Need This Test More Often If . . .

▶ You've had a fracture. (At doctor's discretion.)

▶ You're perimenopausal or menopausal and don't get enough calcium. (Annually.)

▶ You're a postmenopausal woman with risk factors for osteoporosis. (Annually or every few years.)

▶ You're over age 60 and overweight or take estrogen. (Annually or every few years.)

▶ You have osteoporosis. (Every year or two to see if you are responding to treatment. With the information gathered, you and your doctor can decide how to move forward with treatment.)

Breast Cancer Testing

The three basic screening tests for breast cancer are the self-exam, the clinical breast exam, and mammography. Increased use of these techniques, combined with improved treatments, has led to earlier detection of breast tumors and a dramatic improvement in the cure rate for breast cancer.

Breast Self-Exam

About the Test. This is a simple five-minute procedure that you can do at home to check for abnormalities. Countless breast tumors are detected by women who perform self-exams, but they are not a substitute for regular mammography.

How Is It Done? First, do a visual inspection. Stand in front of a mirror with your arms at your sides, checking each breast for any lumps, dimpling, swelling, or new differences in size or shape. Repeat with your arms raised and hands clasped behind your head, elbows pressed forward.

The second part of a breast self-exam involves the careful and systematic palpation of your breasts using one of the three palpation patterns illustrated below—up and down, spiral, or pie-shaped wedges. Be sure to use the same pattern each month. Start by raising your left arm over your head. Using three or four fingers of your right hand, feel for any unusual lumps or thickening. Be sure to use the pads of your fingers (not the tips), and press firmly enough to feel all levels of your breast tissue. Next, feel the area between the breast and underarm, then examine the underarm itself. Squeeze the nipple gently to check for any discharge or fluid. Repeat the steps above on your right breast.

Finally, lie down on your back, your left arm raised and a rolled-up towel or pillow under your left shoulder. Repeat the palpation, as above.

How Often Is It Needed? The American Cancer Society recommends that all women age 20 and older perform breast self-exams monthly. A good time to do it is at the end of your period, when the breasts usually aren't swollen or tender.

BREAST PALPATION PATTERNS

Check your breasts every month using one of these three palpation techniques.

Up and down

Spiral

Proper hand position

Wedges

Clinical Breast Exam

About the Test. This is a physical examination and breast palpation performed by a doctor.

How Is It Done? In a clinical breast exam, the doctor palpates your breasts and under your arms to check for any lumps or changes. Doctors have experience in feeling for tumors and can usually differentiate normal from abnormal lumps. The next time you have a clinical breast exam, ask your doctor to show you how to feel the difference between normal and abnormal lumps so you can learn to detect any suspicious areas.

How Often Is It Needed? Women age 20 and over should get a clinical breast exam every 3 years. Beginning at age 40, clinical breast exams should be performed every year.

Mammography

About the Test. Mammography is currently the best tool available for detecting breast cancer at an early stage, when it is most curable. The technique records x-ray images of the breast on film, which can then be read by a radiologist. Areas of increased density or with calcium deposits may be signs of a tumor and may require a follow-up with a biopsy or other procedure. A mammogram can detect tumors one-quarter of an inch in size, considerably smaller than can be felt by touch. Early detection is critical, because it allows many women the option of being treated with a breast-conserving lumpectomy (surgical removal of just the tumor and some surrounding tissue) rather than more extensive removal of breast tissue.

How Is It Done? Choose a facility that does a high volume of mammograms; the readings tend to be more accurate. You'll undress from the waist up, then sit or stand, while one breast at a time is flattened between two plates. The procedure takes about 15 minutes and may cause some discomfort. Let the technician know about any breast problems you may have or if you are pregnant.

A new technique called digital mammography captures x-ray images on computer rather than on film. It shows promise for improving detection of breast tumors. Because it allows for digital enhancement of the x-rays, even very small tumors can be spotted. It also lowers the number of false-positive results (lesions that look suspicious but turn out to be non cancerous). Another plus for this new technology: The images can easily be e-mailed for review by specialists at distant medical centers.

How Often Is It Needed? For women age 40 and older, a mammogram every 1 to 2 years is recommended. After age 70, your doctor may order them less often.

You'll Need These Tests More Often If . . .
▶ You have had a previous diagnosis of breast cancer.
▶ You have a strong family history of the disease.
▶ You have cysts, areas of calcification, or other signs or symptoms.
▶ ALL OF THE ABOVE: A biannual Pap test and clinical exam; a mammogram at your doctor's discretion.

Related Breast-Screening Tests

Magnetic Resonance Imaging
An MRI is an advanced technique using radio waves and magnetic fields to generate computerized images of the breast. The procedure is costly (although usually covered by insurance) and requires lying still for up to 90 minutes inside the cylindrical MRI machine. (If you're claustrophobic, look for an "open" MRI machine.) A breast MRI can be useful for follow-up if a suspicious area is found during mammography or palpation and for screening women who have had silicone breast implants, which can make mammography difficult.

MRI also helps determine a cancer stage or whether more than one tumor is present—critical in treatment planning.

Ultrasound
Also called sonography, ultrasound uses sound waves to take a 3-D picture of the breast. The skin is covered with a gel, then an instrument called a transducer is passed over the breast. Ultrasound may be useful for evaluating suspicious areas that are hard to see on a mammogram. It may be especially helpful for younger women, whose breast tissue is denser and hence hard

to record on mammograms. Because ultrasound does not involve x-rays, it's commonly used for pregnant women.

Ductal Lavage
A procedure called ductal lavage uses a suction device to retrieve cells from the lining of the milk ducts, where most breast cancers originate. The cells are then examined microscopically for any cancerous changes. The technique is still undergoing testing but may be particularly useful for detecting recurrences in high risk women who have already had breast cancer.

Cholesterol Measurement

Cholesterol Measurement

High levels of the "bad" kinds of cholesterol and other blood fats (lipids) raise your risk for heart attack, stroke, and other major maladies. Specifically, a type of blood fat called low-density lipoprotein (LDL) and fats in the blood called triglycerides, promote buildup of artery-narrowing plaque and increase heart disease risk. Not all types of cholesterol are bad, however. High-density lipoprotein (HDL), or "good" cholesterol actually protects against heart disease. Keeping bad cholesterol levels low and good cholesterol levels high is essential for good health.

About the Test. A cholesterol blood test measures various components of fats in your blood:

- **Total cholesterol.** This is the sum of HDL plus LDL, measured in milligrams (mg) per deciliter (dL) of blood. Experts recommend the level of total cholesterol be kept under 200 mg/dL and suggest that the HDL level within this number be kept at 25% or more of the total.
- **LDL ("bad") cholesterol.** LDL levels should be kept below 100 mg/dL, if possible. Levels ranging from 100 to 129 mg/dL are considered near or above optimal; those between 130 and 159 mg/dL are borderline-high; between 160 and 189, high; and over 190, very high.
- **HDL ("good") cholesterol.** HDL levels of 60 mg/dL or above are considered to be protective against heart disease. Conversely, levels of 40 mg/dL or below put you at high risk.
- **Triglycerides.** Levels of 150 mg/dL or less are considered normal; 150 to 199 are considered

borderline-high; 200 to 499 are considered high; and 500 or more, very high.

How Is It Done? Blood is drawn, usually from your arm, and sent to a lab, where lipid levels are measured. Let your doctor know of any drugs or supplements you may be taking, as some may interfere with test results. Eat your normal diet for one week prior to the test; your doctor will instruct you on fasting 12 to 14 hours before the test. Don't drink alcohol for a day before the test.

How Often Is It Needed? The National Cholesterol Education Program recommends regular cholesterol screening for all people starting at age 20. Most experts suggest you have your cholesterol checked every five years if you are healthy and not at high risk for heart disease. Initial tests should measure total cholesterol as well as levels of HDL, LDL, and triglycerides.

You'll Need This Test More Often If . . .
▶ You are obese and/or physically inactive.
▶ You have diabetes.
▶ You have a family history of heart disease.
▶ You already have high cholesterol.
▶ ALL OF THE ABOVE: You should have your cholesterol checked by a doctor every 3 to 6 months, because you could be at high risk for coronary heart disease. Cholesterol tests can help evaluate the success of weight loss and exercise regimens, as well as the effectiveness of cholesterol-lowering drugs.

Cholesterol Home Monitoring

Various testing kits are available for monitoring your cholesterol levels at home. You prick your finger with a lancet device to draw a drop or two of blood, which is then placed on a special test strip. After a few minutes, the test strip changes color. Matching the color change to a chart gives

you your total cholesterol number.

Getting only your total cholesterol, rather than levels of HDL, LDL, and triglycerides (all of which are important for assessing your overall heart disease risk), is a key drawback to these home tests. A normal result on a home cholesterol

test can give you a false sense of security even if, for instance, your HDL levels are dangerously low. If you already have high cholesterol or are at high risk for heart disease, it is important that you get regular cholesterol tests at your doctor's office, including an assessment of levels of the different types of blood fats.

Colon Testing

Various procedures, including the fecal occult blood test and sigmoidoscopy (*below*), and the colonoscopy and digital rectal exam (*page 360*), are available for detecting cancer and other problems in the colon or rectum, the lowest parts of your digestive tract. Early detection of cancer is essential, offering a high likelihood of cure. It is important not to forego these tests because of embarrassment or unpleasantness. They are critical for saving lives.

Fecal Occult Blood Test (FOB)

About the Test. This is an inexpensive method for detecting hidden (or occult) blood in your feces, which cannot be seen with the naked eye. Blood may be a sign of colon cancer or a precancerous polyp in the gastrointestinal tract. Bleeding gums, ulcers, inflammatory bowel disease, and hemorrhoids are other causes.

How Is It Done? Your doctor will give you a packet for taking samples of your stool at home. Using a wooden applicator, you smear a stool sample on a specimen card on three consecutive days, then promptly drop the samples at your doctor's office or mail them to a lab for analysis.

How Often Is It Needed? Experts recommend that everyone have an annual fecal occult blood test starting at age 50.

Sigmoidoscopy

About the Test. Your doctor performs sigmoidoscopy to check for polyps, cancer, bowel inflammation, hemorrhoids, and other problems in the lower third of your colon.

How Is It Done? At your doctor's office, you will be asked to undress and lie on your side on a table with your knees drawn up, a cloth draped over you for modesty. Your doctor will first perform a digital rectal exam. Then a thin, flexible, lighted viewing tube called a sigmoidoscope is inserted into your anus and rectum and slowly advanced up the lower two feet of your colon to view the walls of your bowel. If polyps are found, they may be removed and sent to a lab for analysis. Sedatives may be given for mild cramping. The procedure takes 10 to 15 minutes. You may have some gas afterward. If you have any fever, bleeding, or pain, call your doctor.

How Often Is It Needed? The American Cancer Society recommends screening with sigmoidoscopy every 3 to 5 years, beginning at age 50. If abnormalities are found, a follow-up colonoscopy may be required.

You'll Need These Tests More Often If . . .
▶ You have had colon cancer.
▶ You have family history of the disease.
▶ ALL OF THE ABOVE: An FOB and sigmoidoscopy before 50; discuss frequency with your doctor.

SIGMOIDOSCOPY/COLONOSCOPY

transverse colon
flexible colonoscope
descending colon
ascending colon
small intestine
end of sigmoidoscope
cecum
sigmoid colon
flexible sigmoidoscope
rectum

A sigmoidoscopy enables the doctor to check your anus, rectum, and lower two feet of colon; a colonoscopy, which uses a longer viewing tube, surveys the entire colon from rectum to cecum.

Colonoscopy

About the Test. Unlike a sigmoidoscopy, which views only the lower portion of your digestive tract, a colonoscopy checks the entire length of the colon. This exam is considered the gold-standard technique for visualizing the colon, but it is expensive. Colonoscopy is performed by a gastroenterologist who looks for ulcers, obstructions, polyps, tumors, inflammation, and other bowel problems.

How Is It Done? In order to clean the bowel and improve viewing, the doctor will give you instructions on fasting, laxatives, and enemas for the day or two preceding the procedure. You will be given a mild intravenous sedative that will make you sleepy and relaxed before the doctor snakes a flexible, lighted viewing tube through your anus and along the entire length of your colon. The procedure is usually painless and takes 30 to 60 minutes. You may be allowed to follow the progress of the scope on a video monitor. A polyp or suspicious area can be removed or a small sample taken (biopsied) for later examination. If you are awake during the procedure, you may experience slight cramping, but this dissi-

pates soon after the procedure is finished. You will feel tired or groggy for several hours afterward, and a friend will need to escort you home from the hospital. If you experience any fever, bleeding, or pain, call your doctor.

How Often Is It Needed? If you have no bowel symptoms and no family history of colon cancer, you should probably have a colonoscopy every 5 to 10 years, beginning at age 50, in place of sigmoidoscopy. A follow-up colonoscopy is required if polyps, tumors, or other abnormal findings are detected via the fecal occult blood test, sigmoidoscopy, or digital rectal exam (*see below*).

You'll Need This Test More Often If . . .
▶ You have ongoing inflammatory bowel problems, such as ulcerative colitis or Crohn's disease. (Annually.)
▶ You have had colon cancer. (Every 1 to 3 years.)
▶ You have had polyps in your bowel. (Every 1 to 3 years.)
▶ You have a history of hereditary polyp disease. (Annually, beginning as early as age 10.)

Digital Rectal Exam

About the Exam. The digital rectal exam (DRE) is performed by your doctor to detect tumors in the rectum, the lower intestine, and (if you're a man) the prostate gland.

How Is It Done? You will be asked to undress and lie on your side, a cloth draped over you for modesty. Your physician will insert a lubricated, gloved finger into your rectum and gently feel for any lumps or abnormal areas. The exam is quick and generally painless.

How Often Is It Needed? People age 50 and over who are otherwise healthy and have no symptoms should get a digital rectal exam every

year. Some experts question the effectiveness of this test for colon cancer screening, because it does not detect most bowel cancers. It is, however, a simple means for assessing the health of the rectum and prostate.

You'll Need This Test More Often If . . .
▶ You have had prostate cancer.
▶ You have had colon cancer.
▶ You have a strong family history of prostate or colon cancer.
▶ ALL OF THE THE ABOVE: A digital rectal exam may be performed earlier than age 50 and possibly more often than once a year, at doctor's discretion.

Genetic Testing

In the fast-moving world of genetics, scientists are uncovering gene mutations that cause or contribute to an array of maladies. This is possible because researchers have now decoded the human genome. Each of its 30,000 genes provides coding for specific proteins that make up the building blocks of the skin, hair, brain, heart, and myriad other body tissues. Gene products also speed up chemical reactions in the body, aiding digestion of food, the beating of the heart, the firing of nerve signals, and countless other processes that help us live, grow, and thrive.

When a gene goes awry, a faulty protein is produced. This will not always cause any problems. Sometimes a defect in a single gene can lead to a serious ailment, such as cystic fibrosis or hemophilia. Single gene defects are often easily traced from generation to generation, as the defective gene is passed from parent to offspring. Geneticists believe many illnesses are caused by multiple gene defects acting in combination with such factors as environmental toxins and poor diet. Unfortunately, few of the genes responsible for complex ailments, such as cancer, Parkinson's disease, and diabetes, have been identified, and their patterns of inheritance remain hard to decipher.

About the Tests. More than 400 genetic tests have been developed for predicting disorders ranging from early-onset Alzheimer's disease and breast cancer to heart disease, sickle-cell anemia, and familial adenomatous polyposis (an inherited condition that leads to colon cancer). Scientists are working to uncover genes that contribute to schizophrenia, high cholesterol, and other forms of cancer, including leukemia, melanoma, and cancers of the thyroid, prostate, ovaries, and kidneys.

A genetic test can help confirm diagnosis of an inherited disease. It can also tell you whether or not you carry certain genes that put you at higher risk for developing an inherited condition. Having a gene, though, is different from having the illness. If you carry the BRCA1 or BRCA2 gene for breast cancer, for example, you have a greater than 50% chance of developing the disease, and your doctor will want to monitor you closely and discuss preventive therapies. This gene does not mean you will inevitably develop breast cancer. In fact, the great majority of women who do get breast cancer do not carry either of these genes. Cancer is caused by many variables.

Genetic tests are most commonly performed to detect known inherited diseases such as sickle-cell anemia and phenylketonuria, which can cause brain damage in newborns. Expectant parents can also screen the fetus for genetic diseases such as Down's syndrome. Gene testing to match genetically similar donors for organ transplants is also common.

How Is It Done? The doctor or technician usually draws a sample of your blood. Sometimes urine, saliva, or other body tissues are taken. The sample is then analyzed for genetic mutations. In some cases, family members may be asked to contribute tissue samples for comparison. The tests can be expensive. Results may not be available for weeks or even months.

Special Considerations

▶ If you have a strong family history of a specific disease, such as colon or breast cancer, your doctor may recommend a genetic test. However, learning that you carry a genetic defect can be emotionally trying, especially if no good treatments for the associated condition are currently available. In addition, some ethicists have raised concerns about potential workplace and insurance discrimination. The decision to undergo a genetic test is a personal one.

▶ If you are considering testing, it is essential that you first speak with a genetic counselor professionally trained to aid you in decision-making and help you interpret test results. To learn more, contact the National Society of Genetic Counselors (610-872-7608 or www.nsgc.org).

Glucose Measurement

About the Test. Glucose tests measure the amount of sugar in your blood and are used to screen for diabetes or assess the effectiveness of diabetes treatments. Persistently high glucose levels are a hallmark of diabetes. Prompt management is required to prevent serious complications.

How Is It Done? Blood sugar (glucose) levels can be measured using various tests. The fasting blood glucose test is simple and inexpensive (usually about $10); you don't eat for 8 to 12 hours before a blood sample is taken. Glucose levels above 125 mg per deciliter of blood (mg/dL) on two occasions indicate diabetes. (Levels below 110 are considered normal, and levels of 110 to 125 indicate potential problems that may lead to diabetes.) A blood glucose test taken two hours after eating (called a postprandial blood glucose test) may be more accurate; a level of 200 or above indicates diabetes. If these tests are inconclusive, an oral glucose tolerance test may be performed. You are given a high-glucose beverage to drink; glucose levels in the blood and urine are measured for several hours afterward.

If you already have diabetes, a hemoglobin A1c test (also called a glycated hemoglobin test) is used to assess whether or not your therapy is effective. It provides a good estimate of average blood glucose values over the previous 8 to 10 weeks. Home monitoring (*see below*) is also important.

How Often Is It Needed? The American Diabetes Association recommends blood glucose testing be performed every 3 years in people age 45 or older.

You'll Need This Test More Often If . . .
▶ **You are obese and/or physically inactive.**
▶ **You have high blood pressure.**
▶ **You have high cholesterol.**
▶ **You are African-American, Hispanic, or Native American.**
▶ **ALL OF THE ABOVE: Glucose testing may be needed earlier than age 45 and more often than every 3 years; discuss frequency with your doctor.**
▶ **You have diabetes. (Home monitoring as often as several times a day for tight control.)**

Home Glucose Monitoring

If you have type 1 diabetes, you may need to monitor your glucose levels at home four or more times a day to ensure blood sugar levels are under tight control.

Many people with type 2 diabetes check their glucose level just once a day. However, testing more frequently than this allows for better control of your blood sugar levels and the disease.

Regardless of what type of diabetes you have, aim for pre-meal glucose levels between 80 and 120 mg/dL and bedtime levels between 100 and 140.

Several types of home test kits are available. The most pop- ular one involves using a special lancing device to draw a drop of blood from your fingertip. (A laser-prick device is available for children.) The blood is placed on a special test strip and read by a meter that gives your glucose levels in less than a minute. To optimize results, test the meter once a month, keep it clean, and use fresh test strips.

Other devices draw minute amounts of blood from your forearm, often less painful than pricking your finger. In addition to measuring glucose, some home monitors measure substances in the blood called ketones, which can build up in the body and cause a life- threatening complication called diabetic ketoacidosis. A home test kit for hemoglobin A1c is now available.

The GlucoWatch Biographer is a battery-powered device you wear on your wrist like a watch. It measures glucose levels by sending painless electrical currents through the skin. After a three-hour warm-up and an initial calibration with a traditional finger stick, the watch can provide a glucose reading every 20 minutes for up to 12 hours, even during sleep (an alarm is triggered if there's a problem). This device should be used only in combination with finger-stick testing.

Hearing Tests

About the Test. Hearing tests are designed to assess hearing loss and detect any structural or nerve damage that may be causing problems. You will listen to tones of varying pitch and volume and be asked to identify words, sometimes in the presence of background noise.

How Is It Done? Hearing tests are usually performed by an audiologist, a specialist in hearing problems. You sit in a soundproof room, wearing headphones or a headband that plays tones or words. Avoid coffee or products that contain caffeine for 4 hours beforehand. Complete testing takes about an hour. Your doctor will review the results afterward.

How Often Is It Needed? Your doctor will screen for any hearing problems during regular checkups or every 1 to 2 years, especially after age 75. If necessary, you will be given information about hearing aids or be referred to a hearing specialist.

Special Considerations
▶ Advanced imaging techniques, such as computed tomography (CT) and magnetic resonance imaging (MRI) of the head, may be required to detect damage to tissues such as the cochlea in the ear. The tests can also help to determine whether or not you could be a candidate for a cochlear implant.
▶ Some inner ear disorders also cause dizziness and/or balance problems, so you may have to undergo tests to assess your balance as well.

Pap Test and Pelvic Exam

About the Test. Named for its inventor, Dr. George Papanicolaou, a Pap test (also called a Pap smear), is a simple, painless, and inexpensive procedure used to screen women for cervical cancer. It is usually performed during a pelvic exam, in which your physician checks your reproductive organs for problems in the uterus, ovaries, and cervix. Because of the widespread use of Pap tests, cervical cancer, once the leading cause of cancer deaths in American women, now ranks seventh. Millions of cases of cervical cancer have been caught early and completely cured thanks to this test.

How Is It Done? You will be asked to disrobe and lie on your back, your feet in stirrups. Your doctor will gently insert an instrument called a speculum to open your vagina and better view the area. For the Pap test, a swab of cells is taken from the cervix and sent to a lab for analysis. Because blood may interfere with the results, the best time to have a Pap test is 2 weeks after the start of your menstrual period.

How Often Is It Needed? The American Cancer Society recommends annual Pap tests for all women at age 18 or when they become sexually active. If the results are normal for 3 years in a row, or if you are over age 65, your doctor may choose to perform the test every 2 or 3 years. The Society also recommends pelvic exams every 3 years for women 18 to 39 years of age, then every year for women 40 and older.

You'll Need These Tests More Often If . . .
▶ Your Pap test results are abnormal or ambiguous. (Pap test every 6 months over the following 18 months, or a colposcopy, which uses a magnifier to look for abnormal tissue.)
▶ You've had cancer of the reproductive tract. (Pap test and pelvic exam annually or more often at doctor's discretion.)
▶ You test positive for the human papilloma virus, which causes most cases of cervical cancer. (Pap test and pelvic exam annually or more often at doctor's discretion.)

PSA (Prostate Specific Antigen) Test

About the Test. Commonly used as a screening test in men to help detect prostate cancer or assess its spread, the PSA test looks for blood levels of prostate specific antigen, a protein produced by prostate cells. High PSA levels may be a sign of prostate cancer, although levels may also be elevated in those with infections, inflammation, or benign enlargement of the prostate (BPH). PSA levels below 4 nanograms per milliliter of blood (ng/ml) are considered normal. A PSA score of 4 to 10 is considered borderline, while levels above 10 are classified as high.

How Is It Done? PSA levels are determined from a blood test, which can be taken during a routine office visit or be specifically arranged. If PSA levels are high, your doctor will take a small tissue sample (biopsy) of the prostate, which will be sent to a lab to be analyzed for signs of prostate cancer.

How Often Is It Needed? Some professional and government groups do not advocate regular PSA testing for most men; they suggest the results are often unreliable and can lead to unnecessary and expensive biopsies and follow-up exams. The American Cancer Society and the American Urological Association, however, recommend annual PSA testing for all men beginning at age 50, including seniors with a life expectancy of at least 10 years.

You'll Need This Test More Often If . . .
▶ You currently have prostate cancer. (Frequent PSA tests helps gauge response to treatment.)
▶ You have a family history of prostate cancer. (PSA testing may be needed before age 50 and can be done more often at doctor's discretion.)
▶ You have prostate problems. (PSA testing may begin before age 50 and can be done more often at doctor's discretion.)

Sexually Transmitted Disease Testing

About the Test. Many infectious agents can cause sexually transmitted diseases (STDs). Human immunodeficiency virus (HIV), the cause of AIDS, has become a worldwide epidemic in recent years. Other common STDs include chlamydia, genital warts, gonorrhea, syphilis, crab lice, hepatitis, and herpes simplex. The best way to find out if you or your partner is infected is to get tested. Signs of an STD include discharge from the vagina or penis, itching in the genital or anal areas, pain, soreness, swelling around the genitals, rashes or sores on the genitals or elsewhere on the body, odors in the genital region, or fever and fatigue. STD tests are designed to identify the infecting organism so antibiotics, antiviral drugs, or other appropriate treatments can be prescribed.

How Is It Done? The type of STD test best for you depends on the type of infection you have. Your doctor may be able to diagnose a condition based on your symptoms. A sample of fluids or cells from the urethra, cervix, throat, or rectum may be taken and sent to a lab for culture and analysis. Some STDs, such as AIDS or hepatitis, can be identified by a blood test. Gonorrhea and chlamydia may be diagnosed by culturing unusual discharges. Crab lice or their tiny white eggs (nits) may be visible on pubic hair.

How Often Is It Needed? If you are sexually active with multiple partners, it is a good idea to have an annual sexual health exam. If you and your partner are monogamous and free of sexually transmitted diseases, no additional testing is needed.

You'll Need This Test More Often If . . .
▶ You are intimate with someone with a known sexually transmitted disease. (Every 3 or 4 months, or at doctor's discretion.)

Skin Self-Exam

About the Exam. Regular examination of your skin is the best way to detect changes that may be cancerous. Even malignant melanoma, the most aggressive and potentially deadly form of skin cancer, is completely curable if caught at an early stage.

How Is It Done? Stand in front of a full-length mirror in a well-lighted room and slowly inspect the entire surface of your skin. Don't forget the soles of your feet, between your toes, under your nails, and the whites of your eyes. A handheld mirror (or the help of a friend) may be useful for examining hard-to-see spots such as the top of your scalp, the back of your neck, and your buttocks. It is important to become familiar with any existing moles or freckles and to monitor them closely for any changes. It is also important to check for any new spots. If you find anything unusual, see your doctor.

How Often Is It Needed? Most people should perform a skin self-examination every 6 months.

Do the Exam Monthly If . . .
► You have light skin.
► You have blond or red hair.
► You have blue or green eyes.
► You have a family history of skin cancer.
► You've had a severe, blistering sunburn as a child or teenager.

See a Dermatologist Often If . . .
► You have had skin cancer (at least annually, or more often at doctor's discretion).
► NOTE: Some women experience mole changes during pregnancy. If you have had skin cancer and are pregnant, be sure to mention your pregnancy to your dermatologist.

The ABCs (and Ds & Es) of Melanoma

While most of your "suspicious" moles will turn out to be noncancerous, it's better to be cautious. If a mole or growth anywhere on your body has one or more of the following signs, show it to a skin doctor (dermatologist) as soon as possible: It could be a malignant melanoma.

Key Signs to Look For
Use this alphabet mnemonic device to help you remember early warning signs:
● **Asymmetry:** One half of the mole does not match the other. Look for any raised or flat patches or bumps that are different on one side of the mole than the other.
● **Borders:** Irregular, jagged, notched, scalloped, or blurred borders.
● **Color:** Variation of color within a mole. Look for dark spots or spots of different colors, including shades of brown, black, red, white, or blue.
● **Diameter:** Any skin lesion wider than a pencil eraser (6 millimeters).
● **Elevation:** If a mole changes in height, especially a sudden elevation of a previously flat mole.

Additional Clues
In addition to the key signs, be aware of any change in the surface texture of a mole, especially scaliness, erosion, oozing, crusting, ulceration, or bleeding. Be sure to keep an eye on changes in the surrounding skin, especially redness and swelling, or changes in sensation, such as itching, tenderness, or pain.

Stress Test

About the Test. The cardiac stress test has become a standard technique for assessing the condition of your heart. Also known as an exercise electrocardiogram (ECG), it provides invaluable information about your heart's rate and rhythm and its ability to pump blood adequately during the stress of exercise.

How Is It Done? Wire leads that record the electrical activity in your heart are attached to your chest; your resting heart rate and rhythm and blood pressure are recorded. You then exercise on a stationary bike or treadmill. Resistance is gradually increased until you reach a preset target heart rate or experience chest pain. The test usually takes about 20 minutes. Wear comfortable shoes, and don't eat, smoke, or drink caffeine or alcohol for several hours beforehand. If you have weak lungs, arthritis, or another condition that makes it problematic for you to exercise, you may instead be given an intravenous drug called dobutamine or another called atropine that mimics the effects of exercise on the heart. Variations of the ECG stress test use injections of radioactive tracers (cardiac nuclear scan) or sound waves (stress echocardiography) to assess heart function during exercise.

How Often Is It Needed? Some doctors order a baseline stress test at around age 40 for men and 50 for women, especially for patients who are about to undertake a new exercise regime.

You'll Need This Test More Often If . . .
► You have had a heart attack.
► You have had an angioplasty.
► You have had bypass surgery.
► ALL OF THE ABOVE: Stress tests may be needed every 6 to 12 months to assess heart function and tolerance for exercise.
► You have heart disease. (Every 6 to 12 months to gauge heart function, tolerance for exercise, and response to various heart medicines.)
► You are about to have major surgery. (Stress test before surgery.)

Testicular Exam

About the Exam. A testicular self-exam is a simple 5-minute procedure men can perform at home to check for any unusual lumps or changes in the testicles that may be a sign of cancer. A clinical testicular exam is performed by a doctor, who will also check for anything abnormal. Early detection of testicular cancer leads to cure in 90% of cases.

How Is It Done? A good time to perform a self-exam is after a warm bath or shower, when the scrotum is relaxed. Gently roll your testes between your fingers, looking and feeling for any hard lumps or smooth, rounded masses. Changes in the size, shape, or texture of the testes may be a sign of cancer or other problems. Bring any abnormal findings to your doctor's attention. At the office, your doctor may perform a thorough inspection and palpation of the testes to detect anything unusual.

How Often Is It Needed? Testicular cancer is fairly rare. When it does occur, it almost always strikes those younger than age 40. Many doctors recommend monthly self-exams in otherwise healthy younger men ages 15 to 40. After age 40, regular testicular exams are not needed.

You'll Need This Test More Often If . . .
► You've had testicular cancer.
► You have a family history of testicular cancer.
► You had an undescended testicle at birth.
► ALL OF THE ABOVE: You should perform monthly testicular self-exams after age 40 on an ongoing basis.

Vision Testing

About the Test. Your primary care doctor or a nurse practitioner might perform a vision test during a routine physical, but you will probably be referred to an M.D. who specializes in eye disorders (ophthalmologist) or a vision specialist (optometrist). These professionals also screen for diseases such as cataracts (clouding of the lens), macular degeneration (a leading cause of blindness), and glaucoma (eyeball pressure that can lead to vision loss).

How Is It Done? The examiner will test the sharpness of your vision, having you read letters of diminishing size (Snellen charts) from a distance of 20 feet. A score of 20/20 means you have normal vision. Your close-up reading ability, peripheral vision, and eye movements will be tested, and you will also be checked for color-blindness and blind spots. It's likely that the examiner will place drops in your eyes to dilate your pupils, making your eyes very sensitive to sunlight for several hours.

How Often Is It Needed? If you don't have any special eye problems, you should have a vision check at least every 5 years up to age 50 and every year or 2 thereafter.

You'll Need a Vision Test More Often If . . .
▶ You wear glasses. (Annually.)
▶ You have optic nerve damage. (More than once a year, at doctor's discretion.)
▶ You have diabetes. (More than once a year, at doctor's discretion.)

Get Frequent Glaucoma Screening If . . .
▶ You're over age 65.
▶ You're African-American and over age 40.
▶ You have a family history of glaucoma.
▶ ALL OF THE ABOVE: You may need screening more than once a year at doctor's discretion.

Vision Check: Should You Still Be Driving?

People age 75 and older have a higher rate of motor vehicle deaths than any other age group, except those under 25. Although driving skills may decline with age for a number of reasons, vision loss is one of the main ones. It's important to be alert for signs of vision problems that could affect your driving.

Although standards differ from state to state, the American Academy of Ophthalmology recommends that licensed drivers have a visual acuity of 20/40 or better (with or without corrective lenses) and an uninterrupted field of peripheral vision of 140° in diameter in one or both eyes. While poor peripheral vision is more likely than visual acuity to predict which older drivers are apt to experience a crash, most states do not test peripheral vision as a license requirement. States usually rely on a test of visual acuity because it's easier to measure.

Unless you have had a recent eye exam, you probably don't know how good your peripheral vision and visual acuity are. By asking yourself a few simple questions about your vision, you can get a good idea about how it may be affecting your driving.
● Do you have problems reading street or highway signs?
● Does glare from the lights of oncoming cars bother you at night?

● Do you have difficulty seeing other cars, pedestrians, lane lines, medians, or curbs? Does this problem get worse at night, dusk, or dawn?

Answering "Yes" to any of these questions may indicate that low vision is affecting your driving. It doesn't necessarily mean you'll have to stop driving, but it does mean you need to make some changes.

Start by scheduling an annual eye exam. Put some limits on the places and times you drive (only during daylight hours). Begin scouting for alternative methods of transportation before you have to stop driving altogether.

Glossary

A

acupuncture Ancient treatment method of traditional Chinese medicine that uses hair-thin needles inserted into the skin at key points to restore healthy energy flow, or *qi*.

acute Term describing a condition lasting two weeks or less; short, severe, nonchronic.

adjuvant chemotherapy Drug treatment typically following cancer surgery to destroy remnant malignant cells.

aerobic exercise Continuous rhythmic exercise using large muscle groups. Aerobics increase the demand for oxygen, elevating the workload of the heart and lungs.

allergen Normally harmless substance that produces allergic reaction in susceptible people. Includes pollen, animal dander, dust mites, cosmetics, and some foods.

alternative medicine Approach to healing, such as herbal therapy or acupuncture, falling outside domain of conventional medicine (*see also integrative medicine*).

amino acids Chemical substances, found in foods and produced in the body, that are used to build proteins.

anaphylactic shock Intense allergic reaction to a drug, food, or venom, producing life-threatening heart and breathing problems.

anesthesia Drug-induced partial or complete loss of sensation, sometimes accompanied by loss of consciousness.

antibiotic Medication that kills or inhibits infection-causing bacteria.

antibiotic resistance Ability of microorganisms to alter their structure and become unresponsive to antibiotics. Most likely to occur after long-term antibiotic use.

antibodies Immune-system chemicals, also called immunoglobulins, that track down and neutralize specific foreign substances (called antigens) in the blood.

antioxidants Substances that protect cells from damaging, highly reactive oxygen molecules called free radicals. Some are produced in the body; others, such as vitamins C and E, are obtained through diet or supplements.

aromatherapy Use of aromatic essential oils, extracted from plants, trees, and herbs, to promote well-being.

artery Blood vessel that carries blood from the heart to various parts of the body.

atherosclerosis Buildup of cholesterol and other substances in artery walls, causing artery stiffness; leads to heart disease, heart attack, stroke, and other ailments.

autoimmune disorder Ailment, such as lupus, in which the body produces antibodies that attack its own tissues.

B

benign Term describing an abnormal growth of cells that is not cancerous.

biofeedback Technique using visual and auditory cues that trains a person wearing electronic sensors to control involuntary body processes, such as heartbeat and blood pressure, and to reduce stress.

biopsy Surgical removal of a small piece of living tissue for microscopic examination.

blood clot Blood cells that have clumped together (coagulated) to form a thick mass.

bodywork Therapies, including acupressure and massage, used to treat illness and promote relaxation. May involve exercise, postural re-education, and body manipulation.

C

carcinoma Malignant growth of surface (epithelial) tissues, such as those in the skin, glands, and internal organs.

catheter Hollow flexible tube that can be inserted into body cavities or vessels to inject drugs or remove fluids.

chemotherapy Treatment or control of disease (usually cancer) through use of chemical agents (drugs) that directly affect diseased cells.

chronic Term describing an illness or condition that persists over a long period.

cognitive-behavioral therapy Psychotherapy that teaches patients to identify and correct thinking processes causing certain behaviors.

collagen Fibrous protein making up the body's main supportive and connective tissues.

congenital Describing a condition present at birth.

conventional medicine Approach to healing commonly practiced in Western countries. A doctor diagnoses a problem and typically treats it with drugs or surgery. Also known as allopathic medicine.

curettage Scraping of a cavity, such as the uterus, to remove tissues or growths, often for analysis.

D-E

defibrillator Device that delivers a brief electric shock to re-establish normal heart contractions.

dietary supplement (*see nutritional supplement*).

dose Amount of medication taken at a single time.

dosage Number and frequency of doses to be taken.

edema Swelling due to excess fluid buildup in tissues.

embolus Abnormal substance (usually a blood clot) circulating in bloodstream.

embolism Sudden blockage of a vessel by an embolus.

endoscopy Procedure using a thin, lighted tube to examine hollow organs, such as the stomach, bladder, or colon.

estrogen Female sex hormone, produced mainly in the ovaries, that helps regulate menstruation, reproduction, and other processes.

estrogen replacement therapy (ERT) Use of synthesized forms of estrogen to counter effects of low estrogen levels after menopause.

extract Pill, powder, liquid, tincture, or other form of an herb or drug that contains a concentrated, and usually standardized, amount of a therapeutic ingredient.

F

fatty acids Building blocks the body uses to make fats;

may be classified as saturated, polyunsaturated, or monounsaturated. The body manufactures many fatty acids; those it cannot produce (essential fatty acids) must be obtained through diet or supplements.

fiber Indigestible plant parts that pass through the digestive system, absorbing water and speeding elimination.

Food and Drug Administration (FDA) U.S. government agency that regulates and monitors the safety of food and drugs (but not nutritional supplements).

free radicals Unstable and highly reactive compounds, usually containing oxygen, which can damage cells.

G-H

gland Organ or tissue that secretes a substance to be used elsewhere in body.

glucose Blood sugar that is an energy source for the body.

guided imagery Conscious use of imagination to create positive healing visualizations.

hemoglobin Oxygen-carrying portion of red blood cells; transports oxygen from lungs to cells and takes carbon dioxide from cells back to lungs to be expelled.

hemorrhage Medical term for "bleeding"; may be internal or external.

herb Plant or plant part—leaf, stem, root, bark, bud, or flower—that can be used medicinally and/or for culinary or other purposes.

high density lipoprotein (HDL) Protein in the blood that collects cholesterol from tissues and delivers it to the

liver for reprocessing or excretion. Also known as "good" cholesterol because it protects the heart from disease.

histamines Chemicals released when an allergic reaction occurs; can cause congestion, itching, and swelling.

hormone replacement therapy (HRT) Administration of estrogen, with or without progesterone, to relieve adverse effects of menopause.

hormones Chemical messengers produced by the glands and carried through the bloodstream; regulate everything from metabolism to response to stress.

I

immune response Body's natural defense system against infectious organisms (including viruses and bacteria) and invasive cancer cells.

immunotherapy Treatment that stimulates or restores ability of the body's immune system to fight off infection and disease or to counter side effects of treatments such as chemotherapy.

inflammation Body's natural response to trauma, toxins, or infection. Injured tissues release substances to increase blood flow to area. White blood cells remove dead tissue and other debris, causing swelling, redness, and pain.

integrative medicine Approach to healing utilizing aspects of both conventional and alternative medicine.

J-K-L

laparoscope Tiny instrument with a light and camera

that's inserted through a small incision for surgical and diagnostic procedures.

laser Device with a powerful, concentrated light beam, used as a surgical cutting tool.

lesion Tissue abnormality from injury or physical alteration (a tumor, mole, or cyst).

lipid Term for blood-borne fat, wax, and fatty compound.

localized Restricted to a particular area; often describes an infection or disease.

low density lipoprotein (LDL) Protein in the blood containing high levels of cholesterol and triglycerides; initiates plaque formation in blood vessels. Also known as "bad" cholesterol.

lumbar Relating to a region of the lower back between the ribs and pelvis.

lymph Fluid containing white blood cells, proteins, and fats that circulates through the body via lymphatic vessels; plays an important role in immune system.

lymph node Normal mass of the lymphatic system found in clusters throughout the body; contains lymphocytes (white blood cells) that filter lymphatic fluid.

M

malignant Term describing a condition that can become progressively worse, even fatal; often refers to tumors that spread to new sites (metastasize).

mast cells Connective tissue cells that release inflammatory substances, such as histamine, during allergic reactions or in response to injury or inflammation.

meditation Mind-body technique that employs quiet contemplation to induce mental and physical tranquility.

membrane Thin, soft layer of tissue that lines, covers, or separates organs or bodily structures.

metabolism Array of chemical reactions enabling the body to convert food into energy to be used or stored.

metastasis Secondary malignant tumor that has spread from a primary cancer site to another area of the body.

microbes Short for microorganisms; single-celled or tiny multicelled organisms (bacteria, viruses, some algae and fungi) that can cause disease.

microgram (mcg) Metric measure of weight used in dosages. There are 1,000 mcg in 1 milligram (mg).

milligram (mg) Metric measure of weight used in dosages. There are 1,000 mg in 1 gram.

mineral Inorganic substance crucial for heart rhythm, bone formation, digestion, and other metabolic processes.

monounsaturated fat Type of fat thought to reduce heart disease risk by lowering LDL ("bad") cholesterol levels.

mucous membrane Pink, shiny, skin-like layer lining lips, mouth, vagina, eyelids, and other body cavities and passages.

N

neurons Cells of the nervous system that transmit and receive messages.

neurotransmitters Various chemicals found in the brain and throughout the body, which relay messages between nerve cells.

node Small, rounded mass of tissue; abnormal nodes are often called nodules.

nonsteroidal anti-inflammatory drug (NSAID) Drug that reduces pain and inflammation by blocking production of hormone-like natural substances called prostaglandins.

nutritional supplement Nutrient synthesized in a lab or extracted from plants or animals and used medicinally.

O-P

occupational therapy (OT) Treatment that helps disabled or injured people relearn muscular coordination and cope with daily tasks.

over-the-counter (OTC) Drug that is sold without a doctor's prescription.

palpate To physically examine the body by touch.

physical therapy (PT) Rehabilitative treatment using therapeutic exercise, massage, and various heat, cold, and electrical therapies to promote recovery from illness, injury, or disability.

phytoestrogens Plant-based estrogen-like compounds that may relieve menopausal symptoms, effects of certain cancers, and other complaints.

placebo Substance containing no medicinal ingredients; used in scientific studies as a control and compared to material under study. Also called a dummy pill.

platelets Small, colorless, disk-shaped bodies found in the blood, integral to clot formation.

plasma Liquid, cell-free portion of blood and lymph.

plaque (arterial) Deposits of fatty substances, such as cholesterol, in inner lining of artery walls. Buildup can lead to atherosclerosis.

plaque (dental) Thin film of saliva, food particles, and bacteria on teeth and tongue.

polyp Usually benign growth (maybe with a stem) that protrudes from the mucous lining of an organ, such as the nose, uterus, or colon.

polyunsaturated fat Type of fat thought to lower heart disease risk by reducing LDL ("bad") cholesterol levels; large amounts may also reduce levels of HDL ("good") cholesterol.

progesterone Female sex hormone, made by ovaries, that regulates menstrual cycle.

Q-R-S

remission Temporary lessening or disappearance of symptoms of a chronic disease.

renal Relating to, or in the region of, the kidneys.

saturated fat A type of fat converted to LDL ("bad") cholesterol and thought to increase heart disease risk. It's found in animal fats (whole milk, butter, meat) and in certain tropical oils (palm, palm kernel, coconut).

sedatives Drugs that produce a tranquilizing effect and calm nervous excitement.

serotonin Amino-acid-like compound found in blood, the digestive tract, and the brain, where it is a principal neurotransmitter.

shunt Surgical passage created between two blood vessels to divert blood from one place to another.

staging Process of classifying the spread and extent of a disease to determine appropriate treatment.

stem cell Unspecialized cell that replicates itself indefinitely. Can produce specialized cells for heart muscle and brain or liver tissue.

stent Mold designed to hold a surgical graft intact. Often used after a heart attack in the form of a tiny tube inserted into a blood vessel to stabilize it and keep it open.

T

tai chi Ancient Chinese exercise regimen using precise motions and breathing to promote balance and relaxation.

testosterone Male sex hormone, produced in the testes, that initiates puberty and helps build muscle and bone.

tincture Liquid made by soaking an herb or its parts in water and ethyl alcohol (such as vodka). Alcohol helps concentrate and preserve herb's active ingredients.

toxin Poisonous substance of animal or plant origin.

tranquilizer Drug that produces a calming or sedative effect without disrupting normal mental activity.

trans fatty acids Fats produced when hydrogen is added to unsaturated fats to make them more solid or shelf-stable (also called hydrogenation). Can act like saturated fats, raising total and LDL ("bad") cholesterol.

trigger point Knot or taut muscle band that forms when muscles fail to relax, making area sensitive to touch. Can be treated with deep massage or drug injections.

triglycerides Main form of fat found in the body. High trigylceride levels in the blood increase likelihood of developing heart disease.

U-Z

ultrasound High-frequency sound waves that create 3-D images; used for diagnosis and treatment.

vaccine Weakened or killed infectious microorganisms or other substances introduced to stimulate immunity and provide protection against certain infectious diseases.

vein Blood vessel that carries blood from various parts of the body to the heart.

virus Tiny infectious agent causing diseases, from minor (colds) to deadly (AIDS).

vitamins Organic substances playing an essential role in regulating cell functions. Most must be ingested, since the body cannot produce them.

wellness Condition of good physical and mental health, maintained by proper diet, exercise, and lifestyle.

x-ray Electromagnetic rays with a short wavelength that pass through tissues to produce a photographic image of body structures for analysis. X-rays with short wavelengths are used medicinally during radiation therapy.

Index

Boldface page numbers indicate major medical entries.
Italic page numbers indicate illustrations.
Hundreds of drugs are featured in this book, but not all could be included in this index. Refer to specific ailment entries for the most complete drug information.

A

Acalculous cholecystitis, 134
Accutane, 21, 22, 277
ACE inhibitors; heart problems, 91–92, 98, 160; high blood pressure, 175
Acetycholine, 28
Acid, stomach. *See* Heartburn; Ulcers
Acne, 20–22. *See also* Rosacea; Skin conditions
Actinic keratoses, 288
Acupressure, 53, 270, 347
Acupuncture, 33, 59; and arthritis, 39; and asthma, 43; and back pain, 53; and bursitis, 69; and carpal tunnel syndrome, 73; and chronic fatigue syndrome, 81; and fibromyalgia, 128; and menopause, 227; and migraines, 231; and multiple sclerosis, 235; and rheumatoid arthritis, 274; and shingles, 279; and stroke, 303; and tinnitus, 313; and TMJ, 307; and tobacco dependence, 317
Additives, food, 229
Aerobic exercise, 35, 37, 119, 127, 133, 172
African Americans, health problems of, 175, 261
Air pollution, 119, 253, 337
Alcohol; and atrial fibrillation, 45; and cirrhosis, 167; and gout, 143, 144, 145; and high blood pressure, 173; and infertility, 181; and osteoporosis, 245; and rosacea, 277; and sleep problems, 189, 292; and tinnitus, 312
Aldactone, 91, 175, 257
Alexander technique, 49
Alginic acid, 162
Allergies, 23–27, 115, 116, 284, 346
Alopecia areata. *See* Hair loss
Alpha-blockers, 175, 264

Alpha hydroxy acid, 338
Alzheimer's disease, 28–29, 141, 221, 223
Ambulatory phlebectomy, 336
Amino acids, 93
Androgen-deprivation therapy, 261
Androgens, 20. *See also* Testosterone
Anemia, 333
Anger, 178
Angina, 94, 96, 97, 175
Angiogenesis inhibitors, 57, 288
Angioplasty, 97, 98, 160, 251, 304
Angiotension II receptor blockers, 175
Antacids, 162, 323
Anti-angiogenic drugs, 219
Anti-arrhythmic drugs, 46
Antibiotics, 284; and acne, 21; and diverticulitis, 111; and Lyme disease, 212; and respiratory problems, 65, 83, 130, 253, 283, 284; and urinary tract infections, 329
Anticholinergics, 234, 248
Anticoagulants, 45, 159
Anticonvulsants, 57, 280
Antidepressants; and back pain, 51; and chronic fatigue syndrome, 79; and fibromyalgia, 125, 127; and stroke, 302
Antihistamines, 24, 25, 190, 263, 327
Antihypertensives, 160, 173, 174, 175
Antimalarial drugs, 210
Antioxidants; and asthma, 43; and cataracts, 77; and eczema, 117; and macular degeneration, 219; and memory loss, 223; and multiple sclerosis, 235; and obesity, 240; and pneumonia, 253; and rheumatoid arthritis, 275
Antiplatelet drug, 97, 302
Antispasmodic drugs, 198, 234, 327
Antiviral medication, 279, 280
Anxiety, 29, 30–33, 49, 277, 313. *See also* Stress
Apples, 43, 71
Arginine, 93, 124, 251
Arnica, 298
Aromatase inhibitors, 63
Aromatherapy, 153
Arthritis, 34–39, 68, 211
Arthritis, rheumatoid, 272–75
Arthroplasty, 38, 39
Arthroscopy, 38, 69
Artificial heart, 92

Artificial insemination (AI), 183
Artificial sweeteners, 229
Aspartame, 229
Aspirin, 84; and atrial fibrillation, 45; and heart problems, 95, 97, 158, 159, 160; and heartburn, 164; and strokes, 302; and tinnitus, 312. *See also* NSAIDs; Low-dose aspirin therapy
Assisted reproductive technologies, 183
Asthma, 23, 40–43, 117, 120, 282
Atherectomy, 251
Atherosclerosis, 94, 109, 122, 176, 250
Athlete's foot, 342, 348
Atrial fibrillation, 44–47, 94
Autoimmune disorders; lupus, 208–10; prostatitis, 266; thyroid disorders, 308–11
Autologen, 340
Azulfidine, 185, 273, 275

B

Back pain, 48–53
Bacteria, 20, 82, 283, 322, 328
Bactrim, 114, 267, 329, 330
Bad breath, 319
Baking soda, 147, 165
Baldness, 150
Bariatric surgery, 240–41
Barrett's esophagus, 161, 163
Basal cell carcinoma, 286, 288. *See also* Skin cancer
Batista procedure, 92
Bee venom, 235
Behavioral therapy. *See* Cognitive-behavior therapy
Benadryl, 25, 117, 190, 284, 346, 347
Benign prostatic hyperplasia (BPH), 262-64, 267
Benzodiazepines, 32, 191, 271
Beta-blockers, 98; and heart problems, 45, 92, 97. 160; and glaucoma, 140; and high blood pressure, 174, 175; and thyroid disorders, 310
Beta-carotene, 66, 77, 117, 219
Bile, 132, 166
Bile-acid sequestrants, 178–79
Biofeedback, 39, 53, 81, 195, 231, 279, 301, 313, 307, 327. *See also* Relaxation techniques
Biologic response modifiers, 274
Biopsy, 55, 59, 60, 287
Biotechnology, 203
Birth control, 329. *See also* Oral contraceptives

Corticosteroids *(continued)* and multiple sclerosis, 233–34; and rheumatoid arthritis, 273; strains and sprains, 297; and TMJ, 307
Cortisone cream, 152, 210
Cosmetic surgery, 277
Cough medicine, 65, 85, 130, 253, 284, 344
Coughing, 64, 65, 118, 252, 344
Coumadin, 45, 95, 302
Counseling, 124, 235, 317
COX-2 inhibitors, 38; and arthritis, 36; and back pain, 51; and bursitis, 69; and carpal tunnel syndrome, 73; and chronic fatigue syndrome, 79; and colon cancer, 88; and gout, 144; and lupus, 210; and Lyme disease, 212; and rheumatoid arthritis, 273, 274; and ulcers, 324
CPAP, 292, 293
CPR (cardiopulmonary resuscitation), 159
Cramps, 184, 194, 256
Cranberry juice, 330
Cravings, 315, 316
Crohn's disease, 184
Cuprimine, 198, 273
Curettage and electrodessication, 288, 289
Cystitis, 328
Cytokines, 272

D

Darvon, 271, 279
DASH diet, 171, 174
Decongestants, 24, 25, 84–85, 130, 263, 294
Deep brain stimulation, 249
Deep-breathing exercises, 39, 225
Deep vein thrombosis, 336
Defibrillator, 159, 160
Dehydration, 104, 145, 344
Dementia, 304
Demerol, 134, 160, 198, 230
Dental implants, 319, 320
Dentures, 319
Depression, 22, 29, 31, 99–103; and erectile dysfunction, 122; and insomnia, 188; and lung cancer, 207; and memory loss, 221; and multiple sclerosis, 234; and PMS, 256; and strokes, 302, 304
Dermabrasion, 22, 339
Dermatitis, 115–17
Detrol, 326
DHEA, 183
Diabetes, 71, 74, 123, 175, 240, 219, 362

Diabetes type 1, 104–106
Diabetes type 2, 107–109
Diarrhea, 184, 185, 192, 195, 344–45
Diathermy, 69
Diet; and coronary heart disease, 95; and depression, 103; and diabetes, 108; and diverticulitis, 111; and high cholesterol, 177; and migraines, 230; and MS, 234; and obesity, 237; and Parkinson's disease, 249; and teeth, 321; and wrinkles, 340
Digestion, 161, 184, 192, 194, 322, 346
Digital rectal exam, 360
Digitalis drugs, 92
Dilation, endoscopic, 165
Discoid lupus, 208, 210
Ditropan, 234, 327
Diuretics, 73, 91, 93, 144, 160, 174–75, 198, 257, 327
Diuril, 175, 198
Diverticulitis, 110–12
DMARDS, 273, 274, 275
Dong quai, 227
Dopamine, 99, 101, 246, 247, 270, 315
Dramamine, 347
Drixoral, 25, 130, 284, 294
Drugs; generic, 309; side effects, 126, 173
Ductal carcinoma, 58, 61
Duodenum, 322
Dust mites, 23, 24, 41, 116
Dysmenorrhea, 256

E

Ear infection, 113–14
Ears; hearing loss, 154–57; tinnitus, 312–13
Earwax, 113, 114, 156, 157, 313
Echinacea, 66, 85, 131, 138, 181, 187
ECT, 100, 103
Eczema, 113, 115–17
Eggs (food), 43, 178
Ejaculations, 267
Elavil, 51, 79, 101, 127, 191, 194, 230, 280, 302, 313, 307
Electroconvulsive therapy (ECT). 100, 103
Electromyography, 73
Emphysema, 118–21
ENADA, 80
Endometrial ablation, 332
Endometriosis, 180
Endorphins, 53, 72, 103, 172, 280
Endoscopic dilation, 165
Endoscopy, 62, 163, 285, 324
Enema, 111
Enzymatic sclerostomy, 142
Epidermal growth factor receptor (EGFR), 88

Epidural block, 280
Epstein-Barr virus, 81, 216
Erectile dysfunction, 122–25, 260, 264
Erythromycin, 21, 212, 253, 276, 277
Esidrix, 175, 198
Esophagus, 161, 163
Essential fatty acids, 117, 235
Essiac, 215
Estrogen, 62, 63, 96, 255; and menopause, 224; and urinary tract infections, 328; and uterine fibroids, 331; and varicose veins, 335
Estrogen replacement therapy, 225. *See also* Hormone replacement therapy
Eucalyptus oil, 282
Evening primrose oil, 235, 257, 275
Evista, 226, 244
Exercise, 36, 42, 63, 72, 112, 120, 113, 142, 181, 194, 222, 248, 250; and back pain, 50; and chronic fatigue syndrome, 78, 80; and heart health, 93, 95, 159, 160; and depression, 103; and diabetes, 106, 107; and fibromyalgia, 127; and high blood pressure, 172–73; and insomnia, 190; and lupus, 209; and lymphoma, 216; and menopause, 226; and multiple sclerosis, 234; and obesity, 238; and PMS, 256; and rheumatoid arthritis, 274; for strains and sprains, 299. *See also* Specific ailments
Exfoliation, 338
Expectorants, 65, 85, 130, 253, 284, 344. *See also* Cough medicine
Extracapsular cataract extraction (ECCE), 76
Extracorporeal shock wave lithotripsy (ESWL), 198
Eye problems, 340; cataracts, 74-77; conjunctivitis, 344; diabetes, 108, 109; glaucoma, 139–42; macular degeneration, 217–20; and shingles, 280; tests, 367. *See also* Vision problems
Eye drops, 26, 141, 225, 310
Eye Movement Desensitization and Reprocessing, 32

F

Facelift, 340
Fad diets, 238
Fallopian tubes, 180

Famvir, 137, 279
Fatigue, 78–81, 212
Fava beans, 247
Fecal occult blood test, 359
Feet, 108, 109, 334
Fever, 345
Fiber, 110, 112, 185, 193–94, 238
Fibroids, 180, 331–33
Fibromyalgia, 125–29
Finasteride, 151, 153
Fish oil, 95, 145, 186, 273
5-alpha reductase, 150, 264
Flavonoids, 66, 71, 145, 243, 324
Flovent, 41, 120
Floxin, 329, 330
Flu, 65, 84, 129–31
Flu shot, 233, 254, 353
Fluids, 112, 120, 254, 330
Fluorescein angiography, 220
Fluorescent lights, 209
Fluoride, 147
Folic acid, 311
Follicle-stimulating hormone (FSH), 182
Food; allergies, 27; and colds, 85; and mood, 102; and PMS, 255–56
Fosamax, 226, 243, 245, 303
Free radicals, 246, 337
Frozen shoulder, 69
Fundoplication, 165
Fungus, 347–48, 283

G

Galantamine, 28, 222–23
Gallstones, 132–35
Gangrene, 251
Gargles, 83, 347
Garlic, 95
Gastric ulcers, 322. *See also* Ulcers
Gastroesophageal reflux disease. *See* GERD
Genasense, 203
Gene therapy, 288
Generalized anxiety disorder, 30. *See also* Anxiety; Stress
Genetic testing, 361
Genital herpes, 136–38
GERD, 161, 165. *See also* Heartburn
Ginger, 87, 285, 346, 347
Gingivitis, 146, 148
Ginkgo biloba, 29, 95, 124, 181, 223, 251
Ginseng, 227
Glaucoma, 74, 139–42, 367
Gleason score, 259
Gleevec, 203
Glioma, 54
Glucophage, 109, 240
Glucosamine, 34, 39, 307

Glucose testing, 105, 362
Goiter, 310, 311
Gonadotropin-releasing hormone agonists, 182, 332
Gout, 143–45
Grapefruit juice, 171
Grave's disease, 310
Green tea, 240
Group therapy, 103
Guided imagery, 43
Gum disease, 146–49. *See also* Teeth; Tooth loss

H

H2 blockers, 162
Hair loss, 150–53
Hand, 70–73
Hattler respiratory catheter, 119
Hay fever, 23, 24, 26, 117, 292
Headaches, 228–31, 345
Hearing aids, 114, 156, 157, 313
Hearing loss, 154–57, 312
Hearing tests, 363
Heart; disorders, 44–47, 94–98, 226; and gum disease, 149; problems, 90–93; stress test, 366
Heart attack, 31, 94, 96, 98, 158–60, 165, 175, 293, 321
Heart failure. *See* Congestive heart failure
Heartbeat, irregular, 44
Heartburn, 161–65. *See also* GERD; Indigestion
Heat therapy, 37, 48, 50, 68, 69, 126, 254, 264, 270, 297, 332
Helminthic parasites, 186
Hemorrhagic stroke, 300, 303
Hemorrhoids, 345–46
Hepatitis, 166–69, 353
Hepatocyte growth factor, 186
Herbs and nutritional supplements; acne, 22; allergies, 27; and Alzheimer's disease, 29; and anxiety, 33; and bronchitis, 66; and chronic fatigue syndrome, 81; and depression, 100, 101; hepatitis, 169; and inflammatory bowel disease, 187; and insomnia, 191; and memory loss, 223; and menopause, 227; and migraines, 231; and PMS, 256, 257; and rheumatoid arthritis, 275; and sinusitis, 285; strains and sprains, 298; and varicose veins, 336. *See also* specific herbs and vitamins
Herniated disk, 52
Herpes, genital, 136–38
Heterocyclics, 101. *See also* Tricyclics

Hiatal hernia, 164
High blood pressure, 170–75. *See also* Blood pressure
High cholesterol, 176–79
High-fiber diet, 185, 226, 311, 333
Hip fractures, 242
Histamine blocker, 36, 163
Histamines, 23, 40, 42
Hodgkin's lymphoma, 214, 216
Homocysteine, 311
Horehound, 66
Hormonal imbalance, 20, 180, 255
Hormone replacement therapy, 60, 62, 224–26; and coronary heart disease, 96; and osteoporosis, 244; and varicose veins, 335
Horse chestnut *seed* extract, 336
Hospice care, 89
Hot flashes, 224, 225, 226
Huperzine A, 29, 223
Hyaluronic acid, 38
Hyperglycemia, 104
Hypertension. *See* High blood pressure
Hyperthyroidism, 308, 310. *See also* Thyroid disorders
Hypnosis, 39, 195, 279
Hypoglycemia, 104, 109
Hypotension, 173
Hypothyroidism, 308. *See also* Thyroid disorders
Hysterectomy, 225, 331, 332, 333

I

Ice. *See* Cold therapy
IgE, 24, 25, 42, 117
Immune-suppressing drugs, 169, 186
Immune system, 66, 345; and asthma, 40; and chronic fatigue syndrome, 78; and colds, 82; and eczema, 115; and genital herpes, 138; and lupus, 208; and multiple sclerosis, 232; and pneumonia, 253; prostatitis, 266; shingles, 278–80; and stress, 84
Immunoglobulin E. *See* IgE
Immunosuppressant drugs, 210
Immunotherapy, 25, 26, 260, 287, 289
Imodium, 186, 194, 344
Implantable cardioverter-defibrillator (ICD), 93
Implants, dental, 318, 319, 320
Impotence, 122–125
In vitro fertilization (IVF), 180, 183
Incision and drainage, 69

Incontinence, 226, 234, 325–27
Inderal, 45, 97, 175, 230, 310
Indigestion, 346. *See also*
    Heartburn
Infections, bacterial, 344, 347;
    colon, 110; conjunctivitis,
    344; ear, 113–14; fungal, 342;
    gallbladder, 132; liver, 166;
    lung, 252; respiratory, 64–66,
    121; sinusitis, 281–85; urinary
    tract, 196, 197, 328–30; viral,
    136, 166, 344; yeast, 348
Inflammatory bowel disease,
    184–88. *See also* Irritable
    bowel syndrome
Influenza. *See* Flu
Ingrown toenail, 348
Inhalers, 41
Insect bites and stings, 23,
    346–47
Insight therapy, 31
Insomnia, 33, 101, 188–91, 224.
    See also Sleep; Sleep apnea
Insulin, 104, 105, 107
Insulin pump, 106
Intercourse, 93, 138, 225, 330
Interferon, 56, 233
Interferon-alpha, 167, 201, 203,
    216, 289, 290
Interpersonal therapy, 102–103
Intestine, large, 86, 110, 184
Intracapsular cataract extraction
    (ICCE), 77
Investigative therapies, 57
Iodine, radioactive, 310
Iron, 271, 333
Irritable bowel syndrome,
    192–95. *See also* Inflammatory
    bowel disease
Ischemic colitis, 195
Ischemic strokes, 300
Isoflavones, 226, 227
Itching, 116, 117, 346, 348

J

Jaundice, 166
Jaw, 305–07
Jet lag, 190, 191
Joints; and arthritis, 34–39, 272;
    bursitis, 67–69; and gout, 143;
    and Lyme disease, 211;
    replacement, 38, 213, 245;
    sprains and strains, 295
Juvenile rheumatoid arthritis,
    275

K

Kava, 31, 189
Kegel exercises, 226, 325–26
Ketoacidosis, 104, 105
Kidney stones, 144, 145, 196–99
Kidneys, 109, 174, 328

Klonopin, 191, 234, 271
Kyphoplasty, 245

L

L-dopa, 247, 249
Lactose intolerance, 192, 193
Laetrile, 215
Laminectomy, 53
Laparoscopic surgery, 134, 135
Large intestine, 86, 110, 184
Laser ablation, 88–89
Laser-assisted uvulopalatoplasty,
    292
Laser photocoagulation, 220
Laser surgery, 21, 22, 56, 77, 96,
    220, 336
Laser therapy, 205, 288, 339, 340
Laser trabeculoplasty, 141–42
Laxatives, 112
Left-ventricular assist device
    (LVAD), 92–93
Legs, 250, 270–71, 334
Leukapheresis, 203
Leukemia, 200–03
Leukeran, 202, 274
Leukotriene antagonists, 26, 41,
    285
Levaquin, 114, 121, 253, 283
Levodopa, 247, 249
Licorice, 117, 174, 324
Lidocaine, 127, 137, 230, 320
Ligaments, 70, 295
Light therapy, 269. *See also*
    Phototherapy; Sunlight
Lipids, 176
Liposuction, 241
Lithothripsy, 198
Liver, 166, 176
Lobular carcinoma, 58
Lomotil, 186, 194, 344
Lotronex, 194, 195
Low blood pressure, 173
Low-dose aspirin therapy, 97,
    177, 251
Low-fat diet, 222, 226, 333
Lumpectomy, 60, 61
Lung cancer, 204–07
Lungs, 118, 121, 252–54
Lupus, 208–10
Lyme disease, 211–13
Lymph nodes, 58, 60, 61, 88,
    289
Lymphatic system, 214–16
Lymphoma, 214–16

M

Maalox, 162, 323
MAbs. *See* Monoclonal antibodies
Macular degeneration, 217–20,
    367
Magnesium, 46, 227, 235, 256,
    271, 313

Magnetic resonance imaging
    (MRI), 73
Malignant melanoma, 286, 365.
    See also Skin cancer
Malocclusion, 305
Mammogram, 215, 225, 357
MAO inhibitors, 33, 102
Marijuana, 235
Marshmallow root, 187
Massage, 53, 69, 153. *See also*
    Relaxation techniques
Mastectomy, 60, 61
Maze procedure, 47
Meat, 197
Meditation, 39, 103, 222, 279.
    See also Relaxation tech-
    niques
Meglitinides, 109
Melanoma, 286, 365. *See also*
    Skin cancer
Melatonin, 81, 190
Melissa cream, 138
Memory loss, 221–23
Men; and cluster headaches, 231;
    and infertility, 182; and osteo-
    porosis, 245; and prostate
    cancer, 258–61
Menopause, 96, 183, 224–27,
    255, 325; and carpal tunnel
    syndrome, 71; and insomnia,
    189; and osteoporosis, 242;
    and urinary tract infections,
    328
Menstrual cycle, 181, 224, 331
Mental fuzziness, 224
Metabolism, 308
Metamucil, 133, 185, 194
Mevacor, 97, 178, 226
Microlipoinjection, 339–40
Migraines, 96, 228–31
Mild cognitive impairment, 221
Milk, 165, 190, 244
Milk thistle, 169
Miscarriage, 181
Mohs micrographic surgery, 288,
    289
Monoclonal antibodies, 56, 186,
    216
Mononucleosis, 81
Mood changes, 224, 257
Mood disorders, 99–103
Motion sickness, 347
Mouthwash, 148, 319, 320
MRI (Magnetic resonance imag-
    ing), 73
Mucus, 64, 120
Mullein flower eardrops, 114
Multiple sclerosis, 232–35
Multivitamins, 81, 130, 187, 216,
    223, 36
Muscle relaxants, 48, 51, 127,
    302

Stanols, 179
Statins, 97, 160, 178, 179
Steam, 83, 254, 283
Stent, 88, 97, 98, 304
Stereotactic localization, 56
Steroids, 25, 38; and acne, 22; and macular degeneration, 219; and rheumatoid arthritis, 273
Sterols, 179
Still's disease, 275
Stinging nettle, 27
Stomach, 322
Stomach shrinking surgery, 240-41
Strains and sprains, 295–99
Strength training, 127, 244
Strep throat, 347
Stress; and insomnia, 188; and irritable bowel syndrome, 192; and migraines, 231; and multiple sclerosis, 233; and rosacea, 277; and TMJ, 306; and wrinkles, 338. *See also* Stress reduction
Stress fractures, 295
Stress incontinence, 325
Stress reduction; and anxiety, 33; and brain tumors, 55; and breast cancer, 63; and congestive heart failure, 93; and coronary heart disease, 95, 96; and eczema, 116; and erectile dysfunction, 124; and fibromyalgia, 125, 127; and genital herpes, 137; and hair loss, 150; and hepatitis, 167; and high blood pressure, 172; and infertility, 182; and inflammatory bowel disease, 187; and insomnia, 190; and irritable bowel syndrome, 195; and leukemia, 201; and lupus, 209; and PMS, 256; and shingles, 279; and sinusitis, 282; and tinnitus, 312; and ulcers, 324. *See also* Relaxation techniques
Stress test, 98, 238, 366
Stroke, 44, 45, 175, 300–04
Sudafed, 25, 130, 284, 294
Sugar, 104
Suicide, 22, 100, 103
Sulfonylureas, 109
Sunlight; and acne, 22; and cataracts, 74, 75, 77; and jet lag, 191; and lupus, 209, 210; and macular degeneration, 219; and psoriasis, 268; and skin cancer, 290; and wrinkles, 337
Superficial thrombophlebitis, 336

Support groups, 237–38
Surgery, obesity, 240–41
Surgical resection, 88
Swank Diet, 234
Swimmer's ear, 113
Swiss ball exercises, 50
Synthroid, 309, 311
Systemic therapy, 62

T

Tagamet, 36, 163, 323
Tai chi, 37, 81, 213. *See also* Relaxation techniques
Tamoxifen, 62–63, 289
Tanning, 287
Tartar, 146, 148, 318
Taxol, 62, 207
Tea, 85, 240, 243, 321, 346, 347
Tea tree oil, 22
Teeth, 318–21. *See also* Gum disease; Tooth loss
Teeth grinding, 306
Temporomandibular joints (TMJ), 305–07
Tendinitis, 298, 299
Tendons, 70
Tenormin, 45, 175
TENS, 52, 271
Testicular exam, 366
Testosterone, 20, 123, 245, 258
Tests, preventive, 350–67
Tetanus booster, 353
Thalamotomy, 249
Thalidomide, 288
Thiazide diuretics, 198
Thiazolidinediones, 186
Thirst, 104
Thoracentesis, 254
Thrombolytic drugs, 159, 301
Thyroid disorders, 71, 308–11
TIAs, 303
Ticlid, 97, 251, 302
Tinnitus, 312–13
TMJ (Temporomandibular joints), 305–07
TNF blockers, 274
Tobacco dependence, 314–17. *See also* Nicotine; Smoking
Toenail fungus, 347–48
Tofu, 189, 226
Tongue, 148
Tooth loss, 318–21. *See also* Gum disease; Teeth
Toothpaste, 147, 319
Tracheostomy, 293
Tranquilizers, 160
Trans fatty acids, 177
Transcutaneous electrical nerve stimulation (TENS), 52, 271
Transient ischemic attacks (TIAs), 303

Transplants, 62, 92, 105, 121, 152, 168–69, 203, 219. *See also* specific organs
Transurethral needle ablation (TUNA), 264
Transvaginal pelvic floor electrical stimulation, 327
Trench mouth, 148
Tricyclics, 32, 127, 234, 279–80, 327. *See also* Heterocyclics
Trigger finger, 298
Trigger-point injections, 127
Triglycerides, 176, 179, 358
Triptans, 229
Tryptophan, 102, 190, 256
TSH, 308, 309
Tumor ablation, 62
Tumors; brain, 54–57; colon, 86–89
Tylenol, 35, 50, 79, 126, 137, 164, 190, 209, 230, 253, 297, 306

U

Ulcerative colitis, 184, 187
Ulcers, 245, 322–24
Ultrasound, 69, 76, 77
Ultraviolet light (UV), 22, 75, 117, 209, 269, 290
Ureter, 196
Ureteroscopy, 199
Urethra, 262, 328
Urge incontinence, 264, 325
Uric acid, 143, 144, 145, 196, 197
Urinary incontinence, 226, 234, 325–27
Urinary tract infection, 110, 196, 197, 328–30
Urination, 262, 266, 267
Urispas, 327, 330
Uterine cancer, 225
Uterine fibroids, 331–33
Uterus, 180, 331–33, 363

V

Vaccines, 353; Alzheimer's disease, 29; brain tumors, 56; cholesterol, 177; flu, 129, 131; hepatitis, 168; herpes, 137; Lyme disease, 212; lymphoma, 216; melanoma, 290; pneumonia, 65, 253–54; psoriasis, 269; shingles, 280; tobacco dependence, 315; ulcers, 324; urinary tract infections, 329
Vaginal dryness, 224
Vaginitis, 348
Valerian, 33, 81, 101, 191
Valium, 32, 51, 234, 307
Valtrex, 137, 279